Chir.
69,- €
'/19

Clinical Care and Rehabilitation in Head and Neck Cancer

Philip C. Doyle
Editor

Clinical Care and Rehabilitation in Head and Neck Cancer

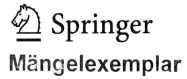

Springer

Mängelexemplar

Editor
Philip C. Doyle
Department of Otolaryngology Head and Neck Surgery and
School of Communication Sciences & Disorders
Western University
London
ON
Canada

ISBN 978-3-030-04701-6   ISBN 978-3-030-04702-3   (eBook)
https://doi.org/10.1007/978-3-030-04702-3

Library of Congress Control Number: 2019934810

This Springer imprint is published by the registered company Springer Nature Switzerland AG
The registered company address is: Gewerbestrasse 11, 6330 Cham, Switzerland

For my children, Katie and Peter,
for my wife Betsy, and
for my brother Jim!

Foreword

Clinical Care and Rehabilitation in Head and Neck Cancer provides a much-needed comprehensive resource for students and clinicians in speech-language pathology as well as in other medical and rehabilitation fields that are engaged in maintaining and restoring function in patients treated for head and neck cancer (HNCa). The editor, Dr. Philip C. Doyle, an internationally recognized authority in this area, has assembled an impressive multidisciplinary group of leading experts to join him in producing chapters that cover the broad range of physical, psychological, social, and communication problems experienced by HNCa patients. The information is clinically oriented, evidence based, and integrated in a way that facilitates current best practices in the interdisciplinary (team-based) care of patients.

The book is divided into three main sections: (1) Head and Neck Cancer and Its Treatment, (2) Treatment-Related Changes: Breathing, Voice, Speech, and Swallowing, and (3) Special Factors in Head and Neck Cancer. The six chapters in the first section contain basic information about the nature of HNCa cancer and provide a solid foundation on the state of the art for treating cancers of the head and neck. In addition to basic information, special attention is devoted to the impact of HNCa and its treatment on the multidimensional aspects of patient function, with an overview of considerations in optimizing the clinical management of these patients.

The second section of the book is comprised of 13 chapters that delve deeply into the impact and effective clinical management and rehabilitation of disturbances/disruptions in breathing, voice, speech, and swallowing that result secondary to the medical treatment of HNCa. Multiple chapters are devoted to methods for restoring voice, speech, and swallowing function for laryngectomy patients. Other chapters focus on the assessment and rehabilitation of speech and swallowing problems in patients treated for cancers of the oral cavity and oropharynx.

The ten chapters in the final section of the book deal with a range of important additional factors and topics associated with the treatment and rehabilitation of HNCa patients – with an emphasis on delineating other sources and types of treatment-related morbidity and the assessment of quality of life and communication participation in HNCa patients.

I heartily congratulate Dr. Doyle and his coauthors on producing such a valuable resource for our field. This is the first book that I know of that systematically addresses all the relevant issues and concerns related to HNCa and its treatment in one source. As such, it provides a comprehensive framework for optimizing the interdisciplinary clinical care of HNCa patients.

Boston, MA, USA   Robert E. Hillman

Preface

The conceptualization and development of this edited book had its origin while I was on sabbatical at Stanford University in early 2016. While working on several project ideas at that time, I became increasingly aware that a number of issues specific to rehabilitation following a diagnosis of head and neck cancer (HNCa) continued to be missing or glossed over in the clinical (rehabilitation) literature. It is widely acknowledged that malignancies of the head and neck and the consequences of treatment frequently impact the most fundamental aspects of human existence. More directly, HNCa and efforts to eliminate it will almost always impact voice and speech production, as well as eating and swallowing. Abnormalities in voice production, and in some instances its complete loss, are common following treatment for laryngeal cancer. Similarly, speech production may be altered across a range of severities in those treated for cancers of the oral cavity and related structures such as the tongue, mandible, maxilla, and pharynx. Regardless of site, treatment of HNCa often impacts myriad facets of one's life and, as a result, may reduce the true "success" of treatment – for example, changes in psychological health, nutritional status, reductions in physical capacity, altered cosmesis, and overall well-being are common.

However, the deficits described above cannot be viewed as isolated, discrete elements. Rather, they are dynamic and highly interactive and, unfortunately, frequently have a significant long-term impact on one's life posttreatment. HNCa and its treatment may reduce one's desire to pursue or continue a variety of personal, vocational, and social roles. These types of changes will always need to be contextualized relative to how the person who is treated for HNCa moves forward to reclaim as normal a life as possible. Consequently, the range and degree of deficits that may be experienced secondary to treatment are often shared by family members and loved ones. Simply stated, the effects of the treatment may at times be devastating with wide-ranging consequences and associated limitations.

Although the historical record and disease statistics for HNCa form what may be described as a relatively small proportion of all malignancies, the functional limitations that occur may be exponential. At present, we are at a very critical threshold where there is an expanding concern regarding increases in the incidence of HNCa. This is most particularly noted relative to oropharyngeal malignancies. In fact, the Centers for Disease Control and Prevention have estimated that the number of people who will be newly diagnosed with HNCa will now double every 10 years. This suspicion becomes even more critical given that an increasing number of those who are newly diagnosed will be substantially younger at the time of diagnosis, will represent emerging shifts in the ratio of men-to-women diagnosed with the disease, and, not insignificantly, will result in the persistent potential for disability over a period of long-term survivorship. While HNCa treatment holds increasing potential for success in eliminating disease, its consequences will persist for decades.

Contemporary rehabilitation efforts for those treated for HNCa increasingly demand that clinicians actively consider and address multiple issues. Beyond the obvious concerns specific to any type of cancer (i.e., the desire for curative treatment), clinical efforts that address physical, psychological, communicative, and social consequences secondary to HNCa treatment are essential components of all effective rehabilitation programs. Comprehensive HNCa rehabilitation ultimately seeks to restore multiple areas of functioning in the context of the disabling effects of treatment. Comprehensive rehabilitation also appreciates the "big picture" relative to each individual. In this regard, rehabilitation often focuses on restoration of function while reducing the impact of residual treatment-related deficits on the individual's overall functioning, well-being, quality of life (QOL), and ultimately, offers a process where the target outcome seeks to optimize survivorship.

Regardless of the treatment method(s) pursued, additional problems beyond those associated with voice, speech, eating, and swallowing frequently exist. For example, posttreatment changes in areas such as breathing, maintaining nutrition, limitations in physical capacity because of surgical ablation and reconstruction, concerns specific to cosmetic alterations and associated disfigurement, and deficits in social participation are common. Those treated for HNCa also may experience significant pain, depression, stigma, and subsequent social isolation. Concerns of this type have led clinicians and researchers to describe HNCa as the most emotionally traumatic form of cancer. It is, therefore, essential that clinicians charged with the care and rehabilitation of those treated for HNCa actively seek to identify, acknowledge, and systematically address a range of physical, psychological, social, and communication problems. The best clinicians are often those who consider an array of issues and are open minded; they are also sensitive to concerns that may not directly be within their area of expertise or professional training. Efforts that seek to integrate a wide range of concerns and areas of functioning may be rewarded with better outcomes.

The book is segmented into three sections, the first covering broad aspects that include treatment, potential complications of surgical treatment, etiological factors, psychological concerns, and the optimization of care. In this section, Chap. 1 by Axel Sahovaler, Dave Yeh, and Kevin Fung offers a succinct presentation of the general principles of treatment for head and neck cancer. Chapter 2, again by Yeh and Sahovaler, along with John Yoo, provides an excellent overview of reconstruction options for oral malignancies. Chapter 3, which I coauthored with Edward Damrose, addresses the complications that may potentially occur and influence rehabilitation efforts. Chapter 4 by Julie Theurer provides an excellent review specific to the human papilloma virus as a causal factor in HNCa. In Chap. 5 which was coauthored by Catherine

Bornbaum and me, we covered the issue of distress following diagnosis and treatment of HNCa. In the last chapter within this section (Chap. 6), Barbara Messing, Elizabeth Ward, and Cathy Lazarus offer information that may guide collaborative efforts and optimize clinical care.

The second and largest section of the book focuses specifically on breathing, voice, speech, and swallowing following treatment. Chapter 7 by Todd Bohnenkamp provides an important review of the respiratory system and speech breathing following laryngectomy. Chapter 8 authored by Bryan Lewis outlines options for improving airway functioning and efficiency post laryngectomy. Chapter 9 by Kathleen Nagle summarizes the current status of the electrolarynx and its clinical application. In Chap. 10, I had the privilege to work with Elizabeth Finchem who is herself a laryngectomee, on the process of teaching esophageal speech. Chapter 11 by Donna Graville, Andrew Palmer, and Rachel Bolognone summarizes the current status of tracheoesophageal (TE) puncture voice restoration. This is followed by Chap. 12 where Jodi Knott describes the clinical process of clinical problem-solving related to TE voice restoration. Chapter 13, authored by Jeff Searl, covers details related to lower and upper airway aerodynamics associated with alaryngeal voice and speech. Chapter 14 was coauthored with Lindsay Sleeth with its focus centering on intelligibility considerations postlaryngectomy. Chapter 15 offers a unique contribution by Jana Childes, Andrew Palmer, and Melanie Fried-Oken which outlines the need for and value of communication support and augmentative methods for those treated for HNCa. Chapter 16 by Gabriela Constantinescu and Jana Rieger provides an overview of the speech deficits that emerge secondary to oral and oropharyngeal cancers. I wrote Chap. 17 with its goal being to outline the methods of documenting voice and speech outcomes in those who are laryngectomized. This section of the book ends with Chap. 18 by Heather Starmer who provides information on swallowing disorders and rehabilitation secondary to laryngeal cancer, while in Chap. 19, Loni Arrese and Heidi Schieve address swallowing issues in those treated for oral and oropharyngeal cancers.

The third and last section of the book is comprised of ten chapters which address topics that previously have not garnered consistent attention or focus in the literature related to HNCa. Chapter 20 which was written by Ann Kearney and Patricia Cavanagh provides a summary of the acute and long-term consequences and side effects of chemoradiation therapy. Chapter 21 authored by Richard Cardoso and Mark Chambers offers comprehensive information on oral and dental considerations in those treated for HNCa. In Chap. 22, Brad Smith provides a very important and accessible summary pertaining to lymphedema and associated clinical considerations. Chapter 23 which I coauthored with Angelo Boulougouris covers the topic of shoulder disability following cancer treatment and neck dissection and its potential influence relative to voice and speech rehabilitation. Once again, Heather Starmer authored Chap. 24 which discusses the critical topic of adherence to treatment and the potential influence it has on posttreatment outcomes. In Chap. 25, Wendy Townsend sheds light on the role of the clinical nurse specialist within the larger context of collaboration specific to management. I authored Chap. 26 with the objective of outlining the need for acquiring practice knowledge and clinical skills, particularly when ready access to such knowledge may be limited. I also coauthored Chap. 27 with Chelsea MacDonald where aspects of well-being and quality of life considerations are identified and explored as a valuable index of treatment outcome. Next, in Chap. 28, Paul Evitts has explored in detail the impact that auditory and visual changes have on listeners and the overall process of verbal communication. Finally, Chap. 29 was written by Tanya Eadie who provides a comprehensive discussion of communication participation and the value of its measurement in those treated for HNCa. Collectively, I believe that these chapters offer new insights into the process of rehabilitation following treatment for HNCa.

In closing, current information suggests that successful clinical outcomes for those with HNCa are more likely to be realized when highly structured, yet flexible interdisciplinary programs of care are pursued. Yet contemporary educational resources that focus not only on management of voice, speech, eating, and swallowing disorders but also address how other deficits influence the larger schema of one's rehabilitation success are essential. Collectively, resources that address these issues and the resultant social implications of HNCa and its treatment can serve to establish a comprehensive framework for clinical care. The present book addresses HNCa rehabilitation through a more expansive conceptual and clinical framework. It was, however, my desire to meet this need in a manner that was relatively seamless and accessible to a large readership. Therefore, the ultimate goal of the present book sought to deliver a systematic, comprehensive, and clinically oriented presentation on a range of topics that will provide the reader with a strong, well-integrated, and empirically driven foundation to optimize the clinical care of those with HNCa.

London, ON, Canada   Philip C. Doyle

Acknowledgments

Over the past two and a half years, it has been an honor and a pleasure to work with those who authored or coauthored chapters within this text. Without hesitation, I did in fact exploit my friendship with several of the authors, namely, Tanya Eadie, Julie Theurer, Jeff Searl, Edward Damrose, Elizabeth Finchem, and Jodi Knott – thank you for accepting my offer to contribute. Although those who wrote chapters have provided information specific to a given, predetermined topic area, none of them ever lost sight of the bigger picture related to my vision of head and neck cancer rehabilitation and the larger aspects that affect the quality of one's survivorship. I am very pleased with what the authors have produced and extend a heartfelt "thanks."

As the editor, I had the wonderful privilege to request contributions from a number of individuals that I have known for many years and interacted with previously, whether it be at the professional, clinical, and/or research level. In considering who I would ask to write, it was my desire to meet two criteria. First, and most importantly, I wanted to identify those individuals who have been shown to have an extensive clinical acumen, a detailed knowledge of the literature related to head and neck cancer (both past and present), or in many cases both, as well as having demonstrated the capacity to work with others. Second, in doing so, I purposefully sought authors (or suggestions for authors) who consider their patients as being more important than their résumés or curriculum vitae. Those who contributed are well recognized for their expertise, but many have often flown under the proverbial radar – not individuals who have sought attention or personal gain, but professionals who just do excellent work and continue to work toward becoming better clinicians. Thank you to all!

Among those who have contributed, several are former graduate students for who I served as their research supervisor – Tanya Eadie, Catherine Bornbaum, and Lindsay Sleeth; one, Chelsea MacDonald, is a current doctoral student, and another, Julie Theurer, is a former student from my program who is now a colleague – needless to say, I am very proud of each of you. Along the way, they have provided a new lens from which I could view clinical questions that have been of longstanding interest to me. And, related to the concept of time passing by, one of the other contributors, Kathleen Nagle, is a student of a former student; thus, a third generation was able to be part of this endeavor. Finally, and despite not having written chapters, two other former students, Adam Day and Marie-Ève Caty, as well as my friend and colleague Joanne Fenn have expanded my thinking in several areas – thank you to all! Finally, several chapters were authored by individuals who I have never met. As the concept for the book was being developed, others who I trusted fully told me that I needed to contact these individuals with a request for their participation given the larger theme of the book; fortunately, they agreed to contribute.

Obviously, as I look back on the more extended evolution of how this book developed, and as I reflect on my own interest in this clinical area, I am constantly reminded that a number of individuals provided morsels of good advice, an open ear, comprehensive tutelage, and constant encouragement over the time of my own undergraduate and graduate education. I will always be indebted to the wonderful teachings of Dr. Marion D. Myerson,[1] Dr. Susan J. Shanks,[2] and Dr. Dennis J. Arnst who patiently offered guidance to me as an undergraduate student at Fresno State University. While a master's student at the University of California, Santa Barbara, Dr. Jeffrey L. Danhauer and Dr. Sanford E. Gerber[3] provided a range of opportunities and support to me, and both provided a gentle kick when it was needed. As a doctoral student at the University of California, San Francisco, Dr. Richard M. Flower[4] not only provided incredible support, but he also provided an academic role model and lived an ethical standard that was unmatched. Lastly, to Dr. Charles G. Reed who early in my career provided an incredibly enriched clinical experience within the Veteran's Administration Hospital at Fort Miley in San Francisco which was a learning environment second to none.

I also have been privileged to work with a group of colleagues in the Department of Otolaryngology Head and Neck Surgery at my current institution; they have always been supportive of my interests and have continuously welcomed my graduate students over many years. Two of these colleagues, Kevin Fung and John Yoo, have become valued friends over the years, and I wish to thank both of them for providing me with the opportunity to work with them as well as allowing me to teach and work with medical students, surgical residents, and fellows in their department.

It goes without saying that as I worked on this book in addition to other writing endeavors over the same period, I have had the luxury of wonderful personal support and wise guidance at home. I wish to specifically acknowledge my wife, Betsy, who patiently endured the time demands that naturally, and sometimes unexpectedly, occurred over the course of this project. Thank you for being patient with me and understanding my need to see this book come to fruition.

Lastly, I am deeply indebted and grateful to my publisher, Springer Nature, for helping to facilitate this project. Thank you to Samantha Lonuzzi for working with me on the initial proposal and helping me to move the idea forward. To my developmental editor, Wade Grayson, thanks for your input, guidance, keen eye, and patience, attributes that made this entire process as

---

[1] Deceased August 10, 2011.

[2] Deceased September 13, 2016.

[3] Deceased May 16, 2017.

[4] Deceased August 8, 2017.

easy as possible; further, thank you for your continued support and good humor along the way. Together, your support and professionalism throughout this process is and always will be appreciated. I hope that the end product is what both of you envisioned it to be.

London, ON, Canada   Philip C. Doyle

Contents

Contributors

Loni C. Arrese, PhD Department of Medicine at the University of Wisconsin School of Medicine and Public Health, Madison, WI, USA

Todd Allen Bohnenkamp, PhD Department of Communication Sciences and Disorders, University of Northern Iowa, Cedar Falls, IA, USA

Rachel K. Bolognone, MS Northwest Center for Voice and Swallowing, Department of Otolaryngology – Head & Neck Surgery, Oregon Health and Science University, Portland, OR, USA

Catherine C. Bornbaum, PhD, MSc Dalla Lana School of Public Health, University of Toronto, Toronto, ON, Canada

Angelo Boulougouris, BA, MA, MSc(PT), PhD Fowler-Kennedy Sports Medicine Clinic, Western University, London, ON, Canada

Richard C. Cardoso, DDS Head and Neck Surgery – Section of Oral Oncology & Maxillofacial Prosthodontics, The University of Texas, MD Anderson Cancer Center, Houston, TX, USA

Patricia W. Cavanagh, MS, CCC-SLP, BCS-S Speech Pathology Section, San Francisco Veterans Affairs Medical Center, San Francisco, CA, USA

Mark S. Chambers, DMD Head and Neck Surgery – Section of Oral Oncology & Maxillofacial Prosthodontics, The University of Texas, MD Anderson Cancer Center, Houston, TX, USA

Jana M. Childes, MS Northwest Center for Voice and Swallowing, Department of Otolaryngology – Head and Neck Surgery, Oregon Health and Science University, Portland, OR, USA

Gabriela Constantinescu, PhD Institute for Reconstructive Sciences in Medicine (iRSM), Misericordia Community Hospital and Department of Communication Sciences and Disorders, Faculty of Rehabilitation Medicine, University of Alberta, Edmonton, AL, Canada

Department of Communication Sciences and Disorders, Faculty of Rehabilitation Medicine University of Alberta, and Institute for Reconstructive Sciences in Medicine (iRSM), Misericordia Community Hospital, Edmonton, AB, Canada

Edward J. Damrose, MD, FACS Department of Otolaryngology, Head and Neck Surgery, Stanford University School of Medicine, Stanford, CA, USA

Philip C. Doyle, PhD, CCC-SLP Voice Production and Perception Laboratory & Laboratory for Well-Being and Quality of Life, Department of Otolaryngology – Head and Neck Surgery and School of Communication Sciences and Disorders, Western University, Elborn College, London, ON, Canada

Tanya L. Eadie, PhD, CCC-SLP Department of Speech and Hearing Sciences, Department of Otolaryngology – Head and Neck Surgery, University of Washington, Seattle, WA, USA

Paul M. Evitts, PhD, CCC-SLP Department of Audiology, Speech-Language Pathology, & Deaf Studies, Towson University, Towson, MD, USA
Department of Otolaryngology – Head and Neck Surgery, Johns Hopkins School of Medicine, Baltimore, MD, USA

Elizabeth A. Finchem Alaryngeal Speech Instructor, Tucson, AZ, USA

Melanie B. Fried-Oken, PhD Departments of Neurology, Pediatrics, Biomedical Engineering, & Otolaryngology & Institute on Development and Disability, Oregon Health & Science University, Portland, OR, USA

Kevin Fung, MD, FRCS(C), FACS Department of Otolaryngology – Head and Neck Surgery, London Health Sciences Centre, Schulich School of Medicine & Dentistry, Western University, London, ON, Canada

Donna J. Graville, PhD Northwest Center for Voice and Swallowing, Department of Otolaryngology – Head & Neck Surgery, Oregon Health and Science University, Portland, OR, USA

Ann Kearney, MA, CCC-SLP, BCS-S Stanford Voice and Swallowing Center, Department of Otolaryngology, Head and Neck Surgery, Stanford University Hospital, Stanford, CA, USA

Jodi Knott, MS, CCC/SLP, BCS-S Department of Speech Pathology and Audiology, University of Texas, MD Anderson Cancer Center, Houston, TX, USA

Cathy L. Lazarus, PhD Icahn School of Medicine at Mount Sinai, Thyroid Head and Neck Research Center, Thyroid Head and Neck Cancer (THANC) Foundation, New York, NY, USA
Department of Otolaryngology Head & Neck Surgery, Mount Sinai Beth Israel, New York, NY, USA

W. J. Bryan Lewis, MS, CCC-SLP Department of Surgery, Walter Reed National Military Medical Center, Bethesda, MD, USA
Uniformed Services University of the Health Sciences, Bethesda, MD, USA

Chelsea MacDonald, MSc Laboratory for Well-Being and Quality of Life in Oncology, Health and Rehabilitation Sciences, Western University, London, ON, Canada

Barbara Pisano Messing, MA, CCC-SLP, BCS-S, FASHA Greater Baltimore Medical Center, The Milton J. Dance, Jr. Head and Neck Center, Johns Hopkins Head & Neck Surgery, Johns Hopkins Voice Center, Baltimore, MD, USA

School of Health and Rehabilitation Sciences, The University of Queensland, Brisbane, QLD, Australia

Kathleen F. Nagle, PhD, CCC-SLP Department of Speech-Language Pathology, Seton Hall University, South Orange, NJ, USA

Andrew D. Palmer, PhD Northwest Center for Voice and Swallowing, Department of Otolaryngology – Head & Neck Surgery, Oregon Health & Science University, Portland, OR, USA

Jana M. Rieger, PhD, MSc, BSc Institute for Reconstructive Sciences in Medicine (iRSM), Misericordia Community Hospital and Department of Communication Sciences and Disorders, Faculty of Rehabilitation Medicine, University of Alberta, Edmonton, AL, Canada

Department of Communication Sciences and Disorders, Faculty of Rehabilitation Medicine University of Alberta, and Institute for Reconstructive Sciences in Medicine (iRSM), Misericordia Community Hospital, Edmonton, AB, Canada

Axel Sahovaler, MD Department of Otolaryngology – Head and Neck Surgery, London Health Sciences Centre, Schulich School of Medicine & Dentistry, Western University, London, ON, Canada

Heidi Schieve, MA, CCC-SLP Otolaryngology, The Ohio State University, Columbus, OH, USA

Jeff Searl, PhD, CCC-SLP Department of Communicative Sciences and Disorders, Michigan State University, East Lansing, MI, USA

Lindsay E. Sleeth, BHSc, MSc South West Local Health Integration Network, London, ON, Canada

Voice Production and Perception Laboratory, Rehabilitation Sciences, Western University, London, ON, Canada

Brad G. Smith, MS, CCC-SLP, CLT Sammons Cancer Center, Baylor Scott & White Insitute of Rehabilitation, Dallas, TX, USA

Heather M. Starmer, MA Department of Otolaryngology – Head and Neck Surgery, Head and Neck Speech and Swallowing Rehabilitation, Stanford Cancer Center, Stanford, CA, USA

Julie A. Theurer, PhD, MClSc School of Communication Sciences and Disorders, Western University, London, ON, Canada

Wendy Townsend, BA, MN Head and Neck Surgical Oncology, London Health Sciences Center, London, ON, Canada

Elizabeth Celeste Ward, BSpThy(Hons), Grad Cert Ed, PhD School of Health and Rehabilitation Sciences, The University of Queensland, Brisbane, QLD, Australia

Centre for Functioning and Health Research (CFAHR), Metro South Hospital and Health Service, Queensland Health, Queensland Government, Brisbane, QLD, Australia

David H. Yeh, MD, FRCSC Department of Otolaryngology – Head and Neck Surgery, London Health Sciences Centre, Schulich School of Medicine & Dentistry, Western University, London, ON, Canada

John Yoo, MD, FRCSC, FACS Department of Otolaryngology – Head and Neck Surgery, London Health Sciences Centre, Schulich School of Medicine & Dentistry, Western University, London, ON, Canada

Part I

Head and Neck Cancer and Its Treatment

General Principles of Head and Neck Cancer Treatment

1

Axel Sahovaler, David H. Yeh, and Kevin Fung

Principles of Head and Neck Cancer Treatment: Basic Concepts

The majority of malignant neoplasms of the head and neck region originate on the mucosa of the upper aerodigestive tract, arising from the oral and nasal cavities, paranasal sinuses, pharynx, and larynx. Squamous cell carcinomas (SCCs) account for nearly 95% of all head and neck cancers (HNCs) in this region, and treatment options for this histologic subtype include combinations of surgery, radiotherapy, and chemotherapy (National Comprehensive Cancer Network, 2017). For the management of head and neck SCC, either surgery or radiotherapy can be used as a primary treatment. Chemotherapy has also proven to have a role when concurrently administered with radiotherapy (Pignon, le Maître, Maillard, & Bourhis, 2009).

As a general rule, and in an effort to minimize the side effects of multiple treatment modalities, a monotherapy approach is preferred to treat head and neck SCC, so long as it does not negatively impact locoregional control or survival. For early-stage cancers, a single modality treatment (surgery or radiotherapy) is usually deemed to be

sufficient to achieve cure, and as a consequence, one of those two options is employed. However, for advanced-stage cancers, monotherapy is insufficient to control the disease. Thus, a combined approach of surgery followed by adjuvant radiation with or without concurrent chemotherapy *or* primary chemoradiotherapy without surgery is used.

Due to the anatomy of the head and neck, surgical resection of many head and neck tumors can result in significant functional impairment. Traditional open surgical approaches can result in severe dysphagia and aspiration, which may result in patients being tracheostomy and/or gastrostomy tube dependent. Consequently, in scenarios where similar oncologic outcomes between surgery and radiotherapy can be achieved, the latter approach has been traditionally preferred as it is thought that radiation treatment might cause less morbidity.

Surgery

Minimally invasive surgical techniques (Fig. 1.1) such as transoral laser microsurgery (TLM) (Jäckel, Martin, & Steiner, 2007) and transoral robotic surgery (TORS) have been introduced as appealing alternatives to the traditional and typically more morbid open approaches (Dowthwaite et al., 2012; Yeh et al., 2015). Using these surgical approaches, access to the tumor site without

A. Sahovaler · D. H. Yeh · K. Fung (✉)
Department of Otolaryngology – Head and Neck Surgery, London Health Sciences Centre, Schulich School of Medicine & Dentistry, Western University, London, ON, Canada
e-mail: kevin.fung@lhsc.on.ca

© Springer Nature Switzerland AG 2019
P. C. Doyle (ed.), *Clinical Care and Rehabilitation in Head and Neck Cancer*,
https://doi.org/10.1007/978-3-030-04702-3_1

disruption of the surrounding anatomical structures (i.e., floor of mouth, pharynx) can be achieved (Fig. 1.2). Additionally, these less inva-

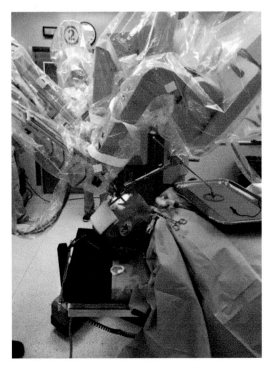

Fig. 1.1 Transoral robotic surgery (TORS) approach. Intraoperative photo with the surgical robot arms positioned before the resection

sive methods serve to minimize functional impairments secondary to cancer treatment (Nichols, Fung, et al., 2013; Yeh et al., 2015). Prospective randomized trials are currently underway in an effort to provide better evidence about these minimally invasive approaches in comparison with other more aggressive surgical approaches (Byrd & Ferris, 2016; Nichols, Yoo, et al., 2013).

Another important aspect of head and neck cancers is that these types of tumors have the potential to metastasize to cervical lymph nodes, resulting in poorer disease prognosis. Thus, in addition to addressing the primary tumor site, treatment of the cervical lymph nodes should be contemplated in all patients with head and neck malignancies. The cervical lymphatic drainage of all head and neck sites is well documented and is divided into six levels on each side of the neck determined by anatomical boundaries (Candela, Kothari, & Shah, 1990; Candela, Shah, Jaques, & Shah, 1990; Shah, 1990; Shah, Candela, & Poddar, 1990) (Fig. 1.3). This nomenclature has helped to divide the cervical lymph nodes in different subgroups and also identify which ones are at greater risk of being involved based on the head and neck tumor site. Consequently, this will mandate which lymphatic region will also require treatment (see Table 1.1).

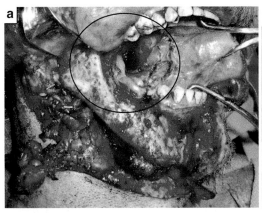
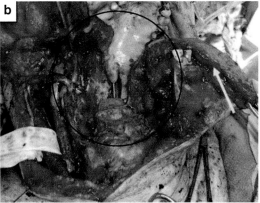

Fig. 1.2 Recurrent base of tongue tumor. (**a**) Intraoperative picture with surgical margins delimitation – *black circle*. Fibro-fatty and lymph node content of the neck (*blue arrow*). (**b**) Transmandibular (TM) approach of the tumor and subsequent postsurgical defect (*black circle*). As can be inferred by the picture, the mandible, right oropharynx, and hypopharynx were resected. The oropharyngeal area can only be approached openly by a TM approach, with significant postoperative functional consequences. (**c**) Postoperative Day 3. A nasogastric tube and a tracheostomy (not shown in the picture) were placed

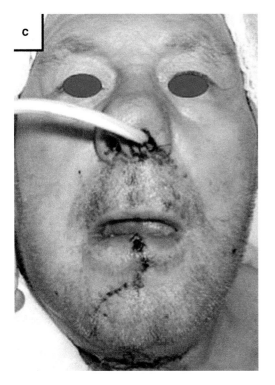

Fig. 1.2   (continued)

Treatment of the neck is performed by a neck dissection which consists of the systematic removal of the lymph nodes and accompanying fibro-fatty tissue of the neck. The decision of whether to perform a lymph node dissection and the extent of such a dissection is based on the risk of spread of the tumor and the presence of clinically or radiographically detectable lymph nodes (Miller, Goldenberg, Education, & Ahns, 2016). If there are no obviously diseased lymph nodes observed either clinically or radiographically, then the term "N0 neck" is utilized. If a patient with HNC has an N0 neck, but the chances of occult metastasis are high (i.e., tumors invading surrounding structures, thick and/or sizable – as a general rule >2 cm – tumors), a *prophylactic*, *elective*, or *selective* neck dissection is performed. This entails resecting only the levels of cervical lymph nodes that drain the primary tumor site (Table 1.1). If there are diseased cervical lymph nodes, the historical recommendation has been to perform a *comprehensive* or *therapeutic* lymphadenectomy which entails the

Fig. 1.3 Lymph node levels of the neck (Memorial Sloan Kettering nomenclature). I: submental (1A) and submandibular nodes (2B); II: upper jugular nodes – 2A, anterior to spinal accessory nerve (SAN) and 2B posterior to SAN; III: mid-jugular nodes; IV: lower jugular nodes; V: posterior triangle group with lower part of SAN chain (5A) and transverse cervical artery chain (5B). Illustration courtesy of Dr. Sam Dowthwaite

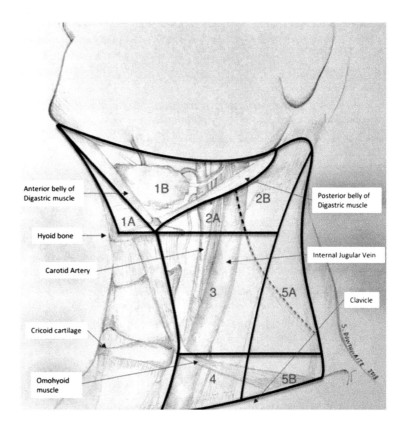

Table 1.1 Lymph nodes at risk depending on primary tumor site

Primary site	Lymph nodes at higher risk for early dissemination
Oral Cavity	I, II, III
Oropharynx	II, III, IV (also retropharyngeal nodes)
Hypopharynx	II, III, IV
Larynx	II, III, IV, VI

removal of all lymph node levels on the affected (ipsilateral) side of the neck. Typically, for lesions that are well lateralized, a unilateral neck dissection can be performed. In contrast, however, for lesions that occupy or cross the midline, bilateral neck dissections are indicated. During the neck dissection, whether it be either prophylactic or therapeutic, it is important for the surgeon to take every effort to preserve cervical functional structures such as the great vessels, nerves, and muscles. Injury to cranial nerves (vagus, hypoglossal, and spinal accessory nerves), as well as damage to the phrenic, lingual, and marginal mandibular nerves, and/or brachial plexus can carry substantial potential for functional and aesthetic negative outcomes.

Radiotherapy

As an alternative to surgery, radiotherapy can be used as primary treatment. It can be applied to both the primary site and to the cervical lymph nodes. This treatment modality, with or without chemotherapy, is broadly referred to as *organ-preserving therapy* (Adelstein et al., 1997; Forastiere et al., 2003, 2013; The Department of Veterans Affairs Laryngeal Cancer Study, 1991). The rationale for this approach is based on premise that similar oncological results can be achieved with radiotherapy as with surgery but with the advantage of conserving the organ versus resecting it. This is paramount in laryngeal and pharyngeal tumors where conserving the organ allows for the possibility to retain speech and swallowing function. However, radiotherapy is not innocuous, and it can lead to significant acute and late toxicities to the tissues surrounding the tumor. Acute side effects include mucosi-

tis, dysphagia, odynophagia, and dermatitis. Late effects comprise soft tissue fibrosis, xerostomia, hypothyroidism, osteoradionecrosis, radiation-induced myelitis, hearing loss, and carotid artery stenosis and even potential carotid artery rupture (see Kearney and Cavanagh, this volume). In addition, radiotherapy can also render patients tracheostomy or gastrostomy tube dependent.

The dose of radiotherapy is relatively standardized but can vary depending on whether it is being used as definitive or adjuvant treatment. If radiation is applied to the main tumor, the adjacent tissues and the cervical lymph nodes are at greater risk of being affected. As a general rule, the main tumor receives maximum dose, whereas the surrounding tissues and the lymph nodes at risk of being compromised receive lower doses. *Intensity-modulated radiation therapy* (*IMRT*) is a modern radiation technique that can restrain the doses of radiation to specific depths and areas. The advantage of this "modulation" is the capability of delivering different radiation doses in order to spare vital structures such as the carotid arteries, brain stem, optic nerves, and orbits and, subsequently, avoiding side effects while still offering improved local control of the disease. It is important to note that radiotherapy cannot be delivered twice to the same region of the head and neck. Body tissues can only tolerate a certain dose of radiation, and delivering more than one course can seriously damage surrounding tissues, exacerbating acute and late toxicities.

Systemic Treatments

Chemotherapy as a single modality is generally not employed in the treatment of HNC, aside from palliation in cases with distant metastasis, or recurrent disease that is not amenable to further surgical resection nor radiotherapy. The scenarios in which chemotherapy is used with curative intent are (1) as primary chemoradiotherapy to enhance the local effects of radiation treatment, (2) as induction (preoperative) chemotherapy to be delivered before definitive treatment with surgery or radiation, and (3) in the adjuvant (postoperative) setting administered concurrently with radiotherapy. The need for radiation alone versus chemoradiation in the postoperative setting is dictated by the presence of adverse pathological features of the specimen. These features would include extracapsular lymph node spread, positive or close surgical margins, multiple lymph nodes affected, or perineural or vascular invasion (Al-Sarraf et al., 1987; Kramer et al., 1987; Pignon et al., 2009). Cisplatin and carboplatin are the most commonly used chemotherapeutic agents in the treatment of HNC (Winquist et al., 2017). Cetuximab, an epidermal growth factor inhibitor has also shown benefits in recurrent or metastatic HNC. Lately, in 2016, immunotherapic agents (pembrolizumab and nivolumab) have been approved for treatment of platinum refractory recurrent or metastatic disease (Harrington et al., 2016; Shetty, 2017). Of note, using systemic therapies concurrent with radiotherapy also results in increased potential for toxicity such as mucositis (Grades 3 and 4), increased rates of gastrostomy placement, cytopenias, acneiform rashes, and hydroelectrolytic disorders (Ang et al., 2014).

Treatment Strategies

The National Comprehensive Cancer Network (NCCN) has outlined acceptable treatment options for cancers of the head and neck (NCCN, 2017). For some head and neck sites, for instance, oral cavity and nasopharynx, there are standard primary treatments such as surgery and chemoradiotherapy, respectively. However, for other sites treatment selection depends on tumor, patient, and physician factors. Tumor factors include location, size, proximity or invasion of vital structures, previous treatment, and the presence and extent of nodal disease. Patient factors comprise of age, medical comorbidities, capability of self-care, family support, rehabilitation potential, and logistical considerations such as access to radiation facility and periodic follow-up. Physician-based factors relate to the expertise of the multidisciplinary treatment group, and this may dictate which treatment modality is offered to the patient. Therefore, treatment decisions are multifactorial with a range of considerations required in the decision-making process. In the sections to follow, we will outline a general approach to treatment of HNC by site of the malignancy.

Oral Cavity

The region described as the oral cavity encompasses the lip, the anterior 2/3 of the tongue, floor of mouth, gingiva, buccal mucosa, retromolar trigone, and the hard palate. Early-stage tumors of the oral cavity (Stages I and II) are equally amenable to being cured by surgical resection or radiotherapy, so a single modality approach is often preferred (Genden et al., 2010; Shah & Gil, 2009). Tumors arising from these oral structures can be easily accessed through the mouth (transoral approach) making surgery a logical option. Surgery offers excellent oncologic outcomes and acceptable function (Shah & Gil, 2009). Side effects of radiotherapy to the oral cavity region can be significant (xerostomia, osteoradionecrosis); therefore, surgery is generally preferred as the primary treatment (Genden et al., 2010).

In order to achieve optimal oncologic control, advanced tumors of the oral cavity (Stages III and IV) are best managed with multimodality therapy (Genden et al., 2010; Shah & Gil, 2009). The typical course of treatment for these disease stages requires upfront surgery, with or without reconstruction (see Yoo, Sahovaler, and Yeh, Chap. 2), followed by either radiation alone or concurrent chemoradiotherapy which is dependent on the tumor margins and other histopathologic findings. More aggressive surgical approaches such as mandibulotomies or a lingual release may be needed to gain exposure to adequately resect the primary tumor (Fig. 1.2b). These procedures increase the morbidity of surgery, and patients are more likely to present with posttreatment dysphagia than to those who require less invasive transoral approach. However, a simple transoral approach is not applicable where tumors are more extensive and, in some cases mandibular resection is needed.

As already mentioned, and similar to other tumor sites, treatment of the neck is necessary in cases where there is clinical or radiological evidence of lymph node involvement (comprehensive neck dissection) or in those patients with high pre-surgical suspicion of occult nodal metastasis in "N0 necks" (prophylactic or selective neck dissection).

Nasal Cavity and Paranasal Sinuses

Sinonasal cancers represent a small portion of the head and neck malignancies and most commonly include SCCs and adenocarcinomas (Robbins et al., 2011). The nasal cavity and paranasal sinuses are contained within bony confines which are in close proximity to the brain and the orbits. This location limits both the ability to perform effective surgery and deliver radiotherapy. For early-stage, well-localized disease, surgery alone represents the standard treatment. Less invasive approaches in the form of endoscopic surgery have gained increasing popularity in achieving satisfactory oncological margins with less morbidity in comparison to more extensive, open approaches (Ong, Solares, Carrau, & Snyderman, 2010).

Radical surgery, either through a transfacial or combined craniofacial approach, followed by postoperative adjuvant radiotherapy is the mainstay treatment of advanced-stage disease. Similarly, surgery and radiotherapy are recommended for unfavorably located tumors that may preclude achieving satisfactory oncological margins when using minimally invasive approaches (Robbins et al., 2011). The majority of these cancers have an insidious course, and they will frequently present with locally advanced disease. If the tumor is unresectable (i.e., invasion of cavernous sinus) or if the resection would lead to unacceptable morbidity (e.g., involvement of both orbits), radiotherapy and concurrent chemoradiotherapy are deemed to be acceptable treatment options. With IMRT, irradiation and toxicity to important structures such as the orbital contents, optic chiasm, and brain can be minimized. Surgical treatment of an N0 neck is rarely indicated in tumors of the nasal cavity and paranasal sinuses because nodal disease is noted at presentation in only 10–20% of patients (Robbins et al., 2011). If there is clinical or radiographic evidence of lymph node involvement, multimodal treatment is recommended.

Nasopharynx

Because nasopharyngeal cancers arise in a head and neck region with rich lymphatic drainage, early regional spread to the retropharyngeal and cervical nodes both unilaterally and bilaterally is common (Ho, Tham, Earnest, Lee, & Lu, 2012). Most cancers of the nasopharynx are radiosensitive, and the nasopharynx has been traditionally surgically inaccessible without causing significant morbidity (King, Ku, Mok, & Teo, 2000). As such, nasopharyngeal carcinomas are treated primarily with radiotherapy with or without chemotherapy (Wee et al., 2005), and surgery is frequently reserved for cases in which there is persistent or recurrent disease after irradiation (Chan, Chow, Tsang, & Wei, 2012; King et al., 2000; Wei, Chan, Ng, & Ho, 2011). Moreover, patients with nasopharyngeal carcinoma commonly present with diffuse cervical lymph node involvement (Wei & Kwong, 2010). Early-stage nasopharyngeal carcinomas (lesions confined to the nasopharynx) with no neck disease can be treated with radiation alone to both the primary site and the cervical lymph nodes at risk. More advanced stages of the disease (lesions outside the nasopharynx or with metastatic lymph nodes) will require primary chemoradiotherapy, a treatment approach that has been shown to improve survival rates (Al-Sarraf et al., 1987).

Oropharynx

There are four different anatomic subsites within the oropharynx: the soft palate, tonsillar region, base of tongue, and posterior pharyngeal wall. For early-stage disease, tumors of the oropharynx can be treated with primary radiotherapy or primary surgery. Because surgical exposure to achieve adequate surgical margins in the oropharynx can result in high morbidity, radiotherapy to the primary site as well as to the cervical lymph nodes at risk is usually favored. Historically, organ-preservation strategies for cancers of the oropharynx resulted in superior functional outcomes with similar oncologic results compared with surgical approaches (Al-Khudari et al., 2013; Holsinger & Ferris, 2015; Hutcheson, Holsinger, Kupferman, & Lewin, 2014; Kelly, Johnson-Obaseki, Lumingu, & Corsten, 2014; More et al., 2013; Yeh et al., 2015).

Recently, transoral laser microsurgery (TLM) and transoral robotic surgery (TORS) have been employed for the surgical treatment of early-stage oropharyngeal carcinoma (Liederbach et al., 2015). These approaches may spare patients the morbidity of traditional open surgical approaches while at the same time ensuring proper oncological margins. There has been a tremendous interest in employing these techniques as the "upfront" treatment of the primary tumor, along with prophylactic treatment of the cervical lymph nodes at risk (Nichols, Fung, et al., 2013). In cases with favorable pathology (negative tumor margins), surgery may be sufficient for oncologic control as a single modality treatment. The current literature would suggest that the oncologic and survival outcomes are similar between the two groups; however, there may be differences in the functional outcomes between primary surgery and primary radiation with ongoing trials attempting to elucidate this question (Dowthwaite et al., 2012; Holsinger & Ferris, 2015; Lee, Park, Byeon, Choi, & Kim, 2014; Monnier & Simon, 2015; Moore et al., 2012; More et al., 2013; Nichols, Yoo, et al., 2013; Yeh et al., 2015).

In advanced-stage disease, multimodality therapy is necessary to optimize the chance of cure. Surgical accessibility to the oropharynx is at times problematic, and surgery does not come without serious potential morbidity. Nevertheless, either minimally invasive transoral or traditional open approaches can be utilized for the upfront surgical management of the primary tumor. At a minimum, a unilateral neck dissection is necessary in all cases of oropharyngeal carcinoma if surgery is deemed to serve as primary method of treatment. With few exceptions, the lymphatic drainage of the oropharynx is bilateral; therefore, bilateral neck dissection will often be necessary. As part of a multimodal approach, radiotherapy is administered in the postoperative setting for advanced-stage disease, with chemotherapy given concurrently in selected cases if the tumor pathology demonstrates unfavorable features (i.e., positive margins or nodal extracapsular extension).

If an organ-preserving treatment strategy is decided on for advanced oropharyngeal tumors, concurrent chemoradiotherapy is the preferred treatment course with surgery reserved as a salvage option. Both approaches, however, are valid, and the decision toward selection of one method over the other is based on a combination of tumor, patient, and physician factors.

Hypopharynx

The hypopharynx is composed by the left and right pyriform sinuses, the posterior pharyngeal wall, and the postcricoid region. Early-stage tumors without nodal involvement (Stages I and II) are commonly treated with primary radiotherapy. In selected small tumors of the hypopharynx, there has been a renewed interest in surgical management using minimally invasive (TLM or TORS) surgical approaches (Lörincz, Busch, Möckelmann, & Knecht, 2015). However, cancers of the hypopharynx are typically diagnosed in advanced stages, and these tumors can spread locally to involve the cervical esophagus and the larynx. The delayed presentation and the potential for early disease extension also increases the likelihood of involvement to the cervical lymph nodes at the time of diagnosis. Traditionally, surgery in the form of a total laryngopharyngectomy, neck dissection, and pharyngeal reconstruction was the preferred initial treatment modality (Takes et al., 2012). With more contemporary evidence demonstrating that organ-preservation strategies do not compromise oncologic outcomes and the fact that they can be delivered with less morbidity than traditional surgical techniques, nonsurgical treatments have gained increasing popularity (Bertino et al., 2016).

With advanced-stage disease, the addition of concurrent chemotherapy to radiotherapy confers a survival benefit (Adelstein et al., 1997; Lee et al., 2008; Lörincz et al., 2015). With the aim of preserving the larynx, concurrent chemoradiotherapy is preferred over traditional surgical approaches, primarily due to less potential side effects. However, if the tumor causes a dysfunctional larynx leading to airway obstruction or if there is frank laryngeal cartilage involvement, the chance of a meaningful laryngeal preservation is poor, and surgery is often recommended through the traditional surgical approach (total laryngopharyngectomy, neck dissection, and pharyngeal reconstruction).

Overall, the treatment for hypopharyngeal cancer frequently results in definitive functional impairments. If surgery is undertaken, this commonly involves laryngopharyngectomy, resulting in a permanent tracheostoma. Both surgical and nonsurgical approaches may, in many cases, result in gastrostomy tube dependency. This is particularly relevant in tumors arising in the posterior pharyngeal wall, smokers, patients who are nonadherent to dysphagia exercise regimens, and patients who were unable to maintain oral intake throughout the treatment (Bhayani et al., 2013; Murono, Tsuji, & Endo, 2015). Oncologic outcomes with hypopharyngeal cancers remain relatively poor, with 5-year overall survival rates of approximately 30–41% (Newman et al., 2014; Zhou, Li, Wei, Qian, & Li, 2015).

Larynx

The larynx encompasses multiple structures including the supraglottis (epiglottis, false vocal folds, ventricles, aryepiglottic folds, and arytenoids), glottis (true vocal cords, including the anterior and posterior commissures), and the subglottis. The location of the tumor has important implications on the treatment options that can be offered. Whereas approximately 75% of glottic

tumors present with localized disease at diagnosis, 70% of supraglottic tumors have advanced disease at presentation (Harris, Bhuskute, Rao, Farwell, & Bewley, 2016). This can be explained by the fact that the supraglottis is drained by a rich lymphatic plexus which predisposes this region to a greater potential for lymphatic spread of disease, with an associated negative impact in survival.

Both surgery and radiotherapy have a role in the contemporary management of laryngeal cancer. Avoiding laryngectomy, both through uses of minimally invasive procedures (TLM or TORS) or with primary radiotherapy, aims to preserve voice and speech and avoids the need for a lifelong tracheostoma. However, larynx conservation will result in a range of vocal changes that have been well documented in the literature (Angel, Doyle, & Fung, 2011; Fung et al., 2001).

For early-stage glottic and supraglottic tumors (Stages I and II and some selected cases of Stage III), both primary radiotherapy and surgery can be used with comparable oncologic outcomes. Surgical options include endoscopic resection with either TLM or TORS or an open larynx-preserving partial laryngectomy (vertical or supraglottic horizontal partial laryngectomies). If the surgical option is selected, neck dissections should be considered for supraglottic tumors due to their propensity to spread to the cervical lymph nodes. In contrast, glottic tumors have a relatively low propensity for regional spread (Johnson, Bacon, Myers, & Wagner, 1994; Pressman, 1956; Pressman, Simon, & Monell, 1960). Specifically, with the treatment of glottic tumors, some studies have demonstrated superior voice outcomes with radiotherapy compared to TLM (Osborn et al., 2011). On the other hand, for recurrences after primary radiotherapy, salvage treatment typically necessitates total laryngectomy, whereas after primary TLM approaches, recurrences can be managed with endoscopic minimally invasive resections (Low et al., 2016).

For advanced glottic carcinomas with favorable features (i.e., low-volume disease, a patent airway, and reliable oncologic follow-up), concurrent chemoradiotherapy can be administered. The findings of the Veterans Affairs Laryngeal Cancer Trial (The Department of Veterans Affairs

Laryngeal Cancer Study, 1991) and the RTOG 91–11(Forastiere et al., 2003, 2013) studies led to the conclusion that survival outcomes with concurrent chemoradiotherapy were comparable to those of primary surgery. However, in the VA Trial, 64% of patients who underwent chemoradiotherapy retained their larynx (The Department of Veterans Affairs Laryngeal Cancer Study, 1991). With the advantage of laryngeal preservation, radiotherapy with concurrent chemotherapy became the preferred treatment modality for advanced-stage laryngeal cancer. If, however, the larynx is dysfunctional at the time of diagnosis (presence of aspiration or airway obstruction), upfront surgery is preferred over organ-preserving treatment. The reasoning for this is that chemoradiotherapy probably will worsen the already impaired laryngeal function, and after the treatment, patients will be left with a nonfunctional larynx, with increased risks of ongoing aspiration and persistent airway symptoms.

Summary

Upper aerodigestive tract malignancies are primarily comprised of squamous cell carcinomas. These types of tumors are amenable to treatment either with surgery or radiation. A fundamental principle in the management of head and neck SCCs is to utilize single modality treatment with early-stage disease and multimodality treatment in advanced-stage disease. Single modality treatment tends to carry less morbidity and lends itself to more optimal functional outcomes for patients. In comparison, advanced-stage tumors require multimodal therapy, consequently conferring greater morbidity and increased potential for a range of functional impairments. For all head and neck sites, there are several acceptable and viable treatment options. Ultimately, the treatment decision will be determined based on multiple factors such as tumor location, patient characteristics, and the philosophy of the treatment group. Overall, treatment of HNC and associated regions can have a significant and permanent negative impact on basic functions such as eating, swallowing, speaking, and breathing. These outcomes

must be considered when deciding upon the preferred treatment strategy.

References

Adelstein, D. J., Saxton, J. P., Lavertu, P., Tuason, L., Wood, B. G., Wanamaker, J. R., … Van Kirk, M. A. (1997). A phase III randomized trial comparing concurrent chemotherapy and radiotherapy with radiotherapy alone in resectable stage III and IV squamous cell head and neck cancer: Preliminary results. *Head & Neck, 19*(7), 567–575.

Al-Khudari, S., Bendix, S., Lindholm, J., Simmerman, E., Hall, F., & Ghanem, T. (2013). Gastrostomy tube use after transoral robotic surgery for oropharyngeal cancer. *ISRN Otolaryngology, 2013*, 190364. https://doi.org/10.1155/2013/190364

Al-Sarraf, M., Pajak, T. F., Marcial, V., Mowry, P., Cooper, J. S., Stetz, J., … Velez-Garcia, E. (1987). Concurrent radiotherapy and chemotherapy with cisplatin in inoperable squamous cell carcinoma of the head and neck. An RTOG Study. *Cancer, 59*(2), 259–265. Retrieved from http://www.ncbi.nlm.nih.gov/pubmed/19123002.

Ang, K. K., Zhang, Q., Rosenthal, D. I., Nguyen-Tan, P. F., Sherman, E. J., Weber, R. S., … Gillison, M. L. (2014). Randomized phase III trial of concurrent accelerated radiation plus cisplatin with or without cetuximab for stage III to IV head and neck carcinoma: RTOG 0522. *Journal of Clinical Oncology, 32*(27), 2940–2950. https://doi.org/10.1200/JCO.2013.53.5633

Angel, D., Doyle, P. C., & Fung, K. (2011). Measuring voice outcomes following treatment for laryngeal cancer. *Expert Review of Pharmacoeconomics & Outcomes Research, 11*(4), 415–420.

Bertino, G., Occhini, A., Almadori, G., Bussu, F., Mura, F., & Micciche, F. (2016). Oncologic outcome of hypopharyngeal carcinoma treated with different modalities at 2 different university hospitals. *Head & Neck.* https://doi.org/10.1002/hed.23938

Bhayani, M. K., Hutcheson, K. A., Barringer, D. A., Roberts, D. B., Lewin, J. S., & Lai, S. Y. (2013). Gastrostomy tube placement in patients with hypopharyngeal cancer treated with radiotherapy or chemoradiotherapy: Factors affecting placement and dependence. *Head & Neck,* 1641–1646. https://doi.org/10.1002/hed.23199

Byrd, J. K., & Ferris, R. L. (2016). Is there a role for robotic surgery in the treatment of head and neck cancer? *Current Treatment Options in Oncology, 17*(6). https://doi.org/10.1007/s11864-016-0405-5

Candela, F. C., Kothari, K., & Shah, J. P. (1990). Patterns of cervical node metastases from squamous carcinoma of the oropharynx and hypopharynx. *Head & Neck, 12*(3), 197–203.

Candela, F. C., Shah, J., Jaques, D. P., & Shah, J. P. (1990). Patterns of cervical node metastases from squamous carcinoma of the larynx. *Archives of Otolaryngology – Head & Neck Surgery, 116*(4), 432–435.

Chan, J. Y. W., Chow, V. L. Y., Tsang, R., & Wei, W. I. (2012). Nasopharyngectomy for locally advanced recurrent nasopharyngeal carcinoma: Exploring the limits. *Head & Neck, 34*(7), 923–928. https://doi.org/10.1002/hed.21855

Dowthwaite, S. A., Franklin, J. H., Palma, D. A., Fung, K., Yoo, J., & Nichols, A. C. (2012). The Role of transoral robotic surgery in the management of oropharyngeal cancer: A review of the literature. *ISRN Oncology, 2012*, 1–14. https://doi.org/10.5402/2012/945162

Forastiere, A. A., Goepfert, H., Maor, M., Pajak, T. F., Weber, R., Morrison, W., … Cooper, J. (2003). Concurrent chemotherapy and radiotherapy for organ preservation in advanced laryngeal cancer. *The New England Journal of Medicine, 349*(22), 2091–2098. https://doi.org/10.1056/NEJMoa031317

Forastiere, A. A., Zhang, Q., Weber, R. S., Maor, M. H., Goepfert, H., Pajak, T. F., … Cooper, J. S. (2013). Long-term results of RTOG 91-11: A comparison of three nonsurgical treatment strategies to preserve the larynx in patients with locally advanced larynx cancer. *Journal of Clinical Oncology, 31*(7), 845–852. https://doi.org/10.1200/JCO.2012.43.6097

Fung, K., Yoo, J. C., Leeper, H. A., Hawkins, S., Heeneman, H., Doyle, P. C., & Venkatesan, V. (2001). Vocal function following radiation for non-laryngeal versus laryngeal tumors of the head and neck. *Laryngoscope, 111*, 1920–1924.

Genden, E. M., Ferlito, A., Silver, C. E., Takes, R. P., Suárez, C., Owen, R. P., … Rinaldo, A. (2010). Contemporary management of cancer of the oral cavity. *European Archives of Oto-Rhino-Laryngology, 267*(7), 1001–1017. https://doi.org/10.1007/s00405-010-1206-2

Harrington, K., Kasper, S., Vokes, E. E., Even, C., Worden, F., Saba, N. F., … Monga, M. (2016). Nivolumab for recurrent squamous cell carcinoma of the head and neck. *The New England Journal of Medicine*, 1–12. https://doi.org/10.1056/NEJMoa1602252

Harris, B. N., Bhuskute, A. A., Rao, S., Farwell, D. G., & Bewley, A. F. (2016). Primary surgery for advanced-stage laryngeal cancer: A stage and subsite-specific survival analysis. *Head & Neck*, 1–7. https://doi.org/10.1002/hed.24443

Ho, F. C. H., Tham, I. W. K., Earnest, A., Lee, K. M., & Lu, J. J. (2012). Patterns of regional lymph node metastasis of nasopharyngeal carcinoma: A meta-analysis of clinical evidence. *BMC Cancer, 12*, 98.

Holsinger, F. C., & Ferris, R. L. (2015). Transoral endoscopic head and neck surgery and its role within the multidisciplinary treatment paradigm of oropharynx cancer: Robotics, lasers, and clinical trials. *Journal of Clinical Oncology, 33*(29), 3285–3292. https://doi.org/10.1200/JCO.2015.62.3157

Hutcheson, K. A., Holsinger, F. C., Kupferman, M. E., & Lewin, J. S. (2014). Functional outcomes after TORS for oropharyngeal cancer: a systematic review.

European *Archives of Oto-Rhino-Laryngology*, 463–471. https://doi.org/10.1007/s00405-014-2985-7

Jäckel, M. C., Martin, A., & Steiner, W. (2007). Twenty-five years experience with laser surgery for head and neck tumors: Report of an international symposium, Göttingen, Germany, 2005. *European Archives of Oto-Rhino-Laryngology, 264*(6), 577–585. https://doi.org/10.1007/s00405-007-0280-6

Johnson, J. T., Bacon, G. W., Myers, E. N., & Wagner, R. L. (1994). Medial vs lateral wall pyriform sinus carcinoma: Implications for management of regional lymphatics. *Head & Neck, 16*(5), 401–405.

Kelly, K., Johnson-Obaseki, S., Lumingu, J., & Corsten, M. (2014). Oncologic, functional and surgical outcomes of primary transoral robotic surgery for early squamous cell cancer of the oropharynx: A systematic review. *Oral Oncology, 50*(8), 696–703. https://doi.org/10.1016/j.oraloncology.2014.04.005

King, W. W. K., Ku, P. K. M., Mok, C. O., & Teo, P. M. L. (2000). Nasopharyngectomy in the treatment of recurrent nasopharyngeal carcinoma: A twelve-year experience. *Head and Neck, 22*(3), 215–222. https://doi.org/10.1002/(SICI)1097-0347(200005)22:3<215::AID-HED2>3.0.CO;2-B

Kramer, S., Gelber, R. D., Snow, J. B., Marcial, V. A., Lowry, L. D., Davis, L. W., & Chandler, R. (1987). Combined radiation therapy and surgery in the management of advanced head and neck cancer: Final report of study 73-03 of the radiation therapy oncology group. *Head & Neck Surgery, 10*, 19–30. Retrieved from http://eutils.ncbi.nlm.nih.gov/entrez/eutils/elink.fcgi?dbfrom=pubmed&id=3449477&retmode=ref&cmd=prlinks%5Cnpapers2://publication/uuid/48E19CB2-6687-4B52-AD6C-B2DBF4AC413F

Lee, M.-S., Ho, H., Hsiao, S., Hwang, J., Lee, C., & Hung, S. (2008). Treatment results and prognostic factors in locally advanced hypopharyngeal cancer. *Acta Oto-Laryngologica, 128*(1), 103–109. https://doi.org/10.1080/00016480701387116

Lee, S. Y., Park, Y. M., Byeon, H. K., Choi, E. C., & Kim, S.-H. (2014). Comparison of oncologic and functional outcomes after transoral robotic lateral oropharyngectomy versus conventional surgery for T1 to T3 tonsillar cancer. *Head & Neck, 36*(8), 1138–1145. https://doi.org/10.1002/hed.23424

Liederbach, E., Lewis, C. M., Yao, K., Brockstein, B. E., Wang, C.-H., Lutfi, W., & Bhayani, M. K. (2015). A contemporary analysis of surgical trends in the treatment of squamous cell carcinoma of the oropharynx from 1998 to 2012: A report from the National Cancer Database. *Annals of Surgical Oncology, 22*(13), 4422–4431. https://doi.org/10.1245/s10434-015-4560-x

Lörincz, B. B., Busch, C. J., Möckelmann, N., & Knecht, R. (2015). Feasibility and safety of transoral robotic surgery (TORS) for early hypopharyngeal cancer: A subset analysis of the Hamburg University TORS-trial. *European Archives of Oto-Rhino-Laryngology, 272*(10), 2993–2998. https://doi.org/10.1007/s00405-014-3259-0

Low, T.-H. H., Yeh, D., Zhang, T., Araslanova, R., Hammond, J. A., Palma, D., … Fung, K. (2016). Evaluating organ preservation outcome as treatment endpoint for T1aN0 glottic cancer. *The Laryngoscope*, 1–6. https://doi.org/10.1002/lary.26317

Miller, M. C., Goldenberg, D., Education, T., & Ahns, N. S. (2016). PRACTICE GUIDELINES AHNS Series: Do you know your guidelines ? Principles of surgery for head and neck cancer: A review of the National Comprehensive Cancer Network guidelines. *Head & Neck*, 1–6. https://doi.org/10.1002/hed.24654

Monnier, Y., & Simon, C. (2015). Surgery versus radiotherapy for early oropharyngeal tumors: A never-ending debate. *Current Treatment Options in Oncology*, *16*(9), 1–13. https://doi.org/10.1007/s11864-015-0362-4

Moore, E. J., Olsen, S. M., Laborde, R. R., García, J. J., Walsh, F. J., Price, D. L., … Olsen, K. D. (2012). Long-term functional and oncologic results of transoral robotic surgery for oropharyngeal squamous cell carcinoma. *Mayo Clinic Proceedings, 87*(3), 219–225. https://doi.org/10.1016/j.mayocp.2011.10.007

More, Y. I., Tsue, T. T., Girod, D. a., Harbison, J., Sykes, K. J., Williams, C., & Shnayder, Y. (2013). Functional swallowing outcomes following transoral robotic surgery vs. primary chemoradiotherapy in patients with advanced-stage oropharynx and supraglottis cancers. *JAMA Otolaryngology. Head & Neck Surgery, 139*(1), 43. https://doi.org/10.1001/jamaoto.2013.1074

Murono, S., Tsuji, A., & Endo, K. (2015). Factors associated with gastrostomy tube dependence after concurrent chemoradiotherapy for hypopharyngeal cancer. *Support Care Cancer*, 457–462. https://doi.org/10.1007/s00520-014-2388-8

National Comprehensive Cancer Network. (2017). Head and Neck Cancers. (Version 02.2017).

Newman, J. R., Connolly, T. M., Illing, E. A., Kilgore, M. L., Locher, J. L., & Carroll, W. R. (2014). Survival trends in hypopharyngeal cancer: A population-based review. *Laryngoscope*, 1–6. https://doi.org/10.1002/lary.24915

Nichols, A. C., Fung, K., Chapeskie, C., Dowthwaite, S. A., Basmaji, J., Dhaliwal, S., … Yoo, J. (2013). Development of a transoral robotic surgery program in Canada. *Journal of Otolaryngology - Head & Neck Surgery = Le Journal D'oto-Rhino-Laryngologie et de Chirurgie Cervico-Faciale, 42*(1), 8. https://doi.org/10.1186/1916-0216-42-8

Nichols, A. C., Yoo, J., Hammond, J. A., Fung, K., Winquist, E., Read, N., … Palma, D. A. (2013). Early-stage squamous cell carcinoma of the oropharynx: Radiotherapy vs. trans-oral robotic surgery (ORATOR)--study protocol for a randomized phase II trial. *BMC Cancer, 13*(1), 133. https://doi.org/10.1186/1471-2407-13-133

Ong, Y. K., Solares, C. A., Carrau, R. L., & Snyderman, C. H. (2010). New developments in transnasal endoscopic surgery for malignancies of the sinonasal tract and adjacent skull base. *Current Opinion in Otolaryngology & Head and Neck Surgery, 18*(2), 107–113. https://doi.org/10.1097/MOO.0b013e3283376dcc

Osborn, H. A., Hu, A., Venkatesan, V., Nichols, A., Franklin, J. H., Yoo, J. H., … Fung, K. (2011). Comparison of endoscopic laser resection versus radiation therapy for the treatment of early glottic carcinoma. *Journal of Otolaryngology - Head & Neck Surgery = Le Journal D'oto-Rhino-Laryngologie et de Chirurgie Cervico-Faciale, 40*(3), 200–204.

Pignon, J., le Maître, A., Maillard, E., & Bourhis, J. (2009). Meta-analysis of chemotherapy in head and neck cancer (MACH-NC): An update on 93 randomised trials and 17,346 patients. *Radiotherapy and Oncology, 92*(1), 4–14. https://doi.org/10.1016/j.radonc.2009.04.014

Pressman, J. J. (1956). LXIII Submucosal Compartmentation of the Larynx. *The Annals of Otology, Rhinology, and Laryngology, 65*(3), 766–771.

Pressman, J. J., Simon, M. B., & Monell, C. (1960). Anatomical studies related to the dissemination of cancer of the larynx. *Transactions-American Academy of Ophthalmology and Otolaryngology. American Academy of Ophthalmology and Otolaryngology, 64*, 628–638.

Robbins, K. T., Ferlito, A., Silver, C. E., Takes, R. P., Strojan, P., Snyderman, C. H., … Suárez, C. (2011). Contemporary management of sinonasal cancer. *Head & Neck, 33*(9), 1352–1365. https://doi.org/10.1002/hed.21515

Shah, J. P. (1990). Patterns of cervical lymph node metastasis from squamous carcinomas of the upper aerodigestive tract. *American Journal of Surgery, 160*(4), 405–409. https://doi.org/10.1016/S0002-9610(05)80554-9

Shah, J. P., Candela, F. C., & Poddar, A. K. (1990). The patterns of cervical lymph node metastases from squamous carcinoma of the oral cavity. *Cancer, 66*(1), 109–113. https://doi.org/10.1002/1097-0142(19900701)66:1<109::AID-CNCR2820660120>3.0.CO;2-A

Shah, J. P., & Gil, Z. (2009). Current concepts in management of oral cancer – Surgery. *Oral Oncology, 45*(4–5), 394–401. https://doi.org/10.1016/j.oraloncology.2008.05.017

Shetty, A. V. (2017). Systemic treatment for squamous cell carcino of the head and neck. *Otolaryngologic Clinics of NA, 50*(4), 775–782. https://doi.org/10.1016/j.otc.2017.03.013

Takes, R. P., Strojan, P., Silver, C. E., Bradley, P. J., Haigentz, M., Wolf, G. T., … Ferlito, A. (2012). Current trends in initial management of hypopharyngeal cancer: The declining use of open surgery. *Head & Neck, 34*(2), 270–281. https://doi.org/10.1002/hed.21613

The Department of Veterans Affairs Laryngeal Cancer Study. (1991). Induction chemotherapy plus radiation compared with surgery plus radiation in patients with advanced laryngeal cancer. The Department of Veterans Affairs Laryngeal Cancer Study Group. *The New England Journal of Medicine, 324*(24), 1685–1690. https://doi.org/10.1056/NEJM199106133242402

Wee, J., Tan, E. H., Tai, B. C., Wong, H. B., Leong, S. S., Tan, T., … Machin, D. (2005). Randomized trial of radiotherapy versus concurrent chemoradiotherapy followed by adjuvant chemotherapy in patients with American Joint Committee on Cancer/International Union Against Cancer Stage III and IV nasopharyngeal cancer of the endemic variety. *Journal of Clinical Oncology, 23*(27), 6730–6738. https://doi.org/10.1200/JCO.2005.16.790

Wei, W. I., Chan, J. Y. W., Ng, R. W. M., & Ho, W. K. (2011). Surgical salvage of persistent or recurrent nasopharyngeal carcinoma with maxillary swing approach: Critical appraisal after 2 decades. *Head & Neck, 33*(7), 969–975. https://doi.org/10.1002/hed.21558

Wei, W. I., & Kwong, D. L. W. (2010). Current Management Strategy of Nasopharyngeal Carcinoma. *Clinical and Experimental Otorhinolaryngology, 3*(1), 1–12. https://doi.org/10.3342/ceo.2010.3.1.1

Winquist, E., Agbassi, C., Meyers, B. M., Yoo, J., Chan, K. K. W., & Head and Neck Disease Site Group. (2017). Systemic therapy in the curative treatment of head and neck squamous cell cancer: A systematic review. *Journal of Otolaryngology - Head & Neck Surgery, 46*(1), 29. https://doi.org/10.1186/s40463-017-0199-x

Yeh, D. H., Tam, S., Fung, K., MacNeil, S. D., Yoo, J., Winquist, E., … Nichols, A. C. (2015). Transoral robotic surgery vs. radiotherapy for management of oropharyngeal squamous cell carcinoma – A systematic review of the literature. *European Journal of Surgical Oncology (EJSO), 41*(12), 1603–1614. https://doi.org/10.1016/j.ejso.2015.09.007

Zhou, J., Li, Y., Wei, D., Qian, Y. E., & Li, W. (2015). Overall survival with and without laryngeal function preservation in 580 patients with hypopharyngeal squamous cell carcinoma. *Oncology Reports*, 3196–3202. https://doi.org/10.3892/or.2015.4313

Surgical Reconstruction for Cancer of the Oral Cavity

David H. Yeh, Axel Sahovaler, and John Yoo

Introduction

The oral cavity marks the beginning of the upper aerodigestive tract. Anatomically, it is the region defined anteriorly by the lips and ending at the junction of the hard and soft palate superiorly, the anterior tonsillar pillars laterally, and the line of the circumvallate papillae inferiorly. The oral cavity is lined with squamous epithelium and interspersed with minor salivary glands. Squamous cell carcinomas make up the vast majority of oral cavity cancers with salivary gland malignancies and other rare pathologies making up the remainder. Cancers of the oral cavity are generally treated with primary surgery with adjuvant radiotherapy for advanced-stage tumors (Genden et al., 2010; Shah & Gil, 2009). Major ablative surgery for oral cavity cancers results in loss of mucosa, submucosa, and muscle and in some cases bone and external skin. These tissue deficiencies may also translate into the loss of core functions depending on the size and location of the tumor (Genden, 2012; Hutcheson & Lewin, 2013). There may also be significant aesthetic implications with ablative surgery such as the compromise of oral competence, as well as alterations of natural soft tissue and skeletal contours. These types of changes may create increases in distress, social withdrawal, and reduced quality of life overall (Bornbaum & Doyle, Chap. 5; Doyle & MacDonald, Chap. 27).

The ideal reconstruction attempts to restore form and function and is dependent on several factors including the location and size of the defect, types of tissue resected, pre- or postoperative radiation/chemotherapy, and patient-specific factors such as overall health and comorbidities (Genden, 2012; Neligan, Gullane, & Gilbert, 2003; Urken et al., 1991). Particularly in the oral cavity, the location and extent of post-surgical defects at different subsites can creat specific disabilities. Therefore, beyond issues of oncologic treatment, the goal of surgical reconstruction is to identify and anticipate these issues and address them before they manifest in the posttreatment period.

Restoration of ablative defects requires reconstitution of mucosal lining and rebuilding of lost elements. There are myriad reconstructive options available depending on the complexity of the defect and range from primary closure, local flaps, and regional flaps, to microvascular free tissue transfers. This chapter is, therefore, structured to provide a practical approach for addressing the most common defect using contemporary options.

D. H. Yeh · A. Sahovaler · J. Yoo (✉)
Department of Otolaryngology – Head and Neck Surgery, London Health Sciences Centre, Schulich School of Medicine & Dentistry, Western University, London, ON, Canada
e-mail: john.yoo@lhsc.on.ca

© Springer Nature Switzerland AG 2019
P. C. Doyle (ed.), *Clinical Care and Rehabilitation in Head and Neck Cancer*,
https://doi.org/10.1007/978-3-030-04702-3_2

Relevant Anatomy and Functions of the Oral Cavity

The major subsites of the oral cavity include the lips, floor of mouth, anterior two-thirds of the tongue, buccal mucosa, upper and lower alveolar ridges, retromolar trigone, and hard palate. Somatosensory innervation is derived from contributions from the second and third divisions of the trigeminal nerve, while taste to the anterior tongue is derived from the lingual nerve. Branchial motor innervation is derived from the third division of the trigeminal nerve to the muscles of mastication, and the facial nerve supplies the buccinators and muscles of facial expression. The hypoglossal nerve innervates the intrinsic and extrinsic musculature of both the oral and oropharyngeal tongue. Although a comprehensive description of the complex neurosensory and neuromuscular anatomy is beyond the scope of this chapter, the outlined motor and sensory information provides a summary of the essential functions that may be lost in the process of surgical resection.

The oral cavity is critical for mastication, speech and articulation, respiration, and oral sensation. Different functional aspects are impacted depending on which subsites of the oral cavity are involved by the cancer resection. For example, the extent of lip resection leads to greater degrees of microstomia, thereby increasing the potential for impairments associated with food intake (Harris, Higgins, & Enepekides, 2012; Strong & Haller, 1996). Resecting the hard palate will leave a communication between the oral and nasal cavities, resulting in varied degrees of hypernasal speech and nasal regurgitation (Genden, Wallace, Okay, & Urken, 2004; Morlandt, 2016; Okay, Genden, Buchbinder, & Urken, 2001). Resections of the floor of mouth and ventral tongue, if not reconstructed, can leave the tongue tethered which may result in poor articulation and mastication (Hutcheson & Lewin, 2013). Because each subsite of the oral cavity plays a unique role in the function of the oral cavity, a clear understanding of the ablative functional deficits is the key to choosing the best option for reconstruction. These decisions are guided by a progressive level of surgical complexity that is referred to as the "reconstructive ladder," a topic that will be addressed in the subsequent section.

The Reconstructive Ladder

The armamentarium of reconstruction techniques is often referred to as the reconstructive ladder, a conceptual term that considers options ranging from simple techniques such as primary closure to progressively more complex procedures. The simplest technique that achieves the requisite goals of surgery should be utilized. Although many techniques may achieve defect closure, when larger resections are necessary, more sophisticated reconstructions are often required to achieve optimal function, appearance, and wound healing.

Under selected situations, the wound is allowed to heal without formal closure. This is known as *healing by secondary intention*; it is the simplest of all techniques, but this method should be used mainly for smaller defects because of wound cicatrization. With *primary closure*, the edges of the wound are approximated to one another, and sutures are used to keep the wound closed. The potential pitfall of primary closure is that it can create undue tension and distort the adjacent tissues with resulting functional consequences. *Skin grafts* are infrequently used in oral cavity reconstruction, but such use can mitigate some limitations that can result from primary closure or healing by secondary intention. A full-thickness skin graft incorporates both epithelium and dermis, while a split-thickness skin graft includes epithelium and various degrees of dermis. When used within the oral cavity, a split-thickness skin graft is preferred due to better take; that is, the graft will heal and merge with adjacent tissue. One example where a split-thickness skin graph is commonly used is in association with maxillectomy when the raw surface is skin grafted to better conform to obturator placement.

Pedicled flaps represent tissue transferred from its native bed (i.e., original site) to an adjacent area while retaining its native vascular supply. Flaps can incorporate varying components of tissue from skin, fascia, and/or muscle. In contemporary head and neck reconstruction, free tissue transfers or what is commonly referred to as *free flaps* have become the workhorse for most major surgical defects and have supplanted most pedicled flaps. The principle of free tissue transfer is to harvest tissue with its vascular pedicle, the tissue's primary blood supply, detach the blood supply, and then transplant the tissue from its native location to the new site of the ablative defect. The continuity of the blood vessels is restored by microvascular anastomosis to blood vessels near to the defect site. The enormous freedom to position the flap unencumbered by the pedicle connection, coupled with the near limitless capacity to harvest varying tissue types of different sizes to match the defect, has made free flaps the preferred reconstruction technique for major defects. Details of reconstructive techniques pertaining to each area of the head and neck will be addressed in the following sections.

Lip

The lips are often overlooked as an oral cavity subsite. However, they are crucial for proper oral function and maintenance of facial aesthetics. Achieving oral competency so as to maintain control of secretions, while maintaining adequate mouth opening, is the primary functional objective when reconstruction is required. The orbicularis oris muscle circumscribes the oral palpebrae and constitutes the major lip muscle. This muscle provides the sphincter function to maintain oral competence. Loss of orbicularis continuity results in oral incompetence. On the other hand, microstomia (reduction in size of the oral aperture) can occur as a consequence of lip resections and might inhibit oral intake; it can, in some instances, make denture placement difficult.

Numerous options exist for lip reconstruction, but the location and extent of the defect typically dictate the type of reconstruction utilized. In general, lip defects can be classified by their location and their relative width. In lip defects that encompass less than one-third of the lip, primary clo-

sure can be achieved without undue microstomia (Harris et al., 2012; Strong & Haller, 1996). Oral competence is maintained, and aesthetics are acceptable. However, as the defect size surpasses one-third of the lip length, the risk of microstomia and its functional implication increases.

Defects that are greater than one-third, but less than two-thirds the width of the lip, can be repaired by borrowing the opposite lip with a lip-switch procedure, referred to at the Abbe or the Estlander techniques (Harris et al., 2012). This involves using a portion of the upper or lower lip (half the defect size) to reconstruct the defect of the opposing lip. The flap is left pedicled on its native labial artery. The flap is elevated and sutured into the defect, while the donor site is closed primarily. The flap is divided in a delayed fashion. This reconstruction maintains excellent oral competence and aesthetics (Fig. 2.1). If the lip commissure is uninvolved, the Abbe flap can be used, whereas if the commissure is involved, the Estlander flap is used. Another option for defects greater than one-third but less than two-thirds the width of the lip is the Karapandzic flap (Harris et al., 2012). Using this flap, bilateral curved circumoral incisions are made at a distance equal to the vertical height of the remaining lip. The benefit of this type of reconstruction is that it mobilizes sensate lip with musculature innervation and with color match that is ideal. However, despite the aforementioned strengths, significant microstomia is an expected sequela of this procedure (Fig. 2.2).

In cases where greater than two-thirds of the lip is resected, reconstruction is achieved with more complex flaps or free tissue transfer. Inevitably, some degree of microstomia and reduced sensation, while achieving acceptable aesthetic outcome, is challenging. Classically, a radial forearm free flap with palmaris tendon flap can be employed for total lip reconstruction. The tendon helps to give support to the lip, while the fasciocutaneous tissue from the forearm recreates the skin of the lip and surrounding skin (Harris et al., 2012; Serletti, Tavin, Moran, & Coniglio, 1997). The disadvantage to this method of reconstruction is the loss of sensation (nerves are not microsurgically addressed), and it will have a

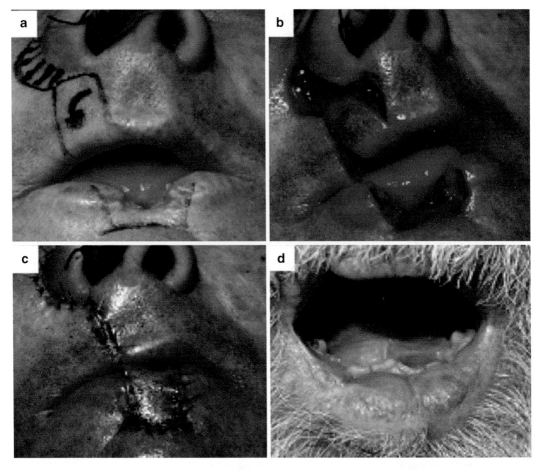

Fig. 2.1 Abbe flap for lip defect: (**a**) 1/3 lower lip defect with intraoperative markings. (**b**) Flap raised based in the labial artery. (**c**) Result of the first stage of the procedure with the pedicle undivided. (**d**) Remote postoperative picture with the pedicle already divided, showing a continent lip without microstomia

significant color mismatch. Despite these limitations, microstomia is not typically observed as a problem with these reconstructions.

Oral Tongue

The standard management of oral tongue cancer is surgical resection with clear tumor margins. After resection of the tumor, the need for surgical reconstruction depends on the location of the resection and size of the resulting defect. The goals of tongue reconstruction are to maximize tongue mobility, to limit tongue tethering, and to restore tongue volume (Chepeha et al., 2016; Hutcheson & Lewin, 2013; Pauloski, 2008).

These objectives ensure that articulation, the ability to move food boluses, and the capacity to clear secretions are optimized. The ideal tongue reconstruction requires premaxillary and palate contact in order to ensure satisfactory speech production. Mobility of the tongue tip past the alveolar ridge helps to further ensure efficient tongue movement and to facilitate clearing of oral secretions (Riemann et al., 2016; Vos & Burkey, 2004).

Resections of less than 1/3 of the tongue may be closed primarily or left to heal by secondary intention. In fact, studies have shown that the functional outcomes of speech and swallowing are superior with primary closure of small tongue defects when compared with pedicled or free flap reconstruction (Vos & Burkey, 2004). For small

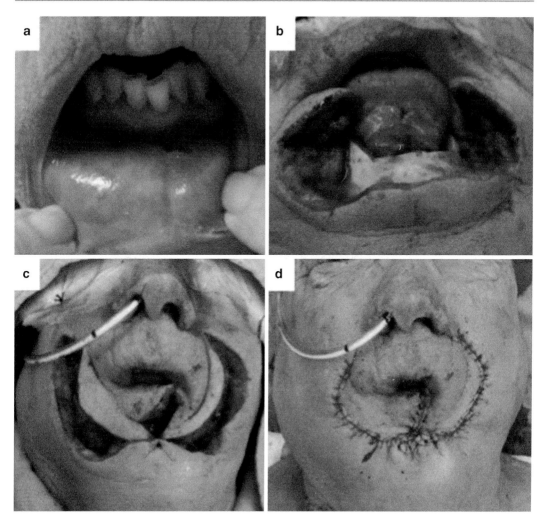

Fig. 2.2 Karapandzic flap for lip defect: (**a**) Carcinoma of the inferior alveolar ridge. (**b**) Postoperative defect consisting in a marginal mandibulectomy and a lip resection encompassing more than one-third but less than two- thirds of the lower lip. (**c**) Karapandzic flap with bilateral circumoral incisions to advance the remaining lower lip. (**d**) Oral continence is reestablished, with normal color match but with significant microstomia

superficial defects of the ventral tongue and floor of mouth, a split-thickness skin graft can be used to decrease tongue tethering (Vos & Burkey, 2004), and this is represented in Fig. 2.3. However, it must be emphasized that even small defects can lead to functional limitations, and, therefore, careful patient/reconstruction selection is required to optimize outcomes.

With larger resections of the tongue, bringing in additional tissue is necessary to achieve the reconstructive goals. If greater than one-third of the tongue is resected, options include pedicled flaps such as the buccinator-based myomucosal flap (Hayden & Nagel, 2013; Rigby & Taylor, 2013; Szeto et al., 2011), the submental island artery flap (Hayden & Nagel, 2013; Howard, Nagel, Donald, Hinni, & Hayden, 2014; Patel, Bayles, & Hayden, 2007; Rigby & Taylor, 2013), or the nasolabial flap represented in Fig. 2.4 (Napolitano & Mast, 2001; Rahpeyma & Khajehahmadi, 2016). In contemporary head and neck surgery, free tissue transfers have become the mainstay of reconstruction for most moderate sized and large tongue defects.

Free flaps are highly reliable and safe in experienced hands and are often the option of

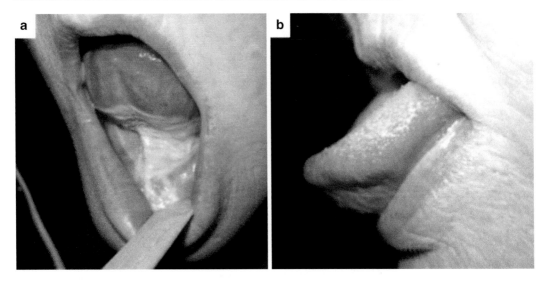

Fig. 2.3 Skin graft for ventral tongue/floor of mouth defect: (**a**, **b**) Remote postoperative picture after a ventral tongue and floor of mouth reconstruction with a skin graft, which obtained adequate tongue mobility and protrusion

choice for all but the simplest of oral cavity defects. Free flaps enable replacement of pliable tissue of ideal volume and surface area. The most common free flap used for tongue defects is the radial forearm free flap due its pliability, flexibility, and ease of elevation from the donor site as shown in Fig. 2.5 (Baas, Duraku, Corten, & Mureau, 2015; Kuriakose, Loree, Spies, Meyers, & Hicks, 2001; Rigby & Taylor, 2013). An additional perceived advantage of the radial forearm flap is its potential to be innervated in order to regain some sensation. Although appealing in concept, the benefits of direct reinnervation between the cutaneous nerve of the forearm and the lingual nerve have been difficult to demonstrate (Kuriakose et al., 2001; Namin & Varvares, 2016). When even greater volumes of tongue are lost such as with subtotal defects, the anterolateral thigh free flap has gained increasing popularity as the preferred reconstructive choice (Chana & Wei, 2004; Park & Miles, 2011; Rigby & Taylor, 2013; Vos & Burkey, 2004. Numerous other free flap options are available and have been used for various defects depending on size of defect and patient body habitus.

Floor of Mouth

The floor of mouth is critical for tongue protrusion, and undue scarring can limit mobility. After surgical resection of very small floor of mouth cancers, healing by secondary intention or through skin grafting may be acceptable options. However, in resections that include deeper musculature or involve significant portions of the ventral tongue, tethering and impaired mobility will occur without reconstruction. For that reason, pedicled flaps or free flaps (Fig. 2.6) are the standards of care with the greatest potential for successful outcomes (Rigby & Taylor, 2013; Vos & Burkey, 2004).

Buccal Mucosa

If resections that involve the buccal mucosa of the oral cavity are not reconstructed, scar contracture can lead to severe trismus, a reduction in jaw opening. Smaller buccal defects can be managed with primary closure, split-thickness skin graft, or pedicled soft tissue flaps such as the submental island artery flap (Genden, Buchbinder, & Urken,

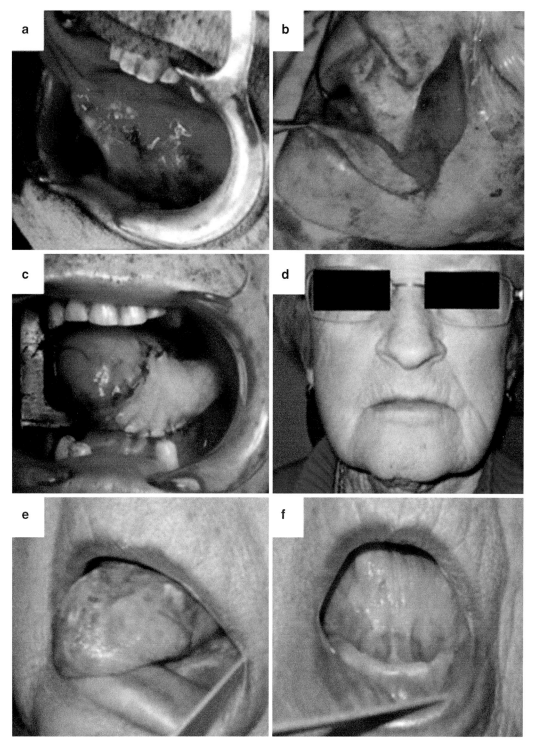

Fig. 2.4 Nasolabial flap for oral tongue defect: (**a**) Left lateral and ventral tongue defect. (**b**) Nasolabial pedicled flap raised showing good reach to the defect. (**c**) Inset of the flap, which is still attached to the pedicle from the skin. (**d–f**) Remote postoperative pictures depicting the scar placed in the nasolabial fold and excellent tongue mobility after the pedicle was divided in a second stage

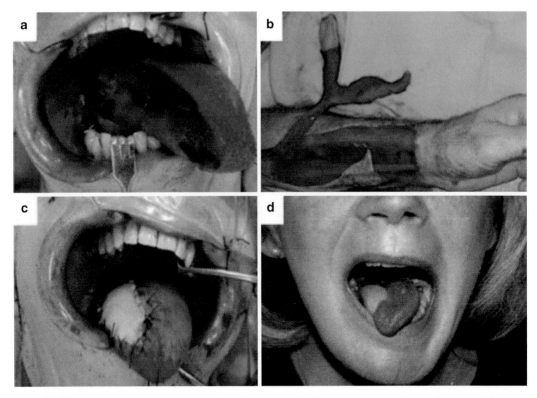

Fig. 2.5 Radial forearm free flap for oral tongue defect: (**a**) Left hemiglossectomy defect after carcinoma of the oral tongue resection. (**b**) Left radial forearm cutaneous free flap raised in situ with a fibroadipose component to add bulk to the reconstruction. (**c**) Immediate inset of the flap. (**d**) Remote picture showing good volume restoration and tongue protrusion

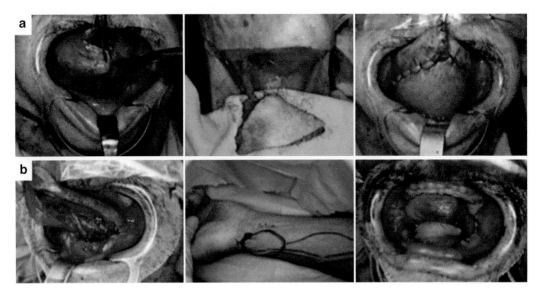

Fig. 2.6 Submental island flap and radial forearm free flap for floor of mouth defects: (**a**) Floor of mouth and ventral tongue defect reconstructed with a submental island flap. (**b**) Similar defect reconstructed with a radial forearm free flap. In both cases the paramount goal is to prevent tongue retraction and tethering, ensuring good mobility

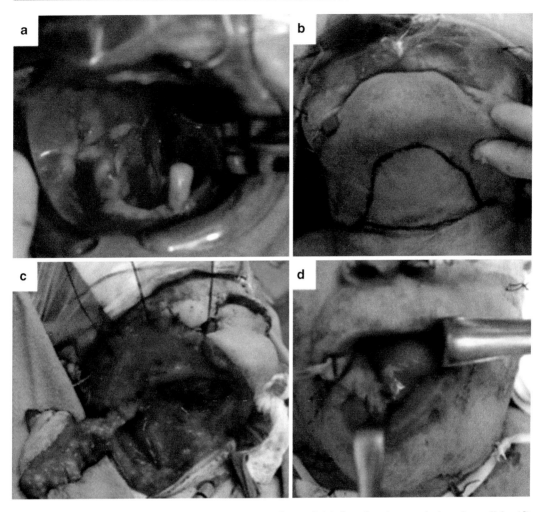

Fig. 2.7 Submental island flap for buccal mucosa defect: (**a**) Carcinoma of the right buccal mucosa which will require a reconstruction to prevent postoperative trismus. (**b**) Intraoperative design of a submental island pedicled flap and (**c**) flap elevation attached to the pedicle. (**d**) Immediate postoperative picture demonstrating good mouth opening

2004; Hayden, Nagel, & Donald, 2014) or the nasolabial flap (Napolitano & Mast, 2001; Rahpeyma & Khajehahmadi, 2016). If a split-thickness skin graft is used for reconstruction, it will require a bolster for several days to secure the graft in position. Otherwise, if the graft becomes displaced, contracture and trismus will result. With larger defects, even with the placement of a split-thickness skin graft, progressive contracture and scar formation can still result with an impact on functioning.

Therefore, for larger defects of the buccal mucosa, pedicled soft tissue flaps such as the submental island artery flap depicted in Fig. 2.7 (Hayden et al., 2014; Hayden & Nagel, 2013; Rigby & Taylor, 2013) or the nasolabial flap (Napolitano & Mast, 2001; Rahpeyma & Khajehahmadi, 2016) can be used to reline the defect. Compared with a split-thickness skin graft, local pedicled flaps are less likely to result in contracture and trismus. Soft tissue free flaps, in particular, the radial forearm free flap (Fig. 2.8), have excellent pliability and is well suited for large buccal reconstruction in order to reduce trismus (Rigby & Taylor, 2013; Vos & Burkey, 2004).

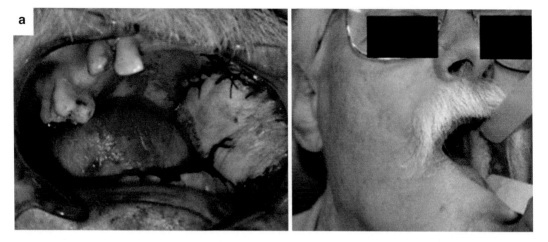

Fig. 2.8 Radial forearm flap for buccal mucosa defect: (**a**) Right buccal mucosa reconstructed with a radial forearm free flap, preventing trismus and scar retraction postoperatively (**b**) Post operative picture showing adequate mouth opening

Upper Alveolar Ridge/Maxilla and Hard Palate

The primary goals of reconstruction of the maxilla and the hard palate include supporting the orbital contents and maintaining separation of the oral and nasal cavities. Other important goals include reconstructing the palatal surface, reconstituting the patency of the lacrimal system, maintaining midface projection, and supporting dental rehabilitation. The extent and location of the defect will dictate the choice of reconstruction method. Reconstruction of the midface is among the most complex in head and neck surgery, and so with respect to this chapter, we will focus only on the hard palate.

The traditional approach for defects of the hard palate has been to employ prosthetic obturators for palatomaxillary defects and still remains an excellent option for many patients (Okay et al., 2001). However, numerous shortcomings were noted with this form of reconstruction especially with larger defects. For example, some limitations include poor retention and instability of the prosthesis, as well as loss of the oronasal prosthetic-tissue seal (see Cardoso & Chambers, Chap. 21). This leads to oronasal fistulae with resultant hypernasal speech and nasal regurgitation.

For non-tooth-bearing hard palate defects that constitute less than one-third of the hard palate, a prosthetic obturator or a local flap can be used for reconstruction. An obturator can be inconvenient for patients as it has to be removed and replaced regularly. The prosthesis-tissue seal can sometimes be a challenge to maintain and may not be acceptable for some patients (Okay et al., 2001). When there is remaining dentition, the prosthesis may be supported by clasps secured to the remaining teeth (Fig. 2.9). The alternative to prosthetic obturators includes pedicled or free flaps. In subtotal defects larger than one-third of the hard palate, either a prosthetic obturator or free tissue transfer with or without bone can be used (Genden et al., 2004). Local pedicled flaps are not large enough to reconstruct these defects. When the alveolar arch remains intact, bony reconstruction is not necessary. It should be noted that soft tissue reconstruction of the hard palate in edentulous patients may result in an inability to retain dentures making dental rehabilitation extremely difficult. In such cases, obturation may be the preferred rehabilitative option. Despite the challenges of these types of defects, functional outcomes are excellent if the oral cavity remains separated from the nasal cavity.

Maxillary defects that include the tooth-bearing alveolus can be reconstructed using a prosthetic obturator, a bone-containing free flap, or a soft tissue flap. With more extensive resections that involve more dentition, the

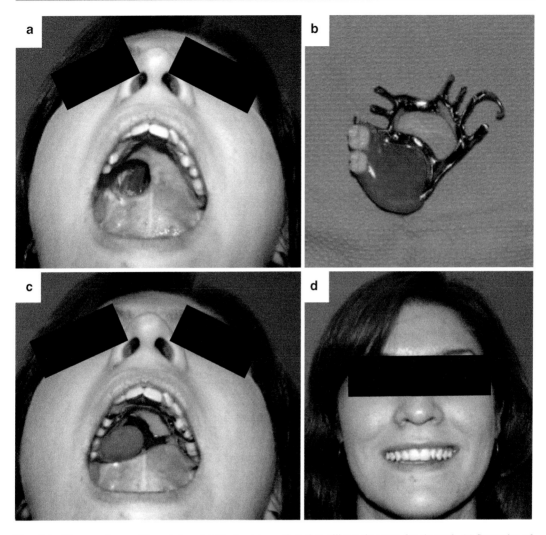

Fig. 2.9 Obturator for maxillary defect: (**a**) Hard palate defect showing communication an oroantral fistula in a non-edentulous patient. (**b**) Custom-made obturator with metal claps that will remain secured to the teeth. (**c**) Separation of the oral and nasal cavity preventing regurgitations and nasal voice with (**d**) cosmetic outcome

prosthetic obturator is less likely to stay in position, and, therefore, a free flap reconstruction may be necessary for successful oronasal separation (Morlandt, 2016). Soft tissue may only provide separation of the oral cavity from the paranasal sinuses and nasal cavity, but it may not provide optimal support for the facial soft tissue. Furthermore, dental rehabilitation is not possible.

Bone flaps may provide excellent facial musculoskeletal support and the potential for future dental rehabilitation through osteointegrated implantation. However, bone flap reconstructions

of the midface are technically more challenging than soft tissue flaps and thus require considerable surgical expertise. Several options for bony reconstructions of the midface including the fibula (Fig. 2.10), scapula, and the iliac crest osteocutaneous free flap have all be well described with excellent results (Brown, Lowe, Kanatas, & Schache, 2017; Clark, Vesely, & Gilbert, 2008; Yoo, Dowthwaite, Fung, Franklin, & Nichols, 2013). Palatomaxillary reconstruction is a challenging aspect of head and neck reconstruction, and a thorough appreciation of biomechanics of the upper jaw and recognition of the critical

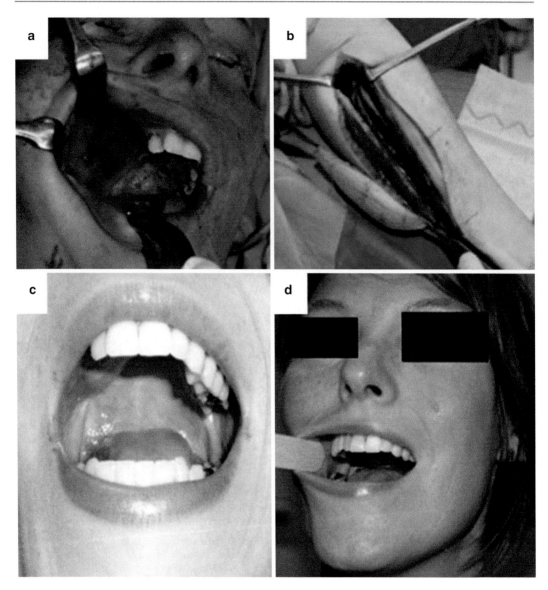

Fig. 2.10 Fibula free flap for maxillary defect: (**a**) Right maxillary defect affecting a tooth-bearing area of the hard palate. (**b**) Fibular free flap elevated with a skin paddle to act as an internal lining. (**c**) Six-month postoperative picture showing good skin mucosalization. (**d**) Five-year postoperative picture with full dental rehabilitation using implants

importance of cosmesis is paramount to achieve a satisfactory reconstruction.

Oromandibular

Tumors of the lower alveolar ridge and retromolar trigone commonly involve the bony mandible. There are two types of mandibular resections that can be performed for tumors in these regions.

Marginal mandibulectomy or rim mandibulectomy removes the overlying soft tissue and the adjacent cortex of the mandible but leaves behind at least 1 cm of mandibular height, thereby maintaining the continuity of the mandible. This can be performed in cases where the tumor involves only the periosteum or superficial cortex of the bone. If a marginal mandibulectomy is performed, the reconstruction requires only soft tissue. Infrequently, the soft tissue can be closed

Fig. 2.11 Lateral mandibular resection without reconstruction: (**a**) Dental panoramic radiography revealing the absence of the left parasymphyseal, angle, and ascending ramus of the mandible left mid-body. (**b**) Photo of the same patient depicting facial asymmetry and (**c**) the latero-deviation of the jaw (also known as "swinging mandible") after no reconstruction

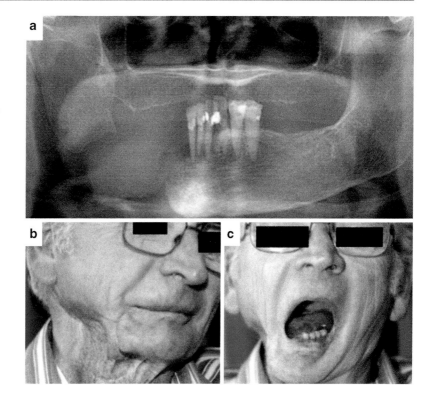

primarily, but in most cases soft tissue flaps are required. Once again, the radial forearm free flap is highly versatile and enables reliable coverage of the exposed bone while restoring mucosal lining. Pedicled flaps may also be used for selected defects. If the bony cortex of the mandible is breached, then a segmental mandibulectomy is required. This results in discontinuity of the mandible which must be restored in most cases.

For segmental oromandibular defects, several reconstructive options are available depending on the location of the mandible defect and patient-specific factors. Segmental defects posterolateral to the mental foramen are considered lateral defects. The most common form of reconstruction is to reconstitute the mandibular bony arch with a vascularized free flap of bone and skin. However, in selected cases the bone segment may be bridged with a metal plate with soft tissue coverage. Historically, lateral defects of the mandible were managed by restoring soft tissue loss but without restoring bony continuity. This resulted in a "swinging mandible" because there were two

free floating discontinuous segments of mandible. The functional and aesthetic implications of this approach were significant. This approach is an uncommon occurrence in contemporary head and neck surgery except in rare circumstances (Fig. 2.11).

Reconstitution of the mandibular arch using a titanium alloy plate coupled with soft tissue coverage is a common approach for the lateral oromandibular defect (Miles, Goldstein, Gilbert, & Gullane, 2010). The addition of a load-bearing reconstruction plate helps to stabilize the two free bone segments and can help to avoid malocclusion, crossbite, pain, and deformity (Wei et al., 2003). Soft tissue coverage can be achieved by regional pedicled flaps such as the pectoralis major myocutaneous flap or, more commonly, free flaps such as the radial forearm or anterolateral thigh.

The ideal reconstruction of soft tissue/bony defects is through composite tissue transfers. The advent of free tissue transfers has allowed numerous options for restoring soft tissue and

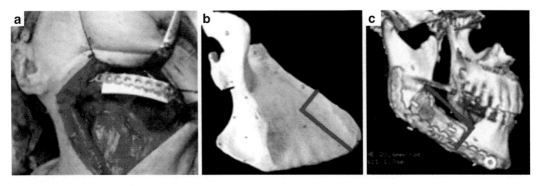

Fig. 2.12 Scapular tip free flap for lateral mandible reconstruction: (**a**) Intraoperative right lateral defect of the mandible with the reconstruction plate inserted. (**b**) Schematic illustrative image of the bone cuts. (**c**) Postoperative CT with 3D reconstruction showing the final result

mandibular arch with a single flap. Restoring bony union not only provides the most stable form of reconstruction but importantly enables dental rehabilitation through osteointegrated implantation. Bone flap options include the fibula (Brown et al., 2017), the scapula (Yoo et al., 2013) which is shown in Fig. 2.12, the radius (Brown et al., 2017), and the iliac crest (Miles et al., 2010; Shnayder et al., 2015) with their respective soft tissue components. Each flap has unique advantages and disadvantages and specific indications; however, the details of those concerns are beyond the scope of the present chapter.

Segmental defects of the mandible that involve the parasymphyseal region are considered anterior defects. In contrast to lateral mandible defects, anterior mandible defects require mandibular arch restoration using vascularized bone. Plate reconstruction is inherently unstable in this location, and it has been associated with an unacceptably high-rate plate extrusion and plate fracture (Wei et al., 2003). As previously described, several options for bone-containing free flaps include the fibula (Fig. 2.13), scapula, radius, iliac crest.

Through-and-Through Defects

In some oral cavity cancers, tumors can enlarge and extend to involve the external skin. Typically, once a tumor involves the external skin, it has reached a substantial size often involving bone and soft tissue which then necessitates a large volume reconstruction. Resection of the tumor and the overlying skin results in what is termed a "through-and-through defect." These are among the most formidable of reconstructive challenges and may require a single complex multi-paddle free flap or a combination of free and pedicled flaps. Due to the volume and size of deficits, at least one free tissue transfer is usually necessary to address the defect. If the defect involves bone and soft tissue, the reconstruction can be achieved with either a single composite free flap containing bone with a large volume of soft tissue or with the use of two flaps, one of which includes bone. Large composite flaps can be based off the subscapular system to include either bone from the lateral border of the scapula or the scapula tip (Fig. 2.14). The bone can be harvested to include multiple paddles of soft tissue. Alternatively, a single free flap can be used to reconstruct the oral cavity defect and a cervicofacial rotation flap, or a pedicled flap with a skin graft can be employed to reconstruct the remaining external skin defect. If a single free flap is insufficient, two free flaps can be used to reconstruct the oral cavity defect and the external skin defect separately.

Summary

The oral cavity is essential for speech, chewing, swallowing, and aesthetics. Achieving the best results in reconstruction after tumor

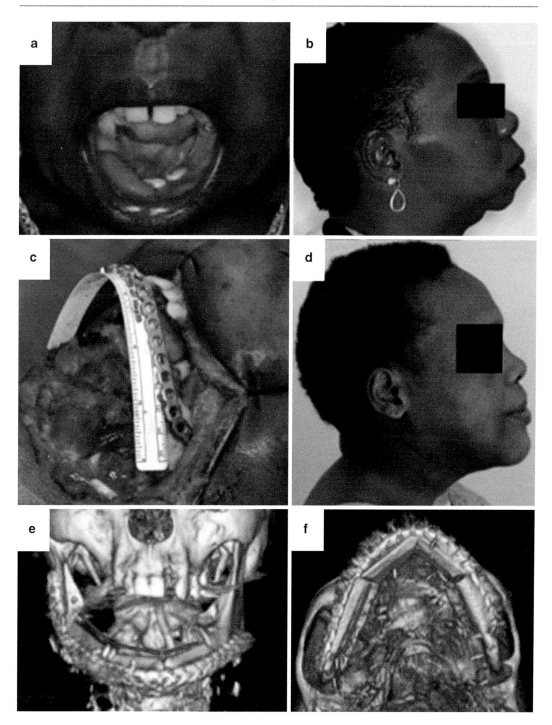

Fig. 2.13 Fibula free flap for anterior and lateral mandible reconstruction: (**a, b**) Preoperative picture showing bone resorption in a patient with osteoradionecrosis of the anterior mandible. (**c**) Intraoperative photo with an angle-to-angle mandibular defect. (**d**) Postoperative image with restitution of the facial contour. (**e, f**) 3D CT scan of the reconstruction with a fibular flap replacing the entire defect

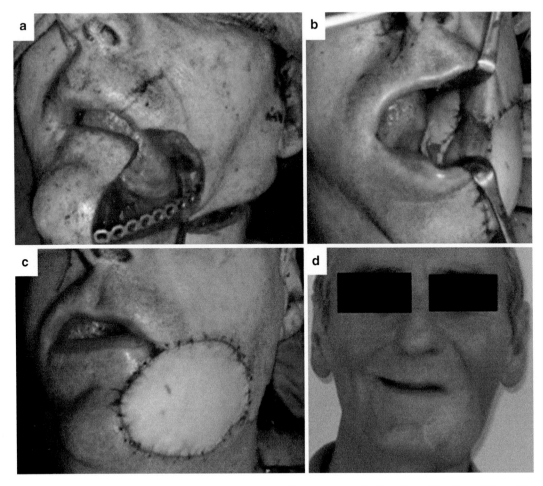

Fig. 2.14 Scapular tip free flap for a through-and-through defect: (**a**) Through-and-through defect after a mandibular tumor invading the skin and the buccal mucosa. (**b, c**) Immediate post-reconstructive picture using a scapular tip free flap with a large skin paddle which covered both the cutaneous and intraoral defect. (**d**) Remote postoperative image with good lip continence and cosmesis

ablation requires a clear understanding of its role in relation to tongue mobility, mastication, oral-nasal competence, and physical appearance. Surgical options include a vast spectrum of operations ranging from primary closure to complex free tissue transfer. Understanding the functional and aesthetic implications of the anatomic defect in conjunction with the unique patient-specific factors is the foundational basis for selecting the appropriate reconstruction.

References

Baas, M., Duraku, L. S., Corten, E. M. L., & Mureau, M. A. M. (2015). A systematic review on the sensory reinnervation of free flaps for tongue reconstruction: Does improved sensibility imply functional benefits? *Journal of Plastic and Reconstructive Aesthetic Surgery, 68*(8), 1025–1035.

Brown, J. S., Lowe, D., Kanatas, A., & Schache, A. (2017). Mandibular reconstruction with vascularised bone flaps: A systematic review over 25 years. *British Journal of Oral and Maxillofacial Surgery, 55*(2), 113–126.

Chana, J. S., & Wei, F.-C. (2004). A review of the advantages of the anterolateral thigh flap in head and neck reconstruction. *British Journal of Plastic Surgery, 57*(7), 603–609.

Chepeha, D. B., Spector, M. E., Chinn, S. B., Casper, K. A., Chanowski, E. J. P., Moyer, J. S., ... Lyden, T. H. (2016). Hemiglossectomy tongue reconstruction: Modeling of elevation, protrusion, and functional outcome using receiver operator characteristic curve. *Head & Neck, 38*(7), 1066–1073.

Clark, J. R., Vesely, M., & Gilbert, R. (2008). Scapular angle osteomyogenous flap in postmaxillectomy reconstruction: Defect, reconstruction, shoulder function, and harvest technique. *Head & Neck, 30*(1), 10–20.

Genden, E. (2012). *Reconstruction of the head and neck: A defect-oriented approach* (1st ed.). New York, NY: Thieme Medical Publishers.

Genden, E. M., Buchbinder, D., & Urken, M. L. (2004). The submental island flap for palatal reconstruction: A novel technique. *Journal of Oral and Maxillofacial Surgery, 62*(3), 387–390.

Genden, E. M., Ferlito, A., Silver, C. E., Takes, R. P., Suárez, C., Owen, R. P., ... Rodrigo, J. P. (2010). Contemporary management of cancer of the oral cavity. *European Archives of Oto-Rhino-Laryngology, 267*(7), 1001–1017.

Genden, E. M., Wallace, D. I., Okay, D., & Urken, M. L. (2004). Reconstruction of the hard palate using the radial forearm free flap: Indications and outcomes. *Head & Neck, 26*(9), 808–814.

Harris, L., Higgins, K., & Enepekides, D. (2012). Local flap reconstruction of acquired lip defects. *Current Opinion in Otolaryngology Head and Neck Surgery, 20*(4), 254–261.

Hayden, R. E., & Nagel, T. H. (2013). The evolving role of free flaps and pedicled flaps in head and neck reconstruction. *Current Opinions in Otolaryngology Head and Neck Surgery, 21*(4), 305–310.

Hayden, R. E., Nagel, T. H., & Donald, C. B. (2014). Hybrid submental flaps for reconstruction in the head and neck: Part pedicled, part free. *Laryngoscope, 124*(3), 637–641.

Howard, B. E., Nagel, T. H., Donald, C. B., Hinni, M. L., & Hayden, R. E. (2014). Oncologic safety of the submental flap for reconstruction in oral cavity malignancies. *Otolaryngology Head and Neck Surgery, 150*(4), 558–562.

Hutcheson, K. A., & Lewin, J. S. (2013). Functional assessment and rehabilitation. How to maximize outcomes. *Otolaryngology Clinics of North America, 46*(4), 657–670.

Kuriakose, M. A., Loree, T. R., Spies, A., Meyers, S., & Hicks, W. L. (2001). Sensate radial forearm free flaps in tongue reconstruction. *Archives of Otolaryngology Head and Neck Surgery, 127*(12), 1463–1466.

Miles, B. A., Goldstein, D. P., Gilbert, R. W., & Gullane, P. J. (2010). Mandible reconstruction. *Current Opinions in Otolaryngology Head and Neck Surgery, 18*(4), 317–322.

Morlandt, A. B. (2016). Reconstruction of the maxillectomy defect. *Current Otorhinolaryngology Reports, 4*(3), 201–210.

Namin, A. W., & Varvares, M. A. (2016). Functional outcomes of sensate versus insensate free flap reconstruction in oral and oropharyngeal reconstruction: A systematic review. *Head & Neck, 38*(11), 1717–1721.

Napolitano, M., & Mast, B. A. (2001). The nasolabial flap revisited as an adjunct to floor-of-mouth reconstruction. *Annals of Plastic Surgery, 46*(3), 265–268.

Neligan, P. C., Gullane, P. J., & Gilbert, R. W. (2003). Functional reconstruction of the oral cavity. *World Journal of Surgery, 27*(7), 856–862.

Okay, D. J., Genden, E., Buchbinder, D., & Urken, M. (2001). Prosthodontic guidelines for surgical reconstruction of the maxilla: A classification system of defects. *Journal of Prosthetic Dentistry, 86*(4), 352–363.

Park, C. W., & Miles, B. A. (2011). The expanding role of the anterolateral thigh free flap in head and neck reconstruction. *Current Opinions in Otolaryngology Head and Neck Surgery, 19*(4), 263–268.

Patel, U., Bayles, S. W., & Hayden, R. E. (2007). The submental flap: A modified technique for resident training. *Laryngoscope, 117*(1), 186–189.

Pauloski, B. R. (2008). Rehabilitation of dysphagia following head and neck cancer. *Physical Medicine and Rehabilitation Clinics of North America, 19*(4), 889–928.

Rahpeyma, A., & Khajehahmadi, S. (2016). The place of nasolabial flap in orofacial reconstruction: A review. *Annals of Medicine and Surgery, 12*(1), 79–87.

Riemann, M., Knipfer, C., Rohde, M., Adler, W., Schuster, M., Noeth, E., ... Stelzle, F. (2016). Oral squamous cell carcinoma of the tongue: Prospective and objective speech evaluation of patients undergoing surgical therapy. *Head & Neck, 38*(7), 993–1001.

Rigby, M. H., & Taylor, S. M. (2013). Soft tissue reconstruction of the oral cavity: A review of current options. *Current Opinions in Otolaryngology Head and Neck Surgery, 21*(4), 311–317.

Serletti, J. M., Tavin, E., Moran, S. L., & Coniglio, J. U. (1997). Total lower lip reconstruction with a sensate composite radial forearm-palmaris longus free flap and a tongue flap. *Plastic and Reconstructive Surgery, 99*(2), 559–561.

Shah, J. P., & Gil, Z. (2009). Current concepts in management of oral cancer – Surgery. *Oral Oncology, 45*(4–5), 394–401.

Shnayder, Y., Lin, D., Desai, S. C., Nussenbaum, B., Sand, J. P., & Wax, M. K. (2015). Reconstruction of the lateral mandibular defect. *JAMA Facial Plastic Surgery, 17*(5), 367–373.

Strong, E. B., & Haller, J. R. (1996). Reconstruction of the lip and perioral region. *Current Opinion in Otolaryngology Head and Neck Surgery, 4*, 267–270.

Szeto, C., Yoo, J., Busato, G.-M., Franklin, J., Fung, K., & Nichols, A. (2011). The buccinator flap: A review of current clinical applications. *Current Opinions in Otolaryngology Head and Neck Surgery, 19*(4), 257–262.

Urken, M. L., Buchbinder, D., Weinberg, H., Vickery, C., Sheiner, A., Parker, R., … Biller, H. F. (1991). Functional evaluation following microvascular oromandibular reconstruction of the oral cancer patient: A comparative study of reconstructed and nonreconstructed patients. *Laryngoscope, 101*(9), 935–950.

Vos, J. D., & Burkey, B. B. (2004). Functional outcomes after free flap reconstruction of the upper aerodigestive tract. *Current Opinions in Otolaryngology Head and Neck Surgery, 12*(4), 305–310.

Wei, F.-C., Celik, N., Yang, W.-G., Chen, I.-H., Chang, Y.-M., & Chen, H.-C. (2003). Complications after reconstruction by plate and soft-tissue free flap in composite mandibular defects and secondary salvage reconstruction with osteocutaneous flap. *Plastic and Reconstructive Surgery, 112*(1), 37–42.

Yoo, J., Dowthwaite, S. A., Fung, K., Franklin, J., & Nichols, A. (2013). A new angle to mandibular reconstruction: The scapular tip free flap. *Head & Neck, 35*(7), 980–986.

Complications Following Total Laryngectomy

3

Edward J. Damrose and Philip C. Doyle

Introduction

There are approximately 12,000 new cases of laryngeal cancer diagnosed annually in the United States, with approximately 4000 total laryngectomy procedures performed (Maddox & Davies, 2012). Men are more commonly affected than women, and squamous cell carcinoma is the most common malignancy encountered. Tobacco and alcohol use expose the larynx to carcinogens which promote tumor development. However, in recent years the incidence of laryngeal cancer has declined secondary to a decrease in smoking rates. Additionally, the rate of total laryngectomy also has seen a decline over the past two decades, potentially as a result of the increased use of chemotherapy combined with radiation therapy (CRT) as an alternative to total laryngectomy (Maddox & Davies, 2012; Hoffman et al., 2006). Total laryngectomy performed following radiation therapy (RT) or CRT is commonly referred to as salvage laryngectomy.

Surgical complications associated with total laryngectomy may be described and grouped in several different ways: early vs late, local vs systemic, functional (deglutition vs respiration vs phonation), and according to the incidence of the specific complications (pharyngocutaneous fistula vs hematoma vs death). But it is important to note that overall complication rates may be increased when total laryngectomy is performed as a salvage operation. This increase in complications is almost certainly due to changes that emerge from the influence of past treatment, whether it be RT or CRT. Similarly, and in the current era where tracheoesophageal puncture (TEP) voice restoration may be often employed, additional consideration related to potential complications may be raised. The use of voice prostheses for postlaryngectomy voice rehabilitation may introduce its own unique set of complications that require monitoring and, if present, immediate management. This chapter seeks to provide the reader with a working framework with which to categorize complications, to understand potential management strategies, and to anticipate when and why these complications may occur. Additionally, while the content of this chapter is focused on medical complications secondary to total laryngectomy, the long-term impact on voice and speech rehabilitation must be considered. Thus, issues pertaining to posttreatment rehabilitation will be addressed.

E. J. Damrose (✉)
Department of Otolaryngology, Head and Neck Surgery, Stanford University School of Medicine, Stanford, CA, USA
e-mail: edamrose@stanford.edu

P. C. Doyle
Voice Production and Perception Laboratory & Laboratory for Well-Being and Quality of Life, Department of Otolaryngology – Head and Neck Surgery and School of Communication Sciences and Disorders, Western University, Elborn College, London, ON, Canada

© Springer Nature Switzerland AG 2019
P. C. Doyle (ed.), *Clinical Care and Rehabilitation in Head and Neck Cancer*,
https://doi.org/10.1007/978-3-030-04702-3_3

Complications

Postoperative complications following total laryngectomy are well recognized (Ganly et al., 2005; Hall et al., 2003). The overall rate of complications is reported to range between 40% and 68% (Hasan et al., 2017; Ganly et al., 2005; Lansaat et al., 2018). Ganly et al. (2005) provide a logical framework for categorizing complications that include those that are local (wound infection, wound dehiscence, flap necrosis, fistula, carotid rupture, or chyle leak), swallowing related (dysphagia or stricture), airway related (lung, trachea, or stoma), and systemic in nature (myocardial infarction, urinary tract infection, pulmonary, renal, or metabolic). Many studies show that the incidence of complications is significantly higher in patients undergoing salvage laryngectomy. Thus, in the current era, clinicians should always be aware that laryngectomy following failed conservative treatment (i.e., RT or CRT) may carry additional risks that require careful observation and monitoring.

Based on a review of the literature, the most common complications encountered include pharyngocutaneous fistula (17–31%), wound infections (9–14%), pneumonia (6%), tracheostomal stenosis (5%), chyle leak (2–5%), and hematoma or hemorrhage (2–6%).[3] Death is rare (0.5%).[4] When laryngectomy necessitates the use of microvascular free flaps for reconstruction, free flap failure necessitating reoperation has been estimated to be around 7% (Hall et al., 2003). Because these types of complications have an impact on recovery and rehabilitation, each will be briefly addressed in the subsequent sections of this chapter.

Pharyngocutaneous Fistula

Pharyngocutaneous fistula (PCF) is the development of a communication between the mucosa-lined pharyngeal component of the aerodigestive tract and the skin. Because of the altered postlaryngectomy anatomy relative to the pharynx and trachea, the emergence of a PCF will result in the cutaneous drainage of saliva with its associated risks. Surgical procedures which result in the disruption of the pharyngeal mucosa, namely, total laryngectomy, Zenker's diverticulectomy, and penetrating neck trauma, among others, may precipitate the development of PCF. The onset of a PCF may be heralded by fever as aerodigestive contents including saliva and food penetrate through the mucosa into the soft tissues of the neck. Clinically, this may appear as erythema or redness of the skin, with accompanying swelling and tenderness. As the subcutaneous collection progresses, drainage of saliva or food products, or appearance of the same in subcutaneous drains, may be observed, and if this occurs, management is required.

PCF is the most common complication associated with total laryngectomy. In fact, it has been estimated to impact up to 30% of all cases, with rates ranging from 5% to 73% depending upon the study (Hasan et al., 2017). Preoperative RT and CRT increase the rate of PCF (Ganly et al., 2005; Hall et al., 2003; Hasan et al., 2017; Lansaat et al., 2018). Concurrent performance of neck dissections and surgery performed within the first year following the completion of RT has also been associated with higher fistula rates (Basheeth, O'Leary, & Sheahan, 2014). Some studies have suggested that a primary TEP may increase the postoperative fistula rate (Emerick et al., 2009), although this suggestion has not been confirmed by other studies (Dowthwaite et al., 2012; Naunheim, Remenschneider, Scangas, Bunting, & Deschler, 2016; Starmer et al., 2009).

Some authors have suggested utilization of flaps (both regional and microvascular flaps) in an effort to incorporate non-irradiated tissue into the repair of the surgical defect or to reinforce the primary closure. Overall the use of such flaps seems to reduce the incidence of PCF (Gil et al., 2009; Patel et al., 2013; Wulff et al., 2015). Malnutrition and hypothyroidism have also been implicated in poor postoperative healing and should be monitored and rectified as needed (Mattioli et al., 2015; Rosko et al., 2018). Time to resumption of oral intake has been traditionally implicated in the development of pharyngocutaneous fistulas. A delay in resuming oral nutritional intake of 7–10 days is usually recommended in patients with no history of radiation and from 14 to 21 days in those patients undergoing salvage laryngectomy. Adherence to these guidelines is of critical importance to efforts that seek to reduce the potential likelihood of the development of a PCF. Regardless of the underlying cause, if a PCF occurs, significant delays in rehabilitation may be observed.

Although concerns related to a change in tissue and the development of a PCF are obviously related to postlaryngectomy healing, several specific issues that impact rehabilitation and quality of life deserve particular mention. For example, should a PCF occur, it will almost certainly delay the resumption of oral intake, increase length of hospitalization and overall cost of care, delay resumption of pulmonary-driven speech, and, most importantly, may be associated with life-threatening complications such as carotid exposure and subsequent rupture.

A PCF also can result in stricture formation at the site following healing, a problem that may have long-term influences on the individual's functional capacity. Stricture formation can lead to chronic dysphagia (Arrese & Schieve, Chap. 19) and impaired postlaryngectomy phonation (either esophageal or tracheoesophageal speech). Should a stricture be present, it may necessitate recurrent dilations or free flap reconstruction to manage if it is severe (Graville, Palmer, & Bolognone, Chap. 11; Knott, Chap. 12). In the event of a stricture, several treatment options can be considered.

Treatment often includes maintaining the patient without permitting them to consume nutrition orally, or what is termed NPO (non per os). In such instances, nutrition must be addressed with a goal of achieving proper alimentation (usually in excess of 2000 calories/day depending upon body weight and albumin). Additionally, the use of antibiotics with demonstrated efficacy against skin and oropharyngeal flora may be required. Finally, the use of pressure dressings, adequate thyroid hormone replacement therapy, and in some cases regional or free microvascular flaps may be necessary in an effort to repair the defect.

Pharyngoesophageal Stricture

Excessive narrowing of the postoperative aerodigestive tract due to scarring and wound contracture is termed a stricture, and its presence may result in impaired deglutition and/or one's inability to generate intrinsic methods of postlaryngectomy alaryngeal speech (Doyle, 1994). Pharyngoesophageal stricture may be a direct complication of total laryngectomy procedures, with a frequency ranging from 10% to 30% (Sweeny et al., 2012). Strictures are often associated with fistula formation and prior radiation. When a fistula forms and subsequently heals, the resultant scar contracture may narrow the aerodigestive tract at the point of origin of the fistula, forming a stricture. Mechanically, the greater the amount of pharyngeal mucosa resected at the time of surgery, the smaller and narrower the lumen of the neopharynx, a procedural factor that can also predispose the region to stricture formation.

Classical dictum has taught that in primary closure of the pharyngeal defect following total laryngectomy, the minimal amount of mucosa to be preserved while still allowing for near normal oral intake is such that primary closure can be accomplished around an 18 French (6 mm) nasogastric tube. In practice, a larger lumen than this is needed for normal oral intake. As a result, approximately 50% of patients with stricture will require serial dilation in order to maintain adequate oral intake (Sweeny et al., 2012). Regional or free microvascular flaps may be required in order to reconstruct severe to total pharyngoesophageal strictures. However, if reconstruction is required, the risk of additional complications is inherently higher. Thus, management decisions may be complex in such cases.

Wound Infection

Wound infections can occur with any surgical procedure and may occur in 5–10% of those who undergo total laryngectomy. Again, prior radiation, hypothyroidism, and poor nutritional status have been implicated in increased rates of infection.

Infection may occur along the suture line, resulting in abscess formation. At times, infection can also involve the tracheostoma resulting in dehiscence, stomal retraction, and ultimately stomal stenosis (see Fig. 3.1). Wound infections may be treated with debridement, antibiotics, and, in those instances when soft tissue loss is extensive, flap reconstruction. A wound culture may be helpful in identifying the causative organism which in turn may help to direct appropriate antibiotic therapy. Figure 3.2a and b illustrates an infection prior to and following treatment with antibiotics, respectively. Although wound infection may most frequently be associated in the

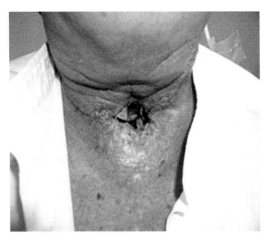

Fig. 3.1 Wound infection involving the stoma of a laryngectomy patient

early postoperative periods, clinicians should always take time to inspect the region. As with most medical issues, early identification may improve outcomes and decrease the likelihood of developing other problems (e.g., PCF).

Chyle Leak

Chyle is a fluid composed of lymph and emulsified fats. It is conveyed through lymphatic channels to the venous circulation, where it is recirculated throughout the body. The thoracic duct is a large lymphatic vessel that conveys up to 75% of the body's lymph (Yu, Ma, Zhang, Wang, & Li, 2010). The thoracic duct enters the junction of the internal jugular and subclavian veins at the base of the left side of the neck (Delaney, Shi, Shokrani, & Sinha, 2017). When this duct is injured, a chyle leak – the extravasation of chyle into the neck or thorax – may ensue. Injury to the thoracic duct and subsequent chyle leak are relatively rare, but it may be seen in 5% of cases and is secondary to performance of a neck dissection, rather than the laryngectomy proper.

Extravasation of chyle at times can reach large volumes in excess of 1000–2000 mL/day. Chyle is rich in triglycerides and fatty acids and, when lost, may result in severe nutritional deficiencies if not replaced. When drains are in place, chyle may appear as a milky or serous fluid within the

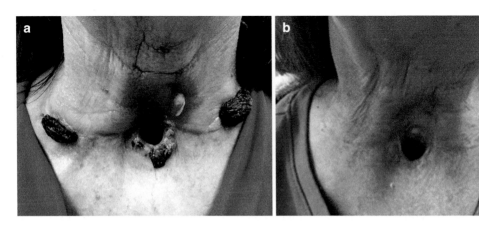

Fig. 3.2 (**a**) Wound infection involving the stoma and suture line of laryngectomy patient. (**b**) Same patient following antibiotic treatment

drains. In the absence of drains, it may collect under the skin and form a fluid collection called a "chyloma." Occasionally, chyle may collect within the thoracic cavity and the pleural space, compressing the lung and leading to respiratory distress (chylothorax). Treatment may include maintenance on a medium-chain fatty acid diet, pressure dressings to the left neck to decrease extravasation of the chyle, the use of intravenous somatostatin or subcutaneous octreotide to decrease chyle production, and/or surgical exploration to ligate the thoracic duct. High-volume leaks (i.e., >1000 mL/day) usually require surgical management, while lower-volume leaks may be managed conservatively (Delaney et al., 2017).

Hemorrhage

Hemorrhage or bleeding may complicate any surgical procedure, and it may occur in approximately 5% of procedures (Hall et al., 2003; Hasan et al., 2017). Bleeding may present as a subcutaneous collection of blood, called a hematoma. An undrained collection of blood may become infected secondarily or may produce soft tissue loss of the overlying skin. A small hematoma can be monitored, but a large hematoma may require surgical drainage. A rapidly expanding hematoma may represent an arterial bleed, and blood loss from such a high-pressure vascular leak can be serious and potentially life-threatening. If drains are in place, the appearance of bright red blood in the drains is usually indicative of a hemorrhage.

Bleeding from a carotid artery potentially may be lethal. It may occur from direct tumor erosion into the carotid artery or from exposure of the carotid artery from loss of overlaying protective soft tissues, as can be seen in a large PCF. When the carotid artery ruptures spontaneously, an event termed a "carotid blowout," the degree of hemorrhage may be massive and quickly lethal. Occasionally, carotid bleeding is heralded by a sudden but brief hemorrhage of bright red blood. As the affected vessel spasms, the loss of blood is halted, although this is temporary. Such a "herald

bleed" may alert the physician to the possibility of an impending "blowout" which will require immediate medical management.

Treatment of a carotid blowout, or any other large vessel bleed, necessitates immediate control of the hemorrhage, usually via pressure, fluid resuscitation, and repair of the injured vessel. Angiography with embolization or placement of a stent may be indicated; in other cases, surgical repair or ligation of the vessel may be needed. If there is exposure of the affected vessel, soft tissue coverage, through the use of either a regional or free microvascular flap, may be needed to prevent the event from recurring.

Tracheal Complications

Total laryngectomy involves creation of a permanent tracheostoma with a union of the upper ring of the trachea to the skin of the anterior neck. The tracheostoma will be present for the remainder of the individual's life, and he will breathe permanently from the new airway as a "neck breather." A widely patent tracheostoma is usually desired to allow ease of respiration and to facilitate placement and maintenance of a TEP voice prosthesis. Complications are rare, usually reported in only 5% of cases. When an airway complication occurs, it principally involves stenosis and less commonly tracheal stenosis, dehiscence, or tracheitis.

Stenosis is a phenomenon typically associated with scarring, and it may be exacerbated by prior radiation, prior tracheostomy placement, or infection. Creation of the tracheostoma under minimal tension, preservation of a complete tracheal ring, and attentive hygiene to the region to minimize superinfection may decrease the risk of stomal stenosis. Techniques that artificially narrow the stoma, with the concept that such maneuvers will better facilitate digital occlusion of the stoma and TEP phonation, are antiquated and should be discouraged. Stomal stenosis can result in difficulty breathing. That is, if there is a reduction in the overall size of the tracheostoma, more airway resistance may occur. If this reduction is significant, inspiration will become more difficult. An added concern related to stenosis is that it can also prevent the placement of or easy access to a TEP voice prosthesis in those who use this method of alaryngeal communication. The latter is especially problematic when devices leak and require urgent replacement. However, it should also be noted that if stenosis is persistent, it will offer continuing challenges for TEP voice prosthesis replacement. Finally, displacement of the TEP voice prosthesis into the distal airway in the setting of stomal stenosis may be life-threatening, as rapid retrieval of the device may prove exceedingly difficult in an emergency situation. Thus, careful consideration of the continued use of TEP voice may need to be re-evaluated in rare instances.

There are a multitude of techniques to manage stomal stenosis. These techniques range from serial dilation using tracheostomy or laryngectomy tubes to surgical enlargement of the stoma, a procedure known as stomaplasty. While the number of techniques described to surgically modify stenosis is beyond the scope of this chapter, it may vary in its complexity from simple resection and recreation of the tracheostoma to preparation and insertion of carefully designed flaps that radially enlarge the diameter of the tracheostoma.

Stomal retrusion, a problem where the tracheostoma sits deep in the anterior neck between the clavicular heads of the sternocleidomastoid (SCM) muscles, presents a challenge for the speech-language pathologist (SLP) and the patient when using baseplates for postlaryngectomy speech and airway heat and moisture exchange (HME) devices (Lewis, Chap. 8). Baseplates may not always sit flush with the skin and, as a consequence, may not completely cover the tracheostoma. If this occurs, leakage around the periphery of the baseplate may take place which may in turn lead to ineffective tracheoesophageal phonation. Surgically, this problem can be mitigated by releasing the clavicular insertions of the SCM muscles and anchoring the trachea to the periosteum of the sternoclavicular heads of the clavicles. This is most easily accomplished at the time of laryngectomy, although it also may be accomplished as a revision procedure if needed. When performed upfront, the patient will be able to utilize a baseplate and HME in the immediate postoperative period, facilitating familiarity and training with the devices for later use.

The Potential Impact of Postlaryngectomy Complications on Voice and Speech Rehabilitation

As outlined and described in prior sections of this chapter, complications associated with total laryngectomy are varied, and they can range in their severity. While some complications may be viewed as relatively minor, others may be life-threatening. Although many of the complications outlined are "medical" in their origin and will require requisite management, all hold the potential to influence voice and speech rehabilitation either from a procedural perspective or relative to the timing of active therapy. Complications, even once they have been managed and resolved, can result in short- and/or long-term changes that can influence how communication intervention is pursued, as well as scheduled follow-up and monitoring. Of the complications addressed previously, four of them have the greatest potential to influence voice and speech rehabilitation decisions. More specifically, PCF, strictures, infections, and tracheal stenosis will almost always require adjustments in alaryngeal speech rehabilitation. However, before specific details and examples are provided, several related concerns deserve explicit mention.

First, as noted within other chapters, the SLP plays an essential role in the team management of those undergoing treatment for laryngeal cancer. Relative to laryngeal cancer, this role ranges from providing service to those who are treated conservatively to those who undergo total laryngectomy either as a primary treatment option or as a salvage procedure. Regardless of the treatment method employed, the patient's history, presence of comorbidities, and/or associated functional limitations must be factored into all decision-making. Information on the surgery itself and type of closure may be quite valuable relative to complications such as a PCF or the presence of a stricture (Walton et al., 2018). Additionally, the course of recovery including the direct consideration of any and all complications that occur cannot be disregarded. This requires that the SLP carefully review the patient's medical chart, seek clarification from other professionals on the team, and acquire explicit information on the type, duration, and aspects of management for any complication experienced. The ability of the SLP to gather such information and weigh its potential impact on voice and speech outcomes is essential. Doing so will serve to inform the clinician about making decisions that may carry increased levels of risk.

Voice and speech rehabilitation at face value would appear to be a relatively simple process, one that does not in and of itself carry great risk to the patient. However, specific types of complications and understanding their cause(s) and the process of how they were managed may guide the clinical rehabilitation process. For example, individuals who are experiencing swallowing difficulties as a consequence of one or more complications may need to have voice and speech management deferred. Swallowing problems may also signal the clinician that the acquisition of intrinsic methods of alaryngeal communication (i.e., esophageal and tracheoesophageal speech) may not be appropriate to pursue at that time. In some instances, alternative methods of communication (Childes, Palmer, & Fried-Oken, Chap. 15) may be required until the problem is fully resolved. Thus, the trajectory of voice and speech rehabilitation will be individualized for all patients, but more importantly, it will be highly individualized for those who have experienced a complication following laryngectomy.

Pharyngeal Cutaneous Fistula. Complications such as a PCF hold the potential for challenges relative to alaryngeal voice and speech rehabilitation. While the literature suggests that the development of a PCF is more common in the early-period postlaryngectomy, at times it may occur well after the completion of surgery and discharge (White et al., 2012). Because the SLP may have the most regular contact with patients in the early time period following discharge, careful observation is necessary. Any indications of the development of a PCF will require immediate referral. While some authors have suggested that conservative methods of management may be quite successful should a PCF develop (White et al., 2012), the SLP must be extremely cautious and avoid any activity that could further traumatize the wound. While this concern might be most prominently noted in relation to TEP voice restoration and prosthesis usage, sizing, and fitting, fistulas may develop in those who have not undergone TEP. Thus, the SLP should carefully visualize patient anatomy at every opportunity and make appropriate referrals if anything suspicious is identified. The array of challenges associated with the occurrence of a PCF in the context of TEP voice restoration will be addressed in further detail in a later section of this chapter. However, a fistula that develops in any patient at any time postlaryngectomy will require medical attention and careful and regular observation.

Stricture. Regardless of the underlying cause, reported changes in swallowing function may influence voice and speech rehabilitation for those seeking to acquire esophageal speech or those who have undergone TEP voice restoration. Postlaryngectomy swallowing deficits have been recognized for many years (Duranceau, Jamieson, Hurwitz, Jones, & Postlethwait, 1976), and the recognition of these types of problems continues today. The presence of a stricture is of particular importance. Narrowing that occurs in the region of the pharyngoesophageal (PE) segment may restrict the ability of the patient who is seeking to acquire esophageal speech. A stricture may influence acquisition in two ways: first it may negatively influence to patient's ability to move air into the esophageal reservoir (insufflation) and one's ability to expel it during the alaryngeal speech process. Failure to acquire esophageal speech may also be influenced by other factors (Doyle & Eadie, 2005); however, a stricture does hold substantial potential to restrict or limit the acquisition of esophageal voicing.

While the presence of a stricture can influence learning of esophageal speech, it may also be detrimental to TEP voice rehabilitation. However, rather than having a direct influence on movement of air into and out of the esophageal reservoir as it occurs with esophageal speech, a stricture for the TEP speaker will most likely be observed in the quality of the voice signal. Given the rather large volumes of pulmonary air that can be moved through the voice prosthesis to continuously supply the esophageal reservoir during expiration, the clinician may detect a strained or effortful voice quality. This type of change in voice quality should not be confused with pharyngoesophageal hypertonicity or "spasm" that was identified initially by Singer and Blom (1980) and documented by others (Lundström, Hammarberg, Munck-Wikland, & Edsborg, 2008: Van Weissenbruch, Kunnen, Van Cauwenberge, Albers, & Sulter, 2000).

With spasm, TEP voicing will cease abruptly; in contrast, a stricture will permit continuous voicing, but the effort required to move air through a narrowed segment of tissue will be increased. Thus, changes in voice quality due to stricture will be a result of a relatively high volume of air being driven through a narrowed PE aperture. Alterations in TE voice quality may also be additionally influenced by prosthesis type, and in some instances, a change in prosthesis may result in some improvement in quality. However, a narrowing of the alaryngeal voicing source will always be subject to interactions between the aerodynamic driving source (the lungs) and the aperture through which that air must flow in order to generate TE voice. Depending on its severity and in addition to changes in vocal quality, a significant stricture may also influence the acoustic features of alaryngeal voice (Robbins, Fisher, Blom, & Singer, 1984), as well as potentially influencing the voicing source with a negative impact on speech intelligibility (Doyle, Danhauer, & Reed, 1988). Consequently, the SLP must understand the dynamic relationship between airflows and pressures and the vibration of tissues that form the new alaryngeal voicing source (Moon & Weinberg, 1987) and how this interaction may

influence speech communication on a more global basis. Because a stricture may create a unique set of challenges for those who have undergone TEP voice restoration, additional details that are specific to that alaryngeal rehabilitation method will be addressed in a later section.

Wound Infection and Healing Problems. It is well recognized that multiple communication options exist for those who undergo total laryngectomy. The clinician's awareness of complications such as those outlined in the present chapter will benefit clinical decision-making and planning. For example, if a significant neck infection has occurred or there has been tissue breakdown, the use of an intraoral artificial larynx should be recommended until the infection is fully treated and recovery has occurred. Similarly, the clinician must also carefully observe their patient in an effort to identify any problems that may be emerging and make appropriate referrals. A brief, yet careful inspection of suture lines, the potential presence of tissue edema, or a change in skin color or vascularity should be performed at the start of each clinical sessions. This would also include simple questioning of the patient relative to pain or discomfort, numbness, or changes in swallowing. If problems are identified, appropriate referrals and follow-up will be required, and adjustments in voice and speech rehabilitation will need to be addressed.

Tracheal Stenosis. As noted, tracheal stenosis can influence both breathing and speech rehabilitation. However, the most substantial rehabilitation challenge in situations where stenosis exists pertains to TEP voice restoration. Because of shrinkage of the trachea, the clinician's ability to actively and easily manipulate a TE puncture voice prosthesis for sizing and fitting will be challenging. If a laryngectomy tube is required to maintain the patency of the airway, cleaning and replacement of the prosthesis can also be problematic. This problem may be exacerbated in situations where the puncture site itself is located in position that is not easily accessed (e.g., a tract that is unusually angled within the trachea or is deeply recessed). In situations of stenosis where a prosthesis needs to be changed, extra care should be taken by the clinician doing the fitting to ensure that it is done in as atraumatic a manner as possible. While tracheal stenosis presents a variety of challenges to the SLP, this type of problem is also made more challenging in an airway that is relatively small in diameter.

Tracheoesophageal Voice Prosthesis (TEP) Complications

Since 1980, tracheoesophageal puncture and voice prosthesis placement have become the mainstay of postlaryngectomy voice restoration in many centers (Singer & Blom, 1980). As with many of the complications noted in this chapter, the potential occurrence of many of them is increased after radiation therapy (Starmer et al., 2009). While voice prosthesis device failure is anticipated, and regular replacement is required, problems with the puncture tract and site itself are variable and present unique challenges to the surgeon and SLP. Following total laryngectomy, the tracheoesophageal wall thins, and the diameter of the tract may enlarge, which can then lead to leakage around or accidental dislodgement of the voice prosthesis (Jiang, Kearney, & Damrose, 2016). An understanding of this process and the potential need for regular resizing of the tract and potentially altering the type of voice prosthesis are important in minimizing potential complications. Thus, it is essential that the clinician have comprehensive knowledge of both clinician procedures associated with TEP voice restoration, as well as the variety of products that are commercially available for use (Graville et al., Chap. 11; Knott, Chap. 12).

Enlargement of the puncture tract with subsequent leakage of saliva around the voice prosthesis increases the risk of aspiration pneumonia threefold (Hutcheson, Lewin, Sturgis, & Risser, 2011). An enlarging puncture site is a problem that can be difficult to manage. While about 80% of patients can be managed with conservative techniques, such as increasing the diameter of the voice prosthesis

(see Knott, Chap. 12), almost 20% will require surgical intervention. However, it is important to note that most patients will require multiple strategies and attempts to resolve the issue successfully (Hutcheson, Lewin, Sturgis, Kapadia, & Risser, 2011). Enlargement of the diameter of the tract appears to be a function of tissue dynamics over time, rather than a result associated with the initial size of the prosthesis placed; in other words, the problem can occur even when using the smallest diameter devices available (Naunheim et al., 2016).

Office-based conservative strategies to resolve leakage around a voice prosthesis are numerous and bely the refractory nature of the problem. These approaches include decreasing the length or increasing the diameter of the device, inclusion of anterior or posterior collars, temporary removal of the device and downsizing of the tract around a small catheter for future resizing, cautery of the tract, placement of a purse-string suture, or injection with a filler to decrease the diameter of the tract. But, regardless of the strategy pursued to remedy the problem, it is essential to acknowledge that if leakage exists, until the problem is resolved, it will necessitate the use of a thickened liquid diet to avoid aspiration. However, as noted, many patients will ultimately require multiple strategies to manage leakage around a voice prosthesis (Brown, Hilgers, Irish, & Balm, 2003; Hutcheson, Lewin, Sturgis, Kapadia, et al., 2011; Hutcheson, Lewin, Sturgis, & Risser, 2011; Jacobs, Delaere, & Vander Poorten, 2008; Knott, Chap. 12; Shuaib, Hutcheson, Knott, Lewin, & Kupferman, 2012).

As noted by Knott (Chap. 12), the use of retention collars to customize the TEP voice prosthesis for the patient with the enlarged tract may be particularly helpful. Lewin et al. (2012) have demonstrated that placement of a single collar, whether tracheal or esophageal, could mitigate leakage around a prosthesis. Some patients may require the placement of devices with consideration of both collars. Collars can be made from 0.020-inch-thick reinforced medical-grade silicone sheeting (Bentec® Medical, Woodland, CA). The central opening for the prosthesis also can be readily created with a 3 mm skin biopsy punch (Acuderm®, Fort Lauderdale, FL).

When conservative options to address leakage are not effective, surgery may be required to definitively close the tracheoesophageal puncture site and the associated fistula tract. A number of techniques and strategies have been described in the literature. In some cases, it may be possible to ligate the tract using a suture (Geyer, Tan, Ismail-Koch, & Puxeddu, 2011). In the majority of cases, healthy non-irradiated tissue will need to be interposed between the esophagus and the trachea in order to seal the fistula. Local flaps, such as the SCM rotational flap, regional flaps such as the deltopectoral flap, or microvascular free flaps such as the radial forearm free flap have all been described with varying degrees of success in repairing an enlarged TEP site fistula (Balasubramanian, Iyer, & Thankappan, 2013; Jaiswal, Yadav, Shankhdhar, Gujjalanavar, & Puranik, 2015; Wreesmann, Smeele, Hilgers, & Lohuis, 2009).

Conclusions

Total laryngectomy is an important surgical procedure in the management of patients with laryngeal cancer. Surgeons and SLPs who elect to treat this unique group of patients need to understand how surgical complications will affect voice and speech rehabilitation decisions and ultimately influence functional outcomes. With the increasing use of chemoradiotherapy as initial treatment, salvage laryngectomy has become increasingly common and with it increased rates of almost every complication, particularly that of pharyngocutaneous fistula. Many of these surgical complications have a direct impact on functional outcomes and, therefore, a patient's quality of life. To achieve the best outcomes for our patients, mitigation of postoperative complications is imperative, and that can only be accomplished through a broad understanding of the potential strategies and therapies available to both the surgeon and the SLP. Finally, careful and regular monitoring of those who undergo total laryngectomy may facilitate the earliest possible identification of complications that may develop in the outpatient population.

References

Balasubramanian, D., Iyer, S., & Thankappan, K. (2013). Tracheoesophageal puncture site closure with single perforator-based deltopectoral flap. *Head & Neck, 35,* E60–E63.

Basheeth, N., O'Leary, G., & Sheahan, P. (2014). Pharyngocutaneous fistula after salvage laryngectomy: Impact of interval between radiotherapy and surgery, and performance of bilateral neck dissection. *Head & Neck, 36,* 580–584.

Brown, D. H., Hilgers, F. J. M., Irish, J. C., & Balm, A. J. M. (2003). Postlaryngectomy voice rehabilitation: State of the art at the millennium. *World Journal of Surgery, 27,* 824–831.

Delaney, S. W., Shi, H., Shokrani, A., & Sinha, U. K. (2017). Management of chyle leak after head and neck surgery: Review of current treatment strategies. *International Journal of Otolaryngology, 2017,* 1–12.

Dowthwaite, S. A., Penhearow, J., Szeto, C., Nichols, A., Franklin, J., Fung, K., & Yoo, J. (2012). Postlaryngectomy pharyngocutaneous fistula: Determining the risk of preoperative tracheostomy and primary tracheoesophageal puncture. *Journal of Otolaryngology Head and Neck Surgery, 41,* 169–175.

Doyle, P. C. (1994). *Foundations of voice and speech rehabilitation following laryngeal cancer.* San Diego, CA: Singular Publishing Group.

Doyle, P. C., Danhauer, J. L., & Reed, C. G. (1988). Listeners' perceptions of consonants produced by esophageal and tracheoesophageal talkers. *Journal of Speech and Hearing Disorders, 53*(4), 400–407.

Doyle, P. C., & Eadie, T. L. (2005). Pharyngoesophageal segment function: A review and reconsideration. In P. C. Doyle & R. L. Keith (Eds.), *Contemporary considerations in the treatment and rehabilitation of head and neck cancer: Voice, speech, and swallowing* (pp. 521–544). Austin, TX: Pro-Ed.

Duranceau, A., Jamieson, G., Hurwitz, A. L., Jones, R. S., & Postlethwait, R. W. (1976). Alteration in esophageal motility after laryngectomy. *American Journal of Surgery, 131*(1), 30–35.

Emerick, K. S., Tomycz, L., Bradford, C. R., Lyden, T. H., Chepeha, D. B., Wolf, G. T., & Teknos, T. N. (2009). Primary versus secondary tracheoesophageal puncture in salvage total laryngectomy following chemoradiation. *Otolaryngology Head and Neck Surgery, 140,* 386–390.

Ganly, I., Patel, S., Matsuo, J., Singh, B., Kraus, D., Boyle, J., … Shah, J. (2005). Postoperative complications of salvage total laryngectomy. *Cancer, 103*(10), 2073–2081.

Geyer, M., Tan, N., Ismail-Koch, H., & Puxeddu, R. (2011). A simple closure technique for reversal of tracheoesophageal puncture. *American Journal of Otolaryngology, 32,* 627–630.

Gil, Z., Gupta, A., Kummer, B., Cordeiro, P. G., Kraus, D. H., Shah, J. P., & Patel, S. G. (2009). The role of pectoralis major muscle flap in salvage total laryngectomy. *Archives of Otolaryngology Head and Neck Surgery, 135,* 1019–1023.

Hall, F. T., O'Brien, C. J., Clifford, A. R., McNeil, E. B., Bron, L., & Jackson, M. A. (2003). Clinical outcome following total laryngectomy for cancer. *ANZ Journal of Surgery, 73*(5), 300–305.

Hasan, Z., Dwivedi, R. C., Gunaratne, D. A., Virk, S. A., Palme, C. E., & Riffat, F. (2017). Systematic review and meta-analysis of the complications of salvage total laryngectomy. *European Journal of Surgical Oncology, 43,* 42–51.

Hoffman, H. T., Porter, K., Karnell, L. H., Cooper, J. S., Weber, R. S., Langer, C. J., … Robinson, R. A. (2006). Laryngeal cancer in the United States: Changes in demographics, patterns of care, and survival. *Laryngoscope, 116*(Pt 2 Suppl 111), 1–13.

Hutcheson, K. A., Lewin, J. S., Sturgis, E. M., Kapadia, A., & Risser, J. (2011). Enlarged tracheoesophageal puncture after total laryngectomy: A systematic review and meta-analysis. *Head & Neck, 33,* 20–30.

Hutcheson, K. A., Lewin, J. S., Sturgis, E. M., & Risser, J. (2011). Outcomes and adverse events of enlarged tracheoesophageal puncture after total laryngectomy. *Laryngoscope, 121,* 1455–1461.

Jacobs, K., Delaere, P. R., & Vander Poorten, V. L. (2008). Submucosal purse-string suture as a treatment of leakage around the indwelling voice prosthesis. *Head & Neck, 30,* 485–491.

Jaiswal, D., Yadav, P., Shankhdhar, V. K., Gujjalanavar, R. S., & Puranik, P. (2015). Tracheoesophageal puncture site closure with sternocleidomastoid musculocutaneous transposition flap. *Indian Journal of Plastic Surgery, 48,* 278–282.

Jiang, N., Kearney, A., & Damrose, E. J. (2016). Tracheoesophageal fistula length decreases over time. *European Archives of Oto-Rhino-Laryngology, 27,* 1819–1824.

Lansaat, L., van der Noort, V., Bernard, S. E., Eerenstein, S. E., Plaat, B. E., Langeveld, T. A., … van den Brekel, M. W. (2018). Predictive factors for pharyngocutaneous fistulization after total laryngectomy: A Dutch Head and Neck Society audit. *European Archives of Oto-Rhino-Laryngology, 275,* 783–794.

Lewin, J. S., Hutcheson, K. A., Barringer, D. A., Croegaert, L. E., Lisec, A., & Chambers, M. S. (2012). Customization of the voice prosthesis to prevent leakage from the enlarged tracheoesophageal puncture: Results of a prospective trial. *Laryngoscope, 122,* 1767–1772.

Lundström, E., Hammarberg, B., Munck-Wikland, E., & Edsborg, N. (2008). The pharyngoesophageal segment in laryngectomees—videoradiographic, acoustic, and voice quality perceptual data. *Logopedics Phoniatrics Vocology, 33*(3), 115–125.

Maddox, P. T., & Davies, L. (2012). Trends in total laryngectomy in the era of organ preservation: A population-based study. *Otolaryngology Head and Neck Surgery, 147,* 85–90.

Mattioli, F., Bettini, M., Molteni, G., Piccinini, A., Valoriani, F., Gabriele, S., & Presutti, L. (2015). Analysis of risk factors for pharyngocutaneous fistula after total laryngectomy with particular focus on nutritional status. *Acta Otorhinolaryngologica Italica, 35,* 243–248.

Moon, J. B., & Weinberg, B. (1987). Aerodynamic and myoelastic contributions to tracheoesophageal voice production. *Journal of Speech, Language, and Hearing Research, 30*(3), 387–395.

Naunheim, M. R., Remenschneider, A. K., Scangas, G. A., Bunting, G. W., & Deschler, D. G. (2016). The effect of initial tracheoesophageal voice prosthesis size on postoperative complications and voice outcomes. *Annals of Otology, Rhinology, and Laryngology, 125,* 478–484.

Patel, U. A., Moore, B. A., Wax, M., Rosenthal, E., Sweeny, L., Militsakh, O. N., … Richmon, J. D. (2013). Impact of pharyngeal closure technique on fistula after salvage laryngectomy. *JAMA Otolaryngology Head and Neck Surgery, 139,* 1156–1162.

Robbins, J., Fisher, H. B., Blom, E. D., & Singer, M. I. (1984). Selected acoustic features of tracheoesophageal, esophageal, and laryngeal speech. *Archives of Otolaryngology, 110*(10), 670–672.

Rosko, A. J., Birkeland, A. C., Bellile, E., Kovatch, K. J., Miller, A. L., Jaffe, C. C., … Spector, M. E. (2018). Hypothyroidism and wound healing after salvage laryngectomy. *Annals of Surgical Oncology, 25,* 1288–1295.

Shuaib, S. W., Hutcheson, K. A., Knott, J. K., Lewin, J. S., & Kupferman, M. E. (2012). Minimally invasive approach for the management of the leaking tracheoesophageal puncture. *Laryngoscope, 122,* 590–594.

Singer, M. I., & Blom, E. D. (1980). An endoscopic technique for restoration of voice after laryngectomy. *Annals of Otology, Rhinology, and Laryngology, 89,* 529–533.

Starmer, H. M., Ishman, S. L., Flint, P. W., Bhatti, N. I., Richmon, J., Koch, W., … Gourin, C. G. (2009). Complications that affect postlaryngectomy voice restoration: Primary surgery vs salvage surgery. *Archives of Otolaryngology Head and Neck Surgery, 135,* 1165–1169.

Sweeny, L., Golden, J. B., White, H. N., Magnuson, J. S., Carroll, W. R., & Rosenthal, E. L. (2012). Incidence and outcomes of stricture formation postlaryngectomy. *Otolaryngology Head and Neck Surgery, 146,* 395–402.

Van Weissenbruch, R., Kunnen, M., Van Cauwenberge, P. B., Albers, F. W., & Sulter, A. M. (2000). Cineradiography of the pharyngoesophageal segment in postlaryngectomy patients. *Annals of Otology, Rhinology & Laryngology, 109*(3), 311–319.

Walton, B., Vellucci, J., Patel, P. B., Jennings, K., McCammon, S., & Underbrink, M. P. (2018). Postlaryngectomy stricture and pharyngocutaneous fistula: Review of techniques in primary pharyngeal reconstruction in laryngectomy. *Clinical Otolaryngology, 43*(1), 109–116.

White, H. N., Golden, B., Sweeny, L., Carroll, W. R., Magnuson, J. S., & Rosenthal, E. L. (2012). Assessment and incidence of salivary leak following laryngectomy. *Laryngoscope, 122*(8), 1796–1799.

Wreesmann, V. B., Smeele, L. E., Hilgers, F. J., & Lohuis, P. J. (2009). Closure of tracheoesophageal fistula with prefabricated revascularized bilaminar radial forearm free flap. *Head & Neck, 31*, 838–842.

Wulff, N. B., Kristensen, C. A., Andersen, E., Charabi, B., Sorensen, C. H., & Homoe, P. (2015). Risk factors for postoperative complications after total laryngectomy following radiotherapy or chemoradiation: A 10-year retrospective longitudinal study in Eastern Denmark. *Clinical Otolaryngology, 40*, 662–671.

Yu, D. X., Ma, X. X., Zhang, X. M., Wang, Q., & Li, C. F. (2010). Morphological features and clinical feasibility of thoracic duct: Detection with nonenhanced magnetic resonance imaging at 3.0 T. *Magnetic Resonance Imaging, 32*, 94–100.

Human Papillomavirus-Related Head and Neck Cancer

Julie A. Theurer

Once a disease that was overwhelmingly characterized by advanced age and extensive use of tobacco and alcohol, the demographic landscape of head and neck cancer (HNCa) now exhibits greater diversity (Ang et al., 2010; Gillison et al., 2008). To a large extent, this diversification is driven by the dramatic increase in virally mediated cancers. Although the incidence of HNCa has declined for various anatomic subsites (i.e., larynx and hypopharynx), this downward epidemiological trend is masked by unbridled growth in the number of oropharyngeal squamous cell cancers (OPSCCs), resulting in increasing incidence of HNCa as a whole (Chaturvedi et al., 2011). It is now well-established that the increasing incidence of OPSCCs is fueled by a dramatic rise in human papillomavirus (HPV)-related cancers (Chaturvedi et al., 2013).

Understanding the impact of HPV-related disease on HNCa incidence is necessary in order for clinicians to more fully grasp the magnitude of disease burden within the HNCa population. Perhaps of greater importance clinically, however, is the need for practitioners to be well-versed in the clinical features, demographic variables, and prognostic ramifications associated with this virally mediated malignancy, one that is now recognized as a distinct disease entity by the field of head and neck oncology. In fact, within the past year, the way in which head and neck oncologists stage OPSCC changed dramatically for patients with HPV-related disease (Lydiatt et al., 2017).

Cancer staging, or the process of describing one's disease severity, is influenced by the magnitude of the primary tumor (T), the extent of disease spread beyond the primary site to lymph nodes (N), and the presence of metastasis (M; American Joint Committee on Cancer [AJCC], 2017a). Early-stage disease (Stage I) represents the least advanced cancers and portends a better prognosis. Late-stage cancers (Stage II–Stage IV) are more advanced, but many are still amenable to treatment. Built on survival outcomes predominantly from patients with HPV-negative disease, early-stage HNCa has been associated with small primary tumors (T1 or >2 cm) and no lymph node involvement (N0). Since most patients with HPV-related disease have lymph node involvement at time of diagnosis, they have historically been staged, and thus treated, as late-stage cancers. In the context of a vastly improved prognosis for HPV-related OPSCC, the HNCa staging system has been revised to incorporate HPV status. Nearly overnight, the staging of a patient with HPV-related T1N2b cancer of the oropharynx (small primary tumor and multiple ipsilateral neck nodes) has been downgraded from a diagnosis of Stage IVa to Stage I cancer (Horne et al., 2016). For the patient, the shift in

J. A. Theurer (✉)
School of Communication Sciences and Disorders, Western University, London, ON, Canada
e-mail: jtheurer@uwo.ca

© Springer Nature Switzerland AG 2019
P. C. Doyle (ed.), *Clinical Care and Rehabilitation in Head and Neck Cancer*,
https://doi.org/10.1007/978-3-030-04702-3_4

staging may be purely semantic; however, this alteration in staging holds great significance in guiding HN oncologists' treatment selection. The oncology treatment guidelines compiled by the National Comprehensive Cancer Network (NCCN) are upheld as the standard of care for the treatment of human malignancies (NCCN, n.d.). The underlying principle of the NCCN Guidelines® ensures that risk of death, disease progression, and/or malignant recurrence is managed optimally, while minimizing the likelihood of treatment-related side effects, allowing patients to "live better lives" (NCCN, n.d.). The NCCN® endorses that early-stage HNCa (i.e., Stage I) can be treated using less toxic and perhaps even single-modality, treatment regimens. In contrast, it is recommended that later-stage disease (i.e., Stage IV), which is associated with greater disease risks, be treated aggressively using multiple modalities (i.e., surgery plus radiation, often in combination with chemotherapy) (Adelstein et al., 2017). Thus, in light of the recently proposed changes to staging of HPV-related disease, a new treatment paradigm for HPV-related OPSCC is set to unfold rapidly.

For several decades, health-care professionals have been strongly encouraged to engage in evidence-based practice, knitting together the best evidence from research with clinical experience, as well as patients' needs and desires, to provide high-quality, patient-centered care. More recently, patients have been empowered to become more educated consumers of health-care services, particularly in relation to cancer care (Palma, 2017). Within this context, clinicians must be increasingly well-versed in the critical differences associated with HPV-related HNCa. Provision of accurate information regarding disease progression and prognosis, and the disease- and treatment-related effects on function and quality of life to this patient population, hinges on one's understanding of the underlying disease. Thus, the purpose of this chapter seeks to provide information regarding the role of human papillomavirus (HPV) in carcinogenesis, its impact on the clinical and morphological features of HNCa, and its implications for patient functioning and quality of life.

Human Papillomavirus

What Is Human Papillomavirus?

Human papillomavirus (HPV) comprises a group of DNA viruses that demonstrate affinity for human epithelial tissue. Exposure to HPV, and subsequently, the development of an HPV infection, commonly occurs through sexual contact. As such, predominant areas of infection include the squamous epithelial tissue of anogenital regions (e.g., cervix, anus, penis, vulva/vagina), the upper aerodigestive tract (UADT; e.g., mouth, pharynx), and esophagus (Khariwala, Moore, Malloy, Gosselin, & Smith, 2015). Greater than 200 HPV types have been identified, with approximately one quarter of these viruses being amenable to transmission through direct sexual contact. Within the group of HPV viruses, subtypes known to induce benign epithelial cell proliferation are characterized as "low-risk" viruses (e.g., HPV-6, HPV-11). Genital warts and upper airway papillomas, or recurrent respiratory papillomatosis (RRP), are attributable to these low-risk HPV strains (Brown, Schroeder, Bryan, et al., 1999; Giuliano et al., 2008). In contrast, "high-risk" virus subtypes (e.g., HPV-16, HPV-18, HPV-31, HPV-33, HPV-35) are associated with malignant transformation of human epithelia. Approximately one dozen of these oncogenic (i.e., cancer-causing) subtypes have been identified and implicated in cancers of the cervix, vagina, vulva, anal canal, and penis, as well as the oropharynx (Jemal et al., 2013).

Who Is Affected by HPV?

Following exposure, HPV DNA "is localized to tumor cell nuclei, is frequently integrated, and is transcriptionally active" (Fakhry & Gillison, 2006, p. 2606). HPV targets and infects keratinocytes within the deepest layer of stratified epithelium; basal keratinocytes in the cervix, other anogenital regions, and the UADT demonstrate particular susceptibility to infection. Valuable information related to HPV infection prevalence has been gathered and reported through the National Health and Nutrition Examination Survey (NHANES) in the United States (Centers for Disease Control and Prevention, National Center for Health Statistics, n.d.). This series of prospective population-based surveys has established that HPV infections are common. In adults (men and women) aged 18–69, overall prevalence of genital infection (including cervical and other anogenital regions) by any HPV type is 43% (McQuillan, Kruszon-Moran, Markowitz, Unger, & Paulose-Ram, 2017). Sex differences in the prevalence of genital HPV infections appear to be negligible, with infection rates of 40–43% in women (Hariri et al., 2011; McQuillan et al., 2017) and approximately 45% in men (McQuillan et al., 2017). Similarly, high-risk HPV types have been identified in 20–29% of women (Hariri et al., 2011; McQuillan et al., 2017) and in 25% of men (McQuillan et al., 2017).

Oral HPV prevalence is considerably lower (i.e., five- to tenfold lower) than rates of genital infection (Gillison, Broutian, et al., 2012; Pickard, Xiao, Broutian, He, & Gillison, 2012). Systematic review of early literature report oral HPV prevalence as approximately 5%, with HPV-16 prevalence of 1.3% (Kreimer et al., 2010). More recent data reveal (1) an overall prevalence of oral HPV infection of 6.9–7.3% (Gillison, Broutian, et al., 2012; McQuillan et al., 2017), (2) higher prevalence in men (11.5%) vs. women (3.3%; McQuillan et al., 2017), and (3) higher prevalence of high-risk vs. low-risk HPV types, with HPV-16 as the most prevalent type (1.0%; Gillison, Broutian, et al., 2012; McQuillan et al., 2017).

The dynamics of HPV infection are not yet well understood. Although HPV infections are relatively common, the majority resolve over time without progression to malignant disease (Hariri et al., 2011). However, reported median times to clearance of infection vary widely, ranging from 3–6 M (D'Souza, Wentz, et al., 2016; Kreimer, Campbell, et al., 2013) to 18–24 M (Louvanto et al., 2013; Rautava et al., 2012). While the majority of oral HPV infections will not result in malignant growth

(Chung & Gillison, 2009), persistent infection by an oncogenic subtype of HPV is a significant predictor of HPV-related tumorigenesis (Hariri et al., 2011; Jemal et al., 2013). In a cohort of individuals with OPSCC, 34.8% demonstrated presence of HPV in pre-diagnosis plasma collection compared to a seropositivity rate of less than 1% in individuals who did not develop a subsequent OPSCC (Kreimer, Johansson, et al., 2013). Further, most individuals experience HPV infection in their second, third, or fourth decades (Kliewer et al., 2009); individuals with HPV-related OPSCCs tend to be diagnosed in their fifth, sixth, or seventh decades (Ang et al., 2010), implicating a protracted time to onset of malignancy in the order of years to decades. Although a precise timeline of progression to malignancy is unknown, it is becoming increasingly clear that HPV infection precedes histopathologic progression to tumorigenesis.

HPV infection prevalence has been shown to be associated with several behavioral variables including sexual practices, tobacco and marijuana use, as well as with demographic characteristics such as age and sex (Gillison, Broutian, et al., 2012; Pickard et al., 2012). Increasing numbers of recent and lifetime oral sex partners, as well as vaginal- and any-sex partners, confer a significant risk for oral HPV infection (Gillison, Broutian, et al., 2012; Pickard et al., 2012). Infection is uncommon among the sexually inexperienced, with an eightfold increase in prevalence documented among individuals reporting sexual experience (Gillison, Broutian, et al., 2012; Pickard et al., 2012). Prevalence is also higher in individuals who report young age at sexual debut, that is, engaging in sex at or prior to age 18 years (Gillison, Broutian, et al., 2012). Data also suggest that infection prevalence increases in a dose-response fashion relative to number of sexual partners and current smoking intensity. Prevalence as high as 20% is identified in those reporting greater than 20 lifetime partners or more than 20 cigarettes smoked per day (Gillison, Broutian, et al., 2012).

Two peaks in infection prevalence have been reported with respect to age: one (7.3%) in individuals aged 30–34 years old and a second higher peak (11.4%) in 60–64-year-olds (Gillison, Broutian, et al., 2012). The second peak may not be fully explained by sexual behavior practices. Rather, it is likely that a combination of factors can explain this phenomenon such as the reactivation of latent infections or an age-related loss of immunity, among others (Garcia-Piñeres et al., 2006). Men tend to exhibit prevalence of oral infection 2–3 times higher than women for all HPV types, including HPV-16 (Gillison, Broutian, et al., 2012; McQuillan et al., 2017). For example, NHANES data reveals an oncogenic HPV prevalence rate of 6.6–6.8% in men compared to 1.2–1.5% in women (Chaturvedi et al., 2015; McQuillan et al., 2017). This prevalence rate contrasts to that associated with anogenital infections which demonstrate similar rates among men and women (McQuillan et al., 2017) and, in some studies, a female preponderance (Khariwala et al., 2015). The increased risk of oral HPV infection in men is likely related to engagement in several high-risk behaviors. For example, men tend to report younger age at sexual debut and significantly higher average numbers of lifetime sex partners (Chaturvedi et al., 2015; D'Souza, Wentz, et al., 2016). Moreover, there is a more robust per-partner increase in oral HPV prevalence in men, with 3–4 times greater risk of oral infection in men compared to women with increasing numbers of partners (Chaturvedi et al., 2015). Other behavioral risk factors for oral HPV infection that occur more frequently in men than women include heavier consumption of alcohol, tobacco, and marijuana (Chaturvedi et al., 2015; D'Souza, Wentz, et al., 2016).

In summary, although oral HPV infection is less prevalent than genital infections, several variables are known to affect one's risk of oral infection. Increasing numbers of sexual partners and younger age at sexual debut are associated with increased prevalence of oral HPV infection. Similarly, age, sex, and high-risk consumptive behaviors also affect rates of oral HPV infection. Importantly, however, the majority of oral HPV infections are unlikely to progress to malignant disease.

How Does HPV Cause Cancer?

The development of human cancers (i.e., carcinogenesis) is attributed to alterations in genes responsible for cell proliferation and/or tumor suppression. Two predominant human tumor suppressor genes include p53 (or TP53), which is located on the 17th chromosome, and Rb, which is located on the 13th chromosome. The proteins associated with the p53 and Rb genes regulate cell cycle arrest (i.e., act as "stop signals" for cell division) and promote DNA repair (Feller, Wood, Khammissa, & Lemmer, 2010; Gillison, 2004). When altered, tumor suppressor genes lose their ability to inhibit cell proliferation. As with most human cancers, carcinogenesis in HNCa is associated with alteration of the p53 and pRb pathways (Gillison, 2004). While disruption of these pathways is responsible for HNCa, the *manner* in which the pathways are altered differs in many complex ways between HPV-related (HPV-positive) and HPV-unrelated (HPV-negative) disease (Fakhry & Gillison, 2006), thus resulting in distinct genetic profiles. Two key molecular differences include inactivation versus mutation of the p53 gene and overexpression versus deletion of the p16 gene in response to altered Rb gene function in HPV-related and HPV-unrelated disease, respectively.[1]

First, HPV-negative disease is accompanied by significantly greater numbers of genetic mutations compared to HPV-positive disease (Agrawal et al., 2011; Stransky et al., 2011). For example, p53 mutations are present in approximately 80% of HPV-negative tumors but are virtually nonexistent in HPV-positive tumors (Agrawal et al., 2011; Stransky et al., 2011). In HPV-negative disease, p53 mutations induced by carcinogen (tobacco and alcohol) exposure lead to decreased expression of genes involved in cell senescence and tumor suppression (Fakhry & Gillison, 2006; Gillison, 2004). However, in HPV-positive tumors, the p53 pathway is not mutated, but

---

[1]For a comprehensive review of the numerous and complex molecular drivers of carcinogenesis that differentiate HPV-positive versus HPV-negative disease, see Gillison (2004).

rather inactivated due to the action of the HPV16 E6 gene. The oncoprotein associated with the E6 gene of HPV targets and destroys the p53 protein, resulting in loss of tumor suppressor function and, ultimately, tumor growth (Fakhry & Gillison, 2006; Gillison, 2004; Kumar et al., 2008). Presumably, the degradation and elimination of p53 that accompanies a viral HPV infection substitutes for the p53 mutations observed in HPV-negative disease (Gillison et al., 2000). A second key difference relates to the variable expression of p16 protein between the two distinct tumor types. That is, in HPV-negative disease, the p16 tumor suppressor gene is inactivated through various genetic and non-genetic modifications and results in lost or diminished expression of the p16 protein (El-Naggar & Westra, 2012; Gillison, 2004). In contrast, HPV-positive cancers demonstrate upregulation of the p16 gene (in response to the action of the HPV16 E7 oncogene), leading to increased expression of the p16 protein (El-Naggar & Westra, 2012; Gillison, 2004). The differential expression of p16 between these two cancers holds great clinical significance: the determination of an oropharyngeal tumor's HPV status often capitalizes on the selective overexpression of p16 in HPV-related disease. While the presence of HPV DNA in the tumor specimen clearly delineates an "HPV-positive cancer," the detection of p16 is often used as a surrogate marker of HPV positivity (Gillison, 2004). Similarly, tumor specimens that do not demonstrate high p16 positivity (and demonstrate other mutation markers) are delineated as "HPV-negative cancer."

p16 Positivity Versus HPV Positivity: What's the Difference?

The presence of high-risk HPV within OPSCCs has become known as an important biomarker of improved clinical outcome (El-Naggar & Westra, 2012). As such, the identification of tumor HPV status has become the standard of care for cancers of the oropharynx because it allows for more accurate patient counselling regarding disease prognosis and may allow for patient inclusion in clinical trials aimed specifically at this virally mediated disease (Finnigan Jr. & Sikora, 2014). Of greater clinical significance, the distinction of HPV-positive disease now impacts an individual's cancer staging (AJCC, 2017b), which can influence decision-making concerning appropriate approaches to disease management.

Methods used commonly to determine HPV status rely on detection of HPV genetic material (in situ hybridization (ISH) or polymerase chain reaction (PCR)-based methods) or the expression of p16 protein (immunohistochemistry (IHC); Seiwert, 2013). The processes by which the presence/integration of viral DNA within tumor cells is obtained (e.g., PCR-based methods or ISH) are technically demanding and expensive, requiring sophisticated laboratory facilities and experienced personnel (El-Naggar & Westra, 2012). In contrast, detecting p16 expression though IHC is relatively simple, inexpensive, and feasible at most health-care centers (El-Naggar & Westra, 2012). Given that p16 overexpression is detectable through more economical and timely methods than HPV DNA, p16 positivity is often used as a surrogate marker for HPV positivity. However, p16 positivity is not a perfect substitute for HPV positivity. Although numerous studies have reported a high correlation between p16 overexpression and HPV DNA detection, the possibility exists that reliance on p16 IHC can overestimate the number of cancers related to HPV. Because elevated p16 expression is not exclusively associated with HPV-driven tumorigenesis, reliance on this diagnostic methodology (rather than HPV DNA detection) is accompanied by an HPV false-positive rate (El-Naggar & Westra, 2012) of 3.8–7.3% (Schlecht et al., 2011; Thavaraj et al., 2011). From a pathologic perspective, the gold standard method for identifying HPV status of OPSCCs would include a combination of p16 IHC with PCR detection of HPV DNA in fresh frozen tumor, although this procedure is not likely feasible in all pathology laboratories (Thavaraj et al., 2011).

Previously, when HPV status did not effectively alter one's disease staging or treatment, the need for clarity between p16 positivity and HPV positivity was less pressing. However, given that the process of disease staging now incorporates the tumor's HPV status, the less-than-perfect correlation between p16 overexpression and HPV positivity deserves acknowledgement. If a "gold standard" approach of combining p16 IHC with PCR detection of HPV DNA remains untenable for the majority of treatment centers, then other tumor morphologic features can corroborate the diagnosis of an HPV-related tumor. For example, the cellular structure of HPV-positive OPSCC tends to be poorly differentiated, nonkeratinizing, and basaloid in appearance compared to the well-differentiated and keratinizing morphology of HPV-negative tumors (Gillison et al., 2000). Taken together, the presence of these morphologic characteristics and the tumor's p16 status will provide a strong indication of the tumor's propensity to be HPV-driven.

Human Papillomavirus-Related Cancers

Historical Perspective of HPV-Related Cancers

From historical reports noting the preponderance of cervical cancers in sex workers compared to those of the general public, and to celibate nuns (Gasparini & Panatto, 2009; zur Hausen, 2009), it has long been hypothesized that a sexually transmitted disease was linked to these genital cancers. Identification of the specific etiologic virus was the subject of substantial study in the 1970s and 1980s (zur Hausen, 1976, 1982). Ultimately, the co-occurrence of benign HPV-related disease (i.e., genital warts or *condylomata acuminata*) with anogenital cancers implicated the papillomavirus as playing a role in the genesis of malignant disease as well. The groundbreaking work of Harold zur Hausen and colleagues provided great insight into the etiologic role of HPV in cervical cancers, establishing the association of low-risk HPV types with benign growths and high-risk HPV types with malignant disease (zur Hausen, 1976, 1982). Evidence of HPV viral DNA in HNCa emerged nearly simultaneously with the discovery of its involvement in anogenital cancers (Syrjänen, Syrjänen, Lamberg, & Pyrhönen, 1983). Similar to the findings in anogenital lesions, benign respiratory papillomas and oral condylomata acuminata were found to contain low-risk HPV-6 and HPV-11, whereas high-risk HPV-16 was identified in UADT cancers (Gissman, Diehl, Schultz-Coulon, & zur Hausen, 1982; Loning et al., 1985). By the beginning of the twenty-first century, the burden of evidence pointed convincingly to an etiologic role of high-risk HPV in a subset of HNCa (Gillison et al., 2000), particularly in tumors of the oropharynx (Niedobitek et al., 1990; Snijders et al., 1992). Current population-based data implicate an HPV infection in causing approximately 600,000 cancers annually, in addition to benign diseases (Arbyn et al., 2012; de Martel, Plummer, Vignat, & Franceschi, 2017). Although the incidence of cervical cancer has been decreasing (likely attributable to HPV vaccination campaigns and standardized screening protocols), the incidences of other HPV-related malignancies continue to rise, including that of OPSCC (Arbyn et al., 2012).

Epidemiology of HPV-Related HNCa

Within two decades, incidence rates for HPV-positive OPSCC in the United States have increased by 225%, while rates of HPV-negative OPSCC have declined by 50% (Chaturvedi et al., 2011). This aggressive shift in incidence is also well-established by Canadian and European data (Habbous et al., 2017; Mehanna, Beech, & Nicholson, 2013; Nichols et al., 2013). HPV has effectively replaced tobacco and alcohol as the major cause of OPSCC in North America and Western Europe (Mehanna et al., 2013), although prevalence of HPV-positive OPSCC remains lower than HPV-negative OPSCC in Eastern Europe and Asia (Mehanna et al., 2016). In the United Kingdom, increasing incidence has been reported for both HPV-positive and HPV-negative OPSCC, as well as malignancies of other head and neck sites (Schache et al., 2016). In spite of these modest population-specific influences on incidence of the disease, the global incidence of HPV-positive OPSCC is expected to surpass the number of cervical cancers in the immediate future (i.e., by the year 2020; Chaturvedi et al., 2011). The HPV-positive OPSCC epidemic will affect health-care provision at numerous levels. First, the volume of patients requiring treatment at tertiary care cancer centers will increase dramatically, placing strain on a system that is already under-resourced (Mundi et al., 2018; van Harten et al., 2015). In turn, greater numbers of individuals will now be exposed to toxic cancer treatments that lead to many serious side effects, placing further strain on the health-care system as patients seek treatment for the physiologic and/or psychosocial sequelae of HNCa treatment.

It is hypothesized that the shifting prevalence of OPSCC by etiology (increasing HPV-positive, decreasing HPV-negative) is driven largely by behavioral variables, which may also account for some of the population-based diversity seen in incidence rates of HNCa. With respect to HPV-negative disease, decreases in incidence may be reflective of documented population-level declines in smoking (Centers for Disease Control and Prevention [CDC], 2011), perhaps the result of successful public health campaigns (Barnoya & Glantz, 2004; Davis, Farrelly, Duke, Kelly, & Willett, 2012). In geographic locations reporting increasing overall incidence of HPV-negative disease, it is hypothesized that rising alcohol consumption rates may be one contributing factor (Schache et al., 2016). Given that HPV infection is known to precede the development of HPV-positive cancers and that exposure to HPV occurs through sexual contact, it follows logically that the increasing incidence of HPV-mediated OPSCCs is attributable to contemporary sexual practices that expose individuals to this sexually transmitted virus. Indeed, increasing rates of sexually transmitted diseases (STDs) have been reported since the 1970s (Health Protection Agency, 2011; Kliewer et al., 2009). The epidemiologic impact of this virally mediated cancer translates into increased diversity in both the demographic and clinical characteristics ascribed to HNCa.

Clinicodemographic Characteristics of HPV-Related HNCa

Historically, a "typical" patient with HNCa would be approximately 60–70 years of age, with a long-standing history of tobacco use, alcohol consumption, and/or betel nut chewing, and would most commonly present with a cancer in the oral cavity, larynx, or hypopharynx. However, increasing numbers of oropharynx cancers are occurring in patients who are appreciably younger, who have more limited or no direct tobacco exposure, and who report a higher number of lifetime sexual partners (Chaturvedi et al., 2011; D'Souza et al., 2007; Gillison, D'Souza, et al., 2008). HPV-related OPSCC tends to occur in patients who are significantly younger (Ang et al., 2010; Chaturvedi et al., 2011; Franceschi, Munoz, Bosch, Snijders, & Walboomers, 1996; Gillison, D'Souza, et al., 2008; Posner et al., 2011), have smaller primary tumor volumes (clinically staged T1/T2 tumors), and have higher performance status scores (Posner et al., 2011). That is, patients with HPV-positive tumors tend to be in good general health and are highly capable of taking care of themselves and engaging in activities of daily living. HPV-positive OPSCCs also occur more frequently in individuals who are male (Chaturvedi et al., 2011; D'Souza et al., 2007), Caucasian (Chaturvedi et al., 2011; Gillison, D'Souza, et al., 2008; Ramer et al., 2016), and of higher socioeconomic status (Gillison, D'Souza, et al., 2008; O'Sullivan et al., 2013).

At time of diagnosis, patients with HPV-positive disease are less likely to present with the constellation of symptoms that typify traditional (i.e., HPV-negative) OPSCC – dysphagia (i.e., difficulty swallowing), odynophagia (i.e., painful swallowing), sore throat, bleeding, and weight loss – symptoms related directly to larger tumor volume and invasiveness of disease at the primary oropharyngeal tumor site (McIlwain, Sood, Nguyen, & Day, 2014; Truong Lam, O'Sullivan, Gullane, & Hui Huang, 2016). In contrast, individuals with HPV-positive OSPCC tend to present with complaints of a neck mass more often than those with HPV-negative OPSCC (McIlwain et al., 2014; Truong Lam et al., 2016), reflective of the higher incidence of lymph node metastasis in HPV-related disease (Paz, Cook, Odom-Maryon, Xie, & Wilczynski, 1997). Consequently, patients with HPV-negative OPSCC tend to have disease staging that reflects larger tumor volumes and lower nodal involvement, while smaller tumor volume and higher nodal involvement associate with HPV-positive OPSCC. Differences in clinicodemographic characteristics are corroborated by distinctive tumor morphology: HPV-positive tumors are predominantly nonkeratinizing, poorly differentiated, and basaloid in appearance, while HPV-negative tumors are more often characterized as moderate to well differentiated and keratinizing (Gillison et al., 2000). Interestingly, these morphologic features correlate with diverging outcomes in HPV-positive versus HPV-negative disease. In HPV-negative disease, poorly differentiated tumors tend to be more aggressive and portend poorer outcomes (Chen et al., 2017). In HPV-positive disease, tumors are commonly poorly differentiated, and yet this morphology is not associated with similar negative outcomes in this patient population (Gillison et al., 2000). These distinct disease- and patient-related characteristics underscore the etiologic uniqueness of these two disease entities.

HPV is present in approximately 20–25% of all diagnoses of HNCa (Gillison et al., 2000; Schwartz et al., 1998) but is identified in >70% of all cancers in the oropharynx (Chaturvedi et al., 2011), demonstrating that HPV-related tumors are more often localized to the oropharynx relative to other HNCa subsites. Within the oropharynx, HPV-positive tumors arise predominantly from the palatine or lingual tonsils compared to other sites, such as the soft palate or pharyngeal walls (Gillison et al., 2000; O'Sullivan et al., 2013; Schwartz et al., 1998). Hypotheses regarding the apparent preferential infection and malignant transformation noted at the oropharyngeal sites of tonsillar tissue espouse a synergy between basal cell access and persistence of infection. In both the palatine and lingual tonsils, basal keratinocytes (which host HPV infections) are exposed naturally, providing the virus unimpeded access to these targeted cells. In contrast, basal keratinocytes in anogenital regions are protected by overlying stratified squamous epithelium, requiring microabrasions to provide viral access (Khariwala et al., 2015). Deep invaginations on the surface of the tonsillar tissue, and the crypts surrounding the palatine tonsils, may further favor capture and entrapment of HPV, enhancing access and prolonging exposure time (Chu, Genden, Posner, & Sikora, 2013; Khariwala et al., 2015). It is also theorized that high-risk HPV-16 demonstrates a genetic propensity to survive in oral keratinocytes, which could enhance infection persistence (Khariwala et al., 2015). Similar to the predominance of high-risk HPV-16 in oral HPV infections, HPV-16 is identified in >90% of oropharynx tumors that stain positive for HPV (D'Souza et al., 2007; Gillison et al., 2000; Kreimer, Clifford, Boyle, & Franceschi, 2005; Schache et al., 2016).

The pathologic role of HPV in other HNCas (i.e., outside of the oropharynx) is unclear. While the virus may be detectable in non-oropharynx tumor specimens, it should not be assumed to have an oncogenic role in these cancers. In one US study, 13.4% of 404 laryngeal cancers contained detectable HPV DNA; however, further analysis (i.e., detection of transcriptionally active E6/E7 oncoproteins) revealed only 1.7% of these cancers were definitively caused by HPV (Taberna et al., 2016). Similar data exist for oral cavity cancers with one study reporting p16 overexpression in 30% of samples but with true HPV positivity confirmed in merely 1% of tumors (Zafereo et al., 2016). Interestingly, analysis of patient- and disease-related variables between individuals with HPV-positive and HPV-negative tumors at non-oropharynx HN subsites fails to reveal group differences relative to patient demographics, carcinogen exposures, clinical characteristics, or survival outcomes (Zafereo et al., 2016). Routine testing for HPV positivity in HNCas outside the oropharynx is not common practice. Furthermore, without evidence of a clear etiologic role, in addition to the lack of distinguishing clinicodemographic characteristics between HPV-related and HPV-unrelated disease outside of the oropharynx, one cannot assume its presence portends good outcome as it does in OPSCC (Lee et al., 2012).

That is, the well-described etiologic role of HPV in OPSCC, in concert with its prognostic impact, necessitates all oropharyngeal tumors be delineated based on HPV status. However, a similar practice is not warranted for other head and neck sites, for which the implications of HPV positivity are not clear.

Current data indicate that HPV-related OPSCCs are 3–5 times more common in men than women (Chaturvedi et al., 2011; D'Souza et al., 2007). In fact, the epidemic-like increase in the incidence of HPV-related OPSCCs has been carried by a dramatic increase within the male population, with only modest increasing incidence noted among women (Chaturvedi et al., 2015). Differential susceptibility and immune system reaction to HPV infection may help explain the male predilection for HPV-related OPSCC (Rettig, Keiss, & Fakhry, 2015). For example, men performing oral sex on women are likely at increased risk for oral acquisition due to the higher prevalence of genital HPV infection in women and an increased viral load maintained in the cervical mucosa (Rettig et al., 2015). Compared to women, and to men who have sex with men, heterosexual men exhibit the highest rates of oral HPV infection. Recent data demonstrate that median clearance times of HPV infection is also significantly longer in men compared to women (D'Souza, Wentz, et al., 2016; Kreimer, Pierce Campbell, et al., 2013), a finding that may account for some of the propensity for greater numbers of HPV-related OPSCCs in men vs. women.

Armed with understanding that oral HPV infection precedes development of HPV-related OPSCC, the risk factors for oral HPV infection are also risk factors for these virally mediated cancers. Sexual behaviors are among the strongest predictors for tumor HPV status (D'Souza et al., 2007; Gillison, D'Souza, et al., 2008; Schwartz et al., 1998). Lifetime number of vaginal and oral sex partners, engagement in casual sex, young age at first intercourse, infrequent use of barriers, history of oral HPV infection, and history of genital warts have been identified as risk factors for HPV-positive OPSCC

(D'Souza et al., 2007; Gillison, D'Souza, et al., 2008). These associations solidify the relationship between OPSCC and the sexually transmitted HPV virus but also imply that the development of HPV-related disease through casual, nonsexual contact (i.e., hugging, closed-mouth kissing) would be atypical (Gillison, Broutian, et al., 2012).

Although HPV in the context of sexual behavior is well-documented, varying relationships have been identified between HPV status and tobacco and alcohol use. Most early reports indicated that HPV-positive disease occurred more frequently in individuals who reported less tobacco exposure and lower alcohol consumption rates (Ang et al., 2010; Gillison et al., 2000; Lindel, Beer, Laissue, Greiner, & Aebersold, 2001); however, more recent NHANES data demonstrate that the incidence of HPV-positive OPSCC in 2007–2008 was significantly higher among "ever" (63%) vs. "never" smokers (37%) in the United States (Chaturvedi, D'Souza, Gillison, & Katki, 2016). Marijuana use has been implicated as an independent predictor of HPV positivity in several retrospective studies (D'Souza et al., 2007; Gillison, D'Souza, et al., 2008). Understanding the clinical and demographic factors that are associated with increased risk for HPV-related OPSCC can greatly aid public health efforts aimed at preventing the underlying sexually transmitted infection and, ultimately, the occurrence of HPV-positive cancers. Yet, for patients already diagnosed with HPV-positive OPSCC, the implications of this viral disease-related to survival- and treatment-related outcomes are of paramount significance.

Impact of HPV Status in HNCa

Disease-Related Outcomes

The greatest significance of knowing a patient's tumor HPV status is that a diagnosis of HPV-related OPSCC portends excellent outcomes compared to those associated with HPV-unrelated disease. Tumor HPV status is a significant predictor of survival in loco-regionally advanced OPSCC (Ang et al., 2010; Fakhry et al., 2008;

Lassen et al., 2009; Posner et al., 2011), with 3-year overall survival (OS) of 82–93% in patients with HPV-positive OPSCC versus 57% in those with HPV-negative OPSCC (Ang et al., 2010; Lin et al., 2013). HPV positivity confers an approximate 50% reduction in all-cause (overall) mortality (O'Rorke et al., 2012) and a 72% reduction in both HNCa- and OPSCC-specific mortality compared to HPV-negative disease (O'Rorke et al., 2012). Progression-free survival (PFS) is also significantly better in patients with HPV-related OPSCC (73.7%) compared to HPV-unrelated OPSCC (43.4%; Ang et al., 2010), with local (94% vs. 80%) and regional control (95% vs. 82%) favoring HPV-related OPSCC at 3 years (O'Sullivan et al., 2013). Improved survival has been linked to multiple variables including younger age at the time of diagnosis, higher performance status, less advanced clinical tumor (T) stage, no tobacco use, fewer comorbidities, increased responsiveness of tumor to chemoradiotherapy (CRT), and lower risk of second primary tumors (Ang et al., 2010; Lin et al., 2013; Lindel et al., 2001).

The potent survival benefit associated with HPV-related disease is maintained across a variety of primary treatment approaches including transoral robotic surgery (TORS) and chemoradiotherapy (CRT) (Salazar et al., 2014). Examination of numerous clinical treatment trials reveals that radiotherapy (RT) administered with a concurrent chemotherapeutic agent results in similar overall survival (2-year OS: 92%; 3-year OS: 88%; 5-year OS: 78%) regardless of whether cisplatin, cetuximab, or carboplatin was the chemotherapy agent employed (Nien et al., 2016). The survival benefit of HPV positivity also holds for median survival following salvage treatment of persistent or recurrent disease (Argiris et al., 2014; Fakhry et al., 2014; Huang et al., 2015). The enhanced prognosis associated with HPV positivity is even evident in patient cohorts with the poorest survival outcomes in HPV-negative disease. For example, HPV-negative disease in African Americans portends worse survival compared to Caucasian individuals with similar disease; however, the impact of race is nullified in HPV-related OPSCC with

similar overall survival across racial groups (Worsham et al., 2013). Although the majority of individuals with HPV-positive OPSCC experience impressive disease response to treatment and outstanding survival outcomes, a small cohort of patients exhibit highly aggressive cancers that are associated with a much poorer prognosis. It is of great interest to be able to identify these anomalous cases to guide appropriate management. The search continues for robust exposure variables and pathologic and radiologic features that might be useful in identifying and classifying this subset of tumors (Kaka et al., 2013). These cases, in which tumors tend to behave more like HPV-negative cancers, tend to be associated with more extensive smoking histories and the presence of greater numbers of genetic mutations (Chung & Gillison, 2009; Khwaia et al., 2016). It has been suggested that radiologic features of extracapsular spread (ECS) and matted/clustered lymph nodes may provide some indication of aggressive disease (Kaka et al., 2013; Spector et al., 2012). These features have been associated with poorer outcomes outside the oropharynx (Maxwell et al., 2013), but their prognostic utility relative to OPSCC, and HPV-positive vs. HPV-negative disease is unclear at present (Kaka et al., 2013; Kharytaniuk et al., 2016; Sinha, Lewis Jr., Piccirillo, Kallogieri, & Haughey, 2012; Spector et al., 2012). Others posit that gross tumor volume may be useful in predicting disease outcomes and suggest that nodal tumor volume may be more predictive of survival outcomes for HPV-positive disease than that of primary tumor volume (Davis et al., 2016; Kubicek et al., 2010).

Unlike the superior OS and PFS outcomes associated with HPV-related disease, the risk of distant metastasis (or distant spread of disease) is similar to HPV-negative OPSCC (Bledsoe et al., 2013). Although rates of distant disease control are high for both HPV-positive and HPV-negative OPSCC, they do not differ significantly at 90% vs. 86%, respectively (O'Sullivan et al., 2013). In contrast to HPV-negative OSPCC, distant metastases also tend to occur later and appear in numerous and unusual sites in HPV-related OPSCC (Huang et al.,

2012; Sinha et al., 2014; Trosman et al., 2015), leading to an increased risk of death between 5 and 10 years posttreatment (Lin et al., 2013). This unique natural history may require alternative surveillance strategies in those treated for HPV-negative tumors that are adept at identifying unusual sites of metastases over a protracted period of time (Trosman et al., 2015).

It is now well-established that the survival benefit conferred by HPV-related disease is moderated significantly by tobacco use. However, it is unlikely that tobacco exposure in this patient cohort contributes strongly to carcinogenesis; rather, it is plausible that smoking history alters the cancer's behavior and its response to treatment. While many patients with HPV-positive OPSCC are non-smokers or have fewer years of tobacco exposure (Gillison, Zhang, et al., 2012), those with a smoking history and those who are current smokers at time of diagnosis experience worse survival than those not currently smoking or without smoking history (Gillison, Zhang, et al., 2012; Hafkamp et al., 2008; Kumar et al., 2008; Maxwell et al., 2012). In all OPSCCs, regardless of p16 status of tumor and treatment type, tobacco use at diagnosis, and during therapy, directly increases the risk of disease recurrence and progression (at both local and distant sites) and ultimately death (Gillison, Zhang, et al., 2012; Maxwell et al., 2012). For each pack-year (py) of smoking, one's hazard ratio of death increases by 1.0% (Gillison, Zhang, et al., 2012). In early-stage HPV-related OPSCC, greater than 10-py smoking history reduces OS from 93% to 70%; for individuals with more advanced HPV-related OPSCC, greater than 10py reduces OS to 46% (Ang et al., 2010).

The significant interaction between HPV status and tobacco use has led to the categorization of three distinct OPSCC risk groups. Patients at low risk of death include those with early-stage HPV-positive OPSCC and <10 py smoking. Patients at intermediate risk of death include those with advanced-stage HPV-positive OPSCC and >10 py smoking or patients with early-stage HPV-negative disease and <10 py smoking. Patients at highest risk of death include those with advanced-stage HPV-negative OPSCC, with

or without >10 py smoking. Of great significance is that OS for patients with HPV-positive OPSCC in the intermediate-risk group mimics that of patients with HPV-unrelated OPSCC (Ang et al., 2010). For all patients with OPSCC, tumor HPV status and tobacco use (< vs. >10 yrs) are the two strongest predictors of OS and PFS (Ang et al., 2010). In fact, the impact of HPV status on outcome is now affecting the way in which OPSCC is staged.

The Changing "Stage"
Management of HNCa is dictated by the extent of disease (e.g., TNM staging) and patient-related factors (e.g., age, performance status, comorbidities), and to a lesser extent, by clinician and patient preferences. In the case of OPSCCs, advanced T-stage results and/or the presence of *any* nodal disease dramatically advances the stage classification of disease (Edge, Byrd, Compton, Fritz, Greene, & Trotti, 2010). Early-stage disease may be treated sufficiently with monotherapy, while advanced-stage disease requires multimodality treatment to achieve acceptable cure rates, as stipulated by NCCN Guidelines® (Adelstein et al., 2017). This paradigm has proved problematic for patients with HPV-related OPSCC, a disease marked by significant nodal disease at time of diagnosis, resulting in the majority of HPV-related OPSCCs being staged as advanced cancers. As such, the current standard of care for OPSCC involves the use of RT, typically with the addition of chemotherapy because of improved survival with multimodal therapy (Blanchard et al., 2011; Pignon et al., 2009). However, increasingly intense treatments come at a cost. More directly, the risk of acute and late treatment toxicities such as mucositis; xerostomia; fibrosis; dysphagia; oto-, neuro-, and nephron-toxicity; and osteoradionecrosis has been elevated to an unacceptable level (Brizel et al., 1998; Eisbruch et al., 2002; Machtay et al., 2008). Hence, the superior prognosis associated with HPV-related OPSCC is often overshadowed by the fact that our most potent treatments are being directed at an ever-younger, "healthier" patient cohort, who face

the very real possibility of severe and debilitating treatment side effects over a much longer period of survivorship than ever before.

Head and neck oncology is now espousing that HPV positivity does not simply modify one's cancer outcome; rather it drives one's outcome (Proceddu, 2016). As an initial step in fully recognizing this "new cancer," the field has advocated for a separate staging system for HPV-related OPSCC to allow for the development of a disease-specific management paradigm (Dahlstrom, Garden, William Jr., Lim, & Sturgis, 2016; Horne et al., 2016; O'Sullivan et al., 2016; Proceddu, 2016). Several compelling studies solidified the need for alternate staging for HPV-positive disease. Using adjusted hazard ratio analysis, O'Sullivan and colleagues proposed alterations to the staging system which ultimately downplay the impact of nodal tumor volume on one's cancer staging (O'Sullivan et al., 2016). Their meticulous retrospective analysis of survival data for greater than 2000 cases of OPSCC demonstrated that small primary tumors, despite the presence of ipsilateral neck lymph nodes (under 6 cm in size or N0-N2b; Edge et al., 2010), could still constitute early-stage (Stage 1) cancer. The recommendations from O'Sullivan et al. have been corroborated using a separate dataset (Horne et al., 2016), which has demonstrated that a risk-adapted staging structure will more accurately stratify patients with HPV-related disease. In response to the burden of evidence, the most recent AJCC cancer staging manual (8th edition), which came into effect in January 2018, incorporates tumor HPV status into the staging paradigm (AJCC, 2017b).

This one, albeit important, alteration to the management of HPV-related OPSCC represents but one step toward acknowledgment of the distinctiveness of this disease group. Treatment choices within the HN oncology team's armamentarium, however, continue to be derived from clinical trials that included all-comers with OPSCC, regardless of one's HPV status; yet at present, high-level evidence to support distinct treatment paradigms for HPV-positive OPSCC is lacking (Masterson et al., 2014). In response to the HPV-driven changes in the AJCC cancer staging system, randomized treatment trials should

no longer stratify participants based on HPV status. Rather, going forward, clinical trials should be designed to target either HPV-positive or HPV-negative disease exclusively (Proceddu, 2016). Currently, numerous clinical trials are aimed at de-escalation[2] of treatment for HPV-related disease in an attempt to decrease the burden of treatment-related toxicities while maintaining excellent survival rates (Masterson et al., 2014; O'Sullivan et al., 2013). These trials are examining the use of (i) less toxic biologic agents concurrent with radiation versus platinum-based chemotherapy, (ii) alternate timing and doses of chemotherapy and radiotherapy, and (iii) minimally invasive techniques, such as transoral surgical approaches (Masterson et al., 2014; Urban, Corry, & Rischin, 2014). As such, it is anticipated that the treatment landscape for HPV-related OPSCC will change dramatically over the next decade, reflecting the largest treatment paradigm shift for HNCa since the movement toward organ preservation techniques in the 1990s (Blanchard et al., 2011; Bourhis et al., 2006; Parsons et al., 2002; Pignon et al., 2009; VA Laryngeal Cancer Study Group, 1991).

In addition to the consideration of less toxic chemotherapy, reduced radiation doses, and primary surgical management, biotherapy is an emerging treatment alternative. Biological approaches, such as the use of antibody therapy or immunotherapy that modifies the immune system's response to HPV and treatment of virally mediated disease, are playing a larger role in treatment considerations (Ferris, Jaffee, & Ferrone, 2010; Masterson et al., 2014). Cetuximab and panitumumab, monoclonal antibodies (mAb) that target epidermal growth factor (EGFR), have been suggested as therapeutic alternatives to historically prominent platinum-based chemotherapy. Highly anticipated results from recently completed (or nearly completed) randomized controlled trials will reveal if targeted bioradia-

---

[2]The main premise of treatment de-escalation is that a reduction in treatment intensity is likely to be accompanied by a reduction in morbidity associated with standard treatment protocols. For a comprehensive review of recent and ongoing de-escalation trials, see Masterson et al. (2014).

tion (cetuximab/panitumumab + radiotherapy) reduces the burden of acute/late toxicity while also maintaining long-term survival (Masterson et al., 2014). Therapies aimed at improving an anti-HPV immune response hold promise to further enhance treatment outcomes in the future (Spanos et al., 2009). To establish best practice in HPV-positive OPSCC, there is a substantial need for randomized controlled trials that directly compare alternative therapies with standard care. The results of several such ongoing studies are highly anticipated over the next 5–10 years (Masterson et al., 2014). Alternatively, work is underway to test the hypothesis that for patients deemed "low risk," based on disease- and patient-related factors, radiation therapy alone may confer high rates of cure while avoiding toxicities associated with the addition of adjuvant chemotherapy (O'Sullivan et al., 2013).

Functional Outcomes and QOL

By and large, patients' posttreatment functioning is strongly dictated by the primary curative treatment techniques employed and the associated potential for complications. As such, the deficits in functional performance and QOL associated with CRT will be common among patients treated for OPSCC, regardless of HPV status. With disease localized to the oropharynx, treatment modalities aimed at the primary tumor bed (and to a lesser extent, nodal disease) can impact the essential role the oropharynx plays in breathing, speech, and swallowing. The myriad treatment-related anatomic and physiologic alterations that influence these UADT functions, as well as the systemic effects of chemotherapy (e.g., oto-, nephro-, and neurotoxicities), have received excellent coverage elsewhere in this text (see Kearney & Cavanagh, Chap. 20). However, even in the context of identical treatment paradigms, there is emerging evidence that patients with HPV-positive OPSCC may exhibit a unique posttreatment profile of higher functional status and superior QOL compared to patients with HPV-negative disease.

Similar to the HPV-associated survival benefit, early evidence suggests that HPV status confers functional benefit as well. For example, rates of dysphagia are similar immediately following CRT regardless of HPV status, but late severe dysphagia occurs more frequently in individuals with HPV-negative OPSCC (Bledsoe et al., 2013). Although the number of feeding tube placements during treatment is similar between patients with HPV-positive and HPV-negative disease (Bledsoe et al., 2013; Rodriguez et al., 2015), those with HPV-positive disease achieve feeding tube independence more quickly (Rodriguez et al., 2015) and are less likely to require oral diet restrictions 6 months posttreatment compared to those with HPV-negative OPSCC (Bledsoe et al., 2013; Naik et al., 2015). A portion of this functional benefit may be attributable to the fact that patients with HPV-negative disease are significantly older than those with HPV-positive OPSCC. While older patients often experience good disease outcomes following standard treatment protocols, they bear a much greater toxicity burden than younger patients, with severe acute and late toxicities occurring in up to 40% and 60% of patients, respectively (Hanasoge et al., 2016).

Prospective evaluation of patient QOL has revealed an interesting profile in those with HPV-positive disease. As might be expected, this younger, "healthier" patient cohort demonstrates superior health-related QOL ratings pretreatment and at 6 and 12 months posttreatment, regardless of treatment modality (Maxwell et al., 2014). Interestingly, the impact of HPV status on QOL is more robust than the effect of treatment modality; QOL ratings are more similar between those treated with primary surgery and primary CRT than between patients with HPV-positive and HPV-negative disease (Maxwell et al., 2014). While it is becoming increasingly understood that those with HPV-related disease begin treatment with superior QOL and also generally attain similar ratings by 12 M posttreatment, it is intriguing to note that they experience a much sharper decline in QOL during/immediately posttreatment compared to those with HPV-negative disease (Ringash et al., 2016; Sharma et al., 2012; Xiao et al., 2017). Further study is needed to elucidate the underpinnings of this pattern of early, significant decline in QOL, which is unique to the HPV-positive OPSCC population.

To date, much of what is known about the relationship between HPV status and functional/QOL outcomes is based on retrospective analyses of data gathered using disparate measurement tools. In order to better appreciate the impact of HPV status on outcome, prospective, objective, and subjective evaluation of functional outcomes and QOL is required. In the meantime, the clinical reality facing HN oncologists is that there is a "burgeoning population" of cancer survivors due, in part, to the increasing incidence of HPV-positive OPSCC (Ringash, 2015). While we await results of HPV-specific treatment trials, at present, our standard treatment of OPSCC continues to lead to high rates of acute and late treatment-related toxicities (Brizel et al., 1998; Eisbruch et al., 2002; Machtay et al., 2008). The search for less toxic, yet equally curative, treatment options is being fueled by patients' post-treatment functioning and QOL. However, early attempts to de-intensify treatment toxicity through the use of alternate biologic agents in place of cytotoxic cisplatinum chemotherapy have demonstrated disappointing results in respect to reducing treatment-induced functional impairments and improving QOL (Ringash et al., 2016; Samuels et al., 2016). Perhaps more promising are the results of minimally invasive transoral surgery techniques and, more specifically, the elimination of adjuvant therapies when using this treatment approach. For those who undergo TORS for early-stage disease, early evidence has demonstrated superior swallowing outcomes with lower rates of enteral feeding for patients with HPV-positive disease (Dowthwaite et al., 2012). The improved swallowing function associated with TORS may also reflect the avoidance of adjuvant primary tumor bed irradiation and/or chemotherapy in these patients (Dowthwaite et al., 2012; Sinha, Pipkorn, Thorstad, Gay, & Haughey, 2016). However, with the proposal of any alternative or emerging treatment paradigm comes the need for empirical data to support not only its efficacy and effectiveness with respect to cancer control but also the demand for data in relation to functional outcomes and QOL. Unfortunately, trials comparing standard care to de-escalation approaches have been mired by many methodological flaws. For example, an early evaluation of radiation therapy plus cetuximab versus cisplatin-based CRT in OPSCC did not incorporate stratification of patients by HPV status (Bonner et al., 2006). This trial demonstrated that radiation therapy plus cetuximab is less toxic than traditional CRT and is likely most effective for tumors of the oropharynx compared to other head and neck sites (Bonner et al., 2006). However, without stratifying by HPV status (and therefore not controlling for the survival benefits associated with HPV positivity), the true impact of the de-escalation strategy on outcomes was obfuscated. Similarly, early studies comparing TORS with the standard of care (i.e., CRT) have used subjective reports of swallowing-related function and QOL to document superior outcomes (Hutcheson, Holsinger, Kupferman, & Lewin, 2015). However, in the absence of concomitant objective outcome measurement, the full impact of TORS vs. CRT on physiologic functioning is unknown. Careful attention is now being paid to the comparison of novel treatments to the current standard of care and to the launching of clinical trials specifically for the population of patients with HPV-related OPSCC.

Patient Education and Counselling

Due in part to the well-documented survival benefit conferred by HPV status, routine testing of all oropharyngeal biopsy specimens for HPV status has recently become a recommended clinical practice (Lacchetti et al., 2013) and is recognized generally as standard of care. This practice standard provides the first opportunity to engage in education and counselling of patients relative to the etiologic role of HPV and for discussion of the implications of HPV status on prognosis and treatment. Clinicians agree that discussing the survival benefit associated with an HPV-positive diagnosis is highly relevant, but beyond sharing this prognostic information, there is less agreement about what should be discussed with patients (Dodd,

Marlow, & Waller, 2016). For example, some clinicians have expressed hesitancy at discussing the viral etiology at length because it is no longer a modifiable risk factor, and that focus on the sexually transmitted nature may exacerbate self-blame and guilt (Dodd et al., 2016). Some hesitancy may also be attributed to a clinician's feeling of unpreparedness to lead such a discussion. Indeed, the etiologic association between sexually transmitted infections (STIs) and cancer that has long been acknowledged by colleagues in gynecologic oncology has caught HN oncologists by surprise in the last decade (Fakhry & D'Souza, 2013).

Head and neck oncologists are now tasked with educating patients about the etiology of this virally mediated cancer, as well as delving into issues of counselling on complex social and behavioral questions outside the realm of oncology (Fakhry & D'Souza, 2013). Compared to their colleagues in gynecologic oncology, it is unlikely that head and neck oncologists have received substantial training in discussing the diagnosis of a STI. A patient-centered approach to education and counselling will most likely put both clinicians and patients at greater ease. Provision of accurate, factual information about HPV, its transmission, the duration of infection, its progression to cancer, and its impact on prognosis and treatment planning is recommended as standard practice (Fakhry & D'Souza, 2013; Finnigan Jr. & Sikora, 2014). Further, expression of one's willingness/openness to address any associated psychosocial impact, especially when requested by the patient (Dodd et al., 2016), will minimize negative psychosocial outcomes and ensure optimal health promotion (Chu et al., 2013). From the cervical cancer literature, it may be possible to extrapolate that the emotional impacts of an HPV-related cancer can led to feelings of self-blame, guilt, depression, confusion, lowered self-esteem, and grappling with relationship and intimacy issues (Chu et al., 2013). Regardless of the etiology of HNCa, this clinical patient population is at risk for experiencing anxiety and distress at time of diagnosis (Bornbaum et al., 2012; De Boer, McCormick, Pruyn, Ryckman, & van den Borne, 1999;

Kugaya et al., 2000). Learning the origin of one's disease may indeed exacerbate (or alleviate) some of the distress associated with a HNCa diagnosis. Through counselling, the oncology team should be prepared to identify patients who would benefit from additional psychosocial care (Bornbaum, Doyle, Skarakis-Doyle, & Theurer, 2013; Chu et al., 2013).

Due to the breadth of concerns related to HNCa treatment, there is always room for improvement in meeting the informational needs of patients with HPV-positive OPSCC. Health-care professionals agree that patients should be informed that their cancer is related to HPV, yet we cannot assume that when this information is conveyed, the etiologic role of HPV is understood completely. In one prospective survey study, most patients (66%) were able to identify that their cancer is/was related to HPV (Milbury, Rosenthal, El-Naggar, & Badr, 2013), but only one third of patients understood that HPV was the cause of their cancer (Milbury et al., 2013), highlighting that the link between the virus and its role in OPSCC is not always clear. In a similar qualitative study, approximately 75% of patients recalled hearing that their tumor was HPV-positive, but only 50% recalled being told that HPV caused their cancer (D'Souza, Zhang, et al., 2016). Patients will undoubtedly react differently to the news that HPV caused their tumor; thus, our provision of information should be tailored to meet each patient's specific needs. When patients' informational needs are met, it can diminish anxiety and distress (Chu et al., 2013; Fakhry & D'Souza, 2013). Overall, the majority of patients report being satisfied with the amount of information that was provided surrounding their HPV-related cancer; however, others indicate that some of their questions went unasked or unanswered (Baxi et al., 2013). To assist in patient education and counselling, Fakhry and D'Souza included a pamphlet within their 2013 publication that answers common patient questions. Thus, health-care providers can supply this pamphlet to patients as a print-based adjunct to their verbal discussion of HPV-related issues.

Public Health Implications

The clinician's role in education about HPV-related issues should not be limited solely to the HN oncology clinic or to patients already diagnosed with this viral cancer. Our advanced understanding of the etiologic role of oral HPV infection in the vast majority of OPSCCs behooves our involvement in raising public awareness about the sinister consequences associated with this STI. Public health education should be aimed at promoting awareness about methods for safeguarding against sexually transmitted infections such as abstinence, as well as safe vaginal and oral sexual practices. Since the sexual revolution in 1960s and 1970s, age at first intercourse has been decreasing, with a consequent increase in lifetime number of sexual partners (Chu et al., 2013). With this trend in sexual activity, it is likely that the incidence of HPV-related OPSCC will continue to increase dramatically for the foreseeable future. Targeting the spread of HPV infection will be a powerful primary preventative strategy toward stemming the HPV-positive OPSCC epidemic. Historically, the public health focus on HPV-related diseases has been limited and aimed (nearly) exclusively at preventing genital warts and cervical cancer (and, to a lesser extent, other anogenital cancers); however, the relationship between HPV and HNCa continues to be shrouded by confusion, ignorance, and misinformation (Chu et al., 2013). The forecasted worldwide incidence shift in HPV-related cancers from a predominance of cervical cancer to HNCa (Chaturvedi et al., 2011) is already emerging, well ahead of predicted timelines (Canadian Cancer Society, 2016a), with dramatic decreases in the incidence of cervical cancers and a concomitant and steady increase in HPV-related OPSCC. Consequently, we are witnessing the transformation of a previously female-predominant disease to one afflicting larger numbers of men. This trend presents a new and wide-ranging challenge. Men tend to demonstrate significantly poorer understanding of HPV compared to women (Chu et al., 2013), likely reflecting both women's familiarity with the causal relationship between HPV and cervical cancer and the novelty of the causal relationship between HPV and HNCa. Similar misperceptions exist the level of health policy, as evidenced by the discrepancy in vaccination recommendations for boys (Canadian Cancer Society, 2016a).

The dramatic decrease in incidence in cervical cancer can be attributed to two important public health prevention strategies: vaccination and screening for premalignant disease. Several HPV vaccines are currently available, and their use is recommended for females between 9 and 26 years of age (as of 2006) and approved (though not recommended) for use in males between 9 and 21 years of age (as of 2009; Ward, Mehta, & Moore, 2016). The most commonly used vaccines include Cervarix®, a bivalent vaccine targeting HPV-16 and HPV-18, and Gardasil®, a quadrivalent vaccine that targets HPV-6, HPV-11, HPV-16, and HPV-18, the only vaccine approved for both use in both males and females (D'Souza & Dempsey, 2011). To be maximally effective, vaccines must be administered prior to sexual debut (Hildesheim & Herrero, 2007); they *are not* effective as a therapeutic if an infection is already present (Hildesheim et al., 2007). Use of these vaccines is recommended to prevent, at minimum, anogenital HPV infections and related dysplasias. By logical extension, these vaccines will also be valuable in preventing oropharyngeal HPV infection (Gillison, Chaturvedi, & Lowy, 2008). Although prevention of OPSCC is not an indication yet recognized by the Federal Drug Administration (FDA), most health-care providers endorse that this will likely be realized in time (Ward et al., 2016). Due to the recent acknowledgement of the etiologic role of HPV in HNCa, pharmaceutical clinical trials designed to evaluate the effect of vaccination on oral HPV infection are lacking, and, hence, vaccine efficacy against oral HPV infection remains unknown (Gillison, Broutian, et al., 2012; Gooi, Chan, & Fakhry, 2016). Retrospective studies examining the incidence of HPV-related OPSCC before and after the introduction of these vaccines will be needed to help elucidate the true utility of vaccination against this disease (D'Souza & Dempsey, 2011).

Unfortunately, the success of vaccination as a primary prevention strategy to stem the spread of HPV infection has been mitigated somewhat by poor population uptake. For example, although HPV vaccines were licensed in United States and recommended in 2006, only 38% of girls and 14% of boys receive the full, three-dose course (Stokley et al., 2014). However, in spite of poor rates of coverage, the data reveal an impact on HPV infections in the United States, with substantial reductions in infection prevalence in young women (Markowitz et al., 2016). Preliminary data from a randomized vaccine trial indicate a significantly lower prevalence of cervical and oral HPV infection in females treated with a bivalent vaccine versus placebo (Herrero et al., 2013); however, it remains premature to predict the definitive impact of HPV vaccination initiatives on the incidence of HPV-related OPSCC (Gooi et al., 2016; Ward et al., 2016). Furthermore, while the vaccines appear to have similar capability to prevent HPV infection in men and women, it is unknown if they will be equally effective at preventing virally mediated cancers that occur in both sexes (Gillison, Chaturvedi, et al., 2008). The full impact of HPV vaccination on HPV-related OPSCC will be slow to emerge due to the slowly emerging recommendation for use in boys, as well as the lack of adherence to vaccination recommendations (even in females), a finding that has been well-documented (Kamerow, 2016).

As a secondary prevention effort against HPV-related malignancies, cervical cancer screening has been available for decades. The use of the Papanicolaou (Pap) test, a sensitive tool for identification and treatment of precancerous cervical conditions, has led to significant reductions in cervical cancer incidence and mortality worldwide (American Cancer Society, 2016; Canadian Cancer Society, 2016b; Hoffman et al., 2003; Sasieni, Castanon, & Cuzick, 2009; Vicus et al., 2014). Without an identifiable premalignant state, no screening mechanism exists for the identification of oropharyngeal lesions (Fakhry, Rosenthal, Clark, & Gillison, 2011). Support is mounting for the use of HPV detection testing for all HPV-related malignancies, even in lieu of the Pap test for cervical cancers (Canadian Cancer Society, 2016b). Although HPV-16 seropositivity (i.e., blood serum positive for HPV pathogens) is associated with risk of OPSCC, the sensitivity, specificity, and predictive value in using this marker to detect an HPV-positive OPSCC are currently unknown (Kreimer, Johansson, et al., 2013). Finally, the utility of HPV-16 seropositivity as a definitive risk marker is further hampered by the lack of a clear understanding of the timeline from seropositivity (i.e., infection) to the development of OPSCC (Kreimer, Johansson, et al., 2013).

Conclusion

Globally, HPV contributes to more than 600,000 cases of cancer each year. In the face of decreasing incidence of cervical cancers, the increasing burden of disease associated with oropharyngeal cancers is particularly distressing. In order to engage in evidence-based, patient-centered care, it is prudent that clinicians be prepared to provide accurate information about HPV-positive OPSCC while acknowledging that which we do not yet know. With respect to HPV, this infection is common among adults and is usually cleared by the immune system with ease. Vaccines have been developed to prevent infection by common HPV strains, including those responsible for benign warts (HPV-6, HPV-11) and those associated with the majority of HPV-related cancers (HPV-16, HPV-18). The true impact of these vaccines on the incidence of oral HPV infection and OPSCC is not yet known. HPV-positive OPSCC is a unique disease that differs from HPV-negative OPSCC in many important ways, including the mechanism of carcinogenesis, clinical and pathological presentation of tumors, patient demographics, and prognosis.

The search for a better understanding of the natural history of oral HPV infection, including delineating the time line between infection and malignancy and under what conditions infections persist, will help establish the utility of premalignant disease screening as a cancer prevention strategy. Further exploration of the mechanism underlying the improved response of HPV-related OPSCC to current treatments will also pave the way for treatment de-intensification and adoption of HPV-specific therapy approaches. Increased attention to standardized measurement of functional outcomes and QOL will underscore if true differences exist in patient functioning and QOL with respect to HPV status. Finally, rigorous and long-term follow-up of patients with HPV-related disease will enable us to predict what the future holds for survivors of a disease that often strikes in the prime of one's life.

References

Adelstein, D., Gillison, M. L., Pfister, D. G., Spencer, S., Adkins, D., Brizel, D. M., et al. (2017). NCCN guidelines insights: Head and neck cancers, version 2.2017. *Journal of the National Comprehensive Cancer Network: JNCCN, 15*(6), 761–770.

Agrawal, N., Frederick, M. J., Pickering, C. R., Bettegowda, C., Chang, K., Li, R. J., et al. (2011). Exome sequencing of head and neck squamous cell carcinomas reveals inactivating mutations in NOTCH1. *Science, 333*(6046), 1154–1157.

American Cancer Society. (2016). *Cancer facts & figures 2016*. Atlanta, GA: American Cancer Society; 2016. Retrieved October 6, 2017 from https://www.cancer.org/content/dam/cancer-org/research/cancer-facts-and-statistics/annual-cancer-facts-and-figures/2016/cancer-facts-and-figures-2016.pdf

American Joint Committee on Cancer. (2017a). Retrieved September 25, 2017, from https://cancerstaging.org/references-tools/Pages/What-is-Cancer-Staging.aspx

American Joint Committee on Cancer. (2017b). Retrieved August 14, 2017, from https://cancerstaging.org/About/news/Pages/Implementation-of-AJCC-8th-Edition-Cancer-Staging-System.aspx

Ang, K. K., Harris, J., Wheeler, R., Weber, R., Rosenthal, D. I., Nguyen-Tan, P. F., et al. (2010). Human papillomavirus and survival of patients with oropharyngeal cancer. *New England Journal of Medicine, 363*, 24–35.

Arbyn, M., de Sanjose, S., Saraiya, M., Sideri, M., Palefsky, J., Lacey, C., et al. (2012). EUROGIN 2011 roadmap on prevention and treatment of HPV-related disease. *International Journal of Cancer, 131*(9), 1969–1982.

Argiris, A., Li, S., Ghebremichael, M., Egloff, A. M., Wang, L., Forastiere, A. A., et al. (2014). Prognostic significance of human papillomavirus in recurrent or metastatic head and neck cancer: An analysis of eastern cooperative oncology group trials. *Annals of Oncology, 25*, 1210–1216.

Barnoya, J., & Glantz, S. (2004). Association of the California tobacco control program with declines in lung cancer incidence. *Cancer Causes & Control, 15*(7), 689–695.

Baxi, S. S., Shuman, A. G., Corner, G. W., Shuk, E., Sherman, E. J., Elkin, E. B., et al. (2013). Sharing a diagnosis of HPV-related head and neck cancer: The emotions, the confusion and what patients want to know. *Head & Neck, 35*(11), 1534–1541.

Blanchard, P., Baujat, B., Holostenco, V., Bourredjem, A., Baey, C., Bourhis, J., et al. (2011). Meta-analysis of chemotherapy in head and neck cancer (MACH-NC): A comprehensive analysis by tumour site. *Radiotherapy & Oncology, 100*(1), 33–40.

Bledsoe, T. J., Noble, A. R., Hunter, G. K., Rybicki, L. A., Hoschar, A., Chute, D. J., et al. (2013). Oropharyngeal squamous cell carcinoma with known human papillomavirus status treated with definitive chemoradiotherapy: Patterns of failure and toxicity outcomes. *Radiation Oncology, 8*, 174.

Bonner, J. A., Harari, P. M., Giralt, J., Azarnia, N., Shin, D. M., Cohen, R. B., … Ang, K. K. (2006). Radiotherapy plus cetuximab for squamous-cell carcinoma of the head and neck. *New England Journal of Medicine, 354*(6), 567–578.

Bornbaum, C. C., Doyle, P. C., Skarakis-Doyle, E., & Theurer, J. A. (2013). A critical exploration of the International Classification of Functioning, Disability, and Health (ICF) framework from the perspective of oncology: Recommendations for revision. *Journal of Multidisciplinary Healthcare, 6*, 75–86.

Bornbaum, C. C., Fung, K., Franklin, J. H., Nichols, A., Yoo, J., & Doyle, P. (2012). A descriptive analysis of the relationship between quality of life and distress in individuals with head and neck cancer. *Supportive Care in Cancer, 20*(9), 2157–2165.

Bourhis, J., Overgaard, J., Audry, H., Ang, K. K., Saunders, M., Bernier, J., et al. (2006). Hyperfractionated or accelerated radiotherapy in head and neck cancer: A meta-analysis. *Lancet, 368*(9538), 843–854.

Brizel, D. M., Albers, M. E., Fisher, S. R., Scher, R. L., Richtsmeier, W. J., Hars, V., et al. (1998). Hyperfractionated irradiation with or without concurrent chemotherapy for locally advanced head and neck cancer. *New England Journal of Medicine, 338*(25), 1798–1804.

Brown, D. R., Schroeder, J. M., Bryan, J. T., et al. (1999). Detection of multiple human papillomavirus types in condylomata acuminate lesions from other healthy and immunosuppressed patients. *Journal of Clinical Microbiology, 37*, 3316–3322.

Canadian Cancer Society. (2016a). Retrieved on August 16, 2017 from http://www.cancer.ca/en/cancer-information/cancer-101/canadian-cancer-statistics-publication/canadian-cancer-statistics-infographics/?region=on.

Canadian Cancer Society. (2016b). Canadian cancer statistics 2016. Special topic: HPV-associated cancers. Retrieved August 16, 2017 from http://www.cancer.ca/~/media/cancer.ca/CW/cancer%20information/

cancer%20101/Canadian%20cancer%20statistics/
Canadian-Cancer-Statistics-2016-EN.pdf?la=en.

Centers for Disease Control and Prevention (CDC). (2011).
Vital signs: Current cigarette smoking among adults
aged ≥ 18 years – United States, 2005-2010. *Morbidity
and Mortality Weekly Report, 60*, 1207–1211.

Centers for Disease Control and Prevention, National
Center for Health Statistics. (n.d.). About the National
Health and Nutrition Examination Survey. Retrieved
August 17, 2017, from http://www.cdc.gov/nchs/
nhanes/about_nhanes.htm

Chaturvedi, A. K., Anderson, W. F., Lortet-Tieulent, J.,
Curado, M. P., Ferlay, J., Franceschi, S., et al. (2013).
Worldwide trends in incidence rates for oral cavity and
oropharyngeal cancers. *Journal of Clinical Oncology,
31*, 4550–4559.

Chaturvedi, A. K., D'Souza, G., Gillison, M. L., & Katki,
H. A. (2016). Burden of HPV-positive oropharynx
cancers among ever and never smokers in the U.S.
population. *Oral Oncology, 60*, 61–67.

Chaturvedi, A. K., Engels, E. A., Pfeiffer, R. M.,
Hernandez, B. Y., Xiao, W., Kim, E., et al. (2011).
Human papillomavirus and rising oropharyngeal can-
cer incidence in the United States. *Journal of Clinical
Oncology, 29*(32), 4294–4301.

Chaturvedi, A. K., Graubard, B. I., Broutian, T., Pickard,
R. K., Tong, Z. Y., Xiao, W., et al. (2015). NHANES
2009-2012 findings: Association of sexual behaviors
with higher prevalence of oral oncogenic human papillomavirus infections in U.S. men. *Cancer Research,
75*(12), 2468–2377.

Chen, P., Yu, W., Huang, J., Xu, H., Li, G., Chen, X., et al.
(2017). Matched-pair analysis of survival in patients
with poorly differentiated versus well-differentiated
glottis squamous cell carcinoma. *Oncotarget, 8*(9),
14770–14776.

Chu, A., Genden, E., Posner, M., & Sikora, A. (2013). A
patient-centred approach to counselling patients with
head and neck cancer undergoing human papillomavirus testing: A clinician's guide. *Oncologist, 18*(2),
180–189.

Chung, C. H., & Gillison, M. L. (2009). Human papillomavirus in head and neck cancer: Its role in pathogenesis and clinical implications. *Clinical Cancer
Research, 15*(22), 6758–6762.

D'Souza, G., & Dempsey, A. (2011). The role of HPV in
head and neck cancer and review of the HPV vaccine.
Preventive Medicine, 53(1 Suppl), S5–S11.

D'Souza, G., Kreimer, A. R., Viscidi, R., Pawlita, M.,
Fakhry, C., Koch, W. M., et al. (2007). Case-control
study of human papillomavirus and oropharyngeal
cancer. *New England Journal of Medicine, 356*(19),
1944–1956.

D'Souza, G., Wentz, A., Kluz, N., Zhang, Y., Sugar, E.,
Youngfellow, R. M., et al. (2016). Sex differences in
risk factors and natural history of oral human papillomavirus infection. *Journal of Infectious Diseases,
213*(12), 1893–1896.

D'Souza, G., Zhang, Y., Merritt, S., Gold, D., Robbins,
H. A., Buckman, V., et al. (2016). Patient experience

and anxiety during and after treatment for an HPV-
related oropharyngeal cancer. *Oral Oncology, 60*,
90–95.

Dahlstrom, K. R., Garden, A. S., William, W. N., Jr., Lim,
M. Y., & Sturgis, E. M. (2016). Proposed staging
system for patients with HPV-related oropharyngeal
cancer based on nasopharyngeal cancer n categories.
Journal of Clinical Oncology, 34(16), 1848–1854.

Davis, K. C., Farrelly, M. C., Duke, J., Kelly, L., &
Willett, J. (2012). Antismoking media campaign and
smoking cessation outcomes, New York state, 2003–
2009. *Preventing Chronic Diseases, 9*, E40. https://
doi.org/10.5888/pcd9.110102

Davis, K. S., Lim, C. M., Clump, D. A., Heron, D. E.,
Ohr, J. P., Kim, S., et al. (2016). Tumor volume as a
predictor of survival in human papillomavirus-positive
oropharyngeal cancer. *Head & Neck, 38*(Suppl1),
1613–1617.

De Boer, M. F., McCormick, L. K., Pruyn, J. F., Ryckman,
R. M., & van den Borne, B. W. (1999). Physical and
psychosocial correlates of head and neck cancer: A
review of the literature. *Otolaryngology – Head and
Neck Surgery, 120*, 427–436.

de Martel, C., Plummer, M., Vignat, J., & Franceschi, S.
(2017). Worldwide burden of cancer attributable to
HPV by site, country and HPV type. *International
Journal of Cancer, 141*, 664–670.

Dodd, R. H., Marlow, L. A. V., & Waller, J. (2016).
Discussing a diagnosis of human papillomavirus oropharyngeal cancer with patients: An exploratory qualitative study of health professionals. *Head & Neck,
38*(3), 394–401.

Dowthwaite, S. A., Franklin, J. H., Palma, D. A., Fung,
K., Yoo, J., & Nichols, A. C. (2012). The role of transoral robotic surgery in the management of oropharyngeal cancer: A review of the literature. *ISRN Oncology,
2012*, 945162. https://doi.org/10.5402/2012/945162

Edge, S. B., Byrd, D. R., Compton, C. C., Fritz, A. G.,
Greene, F. L., & Trotti, A. (Eds.). (2010). *AJCC
cancer staging manual* (7th ed.). New York, NY:
Springer-Verlag.

Eisbruch, A., Lyden, T., Bradford, C. R., Dawson, L. A.,
Haxer, M. J., Miller, A. E., et al. (2002). Objective
assessment of swallowing dysfunction and aspiration after radiation concurrent with chemotherapy
for head-and-neck cancer. *International Journal of
Radiation Oncology, Biology, Physics, 53*(1), 23–28.

El-Naggar, A. K., & Westra, W. H. (2012). p16 overexpression as a surrogate marking for HPV-related
oropharyngeal carcinoma: A guide for interpretative
relevance and consistency. *Head & Neck, 34*, 458–461.

Fakhry, C., & D'Souza, G. (2013). Discussing the diagnosis of HPV-OSCC: Common questions and answers.
Oral Oncology, 49(9), 863–871.

Fakhry, C., & Gillison, M. L. (2006). Clinical implications
of human papillomavirus in head and neck cancers.
Journal of Clinical Oncology, 24(17), 2606–2611.

Fakhry, C., Rosenthal, B. T., Clark, D. P., & Gillison,
M. L. (2011). Associations between oral HPV16
infection and cytopathology: Evaluation of an oropha-

ryngeal "pap-test equivalent" in high-risk populations. *Cancer Prevention Research, 4*(9), 1378–1384.

Fakhry, C., Westra, W. H., Li, S., Cmelak, A., Ridge, J. A., Pinto, H., et al. (2008). Improved survival of patients with human papillomavirus-positive head and neck squamous cell carcinoma in a prospective clinical trial. *Journal of the National Cancer Institute, 100*, 261–269.

Fakhry, C., Zhang, Q., Nruyen-Tan, P. F., Rosenthal, D., El-Naggar, A., Garden, A. S., et al. (2014). Human papillomavirus and overall survival after progression of oropharyngeal squamous cell carcinoma. *Journal of Clinical Oncology, 32*, 3365–3373.

Feller, L., Wood, N. H., Khammissa, R. A. G., & Lemmer, J. (2010). Human papillomavirus-mediated carcinogenesis and HPV-associated oral and oropharyngeal squamous cell carcinoma. Part 1: Human papillomavirus-mediated carcinogenesis. *Head & Face Medicine, 6*, 14–19.

Ferris, R. L., Jaffee, E. M., & Ferrone, S. (2010). Tumor antigen-targeted, monoclonal antibody-based immunotherapy: Clinical response, cellular immunity, and immunoescape. *Journal of Clinical Oncology, 28*, 4390–4399.

Finnigan, J. P., Jr., & Sikora, A. G. (2014). Counseling the patient with potentially HPV-related newly diagnosed head and neck cancer. *Current Oncology Reports, 16*(3), 375.

Franceschi, S., Munoz, N., Bosch, X. F., Snijders, P. J., & Walboomers, J. M. (1996). Human papillomavirus and cancers of the upper aerodigestive tract: A review of epidemiological and experimental evidence. *Cancer Epidemiology, Biomarkers and Prevention, 5*(7), 567–575.

Garcia-Piñeres, A. H., Hildesheim, A., Herrero, R., Trivett, M., Williams, M., Atmetlla, I., et al. (2006). Persistent human papillomavirus infection is associated with a generalized decreased in immune responsiveness in older women. *Cancer Research, 66*(22), 11070–11076.

Gasparini, R., & Panatto, D. (2009). Cervical cancer: From Hippocrates through Rigoni-Stern to zur Hausen. *Vaccine, 27*(1 Suppl), A4–A5.

Gillison, M. L. (2004). Human papillomavirus-associated head and neck cancer is a distinct epidemiologic, clinical, and molecular entity. *Seminars in Oncology, 31*(6), 744–754.

Gillison, M. L., Broutian, T., Pickard, R. K. L., Tong, Z.-Y., Xiao, W., Kahle, L., et al. (2012). Prevalence of oral HPV infection in the United States, 2009-2010. *Journal of the American Medical Association, 307*(7), 693–703.

Gillison, M. L., Chaturvedi, A. K., & Lowy, D. R. (2008). HPV prophylactic vaccines and the potential prevention of noncervical cancers in both men and women. *Cancer, 113*(10 Suppl), 3036–3046.

Gillison, M. L., D'Souza, G., Westra, W., Sugar, E., Xiao, W., Begum, S., et al. (2008). Distinct risk factor profiles for human papillomavirus type 16-positive and human papillomavirus type 16-negative head and neck cancers. *Journal of the National Cancer Institute, 100*, 407–420.

Gillison, M. L., Koch, W. M., Capone, R. B., Spafford, M., Westra, W. H., Wu, L., et al. (2000). Evidence for a causal association between human papillomavirus type 16-positive and human papillomavirus type 16-negative head and neck cancers. *Journal of the National Cancer Institute, 92*(9), 709–720.

Gillison, M. L., Zhang, Q., Jordan, R., Xiao, W., Westra, W., Trotti, A., et al. (2012). Tobacco smoking and increased risk of death and progression for patients with p16-positive and p16-negative oropharyngeal cancer. *Journal of Clinical Oncology, 30*, 2101–2111.

Gissman, L., Diehl, V., Schultz-Coulon, H. J., & zur Hausen, H. (1982). Molecular cloning and characterization of human papilloma virus DNA derived from a laryngeal papilloma. *Journal of Virology, 44*(1), 393–400.

Giuliano, A. R., Tortolero-Luna, G., Ferrer, E., Burchell, A. N., de Sanjose, S., & Kjaer, S. K. (2008). Epidemiology of human papillomavirus infection in men, cancers other than cervical and benign conditions. *Vaccine, 26*(Suppl 10), K17–K28.

Gooi, Z., Chan, J. Y., & Fakhry, C. (2016). The epidemiology of the human papillomavirus related to oropharyngeal head and neck cancer. *Laryngoscope, 126*(4), 894–900.

Habbous, S., Chu, K. P., Lau, H., Schorr, M., Belayneh, M., Ha, M. N., et al. (2017). Human papillomavirus in oropharyngeal cancer in Canada: Analysis of 5 comprehensive cancer centres using multiple imputation. *Canadian Medical Association Journal, 189*, E1030–E1040.

Hafkamp, H., Manni, J., Haesevoets, A., Voogd, A. C., Schepers, M., Bot, F. J., et al. (2008). Marked differences in survival rate between smokers and nonsmokers with HPV16-assocaited tonsillar carcinomas. *International Journal of Cancer, 122*, 2656–2664.

Hanasoge, S., Magliocca, K. R., Switchenko, J. M., Saba, N. F., Wadsworth, J. T., El-Deiry, M. W., et al. (2016). Clinical outcomes in elderly patients with human papillomavirus-positive squamous cell carcinoma of the oropharynx treated with definitive chemoradiation therapy. *Head & Neck, 38*(6), 846–851.

Hariri, S., Unger, E. R., Sternberg, M., Dunne, E. F., Swan, D., Patel, S., et al. (2011). Prevalence of genital human papillomavirus among females in the United States, the National Health and Nutrition Examination Survery, 2003–2006. *Journal of Infectious Diseases, 204*(4), 566–573.

Health Protection Agency. (2011). Trends in genital herpes and genital warts infections, United Kingdom: 2000 to 2009. Retrieved August 17, 2017, from http://webarchive.nationalarchives.gov.uk/20140714092919/, http://www.hpa.org.uk/hpr/archives/2011/hpr1711.pdf

Herrero, R., Quint, W., Hildesheim, A., Gonzalez, P., Struijk, L., Katki, H. A., et al. (2013). Reduced prevalence of oral human papillomavirus (HPV) 4 years after bivalent HPV vaccination in a randomized clinical trial in Costa Rica. *PLoS One, 8*(7), E68329. https://doi.org/10.1371/journal.pone.0068329

Hildesheim, A., & Herrero, R. (2007). Human papillomavirus vaccine should be given before sexual debut for maximum benefit. *Journal of Infectious Diseases, 196*(10), 1431–1432.

Hildesheim, A., Herrero, R., Wacholder, S., Rodriguez, A. C., Solomon, D., Bratti, M. C., et al. (2007). Effect of human papillomavirus 16/18 L1 virus like particle vaccine among young women with preexisting infection: A randomized trial. *JAMA, 298*(7), 743–753.

Hoffman, M., Cooper, D., Carrara, H., Rosenberg, L., Kelly, J., Stander, I., et al. (2003). Limited Pap screening associated with reduced risk of cervical cancer in South Africa. *International Journal of Epidemiology, 32*(4), 573–577.

Horne, Z. D., Glaser, S. M., Vargo, J. A., Ferris, R. L., Balasubramani, G. K., Clump, D. A., et al. (2016). Confirmation of proposed human papillomavirus risk-adapted staging according to AJCC/UICC TNM criteria for positive oropharyngeal carcinomas. *Cancer, 122*(13), 2021–2030.

Huang, S. H., Patel, S., O'Sullivan, B., Shen, X., Weinreb, I., Perez-Ordonez, B., et al. (2015). Longer survival in patients with human papillomavirus-related head and neck cancer after positive postradiation planned neck dissection. *Head & Neck, 37*(7), 946–952.

Huang, S. H., Perez-Ordonez, B., Liu, F. F., Waldron, J., Ringash, J., Irish, J., et al. (2012). Atypical clinical behavior of p16-confirmed HPV-related oropharyngeal squamous cell carcinoma treated with radical radiotherapy. *International Journal of Radiation Oncology, Biology, Physics, 82*(1), 276–283.

Hutcheson, K. A., Holsinger, F. C., Kupferman, M. E., & Lewin, J. S. (2015). Functional outcomes after TORS for oropharyngeal cancer: A systematic review. *European Archives of Otorhinolaryngology, 272*(2), 463–471.

Jemal, A., Simard, E. P., Dorell, C., Noone, A. M., Markowitz, L. E., Kohler, B., et al. (2013). Annual report to the nation on the status of cancer, 1975–2009, featuring the burden and trends in human papillomavirus (HPV)-associated cancers and HPV vaccination coverage levels. *Journal of the National Cancer Institute, 105*(3), 175–201.

Kaka, A. S., Kumar, B., Kumar, P., Wakely, P. E., Jr., Kirsch, C. M., Old, M. O., et al. (2013). Highly aggressive HPV-related oropharyngeal cancer: Clinical, radiologic, and pathologic characteristics. *Oral Surgery, Oral Medicine, Oral Pathology and Oral Radiology, 116*(3), 327–335.

Kamerow, D. (2016). HPV vaccine: Effective but underused in the US. *British Medical Journal, 353*, i2060. https://doi.org/10.1136/bmj.i2060. (Published 14 April 2016).

Khariwala, S. S., Moore, M. G., Malloy, K. M., Gosselin, B., & Smith, R. V. (2015). The "HPV Discussion": Effective use of data to deliver recommendations to patients impacted by HPV. *Otolaryngology - Head and Neck Surgery, 153*(2), 518–525.

Kharytaniuk, N., Molony, P., Boyle, S., O'Leary, G., Werner, R., Heffron, C., et al. (2016). Association of extracapsular spread with survival according to human papillomavirus status in oropharyngeal squamous cell carcinoma and carcinoma of the unknown primary site. *JAMA Otolaryngology - Head and Neck Surgery, 142*(7), 683–690.

Khwaia, S. S., Baker, C., Haynes, W., Spencer, C. R., Gay, H., Thorstad, W., et al. (2016). High E6 gene expression predicts for distant metastasis and poor survival in patients with HPV-positive oropharyngeal squamous cell carcinoma. *International Journal Radiation Oncology, Biology, Physics, 95*(4), 1132–1141.

Kliewer, E. V., Demers, A. A., Elliott, L., Lotocki, R., Butler, J. R., & Brisson, M. (2009). Twenty-year trends in the incidence and prevalence of diagnoses anogenital warts in Canada. *Sexually Transmitted Diseases, 36*(6), 380–386.

Kreimer, A. R., Bhatia, R. K., Messeguer, A. L., Gonzalez, P., Herrero, R., & Giuliano, A. R. (2010). Oral human papillomavirus in health individuals: A systematic review of the literature. *Sexually Transmitted Diseases, 37*, 386–391.

Kreimer, A. R., Clifford, G. M., Boyle, P., & Franceschi, S. (2005). Human papillomavirus types in head and neck squamous cell carcinomas worldwide: A systematic review. *Cancer Epidemiology, Biomarkers & Prevention, 14*(2), 467–475.

Kreimer, A. R., Johansson, M., Waterboer, T., Kaaks, R., Chang-Claude, J., Drogen, D., et al. (2013). Evaluation of human papillomavirus antibodies and risk of subsequent head and neck cancer. *Journal of Clinical Oncology, 31*(21), 2708–2715.

Kreimer, A. R., Pierce Campbell, C. M., Lin, H. Y., Fulp, W., Papenfuss, M. R., Abrahamsen, M., et al. (2013). Incidence and clearance of oral human papillomavirus infection in men: The HIM cohort study. *Lancet, 382*, 877–887.

Kubicek, G. J., Champ, C., Fogh, S., Wang, F., Reddy, E., Intenzo, C., et al. (2010). FDG-PET staging and important of lymph node SUV in head and neck cancer. *Head and Neck Oncology, 2*, 19.

Kugaya, A., Akechi, T., Okuyama, T., Nakano, T., Mikami, I., Okamura, H., et al. (2000). Prevalence, predictive factors, and screening for psychologic distress in patients with newly diagnosed head and neck cancer. *Cancer, 88*, 2817–2223.

Kumar, B., Cordell, K., Lee, J., Worden, F. P., Prince, M. D., Tran, H. H., et al. (2008). EGFR, p16, HPV titer Bcl-xL, and p53, sex, and smoking as indicators of response to therapy and survival in oropharyngeal cancer. *Journal of Clinical Oncology, 26*(19), 3128–3137.

Lacchetti, C., Waldron, J., Perez-Ordonez, B., Kamel-Reid, S., Cripps, C., & Gilbert, R. (2013). *Routine HPV testing in HNSCC (program in evidence-based care evidence-based series no. 5–9).* Toronto, ON: Cancer Care Ontario.

Lassen, P., Eriksen, J. G., Hamilton-Dutoit, S., Tramm, T., Alsner, J., & Overgaard, J. (2009). Effect of HPV-associated p16INK4A expression on response to radiotherapy and survival in squamous cell carcinoma of the head and neck. *Journal of Clinical Oncology, 27*, 1992–1998.

Lee, L. A., Huang, C. G., Liao, C. T., Lee, L. Y., Hsueh, C., Chen, T. C., et al. (2012). Human papillomavirus-16 infection in advanced oral cavity cancer patients is related to an increased risk of distant metastases and poor survival. *PLoS One, 7*(7), e40767. https://doi.org/10.1371/journal.pone.0040767

Lin, B. M., Wang, H., D'Souza, G., Zhang, Z., Fakhry, C., Joseph, A. W., et al. (2013). Long-term prognosis and risk factors among patients with HPV-associated oropharyngeal squamous cell carcinoma. *Cancer, 119*(9), 3462–3472.

Lindel, K., Beer, K. T., Laissue, J., Greiner, R. H., & Aebersold, D. M. (2001). Human papillomavirus positive squamous cell carcinoma of the oropharynx a radiosensitive subgroup of head and neck carcinoma. *Cancer, 92*(4), 805–813.

Loning, T., Ikenberg, H., Becker, J., Gissmann, L., Hoepfer, I., & zur Hausen, H. (1985). Analysis of oral papillomas, leukoplakias, and invasive carcinomas for human papillomavirus type related DNA. *The Journal of Investigative Dermatology, 84*(5), 417–420.

Louvanto, K., Rautava, J., Willberg, J., Wideman, L., Syrjänen, K., Grénman, S., et al. (2013). Genotype-specific incidence and clearance of human papillomavirus in oral mucosa of women: A six-year follow-up study. *PLoS One, 8*, e53413. https://doi.org/10.1371/journal.pone.0053413

Lydiatt, W. M., Patel, S. G., O'Sullivan, B., Brandwein, M. S., Ridge, J. A., Migliacci, J. C., et al. (2017). Head and neck cancers – major changes in the American Joint Committee on Cancer eighth edition cancer staging manual. *CA: A Cancer Journal for Clinicians, 67*, 122–137.

Machtay, M., Moughan, J., Trotti, A., Garden, A. S., Weber, R. S., Cooper, J. S., et al. (2008). Factors associated with severe late toxicity after concurrent chemoradiation for locally advanced head and neck cancer: An RTOG analysis. *Journal of Clinical Oncology, 26*(21), 3582–3589.

Markowitz, L. E., Liu, G., Hariri, S., Steinau, M., Dunne, E. F., & Unger, E. R. (2016). Prevalence of HPV after introduction of the vaccination program in the United States. *Pediatrics, 137*, 1–9.

Masterson, L., Moualed, D., Masood, A., Dwivedi, R. C., Benson, R., Sterling, J. C., et al. (2014). De-escalation treatment protocols for human papillomavirus-associated oropharyngeal squamous cell carcinoma. *The Cochrane Database of Systematic Reviews, 15*(2). https://doi.org/10.1002/14651858.CD010271.pub2

Maxwell, J. H., Ferris, R. L., Gooding, W., Cunningham, D., Mehta, V., Kim, S., et al. (2013). Extracapsular spread in head and neck carcinoma: Impact of site and human papillomavirus status. *Cancer, 119*(18), 3302–3308.

Maxwell, J. H., Kumar, B., Feng, F., Worden, F. P., Lee, J., Eisbruch, A., et al. (2012). Tobacco use in HPV-positive advanced oropharynx cancer patients related to increased risk of distant metastases and tumor recurrence. *Clinical Cancer Research, 16*(4), 1226–1235.

Maxwell, J. H., Mehta, V., Wang, H., Cunningham, D., Duvvuri, U., Kim, S., et al. (2014). Quality of life in head and neck cancer patients: Impact of HPV and primary treatment modality. *Laryngoscope, 124*(7), 1592–1597.

McIlwain, W. R., Sood, A. J., Nguyen, S. A., & Day, T. A. (2014). Initial symptoms in patients with HPV-positive and HPV-negative oropharyngeal cancer. *JAMA Otolaryngology - Head and Neck Surgery, 140*(5), 441–447.

McQuillan, G., Kruszon-Moran, D., Markowitz, L. E., Unger, E. R., & Paulose-Ram, R. (2017). Prevalence of HPV in adults aged 18–69: United States, 2011–2014. *NCHS Data Brief, 280,* 1–8.

Mehanna, H., Beech, T., & Nicholson, T. (2013). Prevalence of human papillomavirus in oropharyngeal and non-oropharyngeal head and neck cancer – a systematic review and meta-analysis of trends by time and region. *Head & Neck, 35*(5), 747–755.

Mehanna, H., Franklin, N., Compton, N., Robinson, M., Powell, N., Biswas-Baldwin, N., et al. (2016). Geographic variation in human papillomavirus-related oropharyngeal cancer: Data from 4 multinational randomized trials. *Head & Neck, 38*(Suppl1), E1863–E1869.

Milbury, K., Rosenthal, D. I., El-Naggar, A., & Badr, H. (2013). An exploratory study of the informational and psychosocial needs of patients with human papillomavirus-associated oropharyngeal cancer. *Oral Oncology, 49*(11), 1067–1071.

Mundi, N., Theurer, J., Warner, A., Yoo, J., Fung, K., MacNeil, D., … Nichols, A. C. (2018). The impact of seasonal operating room closures on wait times for oral cancer surgery. *Current Oncology, 25*(1), 67.

Naik, M., Ward, M. C., Bledsoe, T. J., Kumar, A. M. S., Rybicki, L. A., Saxton, J. P., et al. (2015). It is not just IMRT: Human papillomavirus related oropharynx squamous cell carcinoma is associated with better swallowing outcomes after definitive chemoradiotherapy. *Oral Oncology, 51*, 800–804.

National Comprehensive Cancer Network. (n.d.). About the NCCN Clinical Practice Guidelines in Oncology (NCCN Guidelines (R)). Retrieved August 17, 2017, from https://www.nccn.org/professionals/default.aspx.

Nichols, A. C., Palma, D. A., Dhaliwal, S. S., Tan, S., Theurer, J., Chow, W., et al. (2013). The epidemic of human papillomavirus and oropharyngeal cancer in a Canadian population. *Current Oncology, 20*(4), 212–219.

Niedobitek, G., Pitteroff, S., Herbst, H., Shepherd, P., Finn, T., Anagnostopoulos, I., et al. (1990). Detection of human papillomavirus type 16 DNA in carcinomas of the palatine tonsil. *Journal of Clinical Pathology, 43*(11), 918–921.

Nien, H. H., Sturgis, E. M., Kies, M. S., El-Naggar, A. K., Morrison, W. H., Beadle, B. M., et al. (2016). Comparison of systemic therapies used concurrently with radiation for the treatment of human papillomavirus-associated oropharyngeal cancer. *Head & Neck, 38*(Suppl1), E1554–E1561.

O'Rorke, M. A., Ellison, M. V., Murray, L. J., Moran, M., James, J., & Anderson, L. A. (2012). Human papillomavirus related head and neck cancer survival: A systematic review and meta-analysis. *Oral Oncology, 48*(12), 1191–1201.

O'Sullivan, B., Huang, S. H., Siu, L. L., Waldron, J., Zhao, H., Perez-Ordonez, B., et al. (2013). Deintensification candidate subgroups in human papillomavirus-related oropharyngeal cancer according to minimal risk of distant metastasis. *Journal of Clinical Oncology, 31*(5), 543–550.

O'Sullivan, D., Huang, S. H., Su, J., Garden, A. S., Sturgis, E. M., Dahlstrom, K., et al. (2016). Development and validation of a staging system for HPV-related oropharyngeal cancer by the International Collaboration on Oropharyngeal cancer Network for Staging (ICON-S): A multicenter cohort study. *Lancet Oncology, 17*(4), 440–451.

Palma, D. (2017). *Taking charge of cancer: What you need to know to get the best treatment*. Oakland, CA: New Harbinger Publications.

Parsons, J. T., Mendenhall, W. M., Stringer, S. P., Amdur, R. J., Hinerman, R. W., Villaret, D. B., et al. (2002). Squamous cell carcinoma of the oropharynx: Surgery, radiation therapy, or both. *Cancer, 94*(11), 2967–2980.

Paz, I. B., Cook, N., Odom-Maryon, T., Xie, Y., & Wilczynski, S. P. (1997). Human papillomavirus (HPV) in head and neck cancer: An association of HPV 16 with squamous cell carcinoma of Waldeyer's tonsillar ring. *Cancer, 79*(3), 595–604.

Pickard, R. K. L., Xiao, W., Broutian, T. R., He, X., & Gillison, M. L. (2012). The prevalence and incidence of oral human papillomavirus infection among young men and women, aged 18-30 years. *Sexually Transmitted Diseases, 39*, 559–566.

Pignon, J. P., le Maître, A., Maillard, E., Bourhis, J., & MACH-NC Collaborative Group. (2009). Meta-analysis of chemotherapy in head and neck cancer (MACH-NC): An update on 93 randomised trials and 17,346 patients. *Radiotherapy and Oncology: Journal of the European Society for Therapeutic Radiology and Oncology, 92*(1), 4–14.

Posner, M. R., Lorch, J. H., Goloubeva, O., Tan, M., Schumaker, L. M., Sarlis, N. J., et al. (2011). Survival and human papillomavirus in oropharynx cancer in TAX 324: A subset analysis from an international phase III trial. *Annals of Oncology, 22*(5), 1071–1077.

Proceddu, S. V. (2016). A TNM classification for HPV+ oropharyngeal cancer. *Lancet Oncology, 17*(4), 403–404.

Ramer, I., Varier, I., Zhang, D., Demicco, E. G., Posner, M. R., Misiukiewicz, K., et al. (2016). Racial disparities in incidence of human papillomavirus-associated oropharyngeal cancer in an urban population. *Cancer Epidemiology, 44*, 91–95.

Rautava, J., Willberg, J., Louvanto, K., Wideman, L., Syrjanen, K., Grenman, S., et al. (2012). Prevalence, genotype distribution and persistence of human papillomavirus in oral mucosa of women: A six-year follow-up study. *PLoS One, 7*(8), e42171. https://doi.org/10.1371/journal.pone.0042171

Rettig, E., Keiss, A. P., & Fakhry, C. (2015). The role of sexual behavior in head and neck cancer: Implications for prevention and therapy. *Expert Review of Anticancer Therapy, 15*(1), 35–49.

Ringash, J. (2015). Survivorship and quality of life in head and neck cancer. *Journal of Clinical Oncology, 33*(29), 3322–3327.

Ringash, J., Fisher, R., Peters, L., Trotti, A., O'Sullivan, B., Corry, J., et al. (2016). Effect of p16 status on the quality-of-life experience during chemoradiation for locally advanced oropharyngeal cancer: A substudy of randomized trial trans-tasman radiation oncology group (TROG) 02.02 (HeadSTART). *International Journal of Radiation Oncology, Biology, Physics, 97*(4), 678–686.

Rodriguez, C. P., Adelstein, D. J., Rybicki, L. A., Savvides, P., Saxton, J. P., Koyfman, S. A., et al. (2015). Randomizes phase III study of 2 cisplatin-based chemoradiation regimens in locally advanced head and neck squamous cell carcinoma: Impact of changing disease epidemiology on contemporary trial design. *Head & Neck, 37*(11), 1583–1589.

Salazar, C. R., Smith, R. V., Garg, M. K., Haigentz, M., Jr., Schiff, B. A., Kawachi, N., et al. (2014). Human papillomavirus-associated head and neck squamous cell carcinoma survival: A comparison by tumor site and initial treatment. *Head and Neck Pathology, 8*(1), 77–87.

Samuels, S. E., Tao, Y., Lyden, T., Haxer, M., Spector, M., Malloy, K. M., et al. (2016). Comparisons of dysphagia and quality of life (QOL) in comparable patients with HPV-positive oropharyngeal cancer receiving chemo-irradiation or cetuximab-irradiation. *Oral Oncology, 54*, 68–74.

Sasieni, P., Castanon, A., & Cuzick, J. (2009). Effectiveness of cervical screening with age: Population based case-control study of prospectively recorded data. *British Medical Journal, 339*, b2968. https://doi.org/10.1136/bmj.b2968

Schache, A. G., Powell, N. G., Cuschieri, K. S., Robinson, M., Leary, S., Mehanna, H., et al. (2016). HPV-related oropharynx cancer in the United Kingdom: An evolution in the understanding of disease etiology. *Cancer Research, 76*(22), 6598–6606.

Schlecht, N. F., Brandwein-Gensler, M., Nuovo, G. J., Li, M., Dunne, A., Kawachi, N., et al. (2011). A comparison of clinically utilized human papillomavirus detection methods in head and neck cancer. *Modern Pathology: An Official Journal of the United States and Canadian Academy of Pathology, Inc, 24*(10), 1295–1305.

Schwartz, S. M., Daling, J. R., Doody, D. R., Wipf, G. C., Carter, J. J., Madeleine, M. M., et al. (1998). Oral cancer risk in relation to sexual history and evidence of human papillomavirus infection. *Journal of the National Cancer Institute, 90*(21), 1626–1636.

Seiwert, T. (2013). Accurate HPV testing: A requirement for precision medicine for head and neck cancer. *Annals of Oncology, 24*(11), 2711–2713.

Sharma, A., Mendez, E., Yueh, B., Lohavanichbutr, P., Houck, J., Doody, D. R., et al. (2012). Human papillomavirus-positive oral cavity and oropharyngeal cancer patients do not have better quality-of-life trajectories. *Otolaryngology - Head and Neck Surgery, 146*(5), 739–745.

Sinha, P., Lewis, J. S., Jr., Piccirillo, J. F., Kallogieri, D., & Haughey, B. H. (2012). Extracapsular spread and adjuvant therapy in human papillomavirus-related, p16-positive oropharyngeal carcinoma. *Cancer, 118*(14), 3519–3530.

Sinha, P., Pipkorn, P., Thorstad, W. L., Gay, H. A., & Haughey, B. H. (2016). Does elimination of planned postoperative radiation to the primary bed in p16-positive, transorally-resected oropharyngeal carcinoma associate with poorer outcomes? *Oral Oncology, 61*, 127–134.

Sinha, P., Thorstad, W. T., Nussenbaum, B., Haughey, B. H., Adkins, D. R., Kallogieri, D., et al. (2014). Distant metastasis in p16-positive oropharyngeal squamous cell carcinoma: A critical analysis of patterns and outcomes. *Oral Oncology, 50*(1), 45–51.

Snijders, P. J., Cromme, F. V., van den Brule, A. J., Schrijnemakers, H. F., Snow, G. B., Meijer, C. J., et al. (1992). Prevalence and expression of human papillomavirus in tonsillar carcinomas, indicating a possible viral etiology. *International Journal of Cancer, 51*(6), 845–850.

Spanos, W. C., Nowicki, P., Lee, D. W., Hoover, A., Hostager, B., Gupta, A., et al. (2009). Immune response during therapy with cisplatin or radiation for human papillomavirus-related head and neck cancer. *Archives of Otolaryngology - Head and Neck Surgery, 135*(11), 1137–1146.

Spector, M. E., Gallagher, K. K., Light, E., Ibrahim, M., Chanowski, E. J., Moyer, J. S., et al. (2012). Matted nodes: Poor prognostic marker in oropharyngeal squamous cell carcinoma independent of HPV and EGFR status. *Head & Neck, 34*(12), 1727–1733.

Stokley, S., Jeyarajah, J., Yankey, D., Cano, M., Gee, J., Roark, J., et al. (2014). Human papillomavirus vaccination coverage among adolescents, 2007–2013, and postlicensure vaccine safety monitoring, 2006–2014 – United States. *Morbidity and Mortality Weekly Report, 63*, 620–624.

Stransky, N., Egloff, A. M., Tward, A. D., Kostic, A. D., Cibulskis, K., Sivachenko, A., et al. (2011). The mutation landscape of head and neck squamous cell carcinoma. *Science, 333*(6046), 1157–1160.

Syrjänen, K. J., Syrjänen, S. M., Lamberg, M. A., & Pyrhönen, S. (1983). Human papillomavirus (HPV) involvement in squamous cell lesions of the oral cavity. *Proceedings of the Finnish Dental Society, 79*(1), 1–8.

Taberna, M., Resteghini, C., Swanson, B., Pickard, R. K. L., Jiang, B., Xiao, W., et al. (2016). Low etiologic fraction for human papillomavirus in larynx squamous cell carcinoma. *Oral Oncology, 61*, 55–61.

Thavaraj, S., Stokes, A., Guerra, E., Bibel, J., Halligan, E., Long, A., et al. (2011). Evaluation of human papillomavirus testing for squamous cell carcinoma of the tonsil in clinical practice. *Journal of Clinical Pathology, 64*(4), 308–312.

Trosman, S. J., Koyfman, S. A., Ward, M. C., Al-Khudari, S., Nwizu, T., Greskovich, J. F., et al. (2015). Effect of human papillomavirus on patterns of distant metastatic failure in oropharyngeal squamous cell carcinoma treated with chemoradiotherapy. *JAMA Otolaryngology – Head and Neck Surgery, 141*(5), 457–462.

Truong Lam, M., O'Sullivan, B., Gullane, P., & Hui Huang, S. (2016). Challenges in establishing the diagnosis of human papillomavirus-related oropharyngeal carcinoma. *Laryngoscope, 126*, 2270–2275.

Urban, D., Corry, J., & Rischin, D. (2014). What is the best treatment for patients with human papillomavirus-positive and –negative OPSCC? *Cancer, 120*(10), 1462–1470.

van Harten, M. C., Hoebers, F. J. P., Kross, K. W., van Werkhoven, E. D., van den Brekel, M. W. M., & van Dijk, B. A. C. (2015). Determinants of treatment waiting times for head and neck cancer in the Netherlands and their relation to survival. *Oral Oncology, 51*(3), 272–278.

Veterans Affairs Laryngeal Cancer Study Group. (1991). Induction chemotherapy plus radiation compared with surgery plus radiation in patients with advanced laryngeal cancer. *New England Journal of Medicine, 324*(24), 1685–1690.

Vicus, D., Sutradhar, R., Lu, Y., Elit, L., Kupets, R., Paszat, L., et al. (2014). The association between cervical cancer screening and mortality from cervical cancer: A population based case-control study. *Gynecologic Oncology, 133*, 167–171.

Ward, G., Mehta, V., & Moore, M. (2016). Morbidity, mortality and cost from HPV-related oropharyngeal cancer: Impact of 2-, 4-, and 9-valent vaccines. *Human Vaccines & Immunotherapies, 12*(6), 1343–1347.

Worsham, M. J., Stephen, J. K., Chen, K. M., Mahan, M., Schweitzer, V., Havard, S., et al. (2013). Improved survival with HPV among African Americans with oropharyngeal cancer. *Clinical Cancer Research, 19*(9), 2486–2492.

Xiao, C., Zhang, Q., Nquyen-Tan, P. F., List, M., Weber, R. S., Ang, K. K., et al. (2017). Quality of life and performance status from a substudy conducted within a prospective phase 3 randomized trial of concurrent standard radiation versus accelerated radiation plus cisplatin for locally advanced head and neck carcinoma: NRG Oncology RTOG 0129. *International Journal of Radiation Oncology, Biology, Physics, 97*(4), 667–677.

Zafereo, M. E., Xu, L., Dahlstrom, K. R., Viamonte, C. A., El-Naggar, A. K., Wei, Q., et al. (2016). Squamous cell carcinoma of the oral cavity often overexpresses p16 but is rarely driven by human papillomavirus. *Oral Oncology, 56*, 47–53.

zur Hausen, H. (1976). Condylomata acuminata and human genital cancer. *Cancer Research, 36*(2 pt 2), 794.

zur Hausen, H. (1982). Human genital cancer: Synergism between two virus infections or synergism between a virus infection and initiating events. *Lancet, 2*(8312), 1370–1372.

zur Hausen, H. (2009). Papillomavirus in the causation of human cancers – a brief historical account. *Virology, 384*(2), 260–265.

Distress as a Consequence of Head and Neck Cancer

Catherine C. Bornbaum and Philip C. Doyle

Introduction

Cancer is a disease of multiple types, sites, and etiologies. Worldwide statistics indicate that cancer is a leading cause of death globally and accounted for 8.8 million deaths in 2015 (World Health Organization, 2018). As a disease, the impact of cancer crosses multiple boundaries of human functioning. Even in situations where disease is deemed to be cured, the impact of cancer and its treatment may persist in many ways for the remainder of one's life.

Unfortunately, concerns related to cancer extend beyond the pervasiveness of the disease to also include the myriad consequences that stem from it. Due to the current forms of treatment available (e.g., chemotherapy, radiotherapy, surgery, and multimodality protocols), there are often significant long-term consequences related to the functioning and quality of life of individuals with cancer (Semple, Sullivan, Dunwoody, & Kernohan, 2004). Further, and not unimportantly,

C. C. Bornbaum (✉)
Dalla Lana School of Public Health, University of Toronto, Toronto, ON, Canada
e-mail: catherine.bornbaum@utoronto.ca

P. C. Doyle
Voice Production and Perception Laboratory & Laboratory for Well-Being and Quality of Life, Department of Otolaryngology – Head and Neck Surgery and School of Communication Sciences and Disorders, Western University, Elborn College, London, ON, Canada

additional challenges within the realm of psychosocial functioning will also be experienced by their caregivers (Bornbaum, 2013). One important area that must be considered in the context of cancer and its treatment is the level of distress that it may create.

Irrespective of anatomical site, all individuals with cancer experience some level of distress related to their diagnosis and treatment (NCCN, 2013). Unfortunately, this problem is amplified in those with head and neck cancer (HNCa), a population who exhibits the highest rates of anxiety, depression, and suicide compared with other cancer sites (Kendal, 2006; Misono, Weiss, Fann, Redman, & Yueh, 2008). While the specific reasons underlying the disproportionate rate of suicide and depression in individuals with HNCa are unknown, researchers have speculated that the cause may be attributable to the devastating effect of the disease and its treatment on the quality of life of individuals with HNCa (Misono et al., 2008). The impact of the disease and its treatment on one's appearance and essential functions such as breathing, swallowing, and speech with its associated disruption in communication were also cited as possible factors contributing to the elevated rates of depression and suicide in individuals with HNCa (Misono et al., 2008).

In addition to the concerns of the person with HNCa, it is apparent that the diagnosis of cancer and its accompanying sequelae (e.g., treatment- and disease-related consequences such as

© Springer Nature Switzerland AG 2019
P. C. Doyle (ed.), *Clinical Care and Rehabilitation in Head and Neck Cancer*,
https://doi.org/10.1007/978-3-030-04702-3_5

impaired breathing, speech, and swallowing) may also create varied levels of distress and may represent a significant crisis for family members and significant others (Blood, Simpson, Dineen, Kauffman, & Raimondi, 1994); these individuals are expected to grieve – or rather, respond to the loss (Lev & McCorkle, 1998) – while simultaneously supporting the health and psychosocial well-being of the individual with cancer. Given this level of burden, it is not surprising that partners of those with HNCa report higher levels of anxiety than those with the disease (Vickery, Latchford, Hewison, Bellew, & Feber, 2003). Consequently, it is apparent that elevated distress has the potential to impact not only individuals with HNCa, but also their loved ones and caregivers. However, the larger issue that may emerge in these circumstances is the very real potential that distress will be a persistent challenge in one's long-term functioning. This chapter seeks to provide a review of issues specific to distress following the treatment of head and neck cancer (HNCa).

What is Distress in the Context of Head and Neck Cancer?

Psychosocial distress has been identified as a significant and ongoing problem among individuals diagnosed with cancer. Distress has become so prevalent that the National Comprehensive Cancer Network (NCCN) established a Distress Management Panel to address the issue. The NCCN (2013) has defined distress as:

> …a multi-determined unpleasant emotional experience of a psychological (cognitive, behavioral, emotional), social, and/or spiritual nature that may interfere with the ability to cope effectively with cancer, its physical symptoms and its treatment. Distress extends along a continuum, ranging from common normal feelings of vulnerability, sadness and fears, to problems that can become disabling, such as depression, anxiety, panic, social isolation, and spiritual crisis. (p. 6)

As highlighted by the presence of a "continuum" of distress, there is an inherent distinction to be made between the pathologic experience of distress (e.g., clinical depression, anxiety disorders)

and one's natural response to a catastrophic life event, be that the threat to one's own life or to the life of a loved one. Transitory negative feelings are a normal part of the cancer experience and are to be expected as individuals react to an unanticipated threat, to the potential and actual losses, and to the potential side effects of unpleasant and/or painful treatments (Haman, 2008). Cancer and its treatment often create feelings of uncertainty, anticipated changes to personal roles and functioning, and practical concerns related to medical care and financial well-being. As individuals and caregivers attempt to manage these concerns, they are likely to experience emotions such as sadness, anger, and fear. Data suggest that the majority of individuals will experience brief episodes of sadness or anxiety, insomnia, loss of interest in activities, thoughts of helplessness and hopelessness, or worries about potential catastrophic events such as the loss of life (Haman, 2008).

Since the relationship between individuals with cancer and their caregivers would almost certainly be interrelated, clinicians might wish to acknowledge that both partners may potentially experience negative consequences when the other is distressed (Northouse, Templin, & Mood, 2001; Segrin, Badger, Dorros, Meek, & Lopez, 2007). Therefore, efforts to develop an improved understanding of the factors that contribute to elevated distress in both those with HNCa and their caregivers are essential. Such recognition may have important implications for improving health-related and rehabilitation outcomes in association with HNCa.

Impact of Cancer as a Disease

The diagnosis of HNCa and its treatment carries with it a unique set of challenges that potentially exceed those associated with other sites of cancer (Howren, Christensen, Karnell, & Funk, 2012; Semple, 2001). Additionally, there is the ever-present concern related to the fear of cancer recurrence (Hodges & Humphris, 2009). Irrespective of treatment modality, individuals diagnosed with HNCa will likely face treatment-related challenges in oral communication, emotional expression, social interaction, and/or physical function. Because of the extensive array of potential consequences, the manner in which one learns to adapt or cope with these distressing changes may significantly influence his or her perceived quality of life and level of distress. Collectively, one's ability to cope with distressing changes related to the disease and/or its treatment may impact both short- and long-term health-related outcomes (Elani & Allison, 2011; Horney et al., 2011).

For instance, side effects may include difficulties related to essential functions such as breathing, eating, swallowing, and speech production, in addition to a loss of smell and taste, decreased sensation, sticky saliva, excessive dry mouth, pain, swelling, and facial disfigurement (Bornbaum et al., 2012; Doyle, 1994; Payakachat, Ounpraseuth, & Suen, 2012). Further, some institutions require those individuals receiving chemoradiation treatment to undergo prophylactic extraction of all dentition in an effort to prevent future dental and mandibular problems (Hunter & Jolly, 2013). Moreover, these myriad side effects stemming from complex treatment regimens HNCa often serve to impair daily functioning and one's ability to work or participate fully in avocational activities (Penner, 2009).

Disability and Employment

Research examining work-related disability in those with HNCa revealed that 52% of individuals who were employed at the time of diagnosis were unable to return to work following the completion of treatment (Taylor et al., 2004). Likewise, other researchers have reported a similar inability of individuals with HNCa to return to their previous employment for extended periods of time, if at all (Shone & Yardley, 1991; Taylor et al., 2004; Verdonck-de Leeuw, Van Bleek, Leemans, & de Bree, 2010). Even if those with HNCa are able to return to work following treatment, many have reported having to change their jobs because of poor health and/or physical discomfort related to treatment

consequences (Liu, 2008). When compared with other types of cancer, individuals with HNCa have reported the highest risk of quitting their jobs following treatment for their cancer (Short, Vasey, & Tunceli, 2005). This change in employment status may have significant implications for the financial and psychosocial well-being of these individuals (Taylor et al., 2004). With emerging data that the age of diagnosis for HNCa is increasingly younger, as well as the likelihood that treatment will be successful, one may survive for many decades with these treatment-related deficits.

Loss of Independence

In addition to the impact on one's employment status, further concerns may arise related to one's independence and ability to participate in social activities. This may also impact one's self image and relative value as a person (Crocker & Major, 1989; Schulz, Bookwala, Knapp, Scheier, & Williamson, 1996). To elaborate, research has shown that individuals treated for HNCa often either decrease the frequency of their driving or stop driving altogether during and after treatment because of treatment-related impairments, a potential result of shoulder dysfunction following neck dissection (Boulougouris & Doyle, 2018; Yuen, Gillespie, Day, Morgan, & Burik, 2007). Consequently, daily routines and tasks such as running errands or driving to and from work (if applicable) are disrupted, as those who have been treated for HNCa must increasingly rely on others (e.g., caregivers) for transportation (Yuen et al., 2007). This reliance on others to perform tasks which once symbolized independence (e.g., driving) may result in feelings of dependence and decreased self-worth in those with HNCa. As a result of these myriad concerns, individuals may experience substantial problems within the context of social and family settings. It is not, therefore, difficult to anticipate that the potential for social withdrawal (Doyle, 1994) and subsequent development of anxiety and depression may be observed (Pandey et al., 2007).

Visibility of Illness

Often, these concerns are exacerbated by the very visible side effects of HNCa and its treatment including the potential for physical disfigurement and scarring (Björklund, Sarvimäki, & Berg, 2010; Doyle, 1994). Physical changes secondary to treatment are common with HNCa; thus, there should be the anticipation that some change in body image will also occur. This in turn may lead to isolation and direct challenges to perceived quality of life (Doyle & MacDonald, Chap. 27). Because society tends to place more importance on the head and neck region than any other area of the body (Semple et al., 2004), gender-based considerations are essential. However, the work by Nash, Fung, MacNeil, Yoo, and Doyle (2014) has suggested that although women have been assumed to be more negatively impacted relative to changes in body image, men also demonstrate these concerns.

The emphasis on facial aesthetics and cosmesis may be particularly difficult for those with HNCa because the visible signs of HNCa and its treatment often cannot easily be concealed (Semple et al., 2004). Consequences such as these often prevent those with HNCa the privacy afforded by less visible forms of illness. As a result, those treated for HNCa may experience unwelcomed intrusions such as those associated with insensitive comments or staring (Björklund et al., 2010). These experiences may result in feelings of stigmatization which may then cause additional psychological distress (Doyle, 2005; Fife & Wright, 2000; Lebel et al., 2013). Factors such as these have led researchers to describe HNCa as the most emotionally traumatic form of cancer (Björklund et al., 2010; Koster & Bergsma, 1990).

Impact on Family and Loved Ones

Given that research has demonstrated a relationship between the emotional experiences of individuals with cancer and their caregivers (Northouse et al., 2001) – in essence suggesting that when one individual is distressed (e.g., person with HNCa),

the other individual may also be distressed (e.g., caregiver) – there appears to be a potential to experience emotional trauma as a result of either having or caring for someone with HNCa. Thus, as with any serious illness, others who are close to the person with HNCa may suffer as well. Essentially, the emotional trauma caused by HNCa and its treatment may directly influence the emotional state of caregivers (Hagedoorn, Sanderman, Bolks, Tuinstra, & Coyne, 2008). Importantly, researchers have begun to acknowledge that HNCa not only has enormous consequences for the individual with the disease but also for their loved ones and caregivers, as the entire family dynamic may be disrupted by the disease and its accompanying consequences (Björklund et al., 2010). In this regard, it is equally important to acknowledge the support systems to those impacted by cancer may provide an essential buffer for depression (De Leeuw, De Graeff, Ros, Hordijk, Blijham, & Winnubst, 2000).

De Leeuw et al. have acknowledged that support systems may carry both negative and positive influences for those with HNCa; however, there does appear to be some benefit, or protective effect, of support systems in reducing depression in some individuals. Thus, it would seem important to understand and acknowledge the concerns of both the individual with HNCa and their caregivers since improvements in our understanding of the caregiver experience may promote the identification of meaningful ways to support caregivers. If one wishes to address the true impact of HNCa on the individual, it cannot be done without direct consideration of others; this is most particularly true relative to immediate family members and loved ones. For that reason, those closest to the individual with HNCa cannot be overlooked.

Caregivers

The definition and use of the term "caregiver" have been discussed in the literature for several years (Hunt, 2003). Caregivers have been described as unpaid individuals who participate in the experiences and activities involved in the provision of assistance to a loved one who is unable to provide for themselves (Pearlin, 1994). Recently, authors have utilized the pragmatic suggestion that a caregiver is "who the person says it is" (Hodges & Humphris, 2009; Kissane & Bloch, 2002; Stenberg, Ruland, & Miaskowski, 2010), implying that the caregiver may consist of a blood relative, neighbor, friend, or other individual. Regardless of how the term caregiver is defined or who fulfills the role, providing care for another individual who has been diagnosed with cancer is an experience, shared closely with the recipient of care, which may affect numerous aspects of the caregiver's life.

It has been well established that family members of individuals with cancer are affected by the illness throughout the trajectory of the disease (Stenberg et al., 2010). For instance, the consequences of the disease continue to impact family members well into the survivorship stage for those who survive the illness and into the end of life care for those who do not (McCorkle & Pasacreta, 2001; Stenberg et al., 2010). Family members often provide the primary source of emotional and social support for individuals with cancer. They also serve a key role in how effectively an individual with cancer is able to manage the impact of their illness and its treatment (Zwahlen, Hagenbuch, Jenewein, Carley, & Buchi, 2011). Considering that hospital stays have decreased in length (Cohen, Stock, Andersen, & Everts, 1997; Yueh et al., 2003), individuals with cancer are increasingly left to manage their illness and its side effects at home. As a result, the burden of responsibility for family members has increased; this in turn has made the role of family-based caregiving ever more vital (Stenberg et al., 2010). This shift toward family-based caregiving often requires a reorganization of personal roles and responsibilities on the part of the caregiver. Such reorganization may be necessary to address the needs of the individual with cancer as well as to ensure that the family is still able to function effectively and perform essential tasks (e.g., raising children, paying bills, home maintenance).

The Role of Caregivers

Most often, the spouse or significant other of the individual with cancer fulfills the role of primary caregiver (Mellon, Northouse, & Weiss, 2006). Despite the fact that these loved ones often receive minimal or no preparation, they are frequently tasked with many care-related responsibilities such as the provision of physical care, medication administration, transportation, emotional support, household management, and assistance with activities of daily living (Northouse & McCorkle, 2010). The demand for these tasks to be undertaken is often within a very short period of time following the diagnosis of their loved one's cancer. While family caregivers have historically provided significant contributions to the care of their loved ones, the level of technical, physical, and psychological support currently required of caregivers has reached unparalleled levels in recent years (Given, Given, & Kozachik, 2001). This shift in burden of care toward caregivers results from healthcare system changes which have transferred the delivery of cancer care from an inpatient, hospital-based setting to ambulatory and home-based settings much sooner following treatment than in previous years (Cohen et al., 1997; Given et al., 2001; Yueh et al., 2003). This shift in care settings has translated to an increased level of caregiver involvement in the daily care of the individual with cancer (Given et al., 2001). Thus, since individuals are providing care for those with cancer much sooner following treatment (e.g., surgery), they must also deal with a more acute set of potential issues (e.g., wound care, infection, swallowing problems).

In addition to the disease- and treatment-related factors that caregivers are responsible for (e.g., disease and treatment monitoring, symptom management, medication administration, transportation to appointments), they must also ensure that the responsibilities usually fulfilled by the individual with cancer (e.g., errands, payment of bills, care for minor children, preparation of meals) are addressed. Ensuring the fulfillment of responsibilities may be particularly burdensome when the person with cancer is a spouse or family member, and the household tasks that were formerly shared between two individuals must now be accounted for by the caregiver alone. While this effort to preserve the normal level of family functioning is commendable, it can create feelings of role overload for the caregiver (Northouse & McCorkle, 2010). As the number of illness-related demands increases, caregivers experience numerous physical, psychological, and social consequences that potentially may exceed those experienced by the individual with cancer (Mellon et al., 2006). Moreover, research has demonstrated that as the level of demand on caregivers increases, they are placed at an elevated risk for the development of depression (Braun, Mikulincer, Rydall, Walsh, & Rodin, 2007). This elevated risk poses a problem not only for the caregiver's well-being but also may impact their ability to provide complex care to another when their own physical and mental health is compromised.

A review of the effects of caring for an individual with cancer conducted by Stenberg et al. (2010) identified more than 200 problems and burdens associated with being a caregiver. This large range of concerns included issues related to one's physical health, psychological state, social activities, and practical responsibilities. While the range of physical health concerns was quite extensive, the most commonly reported physical problems according to Stenberg et al. (2010) included pain, fatigue, sleep disturbances, loss of physical strength, loss of appetite, and weight loss; symptoms which would appear to mirror those of depression (Miller & Massie, 2009). Further complicating the situation, caregivers have been shown to prioritize the needs of the individual with cancer over their own (Williams, 2007), thus, leaving minimal time for maintaining activity and exercise, good nutrition, and regular healthcare check-ups. Consequently, caregivers experienced increased health-related concerns such as fatigue and sleep disturbances, which are exacerbated as symptom burden increases and functioning decreases in the individual with cancer (Palos et al., 2011). Symptom burden is a concept that is comprised of both the severity of symptoms and the individual's subjec-

tive perception of the impact of the symptoms on their daily life and level of functioning (Cleeland, 2007). As a result, one could infer that as the level of symptom burden increases in individuals with HNCa, so too does the level of burden in caregivers.

In addition to physical consequences reported by caregivers, they have also reported a diverse range of positive and negative psychological responses to their experience as a caregiver. Specifically, caregivers have described a spectrum of emotions ranging from positive affect such as hopefulness and compassion for others, to negative emotions such as, bitterness, resentment, fear, anger, depression, and anticipatory grief (Williams & Bakitas, 2012). Regarding the ability to fulfill the responsibilities of providing care, some caregivers have noted positive feelings of accomplishment, while others report feeling overwhelmed (Williams & Bakitas, 2012). Upon reflection of the caregiving experience, some individuals have found caregiving to be positive for their self-esteem (Kim, Schulz, & Carver, 2007), while others have found that managing tasks and emotions in the context of caring for a loved one was immensely difficult (Williams & Bakitas, 2012). Given the broad spectrum of emotional responses to the experience of caregiving, it is apparent that the act of providing care to a loved one with cancer is a complex experience that is marked by both positive and negative affect. In these types of situations, recent research has suggested that guided, self-help approaches that seek to facilitate problem-solving may be of benefit (Krebber et al., 2017).

The provision of care for an individual with cancer is often a challenging, disruptive, and time-consuming activity (Williams & Bakitas, 2012). Given the level of burden facing caregivers, it is not surprising that multiple studies report higher levels of anxiety and depression in caregivers than the patients themselves (Mellon et al., 2006; Vickery et al., 2003). This finding is of central importance to understanding the experience of distress in caregivers because it acknowledges the psychological impact of the diagnosis and treatment of the individual with cancer on the caregiver. The experience of illness and treatment is clearly different for caregivers. They are often faced with the very real prospect of losing their partner or loved one. Such a possibility may produce feelings of grief and helplessness because they are unable to take a direct role in combating the cancer (Vickery et al., 2003).

Relative to social consequences, caregivers have frequently reported problems with employment, education, isolation, financial well-being, and the ability to fulfill roles (Stenberg et al., 2010). When a loved one is diagnosed with cancer, understandably, there are changes in the roles, expectations, responsibilities, and relationship dynamics of the family as individuals adjust to the reality of such a diagnosis and impact of the disease (Northouse, Williams, Given, & McCorkle, 2012). Accordingly, the level of burden on caregivers often increases. This increased burden may be particularly evident in caregivers who must balance their caregiving responsibilities with the provision of care for children and/or ailing parents. These individuals may feel overwhelmed with the demands on their time and energy as they try to balance their responsibilities to their loved ones with their own personal and employment-related obligations (Coristine, Crooks, Grunfeld, Stonebridge, & Christie, 2003). Further, caregivers without flexible jobs or employers who can accommodate such needs have often been required to use sick leave and vacation time in order to fulfill their new and potentially rapidly expanding obligations, which may subsequently create an additional level of economic strain (Stenberg et al., 2010). Thus, it is apparent that the social consequences of being a caregiver extend beyond the realm of one's daily social participation in enjoyable activities, to also include the potential limitation of one's future occupational and economic stability.

With regard to the financial burden of caregiving, an American study of the time costs associated with informal caregiving for cancer survivors found that on average, caregivers provided 8.3 hours of care per day for 13.7 months (Yabroff & Kim, 2009). When the economic burden of caregiving was evaluated relative to the value of the caregiver's time providing care, the value of lost employment, and out-of-pocket expenditures

(e.g., transportation, parking, home modifications, cancer care supplies, etc.), the financial costs were considerable, ranging from $31,442 to $91,670, depending on the specific type of cancer (Van Houtven, Ramsey, Hornbrook, Atienza, & van Ryn, 2010). These estimates of time costs and out-of-pocket expenditures highlight the substantial financial burden that often may be experienced by caregivers.

In addition to the financial stressors noted previously, caregivers have reported feelings of isolation (Northouse, Williams, et al., 2012; Williams & Bakitas, 2012). Not only does the work of caregiving disrupt their opportunity to engage socially with others (Stetz & Brown, 2004), but the caregiver's personal needs are often neglected as their focus remains on the needs of the individual with cancer (Schubart, Kinzie, & Farace, 2008). Feelings of isolation and loneliness were particularly significant in caregivers without access to family or friends (Schubart et al., 2008). The inherent difficulty in serving as a caregiver to a loved one with cancer lies in both the overwhelming nature of the role and the fact that despite one's best effort, the individual with cancer may still suffer and possibly succumb to their illness. Thus, the fear of losing a loved one may in and of itself induce tremendous feelings of anticipatory grief in the caregiver.

Caregivers are expected to grieve while simultaneously supporting the physical, psychological, social, and practical needs of their loved one. They must also work to maintain their regular family and employment-related responsibilities while balancing their own fears, anxieties, and concerns for the well-being of their loved one. Research seeking to understand the experience of caregivers has suggested that the provision of care for an individual with cancer may constitute a distressing life experience (Longacre, Ridge, Burtness, Galloway, & Fang, 2012; Roing, Hirsch, & Holstrom, 2008). Since the presence of elevated distress in caregivers has been identified as a factor that may compromise both the physical health and psychological well-being of both caregivers and individuals with cancer (Hagedoorn et al., 2008; Northouse et al., 2001), investigations into the factors which can influence distress may inform our understanding of the caregiver experience. Improved knowledge regarding the factors that contribute to and/or exacerbate distress may help to identify meaningful ways to both detect and possibly alleviate distress in these individuals.

Coping and Adjustment

While most individuals will eventually adapt to the changes brought on by the cancer experience (Vickery et al., 2003), a subset of individuals will experience distress to the extent that adaptive coping is impaired severely enough or long enough to be considered disruptive (Haman, 2008). A few days characterized by tearfulness and decreased interest in regular activities may be viewed as a component of adaptive coping to the changes and losses for both the individual with cancer and the caregiver (Haman, 2008). However, if the symptoms persist for extended periods of time – some sources suggest more than 1 week (Haman, 2008), while others advocate for at least 2 weeks or more (APA, 2000) – problems may arise with social support networks and one's physical well-being and influence even treatment compliance and survival in individuals with cancer (Haman, 2008). Notably, certain symptoms such as suicidal ideation with accompanying plan and intent require immediate intervention, even if the symptoms only last for short periods of time.

Generally, it has been suggested that if distress persists for greater than a week, leads to noncompliance with treatment recommendations (McDonough, Boyd, Varvares, & Maves, 1996), or puts the individual (or others) in danger, intervention is required (Haman, 2008). Ideally, problematic distress in both those with cancer and their caregivers should be identified and addressed in order to avoid negative outcomes such as, fatigue, weight loss, decreased medical compliance, and increased hospital stays (DiMatteo, Lepper, & Croghan, 2000) in those with cancer, and compromised psychological functioning, and changes to the immune system that limit glucose control and increase

cardiovascular vulnerability (Rohleder, Marin, Ma, & Miller, 2009) in caregivers.

Distress in Individuals with Head and Neck Cancer

Normal emotions such as sadness, worry, and fear occur in every person and are undoubtedly exacerbated by a diagnosis of any serious disease such as cancer. Clinical psychiatric disorders such as depression and anxiety do not develop overnight; rather, they are the cumulative outcome along the continuum of mental health that extends beyond normal emotional responses and psychological reactions (Mohan & Pandey, 2002). Research has established that across the trajectory of illness – from initial diagnosis through treatment, termination of treatment, survivorship, or recurrence and palliation – psychosocial distress is evident in approximately 25–45% of those with cancer (Carlson, 2003; Carlson et al., 2004; Singer et al., 2012; Zabora, Brintzenhofeszoc, Curbow, Hooker, & Piantadosi, 2001). Moreover, large-scale studies conducted at the Tom Baker Cancer Centre in Alberta, Canada (Carlson et al., 2004), and the Johns Hopkins Kimmel Cancer Center in Baltimore, Maryland (Zabora et al., 2001), of a representative sample of individuals screened for psychosocial distress detected high levels of fatigue (in nearly 50% of patients), depression (24%), anxiety (24%), and pain (26%), in addition to financial hardship and other challenges. Distress is a common sequela of cancer as a disease and, thus, requires careful clinical consideration.

From a therapeutic perspective, untreated depression has been shown to affect medical compliance, appetite, and wound healing and contribute to increases in length of hospital stays (DiMatteo et al., 2000; Jenkins, Carmody, & Rush, 1998; McDonough et al., 1996). Furthermore, the impact of depression on functions such as sleep, motivation, and energy level is also well documented (Roscoe et al., 2007). By intensifying fatigue and weight loss, depression has the potential to amplify treatment-related side effects for individuals with cancer, contributing to a vicious cycle that may not only worsen depression and overall rates of distress but also negatively influence disease control through decreased medical compliance (DiMatteo et al., 2000).

Relative to the impact of depression on medical compliance, research has demonstrated that depressed individuals with cancer take more breaks in treatment and thus require a greater length of time in order to complete the prescribed treatment protocol (Archer, Hutchison, & Korszun, 2008; Starmer, 2018). These findings have critical implications for individuals with HNCa given that the success of radiation therapy – one of the key forms of treatment for HNCa – is dependent in part on the completion of therapy as close as possible to the prescribed time (Lydiatt, Moran, & Burke, 2009). In consideration of these factors, the chances of survival are likely to be lessened in those individuals who experience depression, when compared to those individuals who are not depressed (Archer et al., 2008). Thus, given the numerous challenges facing an individual with cancer, support from caregivers is essential in order to facilitate successful coping, adjustment, and sometimes even survival (Foster et al., 2005). As a result, understanding the factors that contribute to elevated distress would appear to be an important component to ensuring the optimal well-being of both those with cancer and their caregivers.

Distress in Caregivers

While cancer has been shown to impact the quality of life of caregivers in myriad ways, researchers have recently suggested that the psychological well-being of caregivers is the area most significantly impacted during the initial stages of the caregiving experience (Northouse, Katapodi, Schafenacker, & Weiss, 2012). When the level of demand for care that is placed on caregivers exceeds their available resources (e.g., psychological wherewithal, personal coping mechanisms, social support), caregivers report feeling overwhelmed and distressed (Drabe, Wittmann, Zwahlen, Büchi, & Jenewein, 2012). Distress in

caregivers is problematic for two key reasons: first for the problems that it poses to caregivers personally and second for the consequent impact on the individuals with cancer. Both the personal consequences of distress for caregivers and the resultant impact on those with cancer are discussed hereunder.

Relative to the personal toll of distress on caregivers, research indicates that between 20% and 40% of caregivers experience high levels of distress or depression (Edwards & Clarke, 2004; Longacre et al., 2012). However these incidence rates increased when the individual with cancer demonstrated poor physical functioning, high symptom distress, and advanced disease (Kurtz, Kurtz, Given, & Given, 2004). The prevalence of high emotional distress in caregivers is problematic for multiple reasons. Not only does it compromise their psychological well-being, but highly distressed caregivers may also experience changes to their immune system that can limit glucose control, promote flare-ups in autoimmune diseases, and increase vulnerability to cardiovascular diseases (Rohleder et al., 2009). These biologic consequences of distress increase the potential for the caregiver's own health to suffer and, consequently, impede their ability to provide adequate care to the individual with cancer.

Regarding the impact of caregiver distress on individuals with cancer, research indicates that because of caregivers' negative emotional states and impaired cognitive and physical functioning, caregivers have more difficulty with the effective administration of medication (Lau et al., 2010) and provision of optimal care (Park et al., 2009; van Ryn et al., 2011) to individuals with cancer. With respect to psychological functioning, high levels of anxiety in caregivers have been shown to increase anxiety in the individuals with cancer (Segrin et al., 2007), and longitudinal data suggest that when caregivers are highly distressed, there is a significant negative effect on the long-term adjustment of the individual with cancer (Northouse et al., 2001).

The findings of Northouse et al. (2001) are in line with the work of Hagedoorn et al. (2008) who conducted a meta-analysis of 46 studies that examined distress in couples coping with cancer

(n = 2468 couples). They discovered a significant relationship between distress in caregivers and those with cancer (r = 0.29, p < 0.001) even after controlling for illness-related factors (e.g., disease stage). These findings indicate that both the individual with cancer and their caregiver's emotional responses to the illness were interrelated. These results suggest that individuals with cancer and their caregivers react to the experience of cancer as an "emotional system" and that both the individual and their caregiver(s) should be viewed as the recipients of care from the perspective of health practitioners (Northouse, Katapodi, et al., 2012).

Benefits of Distress Management

Researchers have reported that psychosocial distress is evident in approximately 25–45% of individuals with cancer in North America (Carlson, Waller, Groff, Giese-Davis, & Bultz, 2013; Hurria et al., 2009; Zabora et al., 2001). Similar rates of distress have been reported in Asia (Kim et al., 2013; Lam, Shing, Bonanno, Mancini, & Fielding, 2012), South America (Decat, de Araujo, & Stiles, 2011), Europe (Andreu et al., 2012; Hofsø, Rustøen, Cooper, Bjordal, & Miaskowski, 2012), Africa (Peltzer, Pengpid, & Skaal, 2012), Australia (Dunn et al., 2012), and the Middle East (Omran, Saeed, & Simpson, 2012). The consistency of distress prevalence is interesting given that an individual's perception of their disease varies greatly across cultures (Erbil et al., 1996). For instance, there are a number of documented culture-related variables that may influence distress and perceived quality of life levels among individuals with cancer. These include attitudes and adjustment toward health and illness, perceptions regarding the cause of disease, the role of the physician in one's care, the interaction style between the practitioner and the individual with cancer, the role of one's family, the individual's needs and coping mechanisms, and the personal demographic factors such as one's age and socioeconomic status (Gordon, 1990; Kleinman, 1986; Thomas, Carlson, & Bultz, 2009).

Given the documented cultural differences influencing perception of illness, it is noteworthy that the rates of distress among individuals with cancer remain so consistent globally. Nevertheless, the similar international prevalence rates imply that psychological distress related to cancer is a common, persistent, and universal concern that transcends cultural differences and as a result should be addressed in a clinically meaningful manner. Thus, exploring the unresolved psychological needs of individuals with cancer may provide information that could be generalized to those with cancer across the cultural spectrum.

When the psychological needs of individuals with cancer remain unresolved, these individuals are more likely to visit emergency rooms and make use of community health services (Carlson & Bultz, 2004). This increased service utilization is related to the physical symptoms resulting from psychological distress such as sleep disturbances, headaches, and gastrointestinal symptoms (Carlson & Bultz, 2004; Doyle, Day, Whitney, Myers, & Eadie, 2009). Consequently, these individuals place greater demands on the increasingly scarce time of their healthcare providers. Additionally, clinical studies have demonstrated that certain forms of psychosocial intervention (e.g., cognitive behavioral therapy, psychoeducational interventions) are beneficial to individuals with cancer (Chambers, Pinnock, Lepore, Hughes, & O'Connell, 2011; Fors et al., 2010; Hammerlid et al., 1999; Newell, Sanson-Fisher, & Savolainen, 2002).

For instance, a systematic review conducted by Newell et al. (2002) found that psychosocial interventions involving counseling (either structured or unstructured) and guided imagery have been shown to improve quality of life and the general functioning of individuals with cancer. Furthermore, participants from multiple studies asserted that they would use the psychological resources again and would recommend them to other individuals diagnosed with cancer (Hamilton, Miedema, MacIntyre, & Easley, 2011; Miller et al., 1998). Thus, this information suggests that if psychological distress can be identified early and addressed in a meaningful manner (i.e., lessened or alleviated), then perhaps not only can we improve the overall functioning of individuals with cancer, but we may also be able to reduce the economic burden on the healthcare system that arises as a result of untreated or poorly managed distress.

Several reviews of the literature have noted that psychological therapies may assist individuals in several ways including improving sexual functioning (Penedo et al., 2007); enhancing quality of life, emotional adjustment, and coping skills (Hamilton et al., 2011; Henderson et al., 2011); and increasing physical health and functional adjustment (Penedo et al., 2007). Further, such intervention has been reported to reduce disease- and treatment-related symptoms in individuals with cancer (Hart et al., 2012) and general physical symptoms in caregivers (Birnie, Garland, & Carlson, 2010). Addressing negative psychosocial outcomes such as distress is a critical component to the delivery of comprehensive healthcare. Without the early identification of problematic distress levels, individuals may experience innumerable consequences related to physical, psychological, and social functioning – the core components of one's evaluation of their perceived quality of life. Therefore, these consequences may ultimately result in decreased quality of life for those living with cancer, as well as the well-being and quality of life of their caregivers.

Thus, efforts to support the identification of distress in both individuals with cancer and their caregivers should be undertaken in an effort to inform the individuals charged with their care (and those most suited to assisting them) of when the level of psychosocial concern (e.g., distress) has reached a problematic point and specifically where intervention efforts may be directed in order to be of most benefit. Fortunately, a number of validated instruments have been devised which are capable of assessing the level of an individual's perceived distress and their accompanying multidimensional concerns. The use of these tools in both clinical environments may help to develop a better understanding of not only the prevalence of distress in individuals with HNCa and their caregivers but also the specific problems that these individuals face and the consequent impact of this distress and these perceived problems on their quality of life and daily functioning.

A diagnosis of HNCa carries with it a unique set of treatment-related challenges that influence physical function, social interaction, and emotional expression. Not surprisingly, treatment of HNCa has been associated with some of the highest rates of anxiety, depression, and suicide when compared with other cancer sites (Bjordal & Kaasa, 1995; Kendal, 2006; Misono et al., 2008). These findings suggest that HNCa is highly traumatic psychosocially with a multitude of complex patient concerns emerging.

Relative to the caregiver experience, these individuals are expected to support the physical, psychological, social, and practical needs of their loved one while simultaneously grieving their own losses – both real and anticipated. They must also work to maintain their regular family and employment-related responsibilities while balancing their fears, anxieties, and concerns for the well-being of their loved one. Ultimately, the provision of care for an individual with cancer may be a challenging, disruptive, and time-consuming endeavor (Williams & Bakitas, 2012). Given the level of burden facing caregivers, it is not surprising that multiple studies report higher levels of anxiety and depression in caregivers than in the individuals with cancer (Mellon et al., 2006; Vickery et al., 2003).

Conclusions

Acknowledgment of the "human side" of cancer care is essential to a compassionate and well-managed cancer care program. The time has come for healthcare providers, and the healthcare system at large, to acknowledge the roles of distress and quality of life as fundamental components of healthcare. Through understanding the relationship between distress and modifiable psychosocial factors, tailored interventions may be constructed with the goal of maximizing individual quality of life and reducing personal distress. Given the well-established and significant multidimensional challenges associated with HNCa, the aforementioned findings highlight the critical need to acknowledge, understand, and elucidate psychosocial distress in both those with HNCa and their caregivers.

Psychological distress related to cancer is a persistent and universal concern that transcends cultural differences and as a result must be addressed in a clinically meaningful manner. Despite this acknowledgment, less than 10% of distressed individuals are identified and referred to the appropriate psychosocial resources (Kadan-Lottick, Vanderwerker, Block, Zhang, & Prigerson, 2005). Failure to acknowledge and treat elevated distress among individuals with HNCa jeopardizes treatment outcomes, decreases quality of life, and increases healthcare costs (Zabora et al., 2001). Thus, in order to minimize the overall negative impact of HNCa and address the consequences of its treatment, distress requires careful clinical consideration. Distress may result in reductions in perceived quality of life, and, thus, efforts are encouraged to understand the presence of and variation in distress and quality of life across both individuals with HNCa and their caregivers.

References

Andreu, Y., Galdón, M. J., Durá, E., Martínez, P., Pérez, S., & Murgui, S. (2012). A longitudinal study of psychosocial distress in breast cancer: Prevalence and risk factors. *Psychology & Health, 27*(1), 72–87. https://doi.org/10.1080/08870446.2010.542814

APA. (2000). *Diagnostic and statistical manual of mental disorders – 4th Edition Text Revision (DSM-IV-TR, 2000)*. In A. P. Association (Ed.). Retrieved from http://online.statref.com.proxy1.lib.uwo.ca/Document.aspx?docAddress=4PNCnYvddqP04-isS-3QEw%3d%3d&SessionId=1A9C4CBJVGMKQUIG&Scroll=1&goBestMatch=true&Index=10&searchContext=DSM-IV-TR|c0||10|0|0|0|0|0||c0

Archer, J., Hutchison, I., & Korszun, A. (2008). Mood and malignancy: Head and neck cancer and depression. *Journal of Oral Pathology & Medicine, 37*(5), 255–270. https://doi.org/10.1111/j.1600-0714.2008.00635.x

Birnie, K., Garland, S. N., & Carlson, L. E. (2010). Psychological benefits for cancer patients and their partners participating in mindfulness-based stress reduction (MBSR). *Psycho-Oncology, 19*(9), 1004–1009. https://doi.org/10.1002/pon.1651

Bjordal, K., & Kaasa, S. (1995). Psychological distress in head and neck cancer patients 7–11 years after curative treatment. *Br J Cancer, 71*, 592–597.

Björklund, M., Sarvimäki, A., & Berg, A. (2010). Living with head and neck cancer: A profile of captivity. *Journal of Nursing and Healthcare of Chronic Illness, 2*(1), 22–31. https://doi.org/10.1111/j.1752-9824.2010.01042.x

Blood, G. W., Simpson, K. C., Dineen, M., Kauffman, S. M., & Raimondi, S. C. (1994). Spouses of individuals with laryngeal cancer: Caregiver strain and burden. *Journal of Communication Disorders, 27*, 19–35.

Bornbaum C. (2013). *Measuring the sixth vital sign: A descriptive analysis of distress in individuals with head and neck cancer and their caregivers*. Dissertation. Western University. Available from: https://ir.lib.uwo.ca/cgi/viewcontent.cgi?article=3070&context=etd

Bornbaum, C. C., Fung, K., Franklin, J. H., Nichols, A., Yoo, J., & Doyle, P. C. (2012). A descriptive analysis of the relationship between quality of life and distress in individuals with head and neck cancer. *Support Care Cancer, 20*(9), 2157–2165. https://doi.org/10.1007/s00520-011-1326-2

Boulougouris, A., & Doyle, P. C. (2018). Shoulder dysfunction and disability secondary to treatment for head and neck cancer. In P. C. Doyle (Ed.), *Clinical care and rehabilitation in head and neck cancer*. Cham, Switzerland: Springer.

Braun, M., Mikulincer, M., Rydall, A., Walsh, A., & Rodin, G. (2007). Hidden morbidity in cancer: Spouse caregivers. *Journal of Clinical Oncology, 25*(30), 4829–4834. https://doi.org/10.1200/jco.2006.10.0909

Carlson, L. (2003). Cancer distress screening needs, models, and methods. *Journal of Psychosomatic Research, 55*(5), 403–409. https://doi.org/10.1016/s0022-3999(03)00514-2

Carlson, L., & Bultz, B. (2004). Efficacy and medical cost offset of psychosocial interventions in cancer care: Making the case for economic analyses. *Psycho-Oncology, 13*(12), 837–849. https://doi.org/10.1002/pon.832

Carlson, L. E., Angen, M., Cullum, J., Goodey, E., Koopmans, J., Lamont, L., … Bultz, B. D. (2004). High levels of untreated distress and fatigue in cancer patients. *British Journal of Cancer, 90*, 2297–2304. https://doi.org/10.1038/sj.bjc.6601887

Carlson, L. E., Waller, A., Groff, S. L., Giese-Davis, J., & Bultz, B. D. (2013). What goes up does not always come down: Patterns of distress, physical and psychosocial morbidity in people with cancer over a one year period. *Psycho-Oncology, 22*(1), 168–176. https://doi.org/10.1002/pon.2068

Chambers, S. K., Pinnock, C., Lepore, S. J., Hughes, S., & O'Connell, D. L. (2011). A systematic review of psychosocial interventions for men with prostate cancer and their partners. *Patient Education and Counseling, 85*(2), e75–e88. https://doi.org/10.1016/j.pec.2011.01.027

Cleeland, C. S. (2007). Symptom burden: Multiple symptoms and their impact as patient-reported outcomes.

JNCI Monographs, 2007(37), 16–21. https://doi.org/10.1093/jncimonographs/lgm005

Cohen, J., Stock, M., Andersen, P., & Everts, E. (1997). Critical pathways for head and neck surgery: Development and implementation. *Archives of Otolaryngology Head and Neck Surgery, 123*(1), 11–14. https://doi.org/10.1001/archotol.1997.01900010013001

Coristine, M., Crooks, D., Grunfeld, E., Stonebridge, C., & Christie, A. (2003). Caregiving for women with advanced breast cancer. *Psycho-Oncology, 12*(7), 709–719. https://doi.org/10.1002/pon.696

Crocker, J., & Major, B. (1989). Social stigma and self-esteem: The self-protective properties of stigma. *Psychological Review, 96*(4), 608.

Decat, C. S. A., de Araujo, T. C. C. F., & Stiles, J. (2011). Distress levels in patients undergoing chemotherapy in Brazil. *Psycho-Oncology, 20*(10), 1130–1133. https://doi.org/10.1002/pon.1833

De Leeuw, J. R., De Graeff, A., Ros, W. J., Hordijk, G. J., Blijham, G. H., & Winnubst, J. A. (2000). Negative and positive influences of social support on depression in patients with head and neck cancer: a prospective study. *Psycho-Oncology, 9*(1), 20–28. Retrieved from: https://onlinelibrary.wiley.com/doi/abs/10.1002/(SICI)1099-1611(200001/02)9:1%3C20::AIDPON425%3E3.0.CO;2-Y.

DiMatteo, M. R., Lepper, H. S., & Croghan, T. W. (2000). Depression is a risk factor for noncompliance with medical treatment: Meta-analysis of the effects of anxiety and depression on patient adherence. *Arch Intern Med, 160*, 2101–2107.

Doyle, P. C. (1994). *Foundations of voice and speech rehabilitation following laryngeal cancer*. San Diego, CA: Singular Publishing Group.

Doyle, P. C. (2005). Rehabilitation in head and neck cancer: Overview. In P. C. Doyle & R. L. Keith (Eds.), *Contemporary consideration in the treatment and rehabilitation of head and neck cancer: Voice, speech, and swallowing*. Austin, TX: Pro-Ed.

Doyle, P. C., Day, A., Whitney, H. D., Myers, C., & Eadie, T. L. (2009). The utility of symptom checklists in long-term postlaryngectomy follow-up of tracheoesophageal speakers. *Canadian Journal of Speech-Language Pathology & Audiology, 33*(4), 174–182.

Drabe, N., Wittmann, L., Zwahlen, D., Büchi, S., & Jenewein, J. (2012). Changes in close relationships between cancer patients and their partners. *Psycho-Oncology, 22*, 1344–1352. https://doi.org/10.1002/pon.3144

Dunn, J., Ng, S. K., Holland, J., Aitken, J., Youl, P., Baade, P. D., & Chambers, S. K. (2012). Trajectories of psychological distress after colorectal cancer. *Psycho-Oncology, 22*, 1759–1765. https://doi.org/10.1002/pon.3210

Edwards, B., & Clarke, V. (2004). The psychological impact of a cancer diagnosis on families: The influence of family functioning and patients' illness characteristics on depression and anxiety. *Psycho-Oncology, 13*(8), 562–576. https://doi.org/10.1002/pon.773

Elani, H. W., & Allison, P. J. (2011). Coping and psychological distress among head and neck cancer patients. *Supportive Care in Cancer, 19*(11), 1735–1741. https://doi.org/10.1007/s00520-010-1013-8

Erbil, P., Razavi, D., Farvacques, C., Bilge, N., Paesmans, M., & Van Houtte, P. (1996). Cancer patients psychological adjustment and perception of illness: Cultural differences between Belgium and Turkey. *Supportive Care in Cancer, 4*, 455–461.

Fife, B. L., & Wright, E. R. (2000). The dimensionality of stigma: A comparison of its impact on the self of persons with HIV/AIDS and cancer. *Journal of Health and Social Behaviour, 41*, 50–67.

Fors, E. A., Bertheussen, G. F., Thune, I., Juvet, L. K., Elvsaas, I.-K. Ø., Oldervoll, L., ... Leivseth, G. (2010). Psychosocial interventions as part of breast cancer rehabilitation programs? Results from a systematic review. *Psycho-Oncology, 20*, 909–918. https://doi.org/10.1002/pon.1844

Foster, L. W., McLellan, L. J., Rybicki, L. A., Sassano, D. A., Hsu, A., & Bolwell, B. J. (2005). Survival of patients who have undergone allogeneic bone marrow transplantation. *Journal of Psychosocial Oncology, 22*(2), 1–20. https://doi.org/10.1300/J077v22n02_01

Given, B. A., Given, C. W., & Kozachik, S. (2001). Family support in advanced cancer. *Ca: A Cancer Journal for Clinicians, 51*, 213–231.

Gordon, D. (1990). Embodying illness, embodying cancer. *Culture, Medicine and Psychiatry., 14*(2), 275–297.

Hagedoorn, M., Sanderman, R., Bolks, H. N., Tuinstra, J., & Coyne, J. C. (2008). Distress in couples coping with cancer: A meta-analysis and critical review of role and gender effects. *Psychological Bulletin, 134*(1), 1–30. https://doi.org/10.1037/0033-2909.134.1.1

Haman, K. L. (2008). Psychologic distress in head and neck cancer: Part 1 – review of the literature. *Journal of Supportive Oncology, 6*(4), 155–163.

Hamilton, R., Miedema, B., MacIntyre, L., & Easley, J. (2011). Using a positive self-talk intervention to enhance coping skills in breast cancer survivors: Lessons from a community-based group delivery model. *Current Oncology, 18*(2), e46–e53.

Hammerlid, E., Ahlner-Elmqvist, M., Bjordal, K., Biorklund, A., Evensen, J., Boysen, M., ... Westin, T. (1999). A prospective multicentre study in Sweden and Norway of mental distress and psychiatric morbidity in head and neck cancer patients. *British Journal of Cancer, 80*(5–6), 766–774. https://doi.org/10.1038/sj.bjc.6690420

Hart, S. L., Hoyt, M. A., Diefenbach, M., Anderson, D. R., Kilbourn, K. M., Craft, L. L., ... Stanton, A. L. (2012). Meta-analysis of efficacy of interventions for elevated depressive symptoms in adults diagnosed with cancer. *JNCI Journal of the National Cancer Institute, 104*(13), 990–1004. https://doi.org/10.1093/jnci/djs256

Henderson, V. P., Clemow, L., Massion, A. O., Hurley, T. G., Druker, S., & Hébert, J. R. (2011). The effects of mindfulness-based stress reduction on psychosocial outcomes and quality of life in early-stage breast cancer patients: A randomized trial. *Breast Cancer Research and Treatment, 131*(1), 99–109. https://doi.org/10.1007/s10549-011-1738-1

Hodges, L. J., & Humphris, G. M. (2009). Fear of recurrence and psychological distress in head and neck cancer patients and their carers. *Psycho-Oncology, 18*(8), 841–848. https://doi.org/10.1002/pon.1346

Hofsø, K., Rustøen, T., Cooper, B. A., Bjordal, K., & Miaskowski, C. (2012). Changes over time in occurrence, severity, and distress of common symptoms during and after radiation therapy for breast cancer. *Journal of Pain and Symptom Management., 45*, 980–1006. https://doi.org/10.1016/j.jpainsymman.2012.06.003

Horney, D. J., Smith, H. E., McGurk, M., Weinman, J., Herold, J., Altman, K., & Llewellyn, C. D. (2011). Associations between quality of life, coping styles, optimism, and anxiety and depression in pretreatment patients with head and neck cancer. *Head Neck, 33*(1), 65–71. https://doi.org/10.1002/hed.21407

Howren, M. B., Christensen, A. J., Karnell, L. H., & Funk, G. F. (2012). Psychological factors associated with head and neck cancer treatment and survivorship: Evidence and opportunities for behavioral medicine. *Journal of Consulting and Clinical Psychology, 81*, 299–317. https://doi.org/10.1037/a0029940

Hunt, C. K. (2003). Concepts in caregiver research. *Journal of Nursing Scholarship, 35*(1), 27–32.

Hunter, K. U., & Jolly, S. (2013). Clinical review of physical activity and functional considerations in head and neck cancer patients. *Supportive Care in Cancer, 21*, 1475–1479. https://doi.org/10.1007/s00520-013-1736-4

Hurria, A., Li, D., Hansen, K., Patil, S., Gupta, R., Nelson, C., … Kelly, E. (2009). Distress in older patients with cancer. *Journal of Clinical Oncology, 27*(26), 4346–4351. https://doi.org/10.1200/jco.2008.19.9463

Jenkins, C., Carmody, T. J., & Rush, J. (1998). Depression in radiation oncology patients: A preliminary evaluation. *Journal of Affective Disorders, 50*, 17–21.

Kadan-Lottick, N. S., Vanderwerker, L. C., Block, S. D., Zhang, B., & Prigerson, H. G. (2005). Psychiatric disorders and mental health service use in patients with advanced cancer. *Cancer, 104*(12), 2872–2881.

Kendal, W. (2006). Suicide and cancer: A gender-comparative study. *Annals of Oncology, 18*(2), 381–387. https://doi.org/10.1093/annonc/mdl385

Kim, J.-H., Yoon, S., Won, W.-Y., Lee, C., Lee, C.-U., Song, K. Y., … Kim, T.-S. (2013). Age-specific influences of emotional distress on performance status in cancer patients. *Psycho-Oncology, 22*(10), 2220–2226. https://doi.org/10.1002/pon.3276

Kim, Y., Schulz, R., & Carver, C. S. (2007). Benefit finding in the cancer caregiving experience. *Psychosomatic Medicine, 69*(3), 283–291. https://doi.org/10.1097/PSY.0b013e3180417cf4

Kissane, D., & Bloch, S. (2002). *Family focused grief therapy*. Oxford: Oxford University Press.

Kleinman, A. (1986). Culture, quality of life and cancer pain: Anthropological and cross-cultural perspectives. In V. Ventafridda, F. Van Dam, R. Yanick, &

M. Tamburini (Eds.), *Assessment of quality of life and cancer treatment* (pp. 43–49). New York, NY: Elsevier.

Koster, M. E. T. A., & Bergsma, J. (1990). Problems and coping behaviour of facial cancer patients. *Social Science & Medicine, 30*(5), 569–578. https://doi.org/10.1016/0277-9536(90)90155-L

Krebber, A. M. H., van Uden-Kraan, C. F., Melissant, H. C., Cuijpers, P., van Straten, A., Becker-Commissaris, A., … Verdonck-de Leeuw, I. M. (2017). A guided self-help intervention targeting psychological distress among head and neck cancer and lung cancer patients: Motivation to start, experiences and perceived outcomes. *Supportive Care in Cancer, 25*(1), 127–135.

Kurtz, M. E., Kurtz, J. C., Given, C. W., & Given, B. A. (2004). Depression and physical health among family caregivers of geriatric patients with cancer--a longitudinal view. *Medical Science Monitor: International Medical Journal of Experimental and Clinical Research, 10*(8), CR447–CR456.

Lam, W. W. T., Shing, Y. T., Bonanno, G. A., Mancini, A. D., & Fielding, R. (2012). Distress trajectories at the first year diagnosis of breast cancer in relation to 6 years survivorship. *Psycho-Oncology, 21*(1), 90–99. https://doi.org/10.1002/pon.1876

Lau, D. T., Berman, R., Halpern, L., Pickard, A. S., Schrauf, R., & Witt, W. (2010). Exploring factors that influence informal caregiving in medication management for home hospice patients. *Journal of Palliative Medicine, 13*(9), 1085–1090. https://doi.org/10.1089/jpm.2010.0082

Lebel, S., Castonguay, M., Mackness, G., Irish, J., Bezjak, A., & Devins, G. M. (2013). The psychosocial impact of stigma in people with head and neck or lung cancer. *Psycho-Oncology, 22*(1), 140–152. https://doi.org/10.1002/pon.2063

Lev, E., & McCorkle, R. (1998). Loss, grief, and bereavement in family members of cancer patients. *Seminars in Oncology Nursing, 14*(2), 145–151.

Liu, H.-E. (2008). Changes of satisfaction with appearance and working status for head and neck tumour patients. *Journal of Clinical Nursing, 17*(14), 1930–1938. https://doi.org/10.1111/j.1365-2702.2008.02291.x

Longacre, M. L., Ridge, J. A., Burtness, B. A., Galloway, T. J., & Fang, C. Y. (2012). Psychological functioning of caregivers for head and neck cancer patients. *Oral Oncology, 48*(1), 18–25. https://doi.org/10.1016/j.oraloncology.2011.11.012

Lydiatt, W. M., Moran, J., & Burke, W. J. (2009). A review of depression in the head and neck cancer patient. *Clinical Advances in Hematology & Oncology, 7*(6), 397–403.

McCorkle, R., & Pasacreta, J. V. (2001). Enhancing caregiver outcomes in palliative care. *Cancer Control, 8*(1), 36–45.

McDonough, E., Boyd, J., Varvares, M., & Maves, M. (1996). Relationship between psychological status and compliance in a sample of patients treated for cancer of the head and neck. *Head & Neck, 18*, 269–276.

Mellon, S., Northouse, L. L., & Weiss, L. K. (2006). A population-based study of the quality of life of cancer survivors and their family caregivers. *Cancer Nursing, 29*(2), 120–131.

Miller, K., & Massie, M. J. (2009). Depressive disorders. In J. C. Holland (Ed.), *Psycho-oncology* (pp. 311–318). New York, NY: Oxford University Press.

Miller, M., Boyer, M., Butow, P., Gattellari, M., Dunn, S., & Childs, A. (1998). The use of unproven methods of treatment by cancer patients: Frequency, expectations and cost. *Supportive Care in Cancer, 6*, 337–347.

Misono, S., Weiss, N. S., Fann, J. R., Redman, M., & Yueh, B. (2008). Incidence of suicide in persons with cancer. *Journal of Clinical Oncology, 26*(29), 4731–4738. https://doi.org/10.1200/jco.2007.13.8941

Mohan, T. B., & Pandey, T. I. (2002). Development of a distress inventory for cancer: Preliminary results. *Journal of Postgraduate Medicine, 48*(1), 16–20.

Nash, M. M. (2014). *Body image and quality of life: An exploration among individuals with head and neck cancer*. Electronic Thesis and Dissertation Repository. 2295. https://ir.lib.uwo.ca/etd/2295.

NCCN. (2013). NCCN clinical practice guidelines in oncology: Distress Management 2.2013. Retrieved from http://www.nccn.org/professionals/physician_gls/pdf/distress.pdf

Newell, S. A., Sanson-Fisher, R. W., & Savolainen, N. J. (2002). Systematic review of psychological therapies for cancer patients: Overview and recommendations for future research. *Journal of the National Cancer Institute, 94*(8), 559–584.

Northouse, L., Templin, T., & Mood, D. (2001). Couples' adjustment to breast disease during the first year following diagnosis. *Journal of Behavioral Medicine, 24*(2), 115–136.

Northouse, L., Williams, A. L., Given, B., & McCorkle, R. (2012). Psychosocial care for family caregivers of patients with cancer. Journal of Clinical Oncology, 30(11), 1227–1234. https://doi.org/10.1200/jco.2011.39.5798.

Northouse, L. L., Katapodi, M. C., Schafenacker, A. M., & Weiss, D. (2012). The impact of caregiving on the psychological well-being of family caregivers and cancer patients. *seminars in Oncology Nursing, 28*(4), 236–245. https://doi.org/10.1016/j.soncn.2012.09.006

Northouse, L. L., & McCorkle, R. (2010). Spouse caregivers of cancer patients. In J. C. Holland, W. S. Breitbart, P. B. Jacobsen, M. S. Lederberg, M. J. Loscalzo, & R. McCorkle (Eds.), *Psycho-oncology* (2nd ed., pp. 516–521). New York, NY: Oxford University Press.

Omran, S., Saeed, A. M. A., & Simpson, J. (2012). Symptom distress of Jordanian patients with cancer receiving chemotherapy. *International Journal of Nursing Practice, 18*(2), 125–132. https://doi.org/10.1111/j.1440-172X.2012.02012.x

Palos, G. R., Mendoza, T. R., Liao, K.-P., Anderson, K. O., Garcia-Gonzalez, A., Hahn, K., ... Cleeland, C. S. (2011). Caregiver symptom burden: The risk of caring for an underserved patient with advanced cancer. *Cancer, 117*(5), 1070–1079. https://doi.org/10.1002/cncr.25695

Pandey, M., Devi, N., Thomas, B. C., Vinod Kumar, S., Krishnan, R., & Ramdas, K. (2007). Distress overlaps with anxiety and depression in patients with head and neck cancer. *Psycho-Oncology, 16*(6), 582–586.

Park, S. M., Kim, Y. J., Kim, S., Choi, J. S., Lim, H.-Y., Choi, Y. S., ... Yun, Y. H. (2009). Impact of caregivers' unmet needs for supportive care on quality of terminal cancer care delivered and caregiver's workforce performance. *Supportive Care in Cancer, 18*(6), 699–706. https://doi.org/10.1007/s00520-009-0668-5

Payakachat, N., Ounpraseuth, S., & Suen, J. Y. (2012). Late complications and long-term quality of life for survivors (>5 years) with history of head and neck cancer. *Head & Neck, 35*(6), 819–825. https://doi.org/10.1002/hed.23035

Pearlin, L. (1994). Conceptual strategies for the study of caregiver stress. In E. Light & G. Niederehe (Eds.), *Stress effects on family caregivers of Alzheimer's patients: Research and interventions* (pp. 3–21). New York, NY: Springer.

Peltzer, K., Pengpid, S., & Skaal, L. (2012). Prevalence of psychological distress and associated factors in urban hospital outpatients in South Africa. *South African Journal of Psychiatry, 18*(1), 10–15.

Penedo, F. J., Traegar, L., Dahn, J., Molton, I., Gonzalez, J. S., Schneiderman, N., & Antoni, M. H. (2007). Cognitive behavioral stress management intervention improves quality of life in Spanish monolingual hispanic men treated for localized prostate cancer: Results of a randomized controlled trial. *International Journal of Behavioral Medicine, 14*(3), 164–172.

Penner, J. L. (2009). Psychosocial care of patients with head and neck cancer. *seminars in Oncology Nursing, 25*(3), 231–241. https://doi.org/10.1016/j.soncn.2009.05.008

Rohleder, N., Marin, T. J., Ma, R., & Miller, G. E. (2009). Biologic cost of caring for a cancer patient: Dysregulation of pro- and anti-inflammatory signaling pathways. *Journal of Clinical Oncology, 27*(18), 2909–2915. https://doi.org/10.1200/jco.2008.18.7435

Roing, M., Hirsch, J.-M., & Holstrom, I. (2008). Living in a state of suspension – a phenomenological approach to the spouse's experience of oral cancer. *Scandinavian Journal of Caring Science, 22*(1), 40–47.

Roscoe, J. A., Kaufman, M. E., Matteson-Rusby, S. E., Palesh, O. G., Ryan, J. L., Kohli, S., ... Morrow, G. R. (2007). Cancer-related fatigue and sleep disorders. *The Oncologist, 12*(suppl_1), 35–42. https://doi.org/10.1634/theoncologist.12-S1-35

Schubart, J. R., Kinzie, M. B., & Farace, E. (2008). Caring for the brain tumor patient: Family caregiver burden and unmet needs. *Neuro-Oncology, 10*(1), 61–72. https://doi.org/10.1215/15228517-2007-040

Schulz, R., Bookwala, J., Knapp, J. E., Scheier, M., & Williamson, G. M. (1996). Pessimism, age, and cancer mortality. *Psychology and Aging, 11*(2), 304–310.

Segrin, C., Badger, T., Dorros, S. M., Meek, P., & Lopez, A. M. (2007). Interdependent anxiety and psychological distress in women with breast cancer and their partners. *Psycho-Oncology, 16*(7), 634–643. https://doi.org/10.1002/pon.1111

Semple, C. J. (2001). The role of the CNS in head and neck oncology. *Nursing Standard, 15*(23), 39–42.

Semple, C. J., Sullivan, K., Dunwoody, L., & Kernohan, W. G. (2004). Psychosocial interventions for patients with head and neck cancer: Past, present and future. *Cancer Nursing, 27*(6), 434–441.

Shone, G. R., & Yardley, M. P. J. (1991). An audit into the incidence of handicap after unilateral radical neck dissection. *The Journal of Laryngology and Otology, 105*, 760–762.

Short, P. F., Vasey, J. J., & Tunceli, K. (2005). Employment pathways in a large cohort of adult cancer survivors. *Cancer, 103*(6), 1292–1301. https://doi.org/10.1002/cncr.20912

Singer, S., Krauss, O., Keszte, J., Siegl, G., Papsdorf, K., Severi, E., ... Kortmann, R. D. (2012). Predictors of emotional distress in patients with head and neck cancer. *Head Neck, 34*(2), 180–187. https://doi.org/10.1002/hed.21702

Starmer, H. M. (2018). Factors influencing adherence to treatment for head and neck cancer. In P. C. Doyle (Ed.), *Clinical care and rehabilitation in head and neck cancer*. Cham, Switzerland: Springer.

Stenberg, U., Ruland, C. M., & Miaskowski, C. (2010). Review of the literature on the effects of caring for a patient with cancer. *Psycho-Oncology, 19*(10), 1013–1025. https://doi.org/10.1002/pon.1670

Stetz, K. M., & Brown, M.-A. (2004). Physical and psychosocial health in family caregiving: A comparison of AIDS and cancer caregivers. *Public Health Nursing, 21*(6), 533–540.

Taylor, J. C., Terrell, J. E., Ronis, D. L., Fowler, K. E., Bishop, C., Lambert, M. T., ... Duffy, S. A. (2004). Disability in patients with head and neck cancer. *Archives of Otolaryngology Head and Neck Surgery, 130*, 764–769.

Thomas, B. C., Carlson, L. E., & Bultz, B. D. (2009). Cancer patient ethnicity and associations with emotional distress – the sixth vital sign: A new look at defining patient ethnicity in a multicultural context. *Journal of Immigrant and Minority Health, 11*(4), 237–248.

Van Houtven, C. H., Ramsey, S. D., Hornbrook, M. C., Atienza, A. A., & van Ryn, M. (2010). Economic burden for informal caregivers of lung and colorectal cancer patients. *The Oncologist, 15*(8), 883–893. https://doi.org/10.1634/theoncologist.2010-0005

van Ryn, M., Sanders, S., Kahn, K., van Houtven, C., Griffin, J. M., Martin, M., ... Rowland, J. (2011). Objective burden, resources, and other stressors among informal cancer caregivers: A hidden quality issue? *Psycho-Oncology, 20*(1), 44–52. https://doi.org/10.1002/pon.1703

Verdonck-de Leeuw, I. M., Van Bleek, W.-J., Leemans, C. R., & de Bree, R. (2010). Employment and return to work in head and neck cancer survivors. *Oral Oncology, 46*(1), 56–60.

Vickery, L. E., Latchford, G., Hewison, J., Bellew, M., & Feber, T. (2003). The impact of head and neck cancer and facial disfigurement on the quality of life of patients and their partners. *Head & Neck, 25*(4), 289–296. https://doi.org/10.1002/hed.10206

Williams, A. L., & Bakitas, M. (2012). Cancer family caregivers: A new direction for interventions. *Journal of Palliative Medicine, 15*(7), 775–783. https://doi.org/10.1089/jpm.2012.0046

Williams, L. A. (2007). Whatever it takes: Informal caregiving dynamics in blood and marrow transplantation. *Oncology Nursing Forum, 34*(2), 379–387.

World Health Organization. (2018). Cancer key facts. Accessed 8 May 2018 from: http://www.who.int/news-room/fact-sheets/detail/cancer

Yabroff, K. R., & Kim, Y. (2009). Time costs associated with informal caregiving for cancer survivors. *Cancer, 115*(S18), 4362–4373. https://doi.org/10.1002/cncr.24588

Yueh, B., Weaver, E. M., Bradley, E. H., Krumholz, H. M., Heagerty, P., Conley, A., & Sasaki, C. T. (2003). A critical evaluation of critical pathways in head and neck cancer. *Archives of Otolaryngology Head and Neck Surgery, 129*, 89–95.

Yuen, H. K., Gillespie, M. B., Day, T. A., Morgan, L., & Burik, J. K. (2007). Driving behaviors in patients with head and neck cancer during and after cancer treatment: A preliminary report. *Head & Neck, 29*(7), 675–681. https://doi.org/10.1002/hed.20567

Zabora, J., Brintzenhofeszoc, K., Curbow, B., Hooker, C., & Piantadosi, S. (2001). The prevalence of psychological distress by cancer site. *Psycho-Oncology, 10*, 19–28.

Zwahlen, D., Hagenbuch, N., Jenewein, J., Carley, M. I., & Buchi, S. (2011). Adopting a family approach to theory and practice: Measuring distress in cancer patient-partner dyads with the distress thermometer. *Psycho-Oncology, 20*(4), 394–403. https://doi.org/10.1002/pon.1744

Optimizing Clinical Management of Head and Neck Cancer

Barbara Pisano Messing, Elizabeth Celeste Ward, and Cathy L. Lazarus

Introduction

The complex nature of head and neck cancer (HNC) and it's management presents clinical and service delivery challenges for professionals working with this population. The disease process, along with patient's age, comorbidities, acute and long-term effects of treatment, altered or loss of function, psychosocial factors, financial loss, and the impact on quality of life required optimization of patient care using a multidisciplinary, coordinated, and systematic approach. Historically, multidisciplinary coordinated care teams and services guided by clinical pathways (CP) have not been widely utilized. Patients may have been evaluated by one or some members of the oncology team, thereby potentially lessening the opportunity to receive treatment based on best practice models and without exposure to available research/clinical trials. Therefore, the collective clinical expertise of the MDT provides valuable input during the critical decision-making process to define potiential and resonable treatment options. The impact from HNC treatment and managing treatment side effects has become a significant public health issue because of the magnitude of the loss of function suffered by patients, the cost of service provision, and the high level of clinical expertise required by cancer providers (Gooi et al., 2016; Miller et al., 2016; National Comprehensive Cancer Network, 2017). Of equal importance is input provided by allied health professionals. Unfortunately, allied health professionals are not always included as integral members of the MDT. Referrals for the evaluation and management of anticipated functional problems from HNC treatment(s) may be inconsistent or nonexistent. Referrals to allied health professionals may not be initiated, or the timing of the referral may be significantly delayed contributing to suboptimal patient outcomes.

Current best practice models are increasingly moving away from historical service patterns

B. P. Messing (✉)
Greater Baltimore Medical Center, The Milton
J. Dance, Jr. Head and Neck Center, Johns Hopkins
Head & Neck Surgery, Johns Hopkins Voice Center,
Baltimore, MD, USA

School of Health and Rehabilitation Sciences, The
University of Queensland, Brisbane, QLD, Australia
e-mail: bmessing@gbmc.org

E. C. Ward
School of Health and Rehabilitation Sciences, The
University of Queensland, Brisbane, QLD, Australia

Centre for Functioning and Health Research
(CFAHR), Metro South Hospital and Health Service,
Queensland Health, Queensland Government,
Brisbane, QLD, Australia

C. L. Lazarus
Icahn School of Medicine at Mount Sinai, Thyroid
Head and Neck Research Center, Thyroid Head and
Neck Cancer (THANC) Foundation,
New York, NY, USA

Department of Otolaryngology Head & Neck
Surgery, Mount Sinai Beth Israel,
New York, NY, USA

© Springer Nature Switzerland AG 2019
P. C. Doyle (ed.), *Clinical Care and Rehabilitation in Head and Neck Cancer*,
https://doi.org/10.1007/978-3-030-04702-3_6

towards integrated, systematic management. International clinical guidelines for cancer care advocate for a multidisciplinary team (MDT) approach to HNC management (Cancer Council Victoria, 2015; Clarke, Radford, Coffey, & Stewart, 2016; Cohen et al., 2016; National Comprehensive Cancer Network, 2017; Taylor-Goh, 2017). In fact, integrated and coordinated MDT input is suggested to initiate at the time of diagnosis and during the treatment planning process through to long-term survivorship. This approach is supported by studies which have established that HNC care delivered using a MDT approach results in improved patient outcomes and better survival rates (Friedland et al., 2011; Tsai, Kung, Wang, Huang, & Liu, 2015; Wang et al., 2012). Lassig et al. (2012) recently reported a 30% better survival rate in 388 patients undergoing radiation therapy and treated in an academic setting when compared to a community center facility. Although the authors proposed several factors to explain the improved survival rate for those treated at academic centers (such as technological advantages), they also highlighted the benefits of a MDT, including attendance at tumor board meetings and coordination of complex care during and following treatment (Lassig et al., 2012). Such evidence supports the need for HNC centers to develop and implement care using an integrated MDT best practice models based on clinical practice guidelines or CPs that are designed to direct HNC care before, during, and after treatment. Best practice models of HNC MDTs are provided in this chapter to provide a foundation of learning and to ultimately move practice patterns which will serve to benefit and enhance HNC patients survivorship outcomes.

Head and Neck Cancer Multidisciplinary Team

The goals of the modern MDT approach in HNC management are to "prevent, recognize, and treat" using evidence-based treatment protocols in a timely, appropriate, and patient-centered manner (Friedland et al., 2011; Jamal, Ebersole, Erman, & Chhetri, 2017). Treatment decisions seek curative intent (when possible) with improved patient care, long-term survival, and maximization of functional and QOL outcomes. However, the effects of these treatments typically cause significant acute and long-term functional side effects (e.g., nutrition, dysphagia, pain) and psychosocial issues (e.g., anxiety, depression) that negatively affect quality of life (see Kearney & Cavanagh, Chap. 20 and Bornbaum & Doyle, Chap. 5). Therefore, all medical and allied health professionals on the MDT must be informed, engaged, and integrated into the patient's care to actively seek to manage the effects of treatment.

The MDT needed for HNC care requires a strong collaboration between highly specialized professionals. For example, the MTD generally consists of a head and neck surgeon, plastic and reconstructive surgeon/microvascular surgeon, radiation oncologist, medical oncologist, oral and maxillofacial surgeon, dentist/maxillofacial prosthodontist, pain specialist, pathologist, radiologist/imaging specialist, psychologist, speech pathologist, oncology dietitian, head and neck nurse specialist/nurse coordinator, clinical research coordinator, pharmacist, oncology social worker, physical therapist, occupational therapist, and, more recently, a lymphedema therapist (National Comprehensive Cancer Network, 2017; Taylor-Goh, 2017). The establishment of guidelines and CPs enable the MDT to communicate among themselves, as well as with the patient and his/her family members regarding many aspects of their care. Clinical guidelines and CPs also provide a framework to identify the level of involvement of each professional and to specify treatment planning, recommendations, assessments, tests, imaging, etc. as indicated throughout all stages of a patient's care. The intensity of involvement by any given team member varies accordingly and will necessarily need to be adapted to the patient's specific treatment response and reactions to treatment. It is recommended that patients will be followed by physician and rehabilitation team from pretreatment to 24 months posttreatment, as indicated. The managing physician(s), usually the head and neck surgeon, and the radiation and medical oncologist continue at least up to 5 years posttreatment for oncologic surveillance according to NCCN guidelines (National Comprehensive Cancer Network, 2017).

According to the Oncology Advisory Board: "excellent patient experience, including better coordination and clearer communication, drives clinical outcomes" (Advisory Board, 2015). Team communication and coordination of services is essential and may serve to reduce redundancy of care, improve efficiency, reduce costs, and improve patient outcomes. The collective experience and value of the MDT is needed to provide this level of integrated and timely care. Defining the roles of oncology physicians and other health professionals within the MDT and CP fosters teamwork and collaboration along the time continuum of care process. Patients should be educated about the MDT and CP throughout this process to increase their awareness, engagement, and knowledge of the high level of support available for optimal management of the sequela of treatment (Lawson & Ward, 2014). Each member of the MDT must understand the importance of respecting the clinical contributions and area of expertise of all team members to provide care in an interactive and collaborative manner. Patient input and education on the CP is essential. Best practice patterns encourage members of the MDT to educate patients before, during, and post-treatment on the purpose of the CP, how to follow the plan, and to actively seek input from patients to improve service delivery.

The MDT and Clinical Pathways

Not only does modern cancer care require multidisciplinary input, but it is also recognized as best practice for the MDT to be involved in the patient's care within a CP – at pretreatment as well as during and post-treatment. Clinical pathways in HNC care strive to provide evidence-based algorithms with the goal of organizing patient care in a MDT model that is everevolving, structured, time-based, and efficient (Dautremont et al., 2016). The establishment of CPs provides the MDT and the patient a plan or "road map" to inform, educate, navigate care, and ensure coordinated and integrated service delivery before, during, and after HNC treatment (Friedland et al., 2011). Furthermore, a MDT utilizing clinical practice guidelines as the framework of a CP

model serves to standardize and implement diagnostic and therapeutic evidence-based methods as a best practice, quality-driven approaches to care (Chen et al., 2000; Ellis, 2013; Weed, 1997).

The use of CPs has been shown to provide cost savings while enhancing patient outcomes (Chen et al., 2000). Delivery of MDT services through a coordinated head and neck CP is recognized to maximize results, increase efficiency in care delivery, reduce costs, shorten the length of hospital stay, and improve overall patient outcomes (Dautremont et al., 2016; Prades, Remue, van Hoof, & Borras, 2015). A comprehensive literature review by Prades et al. (2015) of studies from 2005 to 2012 "assessed the impact of MDT on patient outcomes in cancer care," reported that oncology care provided by organized MDTs resulted in better clinical outcomes, and improved multidisciplinary decision-making processes and models of care, supporting the development and use of teams as a minimum standard for best practice care (Prades et al., 2015). Providing HNC care in a multidisciplinary model challenges teams to work cooperatively and stay engaged in the process. The framework and structure of a CP reinforces the need for teamwork to achieve positive clinical outcomes with team engagement.

The Clinical Care Pathway: MDT Management at Diagnosis

The first stage of the HNC CP is diagnosis and planning. As the patient's diagnostic workup and treatment planning occur, the patient and their significant others benefit from the guidance, support, and education provided by all members of the MDT. Aggregate patient information, clinical assessment, imaging results, tumor histology, and staging should be presented to the MDT with all disciplines at the table, often during weekly tumor board discussions, to collectively establish the recommended treatment (Fig. 6.1). Case presentations and discussions at MDT tumor board conferences help the team as a whole to consider all aspects of the patient and their specific situation, and doing so will often influence

Fig. 6.1 Discussion of case information at a multidisciplinary tumor board

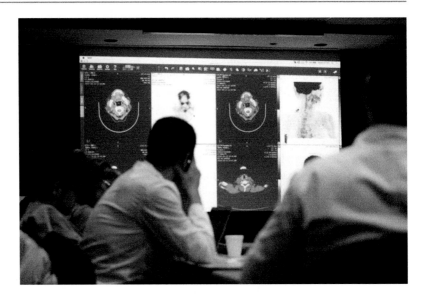

treatment decisions (Bergamini et al., 2016). The complexity of HNC management, where tumor sites are most often in anatomical regions with essential physiological functions (see Sahovaler, Yeh, & Fung, Chap. 1), requires input from the MDT and must be informed by evidence-based practice guidelines to reduce toxicity burden and improve patient survival (Beyzadeoglu, Ozyigit, & Selek, 2015; Gooi et al., 2016).

HNC treatment planning is highly complex and involves consideration of multimodality treatment options of surgery, radiation, and chemotherapy as defined by the National Comprehensive Cancer Network (NCCN) Clinical Practice Guidelines in Oncology (National Comprehensive Cancer Network, 2017) and the American Joint Commission on Cancer (AJCC) staging criteria (Amin et al., 2017). Tumor site, size and locoregional or distant metastasis guide treatment planning decisions using NCCN guidelines (based on AJCC staging classification) for selection of evidence-based HNC management options (Argiris, Karamouzis, Raben, & Ferris, 2008; Gooi et al., 2016; Miller et al., 2016). Physician knowledge of the guidelines, subspecialty clinical expertise, practice preferences, participation in a MDT approach, and practice location may influence treatment decisions (Lewis et al., 2010; Miller et al., 2016).

The Clinical Care Pathway: The MDT and Ongoing Supportive Care

Following diagnostic and treatment planning, clinical care pathways in HNC care involve ongoing input and coordination between the MDT during both the acute treatment phase and ongoing into the posttreatment period. During treatment, regular MDT meetings involving healthcare professionals caring for those patients undergoing primary or adjuvant (chemo) radiotherapy are part of the care pathway in many centers (Fleishman et al., 2007). Team members typically include medical, surgical and radiation oncology nurses, speech pathologists, oncology dieticians, oncology social workers, psychiatrists, psychologists, integrative oncology nursing and music therapists, as well as palliative care physicians with advanced clinical skills and training. During these meetings, one of the team members, often an advanced practice nurse in radiation oncology, reviews information on each patient currently on-treatment, as well as those patients soon to start. These regular meetings, often held weekly, involve discussion and tracking of patient progress during treatment and any evolving issues, such as mucositis, pain, xerostomia, dysphagia, nausea, weight loss, constipation, depression, etc. These sessions also provide a forum for ongoing communication among the professionals regarding patient status and intervention needs. Further, weekly meeting logs are maintained to identify and document follow-up on action plans by the appropriate professionals. Implementation of this type of weekly MDT meeting may result in less duplication of services between disciplines. Also, patients' satisfaction level may increase when informed that their oncology providers communicate with each other on a regular basis regarding the treatment and care they are receiving.

In addition to holding coordinated "on-treatment" meetings, it is essential to establish a "road map" for the patient, caregivers, and team members including planned posttreatment MDT appointments and key events (i.e., imaging, testing, labs, etc). The CP provides clarity for team members, patients, and family members. The structure of a CP should allow for pre-planned visits and interventions (i.e., interventions, imaging, labs, other outcome measures, and functional assessments) from baseline, during treatment, and into the extended long-term period. For example, the "Optimal Care Pathway for HNC" was established to provide a structure for a MDT approach that is accessible to patients and consistent in service delivery. The ultimate goal of the structural pathway is to provide high-quality care using this systematic approach to service provision. The Optimal Care Pathway contains seven critical steps in the patients' journey, including *Step 1*, prevention and early detection; *Step 2*, presentation, initial investigations, and referral; *Step 3*, diagnosis, staging, and treatment planning; *Step 4*, treatment; *Step 5*, care after initial treatment and recovery; *Step 6*, managing recurrent, residual, or metastatic disease; and *Step 7*, end-of-life care. Each step details involvement of all members of the MDT with the caveat that the pathway can be individualized depending on patients' treatment and care needs (Cancer Council Victoria, 2015).

An essential component of CP is to ensure that routine collection of outcome measures are utilized. Outcome measures vary depending on the speciality area of practice. Selection of outcome measures requires the MDT to identify significant and relevant information that is or will be needed to improve patient care. At a minimum, the process requires review of current literature and existing clinical pathways and guidelines, assessment of available tools, and developing consensus among MDT key stakeholders depending on the area of clinical expertise. Furthermore, CP models should be established based on review of validated, theory-based tools and measures. Clinical pathway models should utilize functional assessment protocols and validated clinical outcome measures and incorporate ongoing, long-term follow-up and coordination between the MDT members to maximize patient outcomes and quality of life (Jamal et al., 2017). For example, the United Kingdom National Multidisciplinary Guidelines recommend that all HNC patients should be seen by members of the MDT at "all stages of the patient's journey" and encouraged to follow established intervention pathways to improve patient care and outcomes (Clarke et al., 2016). Ideally, outcome data should be systematically collected at specified time points and integrated into an electronic medical record that will allow data retrieval and analysis across one or many patients over time. Systematic collection of both patient- and clinician-reported outcomes enables the MDT to measure functional changes over time and intervene when problems arise. Changes or problems in swallowing or dysphagia should be monitored by the speech pathologist and evaluated in a timely manner consistent with the CP structure. Dysphagia in HNC and monitoring changes through the CP will be discussed in the following section.

MDT and Clinical Care Pathways: Implementing a Dysphagia Management Pathway

Decline in swallow function significantly contributes to poor nutritional intake negatively impacting health-related QOL. Loss of swallow function and reduced nutritional status can be present from the time of initial diagnosis, become exacerbated during treatment due to related toxicities, and persist long-term for many patients (see Starmer, Chap. 18 and Arrese & Schieve, Chap. 19). Because of this, it is recognized in practice guidelines that swallowing and nutritional status should be assessed pretreatment and continue to be monitored during and post-treatment (Royal College of Speech & Language Therapists, & Taylor-Goh, 2005).

Internationally, countries such as the United States, the Netherlands, the United Kingdom, and Australia have established guidelines for head and neck cancer specifying the importance of including speech and swallow assessments with ongoing follow-up in the management of HNC patients (Gooi et al., 2016; Lawson et al., 2017). The Royal College of Speech and Language Therapists (RCSLT) resource manual for HNC specifies that speech pathologists should provide assessment, evidence-based swallowing interventions, patient education, and psychological support at pretreatment, during treatment, and posttreatment (Taylor-Goh, 2017). In the United States, the National Comprehensive Cancer Network (NCCN) (2017) has recommended the inclusion of speech pathology swallow assessments and follow-up as part of HNC care. However, the specifics of therapy, type, duration, and frequency, is not defined. Additionally, while the American Speech-Language-Hearing Association (ASHA) supports speech pathology interventions in the care of HNC patients through reviews of HNC evidence-based literature, clinical guidelines or recommendations are not provided (Gooi et al., 2016; Lawson et al., 2017). However, ASHA should develop guidelines and establish position statements on HNC management.

Hence, despite support in principle for systematic speech pathology involvement in dysphagia management post-HNC care, there is currently a lack of clarity and consistency in management pathways for the HNC patient (Krisciunas, Sokoloff, Stepas, & Langmore, 2012; Lawson et al., 2017). In particular, HNC standardized protocols using evidence-based swallowing interventions in clinical practice are limited (Krisciunas et al., 2012; Lawson et al., 2017; van den Berg et al., 2016). Existing descrip-

tions of current management of dysphagia following HNC lack in scope and may be highly variable (Krisciunas et al., 2012; Lawson et al., 2017; van den Berg et al., 2016). Therefore, seeking a greater understanding of the critical timing, type, frequency, and intensity of treatment remains a critical need in future research studies given the lack of consistency in HNC dysphagia service delivery across clinicians and institutions (Krisciunas et al., 2012). At present the evidence base remains limited with few studies, small cohorts, heterogeneous groups, and high variability in intervention approaches utilized (inconsistent timing, duration, type of exercises, and the intensity of treatment) (Kraaijenga, van der Molen, van den Brekel, & Hilgers, 2014; Krisciunas et al., 2012; Roe & Ashforth, 2011).

Perhaps the paucity of established or widely accepted speech pathology HNC practice guidelines has led to speech pathologists to traditionally have a reactive, rather than proactive, approach to providing swallowing therapy to those treated for HNC (Lawson et al., 2017). A survey by Krisciunas et al. (Krisciunas et al., 2012) examined the usual practice patterns of speech pathologists working with HNC patients in the United States, and their data revealed that 76% of the respondents received referrals on a "case-by-case basis" without the support of any institutional or departmental policy (Krisciunas et al., 2012). More experienced clinicians (>5 years' experience HNC) were 3.5 times more likely to intervene early and treat patients proactively (Krisciunas et al., 2012). However, over 80% of the clinicians surveyed reported providing treatment after radiation, rather than proactively during treatment (Krisciunas et al., 2012). Data collected should therefore be utilized to drive optimal clinical care and improve function.

Although greater clarity regarding the optimal clinical pathway for dysphagia management is still needed, there are aspects of the clinical pathway of care where there is greater consensus in clinical practice. One of these areas is that related to the issue of dysphagia assessment. Primary to the goal of improving functional outcomes is having the opportunity to provide early and ongoing assessment. This would occur from the point of first presentation to during and posttreatment, a process conducted in a structured, time point-based protocol model to ensure no patient is left behind (Cancer Council Victoria, 2015; Govender, Smith, Gardner, Barratt, & Taylor, 2017; Jamal et al., 2017; Lawson & Ward, 2014). Assessment of swallow function should include a clinical swallow evaluation and an instrumental assessment, either a videofluoroscopic swallow study (VFSS) and/or flexible endoscopic evaluation of swallow (FEES) to assess swallow physiology and severity of dysphagia (Cartmill, Cornwell, Ward, Davidson, & Porceddu, 2012; Leonard & Kendall, 2014). The clinical swallow examination is an important initial element to determine functional oral intake and gain insights into the patient's perspective of their capacity to manage oral intake.

Instrumental assessment, such as VFSS, is then an essential component of a thorough dysphagia assessment, a task that is necessary to identify physiological deficits, the severity of dysphagia, and the risk of aspiration and provide treatment and diet recommendations (Carnaby-Mann, Crary, Schmalfuss, & Amdur, 2012; Eisbruch et al., 2004; Leonard & Kendall, 2014; Manikantan et al., 2009; Perkins, Hancock, & Ward, 2014). This is of particular importance in this clinical population where silent aspiration (i.e., aspiration without overt signs such as coughing) is high. The impact of surgical and radiological interventions requires direct observation of functional swallow issues. Instrumental assessment should be performed at various time points to identify physiological swallowing problems and inform appropriate treatment (Hutcheson & Lewin, 2012). Furthermore, the rate of silent aspiration in HNC patients who are in long-term posttreatment has been understudied and, when reported, most often includes only patients who presented with a swallowing complaint, thereby, missing silent aspirators who remained undiagnosed (Hutcheson & Lewin, 2012; Nguyen et al., 2006). Thus, combined information from clinical and instrumental assessments is necessary for clinical decision-making specific to planning swallowing interventions, using compensatory swallow strategies,

and recommending postural changes. Accurate, timely, and comprehensive assessment and treatment are required to reduce the risk of airway compromise and aspiration pneumonia, as well as to ensure the safest, least restrictive diet necessary to maintain adequate nutrition and hydration before, during, and posttreatment. The optimal course of action necessary to address patients functional needs is to establish and implement care using the structure of a CP with a MDT.

Best practice CPs for dysphagia rehabilitation continue to emerge and are slow to spread despite initial reports related to HNC over the years (Colangelo, Logemann, Pauloski, Pelzer, & Rademaker, 1996; Logemann & Bytell, 1979; McConnel et al., 1994; and others). There has, however, been a body of emerging evidence published in the past 10 years to support the use of early prophylactic management, as an adjunct to the traditional tailored posttreatment rehabilitation. Recent evidence supports that providing prophylactic exercises during and following treatment may improve patients' swallow function, which impacts nutritional status and overall QOL during treatment and long-term (Carnaby-Mann et al., 2012; Carroll et al., 2008; Hutcheson et al., 2013; Kotz et al., 2012; Kraaijenga et al., 2014; Kulbersh et al., 2006; Schindler et al., 2015; van der Molen et al., 2011; van der Molen, van Rossum, Rasch, Smeele, & Hilgers, 2014; Virani, Kunduk, Fink, & McWhorter, 2015). This work is based on the principle that early intervention can contribute to less functional decline, enabling patients to return to an oral diet sooner, leading to less weight loss and shorter and potentially less problematic enteric tube use duration (Carnaby-Mann et al., 2012; Duarte, Chhetri, Liu, Erman, & Wang, 2013; Hutcheson et al., 2013; Kotz et al., 2012; Kraaijenga et al., 2014).

There is positive evidence for early prophylactic swallowing intervention; however, patient adherence to swallowing exercise protocols historically has revealed a low compliance rate and the perception that HNC patients will have limited ability to participate in dysphagia treatment (Krisciunas et al., 2012). In a randomized controlled study of 60 HNC patients undergoing chemoradiation, adherence to prophylactic swallowing exercises showed fairly good adherence (Messing, Ward, Lazarus, et al., 2017). However, adherence rates dropped at 5 weeks during treatment, a finding that was consistent with other studies that reported partial or moderate exercise protocol adherence during treatment (Kotz et al., 2012; Messing, Ward, Lazarus, et al., 2017; Mortensen et al., 2015; van den Berg et al., 2016). Other studies also reported fairly good adherence during the early weeks of treatment with a decline observed later in treatment (Carnaby-Mann et al., 2012; Kraaijenga et al., 2014; Mortensen et al., 2015). Shinn et al. (2013) retrospectively studied adherence rates of 109 oropharyngeal cancer patients undergoing chemoradiation and found that only 13% of participants were fully adherent to swallow exercise protocols while 32% were partially adherent. Reasons for nonadherence included a lack of understanding of the exercise, treatment toxicities (pain, fatigue, nausea), and forgetting to do the exercises (Shinn et al., 2013).

Govender, Wood et al. (2017) studied dysphagia exercise adherence in 13 patients and identified the top reasons for noncompliance as those related to psychological distress (Starmer, Chap. 24), not understanding the exercises, forgetting to do the exercise, not having a system to track completion, feeling overwhelmed, and the common physical barriers of pain and fatigue. Some studies report that compliance was greater by 50% when patients complain of dysphagia (Krisciunas et al., 2012). Interestingly, patients who were prescribed a more intensive and aggressive swallow exercise protocol demonstrate increased compliance (Krisciunas et al., 2012). Acute toxicities experienced by patients during treatment also contribute to the decline in participation or adherence to swallowing exercises. Encouraging patients to continue to perform an evidence-based swallowing exercise protocol during and posttreatment is recommended for management of both early and late effects of treatment on swallow function (Hutcheson et al., 2012, 2013). To increase patients' adherence to performing exercise protocols, the MDT should seek to educate patients on the rationale for and benefits of performing swallowing exercises protocols to optimize and improve patient outcomes.

The complexities of HNC management including tumor factors (tumor size, location, type of treatment), patient factors (comorbidities, adherence, location to treatment center), and clinician factors (experience, support from institution, physician support) all contribute to challenges in establishing best practice and standard protocols (Lawson et al., 2017). The timing of diagnostic and therapeutic intervention, as well as dose/frequency and intensity of treatment, remains highly variable with a predominantly reactive rather than proactive treatment initiation approach (Kraaijenga et al., 2014; Krisciunas et al., 2012; Lawson et al., 2017; Logemann et al., 2008). However, standard of care protocols and best practice guidelines are not yet well established for the HNC patient. Furthermore, patient adherence to exercises remains an ongoing issue regarding what is the minimal required "dose" for positive benefit. For this reason, the importance and potential benefits of using a proactive rather than reactive approach focusing on maintaining adequate oral intake, swallow exercises, compensatory strategies, and maneuvers during and posttreatment are not insignificant and should be a component of HNC management (Hutcheson et al., 2013; Rosenthal, Lewin, & Eisbruch, 2006). When considered together, the issues noted above contribute in part to the difficulty in establishing practice guidelines and standardized treatment protocols for use in HNC management.

Implementation of a Clinical Pathway for Dysphagia Management: Experiences of One Service

Implementing an integrated and systematic MDT head and neck clinical pathway (HNCP) with comprehensive dysphagia management requires timely swallowing evaluations, early/prophylactic and long-term swallow therapy, management of nutritional status, and cancer and treatment-related toxicities requires a significant commitment and investment of resources from health-care professionals, administrative staff and the organization's administration. As recognized through recent research, few clinical services are currently delivering this complete model of care (Kulbersh et al., 2006; Roe & Ashforth, 2011), leading to a recognized "knowledge-to-practice" gap. The Milton J. Dance Jr. Head & Neck Center established a HNC clinical pathway in 2011, known as the Dance Head and Neck Clinical Pathway (D-HNCP). The D-HNCP was implemented following a randomized controlled trial for HNC patients, providing a framework for further development of the pathway (Messing, Ward, Ryniak, et al., 2017). The D-HNCP provides the framework for HNC patients to receive planned MDT appointments and interventions pretreatment, during treatment, to 24 months post-treatment with oncologic surveillance continuing to 5 years post-treatment according to NCCN guidelines.

Within the pathway, routine clinical-reported outcomes (CROs) and patient-reported outcomes (PROs) are collected to monitor patient performance. D-HNCP data are collected and managed using REDCap[1] electronic data capture tools (Harris et al., 2009). REDCap (Research Electronic Data Capture) is a secure, web-based application designed to support data capture for research studies, providing (1) an intuitive interface for validated data entry, (2) audit trails for tracking data manipulation and export procedures, (3) automated export procedures for data downloads to common statistical packages, and (4) procedures for importing data from external sources. Patient demographics and CROs/PROs collected at D-HNCP time points are entered into REDCap. Findings from CROs/PROs as well as patient's subjective complaints serve to help monitor changes, during and posttreatment, in patients' nutritional status, weight, swallowing problems, diet level, and quality-of-life-related issues, which can in turn guide MDT interventions. Success of the D-HNCP, including sustainability, requires frequent team interaction, coordination of care, and the ability to recognize and devise solutions to problems. Comprehensive audits are performed to monitor *both* the MDT's and patients' compliance with scheduling, completion of

D-HNCP time point appointments, and completion of PROs and CROs. Overall, the audits have revealed excellent adherence to the D-HNCP at pretreatment, during treatment, and 1–24-month posttreatment time points. Oncologic surveillence appointments continue past the 24-month time points (5+ years post-treatment) as per NCCN guidelines to monitor patients for potential recurrence, metastasis, or a new primary and to address any posttreatment-related issues (National Comprehensive Cancer Network, 2017). Physicians should be vigilant for any functional issues, such as worsening swallowing problems, weight loss, lymphedema, and mobility issues, which may require referral to the rehabilitation team. Dental recall appointments should continue post-radiation oral and dental care to ensure a healthy oral care regime is maintained (Hancock, Epstein, & Sadler, 2003). A systematic and integrative approach is required to design, implement, and sustain a CP model. Long-term follow of HNC patients proves to be challenging. It is, therefore, important to perform frequent audits to determine reasons for adherence rate changes posttreatment (Messing, Ward, Ryniak, et al., 2017).

Considerations for Implementing Clinical Pathways in HNC Care

Although the benefits of a coordinated MDT CP are not disputed, it is recognized that implementing a CP in today's complex healthcare environment can be fraught with roadblocks and pitfalls. Barriers to adequate treatment are not an isolated problem but multifactorial. Implementation of HNC MDT care within a structured, timely, and organized CP model requires ongoing integrated efforts from all members of the team to maximize functional outcomes and improve overall QOL and long-term survival.

Adherence to the use of established guidelines and clinical pathways in treatment decisions also has been linked to treatment setting, with high-volume centers having better survival outcomes compared to low-volume settings (Lassig et al., 2012; Lewis et al., 2010). Hence, factors specific to the MDT and its capacity to implement and sus-

---

[1] http://www.sciencedirect.com/science/article/pii/S1532046408001226

tain a systematic clinical pathway needs to be addressed. Having a coordinated MDT housed in an established, patient-centered head and neck oncology center with a dedicated team of specialized oncology physicians, nursing, and allied health staff is essential to delivery of a coordinated pathway. However, each member of the MDT must also be a key stakeholder in the development and sustainability of the clinical pathway. Administrative staff are critical to the success of the pathway. Regular ongoing support from administrative staff is necessary to ensure coordination of appointments, tracking time points, scheduling, and conducting patient follow up calls to reschedule missed appointments. Information technology (IT) systems staff and support is also integral to its success. Clinical pathway management, including the implementation of alerts to schedule routine follow-up appointments and reminders for certain assessments and outcome measures to occur at particular time points, can be activated through an electronic medical record system or through other dedicated online electronic database/management systems such as REDCap (Harris et al., 2009). These systems help to provide a visual map of each patient's timeline, identify, and enter all data collected from PRO and CRO measures at designated time points.

Clinical research coordinators or other designated team members help to facilitate monitoring of both the MDT members and patient adherence to the clinical pathway requirements through periodic audits. These audits are essential to ensure that the clinical pathway is sustainable. Early work by Cabana et al. (Cabana et al., 1999) examined the issue of adherence to treatment guidelines and identified numerous physician limitations (lack of awareness, familiarity, agreement, self-efficacy, outcome expectancy, the inertia of previous practice experience, and other external barriers) as contributing to nonadherence to evidence-based guidelines in treatment decision-making (Cabana et al., 1999). Patient noncompliance with physician-recommended treatment based on NCCN guidelines has also been demonstrated to result in treatment deviations or failure to treat in approximately 15% of cancer cases (Lewis et al., 2010; Miller et al., 2016; National Comprehensive Cancer Network, 2017).

Developing a HN clinical pathway requires, in part, organizing a MDT with an experienced and effective leader who is committed to the project and able to identify and recruit champions to unify and move the program into action. Additionally, establishing a HN clinical pathway may require hiring new staff, reassigning or expanding existing job responsiblities, evaluating programmatic resources, and obtaining administrative and financial support from the facility/ cancer service line. The inherent complex nature of a HN clinical pathway requires the engagement of key stakeholders, ongoing and open communication between team members, acceptance of changes as they arise, and an open-mindedness to achieve program sustainability. Some of the potential barriers to the success of the clinical pathway are, as stated above, the complexity of a HN clinical pathway, physician and staff turnover, federal and state local policy changes, program constraints, workload and productivity demands, and patient needs.

Technology: Providing New Opportunities for Enhancing Clinical Pathways in HNC Care

Although there are multiple challenges to implementing clinical care pathways, advances in personal computing/devices and high end-user acceptance of technology-supported healthcare help to facilitate MDT interactions and provide new ways to support and deliver HNC clinical care pathways (Burns, Hill, & Ward, 2014; Cartmill, Wall, Ward, Hill, & Porceddu, 2016; Ward, Wall, Burns, Cartmill, & Hill, 2017). The new era of digital health records, electronic medical records, and integrated database systems now provide a greater opportunity to streamline patient management. Digital medical records help all members of the team have ready and immediate access to assessments conducted by others. Dedicated electronic data management systems within health services can also assist with patient scheduling, sending patient reminders about appointments and follow-ups which can assist and improve patient compliance with their clinical pathway (Wall, Ward, Cartmill, Hill, & Porceddu, 2017a). These systems can also provide prompts for the clinical staff regarding the assessments/outcome measurement required at each assessment time point in the clinical pathway. These built-in system reminders assist all members of the team to remain compliant with routine data collection expectations in accordance with the patient care pathway.

Greater availability of secure, stable videoconferencing platforms has also enhanced opportunities for interactions between MDT members. Videoconference consultations are being used by MDTs to link experts across facilities for case discussions and tumor board meetings (Hazin & Qaddoumi, 2010; Hughes et al., 2012; Olver & Selva-Nayagam, 2000; Savage, Nixon, & MacKenzie, 2007; Stalfors et al., 2001). Exchange of clinical data via digital file transfers enables fast and easy access to second opinions, and remote assistance and expert consultation for imaging and pathology are supporting cancer care in areas without services (Hazin & Qaddoumi, 2010). Medical support via videoconferencing is also being used to support remote and in-home delivery of chemotherapy (Sabesan et al., 2012), as well as regular medical and radiation oncology reviews (Ogawa et al., 2005). Telehealth has also provided opportunity to improve access to services for patients, reducing some of the costs and burden associated with cancer care. Recent evidence has demonstrated successful use of telehealth to provide posttreatment speech pathology services for patients managed for HNC (Burns, Kularatna, et al., 2017; Burns et al., 2012; Collins et al., 2017), with economic analysis revealing clear patient and service benefits (Burns, Kularatna, et al., 2017; Burns, Ward, et al., 2017; Collins et al., 2017).

Other systems, such as computer-based screening programs, have also been demonstrated to allow close monitoring of patient symptoms during HNC management (Wall, Ward, Cartmill, & Hill, 2013). These types of systems provide a fast and efficient way to determine current patient symptom presentation, assist referral into support services when needed, and minimize unnecessary appointments, helping to provide patients with "the right services at the right time" (Wall,

Cartmill, Ward, Hill, Isenring, Byrnes, et al., 2016; Wall, Cartmill, Ward, Hill, Isenring, Porceddu, et al., 2016). Computer programs and apps have also been shown to be viable alternate means for delivery of therapy services. Such systems can help to enable patients to complete rehabilitation components of their care pathway, such as their intensive prophylactic swallowing rehabilitation (Wall et al., 2017a, 2017b), doing so at a time and place that is convenient to them. Finally, Internet-based patient information is used by many patients as a source of education and information sharing for patients with HNC. Though there are ongoing concerns regarding the quality of health information publically available on the Internet, directing patients to good Internet sites can compliment the ongoing education services provided by staff regarding symptoms, side effects, assessments, and other information relevant to the HNC care pathway and provide patients with resources to help their own self-management (Ni Riordain & McCreary, 2009).

Summary

Healthcare providers are continually challenged to obtain the best patient outcomes while reducing costs, hospital length of stay, and readmission rate. Although the complexities of HNC management create inherent barriers to providing care using a MDT approach and structured clinical pathway models, the benefits and necessity are evident and are considered the gold standard of care provision (Prades et al., 2015). Implementing care for HNC patients using a MDT approach and clinical pathway models has been shown to result in positive outcomes both for patients and those team members who provide care (Deneckere et al., 2012; Ellis, 2013; Miller et al., 2016; Prades et al., 2015). Clinical pathway models integrated with electronic medical records are integral to reduce redundancy of documentation and improve communication between care providers, in addition to improving service efficiency and safety. Embracing technology within clinical pathways can also assist in the creation of more efficient ways to monitor patient needs, facilitate access to and between team members, and reduce patient burden.

HNC care delivery using a clinical pathway structure can be challenging requiring vigilance through monitoring, modifications, ongoing staff, and patient education as well as consideration of patient and caregivers needs to ensure successful implementation. However, it is well worth the effort. In the words of a HNC patient, "the team provided an invaluable safety net that I could count during and after my cancer treatments and to this day".

References

Advisory Board. (2015, March 18). *5 myths physicians believe about patient experience.* Advisory Board Company Infographic. Retrieved from https://www.advisory.com/-/media/Advisory-com/Research/PEC/Resources/Posters/5-myths-physicians-believe-about-patient-engagement.pdf.

Amin, M. B., Greene, F. L., Edge, S. B., Compton, C. C., Gershenwald, J. E., Brookland, R. K., ... Winchester, D. P. (2017). The eighth edition AJCC cancer staging manual: Continuing to build a bridge from a population-based to a more "personalized" approach to cancer staging. *CA: A Cancer Journal for Clinicians, 67*(2), 93–99. https://doi.org/10.3322/caac.21388. Retrieved from https://www.ncbi.nlm.nih.gov/pubmed/28094848

Argiris, A., Karamouzis, M. V., Raben, D., & Ferris, R. L. (2008). Head and neck cancer. *Lancet, 371*(9625), 1695–1709. https://doi.org/10.1016/S0140-6736(08)60728-X. Retrieved from https://www.ncbi.nlm.nih.gov/pubmed/18486742

Bergamini, C., Locati, L., Bossi, P., Granata, R., Alfieri, S., Resteghini, C., ... Licitra, L. (2016). Does a multidisciplinary team approach in a tertiary referral centre impact on the initial management of head and neck cancer? *Oral Oncology, 54*, 54–57. https://doi.org/10.1016/j.oraloncology.2016.01.001. Retrieved from https://www.ncbi.nlm.nih.gov/pubmed/26774920

Beyzadeoglu, M., Ozyigit, G., & Selek, U. (2015). *Radiation therapy for head and neck cancers: A case-based review.* Cham: Springer International Publishing.

Burns, C., Hill, A., & Ward, E. C. (2014). Supporting head and neck cancer management: Use of technology. In E. C. Ward & C. J. van As-Brooks (Eds.), *Head and neck cancer: Treatment, rehabilitation and outcomes* (Vol. 2, 2nd ed., pp. 541–568). San Diego, CA: Plural Publishing.

Burns, C. L., Kularatna, S., Ward, E. C., Hill, A. J., Byrnes, J., & Kenny, L. M. (2017). Cost analysis of a speech pathology synchronous telepractice service for patients with head and neck cancer. *Head & Neck, 39*(12), 2470–2480. https://doi.org/10.1002/hed.24916. Retrieved from https://www.ncbi.nlm.nih.gov/pubmed/28963804

Burns, C. L., Ward, E. C., Hill, A. J., Kularatna, S., Byrnes, J., & Kenny, L. M. (2017). Randomized controlled trial of a multisite speech pathology telepractice service providing swallowing and communication intervention to patients with head and neck cancer: Evaluation of service outcomes. *Head & Neck, 39*(5), 932–939. https://doi.org/10.1002/hed.24706. Retrieved from https://www.ncbi.nlm.nih.gov/pubmed/28225567

Burns, C. L., Ward, E. C., Hill, A. J., Malcolm, K., Bassett, L., Kenny, L. M., & Greenup, P. (2012). A pilot trial of a speech pathology telehealth service for head and neck cancer patients. *Journal of Telemedicine and Telecare, 18*(8), 443–446. https://doi.org/10.1258/jtt.2012.GTH104. Retrieved from https://www.ncbi.nlm.nih.gov/pubmed/23209274

Cabana, M. D., Rand, C. S., Powe, N. R., Wu, A. W., Wilson, M. H., Abboud, P. A., & Rubin, H. R. (1999). Why don't physicians follow clinical practice guidelines? A framework for improvement. *JAMA, 282*(15), 1458–1465. Retrieved from https://www.ncbi.nlm.nih.gov/pubmed/10535437

Cancer Council Victoria. (2015, September). *Optimal care – cancer services framework.* Retrieved from http://www.cancervic.org.au/downloads/health-professionals/optimal-care-pathways/Optimal_care_pathway_for_people_with_head_and_neck_cancers.pdf.

Carnaby-Mann, G., Crary, M. A., Schmalfuss, I., & Amdur, R. (2012). "Pharyngocise": Randomized controlled trial of preventative exercises to maintain muscle structure and swallowing function during head-and-neck chemoradiotherapy. *International Journal of Radiation Oncology, Biology, and Physics, 83*(1), 210–219. https://doi.org/10.1016/j.ijrobp.2011.06.1954. Retrieved from http://www.ncbi.nlm.nih.gov/pubmed/22014959

Carroll, W. R., Locher, J. L., Canon, C. L., Bohannon, I. A., McColloch, N. L., & Magnuson, J. S. (2008). Pretreatment swallowing exercises improve swallow function after chemoradiation. *Laryngoscope, 118*(1), 39–43. https://doi.org/10.1097/MLG.0b013e31815659b0. Retrieved from http://www.ncbi.nlm.nih.gov/pubmed/17989581

Cartmill, B., Cornwell, P., Ward, E., Davidson, W., & Porceddu, S. (2012). Long-term functional outcomes and patient perspective following altered fractionation radiotherapy with concomitant boost for oropharyngeal cancer. *Dysphagia, 27*(4), 481–490. https://doi.org/10.1007/s00455-012-9394-0. Retrieved from https://www.ncbi.nlm.nih.gov/pubmed/22362547

Cartmill, B., Wall, L. R., Ward, E. C., Hill, A. J., & Porceddu, S. V. (2016). Computer literacy and health locus of control as determinants for readiness and acceptability of telepractice in a head and neck cancer population. *International Journal of Telerehabilitation, 8*(2), 49–60. https://doi.org/10.5195/ijt.2016.6203. Retrieved from https://www.ncbi.nlm.nih.gov/pubmed/28775801

Chen, A. Y., Callender, D., Mansyur, C., Reyna, K. M., Limitone, E., & Goepfert, H. (2000). The impact of clinical pathways on the practice of head and neck oncologic surgery: The University of Texas M. D. Anderson Cancer Center Experience. *Archives of Otolaryngology – Head & Neck Surgery, 126*(3), 322–326. Retrieved from https://www.ncbi.nlm.nih.gov/pubmed/10722004

Clarke, P., Radford, K., Coffey, M., & Stewart, M. (2016). Speech and swallow rehabilitation in head and neck cancer: United Kingdom National Multidisciplinary Guidelines. *Journal of Laryngology and Otology, 130*(S2), S176–S180. https://doi.org/10.1017/S0022215116000608. Retrieved from https://www.ncbi.nlm.nih.gov/pubmed/27841134

Cohen, E. E., LaMonte, S. J., Erb, N. L., Beckman, K. L., Sadeghi, N., Hutcheson, K. A., ... Pratt-Chapman, M. L. (2016). American Cancer Society head and neck cancer survivorship care guideline. *CA: A Cancer Journal for Clinicians, 66*(3), 203–239. https://doi.org/10.3322/caac.21343. Retrieved from https://www.ncbi.nlm.nih.gov/pubmed/27002678

Colangelo, L. A., Logemann, J. A., Pauloski, B. R., Pelzer, H. J., Jr., & Rademaker, A. W. (1996). T stage and functional outcome in oral and oropharyngeal cancer patients. *Head & Neck: Journal for the Sciences and Specialties of the Head and Neck, 18*(3), 259–268.

Collins, A., Burns, C. L., Ward, E. C., Comans, T., Blake, C., Kenny, L., ... Best, D. (2017). Home-based telehealth service for swallowing and nutrition management following head and neck cancer treatment. *Journal of Telemedicine and Telecare, 23*(10), 866–872. https://doi.org/10.1177/1357633X17733020. Retrieved from https://www.ncbi.nlm.nih.gov/pubmed/29081270

Dautremont, J. F., Rudmik, L. R., Nakoneshny, S. C., Chandarana, S. P., Matthews, T. W., Schrag, C., ... Dort, J. C. (2016). Understanding the impact of a clinical care pathway for major head and neck cancer resection on postdischarge healthcare utilization. *Head & Neck, 38*(Suppl 1), E1216–E1220. https://doi.org/10.1002/hed.24196. Retrieved from https://www.ncbi.nlm.nih.gov/pubmed/26382252

Deneckere, S., Euwema, M., Van Herck, P., Lodewijckx, C., Panella, M., Sermeus, W., & Vanhaecht, K. (2012). Care pathways lead to better teamwork: Results of a systematic review. *Social Science and Medicine, 75*(2), 264–268. https://doi.org/10.1016/j.socscimed.2012.02.060. Retrieved from https://www.ncbi.nlm.nih.gov/pubmed/22560883

Duarte, V. M., Chhetri, D. K., Liu, Y. F., Erman, A. A., & Wang, M. B. (2013). Swallow preservation exercises during chemoradiation therapy maintains swallow function. *Otolaryngology and Head and Neck Surgery, 149*(6), 878–884. https://doi.org/10.1177/0194599813502310. Retrieved from https://www.ncbi.nlm.nih.gov/pubmed/23981953

Eisbruch, A., Schwartz, M., Rasch, C., Vineberg, K., Damen, E., Van, A., ... Balm, A. J. (2004). Dysphagia and aspiration after chemoradiotherapy for head-and-neck cancer: Which anatomic structures are affected and can they be spared by IMRT? *International Journal of Radiation Oncology, Biology, and Physics, 60*(5), 1425–1439. https://doi.org/10.1016/j.ijrobp.2004.05.050. Retrieved from http://www.ncbi.nlm.nih.gov/pubmed/15590174

Ellis, P. G. (2013). Development and implementation of oncology care pathways in an integrated care network: The via oncology pathways experience. *Journal of Oncology Practice, 9*(3), 171–173. https://doi.org/10.1200/JOP.2013.001020. Retrieved from https://www.ncbi.nlm.nih.gov/pubmed/23942503

Fleishman, S. C. E., Arthur, D., Ball, K., Bennett, B., Escala, S., Fred, B., ... Harrison, L. (2007, November). *Streamlining care for patients receiving combined radiation therapy and chemotherapy for head and neck cancer: Putting all the ducks in a row.* Poster presented at the ASTRO-ASCO combined head and neck conference, Palm Springs, CA.

Friedland, P. L., Bozic, B., Dewar, J., Kuan, R., Meyer, C., & Phillips, M. (2011). Impact of multidisciplinary team management in head and neck cancer patients. *British Journal of Cancer, 104*(8), 1246–1248. https://doi.org/10.1038/bjc.2011.92. Retrieved from https://www.ncbi.nlm.nih.gov/pubmed/21448166

Gooi, Z., Fakhry, C., Goldenberg, D., Richmon, J., Kiess, A. P., & Education Committee of the American Head & Neck, Society. (2016). AHNS series: Do you know your guidelines? Principles of radiation therapy for head and neck cancer: A review of the National Comprehensive Cancer Network guidelines. *Head & Neck, 38*(7), 987–992. https://doi.org/10.1002/hed.24448. Retrieved from https://www.ncbi.nlm.nih.gov/pubmed/27015108

Govender, R., Smith, C. H., Gardner, B., Barratt, H., & Taylor, S. A. (2017). Improving swallowing outcomes in patients with head and neck cancer using a theory-based pretreatment swallowing intervention package: Protocol for a randomised feasibility study. *BMJ Open, 7*(3), e014167. https://doi.org/10.1136/bmjopen-2016-014167. Retrieved from https://www.ncbi.nlm.nih.gov/pubmed/28348190

Govender, R., Wood, C. E., Taylor, S. A., Smith, C. H., Barratt, H., & Gardner, B. (2017). Patient experiences of swallowing exercises after head and neck cancer: A qualitative study examining barriers and facilitators using behaviour change theory. *Dysphagia, 32*(4), 559–569. https://doi.org/10.1007/s00455-017-9799-x. Retrieved from https://www.ncbi.nlm.nih.gov/pubmed/28424898

Hancock, P. J., Epstein, J. B., & Sadler, G. R. (2003). Oral and dental management related to radiation therapy for head and neck cancer. *Journal of the Canadian Dental Association, 69*(9), 585–590.

Harris, P. A., Taylor, R., Thielke, R., Payne, J., Gonzalez, N., & Conde, J. G. (2009). Research electronic data capture (REDCap)--a metadata-driven methodology and workflow process for providing translational research informatics support. *Journal of Biomedical Information, 42*(2), 377–381. https://doi.org/10.1016/j.jbi.2008.08.010. Retrieved from https://www.ncbi.nlm.nih.gov/pubmed/18929686

Hazin, R., & Qaddoumi, I. (2010). Teleoncology: Current and future applications for improving cancer care globally. *The Lancet Oncology, 11*(2), 204–210. https://doi.org/10.1016/S1470-2045(09)70288-8. Retrieved from https://www.ncbi.nlm.nih.gov/pubmed/20152772

Hughes, C., Homer, J., Bradley, P., Nutting, C., Ness, A., Persson, M., … Thomas, S. (2012). An evaluation of current services available for people diagnosed with head and neck cancer in the UK (2009-2010). *Clinical Oncology, 24*(10), e187–e192. https://doi.org/10.1016/j.clon.2012.07.005. Retrieved from https://www.ncbi.nlm.nih.gov/pubmed/22858437

Hutcheson, K. A., Bhayani, M. K., Beadle, B. M., Gold, K. A., Shinn, E. H., Lai, S. Y., & Lewin, J. (2013). Eat and exercise during radiotherapy or chemoradiotherapy for pharyngeal cancers: Use it or lose it. *JAMA Otolaryngology. Head & Neck Surgery, 139*(11), 1127–1134. https://doi.org/10.1001/jamaoto.2013.4715. Retrieved from http://www.ncbi.nlm.nih.gov/pubmed/24051544

Hutcheson, K. A., & Lewin, J. S. (2012). Functional outcomes after chemoradiotherapy of laryngeal and pharyngeal cancers. *Current Oncology Reports, 14*(2), 158–165. https://doi.org/10.1007/s11912-012-0216-1. Retrieved from http://www.ncbi.nlm.nih.gov/pubmed/22249533

Hutcheson, K. A., Lewin, J. S., Barringer, D. A., Lisec, A., Gunn, G. B., Moore, M. W., & Holsinger, F. C. (2012). Late dysphagia after radiotherapy-based treatment of head and neck cancer. *Cancer, 118*(23), 5793–5799. https://doi.org/10.1002/cncr.27631. Retrieved from https://www.ncbi.nlm.nih.gov/pubmed/23640737

Jamal, N., Ebersole, B., Erman, A., & Chhetri, D. (2017). Maximizing functional outcomes in head and neck cancer survivors: Assessment and rehabilitation. *Otolaryngologic Clinics of North America, 50*(4), 837–852. https://doi.org/10.1016/j.otc.2017.04.004. Retrieved from https://www.ncbi.nlm.nih.gov/pubmed/28606600

Kotz, T., Federman, A. D., Kao, J., Milman, L., Packer, S., Lopez-Prieto, C., … Genden, E. M. (2012). Prophylactic swallowing exercises in patients with head and neck cancer undergoing chemoradiation: A randomized trial. *Archives of Otolaryngology – Head & Neck Surgery, 138*(4), 376–382. https://doi.org/10.1001/archoto.2012.187. Retrieved from https://www.ncbi.nlm.nih.gov/pubmed/22508621

Kraaijenga, S. A., van der Molen, L., van den Brekel, M. W., & Hilgers, F. J. (2014). Current assessment and treatment strategies of dysphagia in head and neck cancer patients: A systematic review of the 2012/13 literature. *Current Opinion in Supportive and Palliative Care, 8*(2), 152–163. https://doi.org/10.1097/SPC.0000000000000050. Retrieved from http://www.ncbi.nlm.nih.gov/pubmed/24743298

Krisciunas, G. P., Sokoloff, W., Stepas, K., & Langmore, S. E. (2012). Survey of usual practice: Dysphagia therapy in head and neck cancer patients. *Dysphagia,*

27(4), 538–549. https://doi.org/10.1007/s00455-012-9404-2. Retrieved from https://www.ncbi.nlm.nih.gov/pubmed/22456699

Kulbersh, B. D., Rosenthal, E. L., McGrew, B. M., Duncan, R. D., McColloch, N. L., Carroll, W. R., & Magnuson, J. S. (2006). Pretreatment, preoperative swallowing exercises may improve dysphagia quality of life. *Laryngoscope, 116*(6), 883–886. https://doi.org/10.1097/01.mlg.0000217278.96901.fc. Retrieved from https://www.ncbi.nlm.nih.gov/pubmed/16735913

Lassig, A. A., Joseph, A. M., Lindgren, B. R., Fernandes, P., Cooper, S., Schotzko, C., … Yueh, B. (2012). The effect of treating institution on outcomes in head and neck cancer. *Otolaryngology and Head and Neck Surgery, 147*(6), 1083–1092. https://doi.org/10.1177/0194599812457324. Retrieved from https://www.ncbi.nlm.nih.gov/pubmed/22875780

Lawson, N., Krisciunas, G. P., Langmore, S. E., Castellano, K., Sokoloff, W., & Hayatbakhsh, R. (2017). Comparing dysphagia therapy in head and neck cancer patients in Australia with international healthcare systems. *International Journal of Speech-Language Pathology, 19*(2), 128–138. https://doi.org/10.3109/17549507.2016.1159334. Retrieved from https://www.ncbi.nlm.nih.gov/pubmed/27093099

Lawson, N. R., & Ward, E. C. (2014). Patient support and multidisciplinary management. In E. C. Ward & C. J. van As-Brooks (Eds.), *Head and neck cancer: Treatment, rehabilitation and outcomes* (Vol. 2, 2nd ed., pp. 447–492). San Diego, CA: Plural Publishing.

Leonard, R., & Kendall, K. (2014). Anatomy and physiology of deglutition. In R. Leonard & K. Kendall (Eds.), *Dysphagia assessment and treatment planning: A team approach.* San Diego, CA: Plural Publishing.

Lewis, C. M., Hessel, A. C., Roberts, D. B., Guo, Y. Z., Holsinger, F. C., Ginsberg, L. E., … Weber, R. S. (2010). Preferral head and neck cancer treatment: Compliance with national comprehensive cancer network treatment guidelines. *Archives of Otolaryngology – Head & Neck Surgery, 136*(12), 1205–1211. https://doi.org/10.1001/archoto.2010.206. Retrieved from https://www.ncbi.nlm.nih.gov/pubmed/21173369

Logemann, J. A., & Bytell, D. E. (1979). Swallowing disorders in three types of head and neck surgical patients. *Cancer, 44*(3), 1095–1105. Retrieved from https://www.ncbi.nlm.nih.gov/pubmed/476587.

Logemann, J. A., Pauloski, B. R., Rademaker, A. W., Lazarus, C. L., Gaziano, J., Stachowiak, L., … Mittal, B. (2008). Swallowing disorders in the first year after radiation and chemoradiation. *Head & Neck, 30*(2), 148–158. https://doi.org/10.1002/hed.20672. Retrieved from https://www.ncbi.nlm.nih.gov/pubmed/17786992

Manikantan, K., Khode, S., Sayed, S. I., Roe, J., Nutting, C. M., Rhys-Evans, P., … Kazi, R. (2009). Dysphagia in head and neck cancer. *Cancer Treatment Reviews, 35*(8), 724–732. https://doi.org/10.1016/j.

ctrv.2009.08.008. Retrieved from http://www.ncbi.nlm.nih.gov/pubmed/19751966

Mcconnel, F. M., Logemann, J. A., Rademaker, A. W., Pauloski, B. R., Baker, S. R., Lewin, J., … Graner, D. (1994). Surgical variables affecting postoperative swallowing efficiency in oral cancer patients: a pilot study. *The Laryngoscope, 104*(1), 87–90.

Messing, B., Ward, E. C., Ryniak, K., Kim, M., Silinonte, J., Differding, J., … Lazarus, C. (2017, March). *A clinical pathway for swallowing services for patients with head and neck cancer: A service implementation evaluation.* Dysphagia Research Society Meeting. Poster presentation. Portland, OR: Dysphagia Research Society.

Messing, B. P., Ward, E. C., Lazarus, C. L., Kim, M., Zhou, X., Silinonte, J., … Califano, J. (2017). Prophylactic swallow therapy for patients with head and neck cancer undergoing chemoradiotherapy: A randomized trial. *Dysphagia, 32*(4), 487–500. https://doi.org/10.1007/s00455-017-9790-6. Retrieved from https://www.ncbi.nlm.nih.gov/pubmed/28444488

Miller, M. C., Goldenberg, D., & Education Committee of American Head & Neck Society. (2016). Do you know your guidelines? An initiative of the American Head and Neck Society's Education Committee. *Head & Neck, 38*(2), 165–167. https://doi.org/10.1002/hed.24104. Retrieved from https://www.ncbi.nlm.nih.gov/pubmed/25919964

Mortensen, H. R., Jensen, K., Aksglaede, K., Lambertsen, K., Eriksen, E., & Grau, C. (2015). Prophylactic swallowing exercises in head and neck cancer radiotherapy. *Dysphagia, 30,* 304–314. https://doi.org/10.1007/s00455-015-9600-y. Retrieved from http://www.ncbi.nlm.nih.gov/pubmed/25690840

National Comprehensive Cancer Network. (2017). *NCCN clinical practice guidelines in oncology (NCCN guidelines ®) head and neck cancers version 2.2017.* Retrieved from https://www.nccn.org/professionals/physician_gls/f_guidelines.asp.

Nguyen, N. P., Moltz, C. C., Frank, C., Vos, P., Smith, H. J., Karlsson, U., … Sallah, S. (2006). Evolution of chronic dysphagia following treatment for head and neck cancer. *Oral Oncology, 42*(4), 374–380. https://doi.org/10.1016/j.oraloncology.2005.09.003. Retrieved from http://www.ncbi.nlm.nih.gov/pubmed/16314138

Ni Riordain, R., & McCreary, C. (2009). Head and neck cancer information on the internet: Type, accuracy and content. *Oral Oncology, 45*(8), 675–677. https://doi.org/10.1016/j.oraloncology.2008.10.006. Retrieved from https://www.ncbi.nlm.nih.gov/pubmed/19095486

Ogawa, Y., Nemoto, K., Kakuto, Y., Seiji, H., Sasaki, K., Takahashi, C., … Yamada, S. (2005). Construction of a remote radiotherapy planning system. *International Journal of Clinical Oncology, 10*(1), 26–29. https://doi.org/10.1007/s10147-004-0446-9. Retrieved from https://www.ncbi.nlm.nih.gov/pubmed/15729597

Olver, I. N., & Selva-Nayagam, S. (2000). Evaluation of a telemedicine link between Darwin and Adelaide to facilitate cancer management. *Telemedicine Journal, 6*(2), 213–218. https://doi.org/10.1089/107830200415144. Retrieved from https://www.ncbi.nlm.nih.gov/pubmed/10957733

Perkins, K. A., Hancock, K. L., & Ward, E. C. (2014). Speech and swallowing following laryngeal and hypopharyngeal cancer. In E. C. Ward & C. J. van As-Brooks (Eds.), *Head and neck cancer: Treatment, rehabilitation, and outcomes* (2nd ed., pp. 173–240). San Diego, CA: Plural Publishing.

Prades, J., Remue, E., van Hoof, E., & Borras, J. M. (2015). Is it worth reorganising cancer services on the basis of multidisciplinary teams (MDTs)? A systematic review of the objectives and organisation of MDTs and their impact on patient outcomes. *Health Policy, 119*(4), 464–474. https://doi.org/10.1016/j.healthpol.2014.09.006. Retrieved from https://www.ncbi.nlm.nih.gov/pubmed/25271171

Roe, J. W., & Ashforth, K. M. (2011). Prophylactic swallowing exercises for patients receiving radiotherapy for head and neck cancer. *Current Opinion in Otolaryngology & Head and Neck Surgery, 19*(3), 144–149. https://doi.org/10.1097/MOO.0b013e3283457616. Retrieved from http://www.ncbi.nlm.nih.gov/pubmed/21430531

Rosenthal, D. I., Lewin, J. S., & Eisbruch, A. (2006). Prevention and treatment of dysphagia and aspiration after chemoradiation for head and neck cancer. *Journal of Clinical Oncology, 24*(17), 2636–2643. https://doi.org/10.1200/JCO.2006.06.0079. Retrieved from https://www.ncbi.nlm.nih.gov/pubmed/16763277

Sabesan, S., Larkins, S., Evans, R., Varma, S., Andrews, A., Beuttner, P., … Young, M. (2012). Telemedicine for rural cancer care in North Queensland: Bringing cancer care home. *The Australian Journal of Rural Health, 20*(5), 259–264. https://doi.org/10.1111/j.1440-1584.2012.01299.x. Retrieved from https://www.ncbi.nlm.nih.gov/pubmed/22998200

Savage, S. A., Nixon, I., & MacKenzie, K. (2007). Teleconferencing in the management of head and neck cancer. *Clinical Otolaryngology, 32*(2), 130–132. https://doi.org/10.1111/j.1365-2273.2007.01329.x. Retrieved from https://www.ncbi.nlm.nih.gov/pubmed/17403234

Schindler, A., Denaro, N., Russi, E. G., Pizzorni, N., Bossi, P., Merlotti, A., … Murphy, B. (2015). Dysphagia in head and neck cancer patients treated with radiotherapy and systemic therapies: Literature review and consensus. *Critical Reviews in Oncology/Hematology, 96*(2), 372–384. https://doi.org/10.1016/j.critrevonc.2015.06.005. Retrieved from https://www.ncbi.nlm.nih.gov/pubmed/26141260

Shinn, E. H., Basen-Engquist, K., Baum, G., Steen, S., Bauman, R. F., Morrison, W., … Lewin, J. S. (2013). Adherence to preventive exercises and self-reported swallowing outcomes in post-radiation head and neck cancer patients. *Head & Neck, 35*(12), 1707–1712.

https://doi.org/10.1002/hed.23255. Retrieved from http://www.ncbi.nlm.nih.gov/pubmed/24142523

Stalfors, J., Edstrom, S., Bjork-Eriksson, T., Mercke, C., Nyman, J., & Westin, T. (2001). Accuracy of tele-oncology compared with face-to-face consultation in head and neck cancer case conferences. *Journal of Telemedicine and Telecare, 7*(6), 338–343. https://doi.org/10.1258/1357633011936976. Retrieved from https://www.ncbi.nlm.nih.gov/pubmed/11747635

Taylor-Goh, S. (2005). Royal College of Speech & Language Therapists Clinical Guidelines [Electronic Version]. On WWW at http://www.rcslt.org/resources/clinicalguidelines.

Taylor-Goh, S. (2017). *Royal College of Speech & Language Therapists clinical guidelines*. London: Routledge.

Tsai, W. C., Kung, P. T., Wang, S. T., Huang, K. H., & Liu, S. A. (2015). Beneficial impact of multidisciplinary team management on the survival in different stages of oral cavity cancer patients: Results of a nationwide cohort study in Taiwan. *Oral Oncology, 51*(2), 105–111. https://doi.org/10.1016/j.oraloncology.2014.11.006. Retrieved from https://www.ncbi.nlm.nih.gov/pubmed/25484134

van den Berg, M. G., Kalf, J. G., Hendriks, J. C., Takes, R. P., van Herpen, C. M., Wanten, G. J., … Merkx, M. A. (2016). Normalcy of food intake in patients with head and neck cancer supported by combined dietary counseling and swallowing therapy: A randomized clinical trial. *Head & Neck, 38*(Suppl 1), E198–E206. https://doi.org/10.1002/hed.23970. Retrieved from https://www.ncbi.nlm.nih.gov/pubmed/25533021

van der Molen, L., van Rossum, M. A., Burkhead, L. M., Smeele, L. E., Rasch, C. R., & Hilgers, F. J. (2011). A randomized preventive rehabilitation trial in advanced head and neck cancer patients treated with chemoradiotherapy: Feasibility, compliance, and short-term effects. *Dysphagia, 26*(2), 155–170. https://doi.org/10.1007/s00455-010-9288-y. Retrieved from http://www.ncbi.nlm.nih.gov/pubmed/20623305

van der Molen, L., van Rossum, M. A., Rasch, C. R., Smeele, L. E., & Hilgers, F. J. (2014). Two-year results of a prospective preventive swallowing rehabilitation trial in patients treated with chemoradiation for advanced head and neck cancer. *European Archives of Oto-Rhino-Laryngology, 271*(5), 1257–1270. https://doi.org/10.1007/s00405-013-2640-8. Retrieved from http://www.ncbi.nlm.nih.gov/pubmed/23892729

Virani, A., Kunduk, M., Fink, D. S., & McWhorter, A. J. (2015). Effects of 2 different swallowing exercise regimens during organ-preservation therapies for head and neck cancers on swallowing function. *Head & Neck, 37*(2), 162–170. https://doi.org/10.1002/hed.23570. Retrieved from https://www.ncbi.nlm.nih.gov/pubmed/24347440

Wall, L. R., Cartmill, B., Ward, E. C., Hill, A. J., Isenring, E., Byrnes, J., … Porceddu, S. V. (2016). "ScreenIT": Computerized screening of swallowing, nutrition and distress in head and neck cancer patients during (chemo)radiotherapy. *Oral Oncology, 54*, 47–53. https://doi.org/10.1016/j.oraloncology.2016.01.004. Retrieved from https://www.ncbi.nlm.nih.gov/pubmed/26803342

Wall, L. R., Cartmill, B., Ward, E. C., Hill, A. J., Isenring, E., & Porceddu, S. V. (2016). Evaluation of a weekly speech pathology/dietetic service model for providing supportive care intervention to head and neck cancer patients and their carers during (chemo)radiotherapy. *Support Care Cancer, 24*(3), 1227–1234. https://doi.org/10.1007/s00520-015-2912-5. Retrieved from https://www.ncbi.nlm.nih.gov/pubmed/26304158

Wall, L. R., Ward, E. C., Cartmill, B., & Hill, A. J. (2013). Technology-assisted screening of patient-reported functional outcomes in the head and neck cancer population: What's the evidence? *OA Cancer, 1*(2), 1–7.

Wall, L. R., Ward, E. C., Cartmill, B., Hill, A. J., & Porceddu, S. V. (2017a). Adherence to a prophylactic swallowing therapy program during (chemo)radiotherapy: Impact of service-delivery model and patient factors. *Dysphagia, 32*(2), 279–292. https://doi.org/10.1007/s00455-016-9757-z. Retrieved from https://www.ncbi.nlm.nih.gov/pubmed/27844152

Wall, L. R., Ward, E. C., Cartmill, B., Hill, A. J., & Porceddu, S. V. (2017b). Examining user perceptions of SwallowIT: A pilot study of a new telepractice application for delivering intensive swallowing therapy to head and neck cancer patients. *Journal of Telemedicine and Telecare, 23*(1), 53–59. https://doi.org/10.1177/1357633X15617887. Retrieved from https://www.ncbi.nlm.nih.gov/pubmed/26670210

Wang, Y. H., Kung, P. T., Tsai, W. C., Tai, C. J., Liu, S. A., & Tsai, M. H. (2012). Effects of multidisciplinary care on the survival of patients with oral cavity cancer in Taiwan. *Oral Oncology, 48*(9), 803–810. https://doi.org/10.1016/j.oraloncology.2012.03.023. Retrieved from https://www.ncbi.nlm.nih.gov/pubmed/22534006

Ward, E. C., Wall, L. R., Burns, C. L., Cartmill, B., & Hill, A. J. (2017). Application of telepractice for head and neck cancer management: A review of speech language pathology service models. *Current Opinion in Otolaryngology & Head and Neck Surgery, 25*(3), 169–174. https://doi.org/10.1097/MOO.0000000000000357. Retrieved from https://www.ncbi.nlm.nih.gov/pubmed/28319481

Weed, D. T. (1997). Clinical pathways for the care of patients with head and neck cancer. *Current Opinion in Otolaryngology & Head and Neck Surgery, 5*(2), 67–72.

Part II

Treatment Related Changes: Breathing, Voice, Speech and Swallowing

Postlaryngectomy Respiratory System and Speech Breathing

Todd Allen Bohnenkamp

The biological function of the respiratory system is to maintain stable blood gas values during changing homeostatic demands (e.g., changing posture, walking, exercising, sleeping, increased cognitive load, speaking) by exchanging oxygen (O_2) from the air into the blood supply and removing carbon dioxide (CO_2) efficiently (Hugelin, 1986; Shea, 1996; von Euler, 1997; West, 2013). Maintaining this balance requires the seamless integration of automatic and voluntary control systems for respiration. Changes in the upper airway in speakers following a total laryngectomy subsequently alter how clinicians and researchers approach respiration, as well as their production of alaryngeal speech (see Lewis, Chap. 8, and Searl, Chap. 13). Many of these speakers are older, have a past medical history of smoking, and are likely to suffer from some degree of chronic obstructive pulmonary disease (COPD). To compound matters, upper airway changes following laryngectomy likely result in compensatory alterations to breathing. The removal of laryngeal afferent input, greater upper airway resistance, and possible respiratory compromise may affect the flexibility necessary for maintaining homeostasis and for achieving proficient alaryngeal speech (Bohnenkamp, Forrest,

Klaben, & Stager, 2012; Bohnenkamp, Forrest, Klaben, & Stager, 2011; Bohnenkamp, Stowell, Hesse, & Wright, 2010; Donnelly, 1991; Fontana, Pantaleo, Lavorini, Mutolo, Polli, & Pistolesi, 1999; Hida, 1999; Lee, Loudon, Jacobson, & Stuebing, 1993; Sant'Ambrogio, Matthew, Fisher, & Sant'Ambrogio, 1983).

Each alaryngeal speech option varies in its reliance on the respiratory system. Speakers who use an electrolarynx (EL) have a decoupled phonatory and respiratory system, whereas speakers who rely on esophageal speech (ES) may be required to have fine control of the respiratory system depending upon the method of esophageal charging for phonation (e.g., inhalation or injection method). Speakers who use tracheoesophageal speech (TE) as their primary mode of communication are most likely to encounter difficulties with speech associated with respiratory changes (see Graville, Palmer & Bolognone, Chap. 11).

The reliance on the respiratory system for speech in all speakers is influenced by many factors. These unavoidable factors include the influence of sensory input, the balance between the voluntary and involuntary control systems, and maintaining the balance of O_2 and CO_2 in the body. These are all manipulated differently by respiratory demand and speech task (e.g., rest breathing, speech, and oral reading). In the case of speakers with a total laryngectomy, the disconnect of the upper airway and removal of the larynx, age-related changes in the respiratory system, and

T. A. Bohnenkamp (✉)
Department of Communication Sciences and Disorders, University of Northern Iowa, Cedar Falls, IA, USA
e-mail: todd.bohnenkamp@uni.edu

© Springer Nature Switzerland AG 2019
P. C. Doyle (ed.), *Clinical Care and Rehabilitation in Head and Neck Cancer*,
https://doi.org/10.1007/978-3-030-04702-3_7

smoking-related illness will combine with the aforementioned factors to result in adaptations and compensations to breathing to produce speech. This chapter will provide a background on how respiration and the consequences of total laryngectomy affect breathing in these individuals and how these changes may influence alaryngeal speech.

The Importance of Laryngeal Afference

Total laryngectomy results in the removal of the larynx and superior laryngeal nerve (SLN) of cranial nerve (CN) X (vagus). Subsequently, speakers with a total laryngectomy regardless of past smoking history may experience altered breathing and respiratory patterns. The SLN may influence the timing and firing rate of the respiratory muscles (Fontana et al., 1999), a process which aids in maintaining airway integrity. Airflow, pressure, mucosal temperature, and stretch receptor sensation are altered due to the loss of laryngeal afferent input, which comprises 1/3 of all afferent input from the tracheobronchial tree (Donnelly, 1991; Fontana et al., 1999; Sant'Ambrogio et al., 1983). Though the influence of afferent input may be overstated relative to breath-to-breath control, this afferent input is robust and will terminate any respiratory drive during aspiration in individuals with an intact larynx. In addition, this feedback allows individuals to manipulate air pressure differences within 1–2 cm H_2O during both breathing and speech (Shea, 1996; Davis, Zhang, Winkworth, & Bandler, 1996). In the normal laryngeal system, the posterior cricoarytenoid muscles (PCA), oblique and transverse interarytenoid (IA) muscles, and lateral cricoarytenoid muscles (LCA) are active to valve airflow both during inspiration and during expiration. Specifically, IA and LCA are active during expiration to improve gas exchange by slowing expiratory airflow (Dick, Orem, & Shea, 1997). Ohala (1990), Warren (1996), and Wyke (1983) have stated that this may influence how an individual manipulates the respiratory system for speech.

Automatic and Voluntary Neural Control of Respiration

The neural and blood gas disruptions in speakers with respiratory compromise have received little inquiry by speech-language pathology, though they are likely to affect speakers with a total laryngectomy and are implicated in other communication disorders (Duffy, 1995; Kaneko, Zivanovic, Hajek, & Bradley, 2001; Khedr, Shinaway, Khedr, Aziz Ali, & Awad, 2000; Terao et al., 2001; Wessendorf, Teschler, Wang, Konietzko, & Thilman, 2000). The automatic control of the respiratory system responds to metabolic and blood gas changes by altering air flow resistance and respiratory muscle activity. This is accomplished via central pattern generators within the pons (Hugelin, 1986; von Euler, 1997). An example of an automatic response would be to manipulate the depth or rate of breathing to regulate increased levels of carbon dioxide in the blood. Conversely, the voluntary system is often responsible during increased levels of activity (e.g., during speech and exercise). This active process is accomplished by modulating inspiratory and expiratory durations based on afferent air pressure signals in the tracheobronchial and pulmonary airways (Davis et al., 1996; Garrett & Luschei, 1987; Testerman, 1970). Each control system is dependent upon neural signaling from CN IX and X, which transmit information regarding blood gas levels in the aortic blood flow and the status of the stretch receptors (e.g., respond to lung inflation, vibration, inspiratory/expiratory effort, lung volume changes, degree of expiratory or inspiratory effort, and resistance to airflow) in the lungs (Guz, 1997; Shea, 1996). The stretch receptors are the primary inputs that contribute to the perception of shortness of breath, or what is termed dyspnea (Homma, Obata, Sibuya, & Uchida, 1984).

Involuntary and Voluntary Neural Control of Respiration: Speech

Maintaining appropriate O_2 and CO_2 values differ by activity. Specifically, the demands during speech on that maintenance are greater than that during resting tidal breathing but much less than during exercise. Both demands result in increased CO_2 levels in the blood, which results in stimulation to increase either depths of inspiration, use of a greater amount of vital capacity (VC; i.e., greater inspiratory volumes and expirations into a speaker's functional residual capacity; FRC), or increasing respiratory rate to balance blood gases. These adaptations to demands require an integration of motor intent and sensory feedback wherein the voluntary control system is primarily responsible as it overrides our involuntary respiratory system's automatic control drive to breathe.

CO_2 levels increase for short amounts of time during speech, which requires the use of the voluntary system by speakers to ignore hypercapnia (i.e., increased partial pressures of carbon dioxide in the blood; PCO_2). They must complete the utterance and then return to resting chemostatic values via hyperventilation (Hoit & Lohmeier, 2000). In contrast to the response to CO_2, speakers will ignore reduced O_2 levels in the blood to maintain communication, even during instances when completing rigorous exercise (Bunn & Mead, 1971; Hoit & Lohmeier, 2000; Phillipson, McClean, Sullivan, & Zamel, 1978; Russell, Cerny, & Stathopoulos, 1998; Shea, 1996). Eventually, a speaker can no longer maintain the ability to override the need to breathe, which results in breathing for gas exchange and reducing airflows needed for speech by 55% (Doust & Patrick, 1981).

Previous research has indicated that speech is perhaps a more robust voluntary activity than other motor activities. For example, speakers are less likely to complain of the effects of hypercapnia while completing a speech task than while under the same hypercapnic conditions at rest (Phillipson et al., 1978). The voluntary system allows speakers to ignore the hypercapnic stimulus until chemical gas values are much more compromised. However, in contrast to a speech task, Corfield, Roberts, Guz, Murphy, and Adams (1999) reported that individuals in slight hypercapnia demonstrated difficulty manually moving a joystick to track a cursor on a computer screen. Therefore, the complex motor act of speech

which includes the integration of language, articulation, phonation, and respiration may not be as vulnerable to the effects of hypercapnia as a simple motor tracking task is to even slight hypercapnia. Alaryngeal speakers with COPD, though compromised, may not demonstrate the chronic effects of hypercapnia due to their ability to overcome the need to breathe to complete the message.

Speech Breathing in Laryngeal Speakers

An explanation of the similarities and differences between the two theories of speech breathing (i.e., the classic; Draper, Ladefoged, & Whitteridge, 1959; contemporary; Hixon, Goldman, & Mead, 1973; Hixon, Mead, & Goldman, 1976) is beyond the scope of this chapter; however, there are numerous aspects of respiratory control in speakers who undergo a total laryngectomy that differ from typical speakers. Both theories reported that speech requires the coordination of active muscular manipulation of the system (e.g., diaphragm, abdominal muscle contraction, external and internal intercostal contraction, etc.) combined with the inherent amount of relaxation forces available to speakers such as those related to tissue elasticity and recoil and gravity (Draper et al., 1959; Hixon et al., 1973, 1976).

The two theories of speech breathing diverge primarily in their explanation of abdominal muscle activity. The classic theory argues that the abdominal musculature is not needed until the ends of utterances, whereas the contemporary theory stated that abdominal activity is needed prior to and throughout speech. The contemporary view posited that simultaneous internal and external intercostal activity during speech combines with relaxation forces to produce speech.

Typical speech requires deeper inspirations and expirations in addition to increased muscle activity in the chest wall in contrast to what is required in quiet tidal breathing (Draper et al., 1959; Hixon et al., 1973, 1976). Speakers rely primarily on rib cage musculature to inspire to greater percent of their vital capacities (%VC) to provide the relaxation forces needed for speech. Inspiration is always active, but tidal breathing at rest relies on passive forces of the rib cage for expiration. The contemporary view reported that the %VC needed for tidal breathing lies in the middle ranges between 45%VC and 36%VC (i.e., approximate resting expiratory level in typical individuals; REL). Speech, in contrast, occurs between 60%VC and 36%VC (Hixon et al., 1973, 1976). Further, speech is terminated at or near REL which improves speech efficiency and reduces effort. Once a speaker speaks past their REL into their FRC, all expiratory force then becomes active or muscular in nature in an effort to overcome the negative forces of inspiration. This all occurs as speech is almost exclusively initiated and terminated at grammatically appropriate sentence of phrase boundaries, which are likely preplanned and influenced by the utterance length and complexity in addition to the balancing of metabolic demands with speech.

Draper and colleagues had earlier argued in the classic theory of speech breathing that abdominal activity was not required until the speaker reaches lower %VC at the ends of utterances and that there was no need for overlap of activity of the inspiratory and expiratory muscles of the rib cage (i.e., external and internal intercostal muscles). In contrast, to produce the pressures needed for speech, Hixon and colleagues had argued in the contemporary theory that constant abdominal activation is present prior to and during speech and that this results in a generally predictable pattern of chest wall configuration for speech (Hixon et al., 1973, 1976). This general speech configuration change consists of expiratory (inward) abdominal movement followed by rib cage expansion (elevation and reduction of the space between ribs). Hixon and colleagues further contradicted the original Draper et al. argument by reporting the co-contraction, or overlap of activity, of the inspiratory and expiratory muscles of the rib cage muscles during speech to allow for quick and subtle changes to air flows and pressures (i.e., net-zero posture). Interestingly, Ladefoged and Loeb (2002) later reported that, in fact, the rectus abdominis is active prior to and throughout speech utterances and there is a general acceptance that abdominal contraction is essential during speech.

Whereas previous researchers have suggested that the abdominal contraction and rib cage configuration prior to speech are a predictable and relatively invariable oppositional speech-specific process in males (90% of the time; Baken & Cavallo, 1981; Baken, Cavallo, & Weissman, 1979; Cavallo & Baken, 1985), others argued there is no standard or predictable process (Hixon, 1988; McFarland & Smith, 1992; Wilder, 1983). The lack of a predictable posturing allows for flexibility in the production of volumes, flows, and pressures for speech depending on utterance demands. Wilder (1983) reported that a predictable response was present in only 32% of typical healthy female speakers, suggesting that prephonatory posturing is likely to differ by sex of the speaker. This provides adaptability, to the variability of speech task and glottal configuration (Iwarsson, 2001; McFarland & Smith, 1992). Taken together, these findings indicate that control of the chest wall for speech breathing is likely to be flexible and adaptive and will vary by sex and task. This suggests that control of the chest wall will be altered in alaryngeal speakers due to the many changes to the upper airway following a total laryngectomy.

Speech Task

It is well documented that speaking task influences breathing behaviors in typical speakers (Goldman-Eisler, 1968; Goldman-Eisler, 1961; Winkworth, Davis, Adams, & Ellis, 1995; Winkworth, Davis, Ellis, & Adams, 1994) and these differences are likely to be exacerbated in alaryngeal speakers. Speakers will regularly hyperventilate on inspiration following the completion of an utterance to balance blood gas values; however, speech research indicates that these inspirations are more likely to be influenced by the length and complexity of an upcoming utterance rather than recovering from a previous utterance (Goldman-Eisler, 1961, 1968). These inspirations that match length of an utterance argue for a preplanning of speech at the level of the respiratory system. This preplanning can differ by task, specifically in relation to oral reading and spontaneous speech. Winkworth et al. (1994) and Winkworth et al. (1995) reported that inspirations are taken at linguistically appropriate boundaries (e.g., clause boundary, sentence) during both spontaneous speech and oral reading. These inspirations are speaker-specific during spontaneous speech but are determined by text during oral reading. The dynamic nature of spontaneous speech may, therefore, necessitate online adjustments by the respiratory system, whereas oral reading requires inspirations taken to match an unknown, upcoming utterance length. When evaluating utterance length and respiratory behaviors, it is important to understand that speakers behave differently when generating spontaneous speech and oral reading. This is especially so in speakers with respiratory compromise, as well as alaryngeal speakers who may further alter their breathing patterns (Lee et al., 1993). When considering the three primary alaryngeal modes, electrolaryngeal, esophageal, and TE speech, TE speakers are the most likely to encounter these issues because of their use of pulmonary air support and their need to overcome the inherent resistance increases in the neoglottis and TE puncture prosthesis. This information is valuable in the assessment of an alaryngeal speaker's breathing patterns because the speech tasks are not interchangeable and are not comparable. These task changes are also influenced by the expected age-related changes in breathing.

Age

Age is an unavoidable influence on the respiratory system. It can be difficult to determine what causes respiratory changes and whether they are an expected process due to aging and/or if they are combined with injury, smoking, and environmental factors. Changes in the respiratory system might be functional, structural, mechanical, or related to ventilation/perfusion/diffusion and nervous system changes (Ayres, 1990; Chan & Welsh, 1998; Janssens, Pache, & Nicod, 1999; Hoit & Hixon, 1987) and, consequently, are

likely to affect people who have undergone a total laryngectomy.

The interaction of passive and active (muscular) forces for speech is altered as age-related changes result in reduced elasticity, thorax stiffening, respiratory muscle weakness, loss of cross-sectional intercostal muscles tissue, and increased use of high lung volumes to create relaxation forces (Brown & Hasser, 1996; Dhar, Shastri, & Lenora, 1976; Kahane, 1980; McKeown, 1965; Pierce & Ebert, 1965; Tolep & Kelsen, 1993). Older speakers have fewer alveoli and fewer capillaries per alveolus which results in a subsequent loss of airway tissue and contributes to the reduction in elasticity. This also may result in changes in gas exchange and air trapping from collapse of the small airways, namely, bronchioles (Janssens et al., 1999). For example, 60-year-old males can expend 20% more energy during tidal breathing than do 20-year-olds (Janssens et al., 1999). Thus, age-related declines in breathing might be exacerbated following a total laryngectomy, especially considering the age of a typical speaker with a laryngectomy.

The physiological response to muscle atrophy secondary to age is that there is a concomitant reduction in the individual's VC (Hoit & Hixon, 1987; Kendall, 2007; Sperry & Klich, 1992). Vital capacities are reduced by up to 1 L in older speakers as a result of calcification of intercostal and vertebral joints (Crapo, 1993; Murray, 1986). Hoit and Hixon (1987) reported that residual volume (i.e., dead space which is unusable during respiration) also increases with age. As a result of the increased muscular effort necessary for successful compensation, older adults may have less physical reserve to deal with illness when it occurs. These age-related differences may make the effects of a disease state more pronounced, especially in older speakers with COPD, as well as creating likely alternations in alaryngeal speakers (Crapo, 1993).

Respiratory Compromise

COPD is characterized by dyspnea (discomfort during breathing), altered O_2 and CO_2 values due to ventilation-perfusion mismatch, excessive secretions, hypertrophy of mucous glands, and narrowing of airways within the lungs (West, 2013). It is a disease that is assumed during life and confirmed only following death. Though COPD is often associated with a past history of smoking, not all who present with COPD have a history of smoking. Speakers with severe COPD may demonstrate breathlessness, shorter utterance lengths, and poor ability to control speaking loudness (Lee et al., 1993). Additionally, speakers with COPD may be hypercapnic at rest (Hida, 1999) and only worsen with increased activity due to a ventilation-perfusion mismatch.

The ventilation-perfusion mismatch is due to the destruction of the walls of the alveoli and the capillary bed, thereby, reducing both blood flow surrounding the alveoli and subsequent gas exchange. The inability for O_2 to enter the arterial blood and for CO_2 to leave the venous blood flow may result in increased levels of CO_2 in the blood. This may be viewed as a maladaptive compensation because COPD speakers are more likely to prefer to function in this mild hypercapnic state versus increasing the work of breathing during inspiration to increase O_2 (West, 2013). Subsequently, speakers with COPD are likely to alter their breathing for speech. An alteration in response to the reduction in relaxation forces would be to increase muscular activity of the rib cage and abdomen to complete gas exchange (Sharp, Goldberg, Druz, Fishman, & Danon, 1977). Examples of these alterations include lip pursing, altering the rate and depth of inspirations, and recruiting extraneous chest wall activity (Lee et al., 1993; Hida, 1999). Speakers with a total laryngectomy are not able to adapt by using lip pursing due to the loss of airflow through the upper airway as a strategy and would be left with chest wall manipulation as a strategy. The chronic hypercapnic state in these speakers could result in a constant level of discomfort during breathing and speech. Typical speakers routinely demonstrate slightly higher CO_2 levels during utterance and subsequently have to recover, or hyperventilate, following speech production to maintain O_2 and CO_2 values (Hoit & Lohmeier, 2000; Russell et al., 1998); speakers with a laryngectomy may experience exacerbated discomfort.

Speakers with COPD have reduced VC, elevated REL, produce fewer syllables per breath group, increase their abdominal activity during both rest and speech, and produce increased expiratory flows (Lee et al., 1993). The result is that speakers with COPD maintain adequate gas exchange by shortening utterances and increasing the number of inspirations. Because of the effects of COPD on reducing elasticity in the respiratory system, speakers with COPD do not benefit by increasing their %VC at initiation. Instead, they produce increased expiratory flows, which results in their speaking well past their REL into FRC. This results in abnormal thoracoabdominal motion, with increased anterior-posterior dimensions of the thorax and paradoxical activity of the abdomen and rib cage during both rest breathing and maximal voluntary ventilation. This subsequently increases the likelihood of increased effort and probably recruitment of accessory muscles of respiration (Sharp et al., 1977) with its own negative consequences on both gas exchange and speech production.

Previous research has attempted to mimic the effects of COPD by placing typical healthy speakers in slightly hypercapnic states. This forces speakers to balance speech demands with their metabolic demands. Under these conditions, they respond by increasing %VC at speech initiation and terminating at increased VC. This is contradictory to how speakers with COPD respond. The lack of elasticity and the physiologic damage caused by COPD preclude these types of adjustments for both speech initiation and its termination. Speakers in a hypercapnic state produce fewer syllables per breath group and use increased chest wall activity. These speakers report difficulty maintaining linguistic boundaries during speech, but the fact that they attempted to maintain this structure indicates that linguistic effects are quite strong, even in high respiratory drive demands during oral reading (Bailey & Hoit, 2002). Based on their findings, Bailey and Hoit posited two models that could influence breathing. The first model is that metabolic needs and linguistic needs alternate during a breathing cycle (e.g., at one moment, metabolic needs predominate, whereas linguistic needs dominate at others). In contrast, the second model suggests the possibility that both speech and metabolic demands are adjusted simultaneously. However, both models acknowledge that linguistic and metabolic demands are important determinants of speech breathing.

Respiratory Changes Following a Total Laryngectomy

There is the likelihood that speakers with a total laryngectomy will present with COPD, with previous authors reporting rates anywhere between 70% and 81% (Ackerstaff, Hilgers, Balm, & Tan, 1998; Ackerstaff, Hilgers, Balm, & Van Zandwijk, 1995; Ackerstaff, Hilgers, Meeuwis, Knegt, & Weenink, 1999; Ackerstaff, Souren, van Zandwijk, Balm, & Hilgers, 1993; Hess, Schwenk, Frank, & Loddenkemper, 1999; Todisco, Maurizi, Paludetti, Dottorini, & Merante, 1984). To worsen matters for these individuals, pulmonary function testing is not likely to be included in standard assessment protocol in head and neck cancer patients and/or speakers with a laryngectomy (Matsuura et al., 1995). One explanation for the lack of testing is that there is inherent difficulty in the measurement of respiratory function for speakers via the tracheostoma; thus, it is clear that a need exists for improved approaches to assessment (Castro, Dedivitis, & Macedo, 2011).

VCs following a total laryngectomy are often less than 100% of their predicted value (Ackerstaff et al., 1998; Usui, 1979). Reports of VC as low as 2.5 L are common in laryngectomized speakers, a volume that is approximately 50% of that expected for adult males (Ackerstaff et al., 1998). Reduced functional expiratory volume, reduced maximum expiratory flow, peak and mean expiratory flows, and reduced residual volume are all expected in the first year following the total laryngectomy (Ackerstaff et al., 1995; Gregor & Hassman, 1984; Hess et al., 1999; Todisco et al., 1984; Togawa, Konno, & Hoshino, 1980; Usui, 1979).

Pre-laryngectomy smoking behaviors are most likely to influence respiratory health following the removal of the larynx (Ackerstaff et al., 1995; Gregor & Hassman, 1984; Hess et al., 1999; Todisco et al., 1984; Togawa et al., 1980; Usui, 1979); further, this is the primary predictor of an individual's long-term survival. Interestingly, pulmonary function improves immediately following laryngectomy and will stabilize within the first 5 months post-laryngectomy. However, there is an overall detrimental effect on quality of life and ability to maintain a healthy lifestyle (see Doyle & MacDonald, Chap. 27), with reports indicating that only about 8.5% of patients with a laryngectomy meet the physical activity guidelines of the American Cancer Society (Sammut, Ward, & Patel, 2014). This is likely to occur in speakers who have a past history of smoking, but may not apply to those who are younger and/or were of the small number of those who are laryngectomized as a result of the human papilloma virus (HPV) (see Theurer, Chap. 4).

Changes in pulmonary function are common following removal of the larynx but are not always simply related to premorbid smoking habits. For instance, the removal of the larynx and disconnection of the upper airway via the tracheostoma lead to an increased risk of infection by reducing the ciliary beat in the trachea (Todisco et al., 1984). Bacteria levels in the tracheobronchial tree increase up to 5 months post-laryngectomy and then plateau. This increase in bacteria and resulting infections may be an underlying factor in post-laryngectomy respiratory symptoms (Donnelly, 1991; Todisco et al., 1984). Additionally, the loss of the true vocal folds and larynx with the resultant need to breathe through a tracheostoma impairs resting breathing and tissue oxygenation saturation. However, the use of a humidity and moisture exchanger (HME) will help remedy these issues (see Lewis, Chap. 8).

Alaryngeal speakers are presented with a number of developmental and acquired physical changes that will affect speech. The effects of aging, respiratory compromise, and the loss of laryngeal sensation may theoretically influence breathing in speakers following a total laryngectomy, particularly the breath-to-breath control or timing of the firing of the muscles needed for forced expiration. In addition, the lack of airflow, pressure, mucosal temperature, and stretch receptor sensation due to loss of laryngeal input might alter breathing and gas exchange in these speakers. The likelihood that these speakers will suffer from COPD indicates that gas exchange and discomfort during speech may be present. Speakers who suffer from COPD are likely to manipulate the respiratory system differently than what has been reported in typical speakers placed in a hypercapnic state. Alaryngeal speakers have to overcome these respiratory influences and changes for speech. Specifically, TE speakers are the most likely to have to overcome upper airway and changes due to respiratory compromise, in addition to overcoming the increased resistance in the voice prosthesis and PE segment (see Childes, Palmer & Fried-Oken, Chap. 15). However, EL speakers and ES speakers must also adapt to these changes.

Speech Breathing in Alaryngeal Speakers

The three most common types of alaryngeal speech differ in the demands placed on the respiratory system. Speech using the electrolarynx does not require pulmonary air support, and there is a subsequent decoupling of respiratory and phonatory systems. Because of the nature of the phonatory source in EL speakers, there is no demand to maintain similar lung volumes at initiations and termination of speech as laryngeal speakers. Additionally, there is no linguistic or physiological demand to take inspirations at appropriate locations during speech or oral reading; however, the respiratory system is influenced and manipulated throughout speech in these speakers. Esophageal speech, in contrast, does not require pulmonary air support to vibrate the PE segment, but rather air is injected or inhaled into the esophagus for subsequent alaryngeal phonation which may require manipulation of the chest wall (DiCarlo, Amster, & Herer, 1955;

Isshiki & Snidecor, 1965). The effects of a total laryngectomy on alaryngeal speech are most likely to be demonstrated in TE speech. The ability to rely on pulmonary air support is the perceived advantage over EL and ES speech (Robbins, Fisher, Blom, & Singer, 1984); however, the placement of a voice prosthesis can increase resistance to airflow by up to three times that of the larynx, with resistances as high as 7.5 times that of laryngeal speakers when including the pharyngoesophageal segment (Weinberg, Horii, Blom, & Singer, 1982; Weinberg & Moon, 1982; Weinberg & Moon, 1986). This changes how speakers manipulate lung volumes as well as rib cage and abdominal configurations to overcome the anecdotal reports of effortful speech.

Electrolaryngeal Speakers

Pulmonary support is not required for electrolaryngeal speech; however, different chest wall configurations in these speakers can help shed light on the effects of a laryngectomy on respiration and alaryngeal speech. EL speakers' lung volumes at initiation and termination of speech during both spontaneous speech and oral reading are similar to that of tidal breathing, and their %VC are similar to what has been previously reported in laryngeal speakers as optimal for speech ((60–36%VC); Hixon et al., 1973, Hixon et al., 1976). The reports of similar %VCs provided in Table 7.1 are misleading in that people with a total laryngectomy are likely to demonstrate elevated REL (~45%VC; Bohnenkamp et al., 2012; Bohnenkamp et al., 2011; Bohnenkamp et al., 2010; Todisco et al., 1984; Togawa et al., 1980; Usui, 1979). Subsequently, interpretation of the termination lung volumes that are similar to typical speakers is likely due to EL speakers speaking past REL and into their FRC, similar to what has been reported in COPD speakers (see Table 7.1). EL speakers, if driven by metabolic demands, would likely choose to terminate expiration closer to 45%VC in contrast to 36%VC (Hixon et al., 1973, 1976).

Though not necessary, the rib cage and abdomen both expand during inspiration and contract

Table 7.1 Summary of mean percentage and standard deviation (SD) of vital capacity at initiation and termination during speech, oral reading, and tidal breathing

Speech mode	Speech	Oral reading	Tidal breathing
EL[1]			
Initiation	60.58 (6.34)	55.49 (7.52)	59.18 (6.51)
Termination	37.39 (7.98)	41.81 (5.95)	44.91 (9.56)[a]
TE[2,3]			
Initiation	67.51 (12.01)	72.74 (14.59)	61.51 (14.23)
	53.00 (8.00)	54.00 (7.00)	53.00 (7.00)[a]
Termination	36.36 (9.88)	36.37 (9.61)	46.16 (8.52)
	35.00 (10.00)	39.00 (8.00)	39.00 (8.00)[a]

Sources: Adapted from [1]Bohnenkamp et al. (2010); [2]Bohnenkamp et al. (2011); [3]Ward et al. (2007)
[a]Represents resting expiratory level

during expiration during speech (Bohnenkamp et al., 2010; Stepp, Heaton, & Hillman, 2008). This is interesting because of the contradictions and lack of consensus in previous literature as to whether speakers have a predictable posturing behavior prior to speech (Baken & Cavallo, 1981; Baken et al., 1979; Cavallo & Baken, 1985; Hixon, 1988; McFarland & Smith, 1992; Wilder, 1983). In the first 4 months following surgery, EL speakers demonstrate chest wall posturing similar to that of typical speakers (Stepp et al., 2008).

Over time, EL speakers will posture their chest wall less than half of the time during speech and oral reading tasks, and, likely to improve efficiency, any chest wall movement associated with speech more closely resembles tidal breathing or resembles a decoupling of abdominal contraction (Bohnenkamp et al., 2010; Stepp et al., 2008). Typical kinematic behaviors are firmly established throughout adulthood; however, the lack of posturing of the abdominal wall prior to speech indicates that perhaps an EL speaker's ventilatory control during speech is less likely to follow typical movements in the absence of respiratory demand. Their chest wall movements are similar to what would be demonstrated during tidal breathing and speech and have little effect on effort in these speakers (Table 7.2).

Further support for this decoupling in EL speakers is demonstrated in the timing of their activation of the electrolarynx with speech inspirations. Please see Table 7.3. Stepp et al. (2008) reported that EL speakers are less likely to activate the electrolarynx at the onset of expiration prior to speech. This is in contrast to that of

Table 7.2 Summary of mean percentage of maximal rib cage (%RC) and maximal abdominal (%Ab) use and standard deviation (SD) during speech, oral reading, and tidal breathing

Speech mode	Speech	Oral reading	Tidal breathing
EL[1]			
%RC	32.12 (16.83)	22.99 (15.80)	26.79 (16.42)
%Ab	22.51 (9.12)	16.02 (11.24)	12.87 (7.77)
TE[2]			
%RC	31.44 (16.72)	39.76 (16.30)	33.43 (22.09)
%Ab	33.40 (11.06)	36.95 (21.70)	12.51 (9.77)

Sources: Adapted from [1]Bohnenkamp et al. (2010); [2]Bohnenkamp et al. (2012)

laryngeal speakers who initiate speech on expiration. Instead, Stepp et al. reported that EL speakers are more likely to initiate the electrolarynx before peak inspiration and the onset of expiration 8–64% of the time during counting tasks and 10–44% during oral reading of the Rainbow Passage. There were individual differences by participant, but half of their EL speakers inspired during speech over 30% of the time. They were significantly more likely to inspire during speech production than ES and TE speakers. In addition, inspirations during speech production increased with increased time post-laryngectomy with one participant increasing their inspiration during speech from 19% at 4 months post-laryngectomy to 64% at 12 months. This is similar to the findings of Bohnenkamp et al. (2010) who reported that their electrolaryngeal speakers activated the

Table 7.3 Summary of mean percentage of inspirations at appropriate locations during speech and oral reading and standard deviation (SD) in EL and TE speakers

Speech mode	Speech	Oral reading
EL[1]		
All breaths	56.66 (19.76)	41.75 (12.00)
Only appropriate locations	82.03 (11.89)	80.41 (26.45)
EL pauses match inspirations	59.68 (22.47)	46.04 (26.82)
EL pauses match linguistically appropriate locations	50.29 (22.17)	36.58 (15.18)
TE[2]		
All breaths	79.30 (7.19)	77.63 (16.33)
Consistency across readings		63.67 (17.67)
Typical speakers		
All breaths	67.00 (N/A)[3]	90.00 (N/A)[4]
Consistency across readings		88.75 (6.96)[4]

Sources: Adapted from [1]Bohnenkamp et al. (2010); [2]Bohnenkamp et al. (2012); [3]Winkworth et al. (1995); Winkworth et al. (1994)

Table 7.4 Summary of mean and standard deviation (SD) of temporal measures of speech and oral reading in alaryngeal speakers compared to previous reports in typical laryngeal speakers

Speech mode	Speech	Oral reading
EL[1]		
Syllables/breath	7.45 (3.30)	8.10 (3.12)
Utterance length(s)	2.30 (1.24)	2.17 (0.97)
TE[2]		
Syllables/breath	11.27 (3.31)	12.98 (5.34)
Utterance length(s)	2.60 (1.00)	2.97 (1.06)
Typical		
Syllables/breath (50 yo)[3]	18.20 (5.68)	
Syllables/breath (75 yo)[3]	12.54 (2.41)	
Syllables/breath (~66 yo)[4]		17.50 (3.66)
Utterance length (s)	3.84 (2.05)[5]	3.36 (1.39)[6]

Sources: Adapted from [1]Bohnenkamp et al. (2010); [2]Bohnenkamp et al. (2012); [3]Hoit and Hixon (1987); [4]Solomon and Hixon (1993); [5]Winkworth et al. (1995); [6]Winkworth et al. (1994)

electrolarynx prior to onset of expiration 62% of the time during spontaneous speech (range = 16–83%) and 58% of the time during reading (range = 10–96%). Similar to Stepp et al., as time post-laryngectomy increased, EL speakers were more likely to inspire during speech production (Doyle, 2005). In the absence of the physiological need for expiration for speech production, EL speakers appear to rely on a speech breathing pattern that more closely resembles tidal breathing (see Nagle, Chap. 9). This might prove more comfortable or efficient and demonstrates the likelihood that they decouple speech demands from respiratory system control.

EL speakers are similar to laryngeal speakers in that they inspire at grammatically appropriate locations during spontaneous speech (Winkworth et al., 1995). This is interesting, considering that these speakers can mark grammatical boundaries using the on-off control of the electrolarynx versus inspirations and inspiratory pauses; however,

they do not maintain this similarity during oral reading tasks. Bohnenkamp et al. (2010) reported that EL speakers were much less likely to inspire at grammatically appropriate locations during oral reading, which might indicate that oral reading requires less cognitive effort along with a lack of the physiological need to mark pauses. EL speakers do not have the limitations of having to balance linguistic demands of oral reading and speech and could demonstrate longer utterances than laryngeal and TE speakers; however, they produce utterance lengths shorter than what has been reported in typical and TE speakers (Ward et al., 2007; Winkworth et al., 1994; Winkworth et al., 1995). Please see Table 7.4. As previously discussed, speech breathing is a complex activity in laryngeal speakers; however, EL speakers demonstrate a complexity of a different sort in that they decouple their control of the respiratory system and demonstrate variable and unpredictable responses to loss of a physiological phonatory source.

Esophageal Speakers

Esophageal speech does not require pulmonary air support to vibrate the PE segment, but rather, air is injected or inhaled into the esophagus for alaryngeal phonation (see Doyle & Finchem, Chap. 10). There is little research related to the speech breathing behaviors of ES speakers. ES speakers do coordinate their inspiratory movements with both injection and inhalation methods of esophageal insufflation (DiCarlo et al., 1955). DiCarlo et al. investigated how ES speakers manipulated the respiratory system for speech during tidal breathing and while oral reading. The ES speakers used greater rib cage and abdominal movement during tidal breathing, which the authors suggested were likely due to the effects of COPD. In general, ES speakers used inspiratory and expiratory chest wall movements similar to laryngeal speakers during speech, though the amplitudes of chest wall movement during speech in ES speakers were less than seen in laryngeal speakers. The esophageal speakers who were rated as most intelligible used chest wall movements that were most similar to those of typical speakers, whereas poor speakers demonstrated dyscoordination of the inspiratory and injection activity with both the inspiratory and expiratory phases. As would be expected, all ES speakers demonstrated shorter utterance lengths than laryngeal speakers.

Tracheoesophageal Speakers

The effects of a total laryngectomy on respiration in alaryngeal speech are most likely to be demonstrated in TE speech. The ability to use pulmonary air for TE speech is the perceived advantage over EL and ES speech to overcome the anecdotal reports of effortful speech. Highly intelligible (90%) TE speakers initiate and terminate spontaneous speech similar to laryngeal speakers (Bohnenkamp et al., 2012; Bohnenkamp et al., 2011; Ward et al., 2007). The termination of speech near 36%VC in TE speech is misleading because speakers who undergo a laryngectomy have elevated REL (i.e., approximately 9%

higher). Bohnenkamp et al. (2011) reported that speakers terminated speech at levels 10% lower than their REL (35–45%VC) and exclusively spoke well below REL to complete utterances. Ward et al. did not state whether their speakers consistently spoke past REL. Whether these behaviors would be similar in alaryngeal speakers with low intelligibility warrants investigation.

The middle range of lung volumes (60–35%VC) reported in typical speakers is thought to be the optimal configuration for speech; however, TE speakers have reduced passive forces available to them for speech due to the elevated REL. As such, TE speakers use breathing behaviors that are closely related to what has been reported in older speakers, as well as speakers with COPD (Hoit & Hixon, 1987; Lee et al., 1993). TE speakers terminate speech at low lung volumes into FRC versus their inspiring to higher %VC because of the increased effort involved. TE speakers seem to prefer to overcome PE segment and TE puncture voice prosthesis resistance by increasing muscular effort at the ends of utterances, as opposed to increasing inspirations at the beginning. In addition, these speakers may not initiate speech at %VC as a way to control for comfortable loudness (see Table 7.1).

If diagnosed with COPD, TE speakers are likely to use more rib cage activity during oral reading than is used for spontaneous speech (Bohnenkamp et al., 2012). In fact, TE speakers with COPD used 49% of their maximal rib cage movement while reading orally, whereas they relied on only 34% of maximal rib cage movement for speech. This agrees with reports that respiratory difficulties associated with COPD include the loss of elasticity in the respiratory system resulting in the need for increased muscle activity. The use of a greater amount of rib cage activity during expiration is contradictory to the physiologically efficient use by healthy older speakers of taking deeper inspirations for speech.

Abdominal activity during speech in tracheoesophageal speakers is similar during both oral reading (37% of maximum) and speech (33% or maximum), and both instances are considerably higher than previous reports of 7–10% of maximal abdominal movement in laryngeal speakers

(Hoit & Hixon, 1987). TE speakers do contract the abdominal wall prior to phonation nearly 100% of the time. This is likely due to the need to maintain adequate pressures in the trachea needed to force both the TE puncture voice prosthesis and PE segment open for comfortable and efficient speech. However, there is the probability that these active compensations may to lead to fatigue, even if increased effort in the abdominal wall is the most efficient and optimal configuration of the chest wall for TE speakers (see Table 7.2).

The Relationship of Speech Intelligibility and Temporal Measures of Speech

TE speakers produce similar rates of speech compared to typical speakers and are likely to take inspirations at grammatically appropriate locations during speech and oral reading. Though TE speakers' speaking rate is comparable to laryngeal speakers' rates, TE speakers produce fewer syllables per breath group and produce utterances that are approximately two-thirds as long as what would be expected in laryngeal speakers (Bohnenkamp et al., 2012; Bohnenkamp et al., 2011). Please see Tables 7.3 and 7.4. It has been argued that intelligibility in TE speakers could be acoustic-related, indicating a lack of power in the phonatory source that results in reduced formant frequencies (D'Alatri, Bussu, Scarano, Paludetti, & Marchese, 2012). But there is also the likelihood that intelligibility is influenced by the speakers' shorter utterance length regardless of their ability to use grammatically appropriate inspiration patterns. One explanation may be that TE speakers may address concerns regarding intelligibility by shortening utterances and inspiring at times which are grammatically appropriate during speech. Oral reading requires TE speakers to rely on punctuation to mark inspiratory locations and pauses. Subsequently, TE speakers will inspire to a perceived appropriate %VC and terminate speech at lower %VC to complete the utterance. The alternative would be that these speakers are forced to reduce the number of syllables produced per breath group to balance metabolic demands. Therefore, TE speakers appear to preplan their utterances to make use of the amount of air available to them. This is not the case during oral reading, wherein the grammatical structure is specified by the passage's linguistic construction. TE speakers must adapt their respiratory control to the structure of the utterance. This is accomplished primarily by initiating speech at a high lung volume and speaking into FRC, with the only other alternative to take inspirations when physiologically necessary (Bohnenkamp et al., 2012).

Conclusions

The demands placed on alaryngeal speakers differ by their mode of communication. EL speakers, who have the least need for respiratory control for speech, continue to manipulate the system as if timing for speech. However, this speech-related behavior appears to change with increasing post-laryngectomy time as speakers begin decoupling respiration from speech to most efficiently produce speech with the least demand on the system. It is likely that ES speakers continue to manipulate the chest wall similar to laryngeal speakers, depending upon their method of charging air into the esophagus. There is, however, a dearth of research in this population which indicates that much more can be done. TE speech production might be very demanding on the respiratory system, even in intelligible speakers. Alaryngeal speakers' use of greater lung volumes during speech and oral reading and consistently speaking into FRC influences their ability to place grammatically appropriate inspirations during speech and oral reading. Targeting utterance length and specifying locations of inspirations may be viable therapy goals for these speakers.

Finally, TE speech is viewed very favorably in that it allows speakers to use pulmonary air support and subsequently produce longer utterances which may improve their communication effectiveness. However, the literature also indicates that TE speech is effortful and that EL and ES speech remain viable approaches to speech rehabilitation, especially in those who suffer a severely compromised respiratory system. It is, therefore, essential that clinicians understand that there is a physiological cost associated with speech breathing in all three alaryngeal speech modes. Complex control of the respiratory system in typical healthy laryngeal speakers is influenced by numerous predictable factors such as age and speech task. The remarkable communication challenges faced by alaryngeal speakers (often with respiratory compromise such as that related to COPD) and their ability to communicate effectively, regardless of speech mode, speak to a robust physiological system that is very adaptive to change and can maintain functionality under severely increased physical and communicative challenges.

Acknowledgment I wish to thank Laura Murray, Ph.D., for her mentoring and friendship. She instilled the importance of understanding the neurology of respiration early in my doctoral studies. This chapter would not have been possible without her early guidance.

References

Ackerstaff, A. H., Hilgers, F. J., Balm, A. J., & Tan, I. B. (1998). Long-term compliance of laryngectomized patients with a specialized pulmonary rehabilitation device: Provox stomafilter. *Laryngoscope, 108*, 257–260.

Ackerstaff, A. H., Hilgers, F. J., Balm, A. J., & Van Zandwijk, N. (1995). Long-term pulmonary function after total laryngectomy. *Clinical Otolaryngology and Allied Sciences, 20*, 547–551.

Ackerstaff, A. H., Hilgers, F. J., Meeuwis, C. A., Knegt, P. P. M., & Weenink, C. (1999). Pulmonary function pre- and post-total laryngectomy. *Clinical Otolaryngology, 24*, 491–494.

Ackerstaff, A. H., Souren, T., van Zandwijk, N., Balm, A. J., & Hilgers, F. J. (1993). Improvements in the assessment of pulmonary function in laryngectomized patients. *Laryngoscope, 103*, 1391–1394.

Ayres, J. G. (1990). Late onset asthma. *British Medical Journal, 300*, 1602–1603.

Bailey, E. F., & Hoit, J. D. (2002). Speaking and breathing in high respiratory drive. *Journal of Speech, Language and Hearing Research, 45*, 89–99.

Baken, R. J., & Cavallo, S. A. (1981). Prephonatory chest wall posturing. *Folia Phoniatrica, 33*, 193–203.

Baken, R. J., Cavallo, S. A., & Weissman, K. L. (1979). Chest wall movements prior to phonation. *Journal of Speech and Hearing Research, 22*, 862–871.

Bohnenkamp, T. A., Forrest, K. M., Klaben, B. K., & Stager, J. M. (2011). Lung volumes used during speech breathing in tracheoesophageal speakers. *Annals of Otology, Rhinology, & Laryngology, 120*, 550–558.

Bohnenkamp, T. A., Forrest, K. M., Klaben, B. K., & Stager, J. M. (2012). Chest wall kinematics during speech breathing in tracheoesophageal speakers. *Annals of Otology, Rhinology, & Laryngology, 121*, 28–37.

Bohnenkamp, T. A., Stowell, T., Hesse, J., & Wright, S. (2010). Speech breathing in speakers who use an electrolarynx. *Journal of Communication Disorders, 43*, 199–211.

Brown, M., & Hasser, E. (1996). Complexity of age-related change in skeletal muscle. *Journals of Gerontology Series A: Biological Sciences and Medical Sciences, 51*, 117–123.

Bunn, J. C., & Mead, J. (1971). Control of ventilation during speech. *Journal of Applied Physiology, 31*, 870–872.

Castro, M. A., Dedivitis, R. A., & Macedo, A. G. (2011). Evaluation of a method for assessing pulmonary function in laryngectomees. *Acta Otorhinolaryngologica Italica, 31*, 243–247.

Cavallo, S. A., & Baken, R. J. (1985). Prephonatory laryngeal and chest wall dynamics. *Journal of Speech and Hearing Research, 28*, 79–87.

Chan, E. D., & Welsh, C. H. (1998). Geriatric respiratory medicine. *Chest, 114*, 1704–1733.

Corfield, D. R., Roberts, C. A., Guz, A., Murphy, K., & Adams, L. (1999). Modulation of the corticospinal control of ventilation by changes in reflex drive. *Journal of Applied Physiology, 87*, 1923–1930.

Crapo, R. O. (1993). The aging lung. In D. A. Mahler (Ed.), *Pulmonary disease in the elderly patient* (Vol. 63, pp. 1–21). New York, NY: Marcel Dekker.

D'Alatri, L., Bussu, F., Scarano, E., Paludetti, G., & Marchese, M. R. (2012). Objective and subjective assessment of tracheoesophageal prosthesis voice outcome. *Journal of Voice, 26*, 607–613. https://doi.org/10.1016/j.jvoice.2011.08.013

Davis, P. J., Zhang, S. P., Winkworth, A., & Bandler, R. (1996). Neural control of vocalization: Respiratory and emotional influences. *Journal of Voice, 10*, 23–38.

Dhar, S., Shastri, S. R., & Lenora, R. A. K. (1976). Aging and the respiratory system. *Medical Clinics of North America, 60*, 1121–1139.

DiCarlo, L. M., Amster, W. W., & Herer, G. R. (1955). *Speech after laryngectomy*. Syracuse, NY: Syracuse University Press.

Dick, T. E., Orem, J. M., & Shea, S. A. (1997). Behavioral control of breathing. In R. G. Crystal, J. B. West, E. R. Weibel, & P. J. Barnes (Eds.), *The lung: Scientific foundations* (2nd ed., pp. 1821–1837). Baltimore, MD: Lippincott-Raven.

Donnelly, D. F. (1991). Laryngeal reflexes: Integrated and cellular aspects. In G. G. Haddad & J. P. Farber (Eds.), *Developmental neurobiology of breathing* (Vol. 53, pp. 271–278). New York, NY: Marcel-Dekker.

Doust, J. H., & Patrick, J. M. (1981). The limitation of exercise ventilation during speech. *Respiration Physiology, 46*, 137–147.

Doyle, P. C. (2005). Clinical procedures for training use of the electronic artificial larynx. In P. C. Doyle & R. L. Keith (Eds.), *Rehabilitation following treatment for head and neck cancer: Voice, speech, and swallowing*. Austin, TX: Pro-Ed Publishers.

Draper, M. H., Ladefoged, P., & Whitteridge, D. (1959). Respiratory muscles in speech. *Journal of Speech and Hearing Research, 2*, 16–27.

Duffy, J. (1995). *Motor speech disorders: Substrates, differential diagnosis, and management*. New York, NY: Mosby.

Fontana, G. A., Pantaleo, T., Lavorini, F., Mutolo, D., Polli, G., & Pistolesi, M. (1999). Coughing in laryngectomized patients. *American Journal of Respiratory and Critical Care Medicine, 160*, 1578–1584.

Garrett, J. D., & Luschei, E. S. (1987). Subglottic pressure modulation during evoked phonation in the anesthetized cat. In T. Baer, C. Sasaki, & K. Harris (Eds.), *Laryngeal function in phonation and respiration* (pp. 139–153). Boston, MA: College Hill Press.

Goldman-Eisler, F. (1961). Continuity of speech utterance, its determinants and its significance. *Language and Speech, 4*, 220–231.

Goldman-Eisler, F. (1968). *Psycholinguistics: Experiments in spontaneous speech*. Ann Arbor, MI: Academic Press.

Gregor, R. T., & Hassman, E. (1984). Respiratory function in post-laryngectomy patients related to stomal size. *Acta Otolaryngologica, 97*, 177–183.

Guz, A. (1997). Brain, breathing and breathlessness. *Respiration Physiology, 109*, 197–204.

Hess, M. M., Schwenk, R. A., Frank, W., & Loddenkemper, R. (1999). Pulmonary function after total laryngectomy. *The Laryngoscope, 109*, 988–994.

Hida, W. (1999). Role of ventilatory drive in asthma and chronic obstructive pulmonary disease. *Current Opinion in Pulmonary Medicine, 5*, 339–343.

Hixon, T. J. (1988). Comment on Cavallo and Baken (1985). *Journal of Speech, Language, and Hearing Research, 31*, 726–728.

Hixon, T. J., Goldman, M. D., & Mead, J. (1973). Kinematics of the chest wall during speech production: Volume displacements of the rib cage, abdomen, and lung. *Journal of Speech and Hearing Research, 16*, 78–115.

Hixon, T. J., Mead, J., & Goldman, M. D. (1976). Dynamics of the chest wall during speech production: Function of the thorax, rib cage, diaphragm, and abdomen. *Journal of Speech and Hearing Research, 19*, 297–356.

Hoit, J. D., & Hixon, T. J. (1987). Age and speech breathing. *Journal of Speech, Language, and Hearing Research, 30*, 351–366.

Hoit, J. D., & Lohmeier, H. L. (2000). Influence of continuous speaking on ventilation. *Journal of Speech, Language, and Hearing Research, 43*, 1240–1251.

Homma, I., Obata, T., Sibuya, M., & Uchida, M. (1984). Gate mechanism in breathlessness caused by chest wall vibration in humans. *Journal of Applied Physiology: Respiratory, Environmental and Exercise Physiology, 56*, 8–11.

Hugelin, A. (1986). Forebrain and midbrain influences on respiration. In *Handbook of physiology, the respiratory system* (Vol. 2). Bethesda, MD: American Physiological Society.

Isshiki, N., & Snidecor, J. C. (1965). Air intake and usage in esophageal speech. *Acta Otolaryngologica, 59*, 559–574.

Iwarsson, J. (2001). Effects of inhalatory abdominal wall movement on vertical laryngeal position during phonation. *Journal of Voice, 15*(3), 384–394.

Janssens, J. P., Pache, J. C., & Nicod, L. P. (1999). Physiological changes in respiratory function associated with ageing. *European Respiratory Journal, 13*, 197–205.

Kahane, J. C. (1980). Age-related histological changes in the human male and female laryngeal cartilages: Biological and functional implications. In V. Lawrence (Ed.), *Transcripts of the ninth symposium: Care of the professional voice*. New York, NY: The Voice Foundation.

Kaneko, Y., Zivanovic, V., Hajek, V., & Bradley, T. D. (2001, November 11). *Sleep apnea in stroke patients predicts worse functional status and longer hospitalization*. Paper presented at: Annual Meeting of the American Heart Association, Anaheim, CA.

Kendall, K. (2007). Presbyphonia: A review. *Current Opinion in Otolaryngology & Head and Neck Surgery, 15*, 137–140.

Khedr, E. M., Shinaway, O. E., Khedr, T., Aziz Ali, Y. A., & Awad, E. M. (2000). Assessment of corticodiaphragmatic pathway and pulmonary function in acute ischemic stroke patients. *European Journal of Neurology, 7*, 323–330.

Ladefoged, P., & Loeb, G. (2002). *Preliminary studies on respiratory activity in speech*. Unpublished manuscript, University of California-Los Angeles.

Lee, L., Loudon, R. G., Jacobson, B. H., & Stuebing, R. (1993). Speech breathing in patients with lung disease. *American Review of Respiratory Disease, 147*, 1199–1206.

Matsuura, K., Ebihara, S., Yoshizumi, T., Asai, M., Hayashi, R., Shizuka, T., & Uchiyama, K. (1995). Changes in respiratory function before and after laryngectomy. *Nippon Jibiinkoka Gakkai Kaiho, 98*, 1097–1103.

McFarland, D. H., & Smith, A. (1992). Effects of vocal task and respiratory phase on prephonatory chest wall movements. *Journal of Speech and Hearing Research, 35*, 971–982.

McKeown, F. (1965). *Pathology of the aged*. London: Butterworths.

Murray, J. F. (1986). Aging. In J. F. Murray (Ed.), *The normal lung*. Philadelphia, PA: W. B. Saunders.

Ohala, J. J. (1990). Respiratory activity in speech. In W. J. Hardcastle & A. Marchal (Eds.), *Speech production and speech modelling. Vol. 55. Series D: Behavioural and social science* (pp. 23–53). Boston, MA: Kluwer Academic Publishers.

Phillipson, E. A., McClean, P. A., Sullivan, C. E., & Zamel, N. (1978). Interaction of metabolic and behavioral respiratory control during hypercapnia and speech. *American Review of Respiratory Disease, 117*, 903–909.

Pierce, J. A., & Ebert, R. V. (1965). Fibrous network of the lung and its change with age. *Thorax, 20*, 469–476.

Robbins, J., Fisher, H. B., Blom, E. C., & Singer, M. I. (1984). A comparative acoustic study of normal, esophageal, and tracheoesophageal speech production. *Journal of Speech and Hearing Disorders, 49*, 202–210.

Russell, N. K., Cerny, F. J., & Stathopoulos, E. (1998). Effects of varied vocal intensity on ventilation and energy expenditure in women and men. *Journal of Speech, Language, and Hearing Research, 41*, 239–248.

Sammut, L., Ward, M., & Patel, N. (2014). Physical activity and quality of life in head and neck cancer survivors: A literature review. *International Journal of Sports Medicine, 35*, 794–799.

Sant'Ambrogio, G., Matthew, O. P., Fisher, J. T., & Sant'Ambrogio, F. B. (1983). Laryngeal receptors responding to transmural pressure, airflow, and local muscle activity. *Respiratory Physiology and Neurobiology, 54*, 317–330.

Sharp, J. T., Goldberg, N. B., Druz, W. S., Fishman, H. C., & Danon, J. (1977). Thoracoabdominal motion in chronic obstructive pulmonary disease. *American Review of Respiratory Disease, 115*, 47–56.

Shea, S. A. (1996). Behavioural and arousal-related influences on breathing in humans. *Experimental Physiology, 81*, 1–26.

Solomon, N. P., & Hixon, T. J. (1993). Speech breathing in Parkinson's disease. *Journal of Speech and Hearing Research, 36*, 294–310.

Sperry, E. E., & Klich, R. J. (1992). Speech breathing in senescent and younger women during oral reading. *Journal of Speech and Hearing Research, 35*, 1246–1255.

Stepp, C. E., Heaton, J. T., & Hillman, R. E. (2008). Postlaryngectomy speech respiration patterns. *Annals of Otology, Rhinology & Laryngology, 117*, 557–563.

Terao, Y., Ugawa, Y., Enomoto, H., Furubayashi, T., Shiio, Y., Machii, K., … Kanazawa, I. (2001). Hemispheric lateralization in the cortical motor preparation for human vocalization. *The Journal of Neuroscience, 21*, 1600–1609.

Testerman, R. L. (1970). Modulation of laryngeal activity by pulmonary changes during vocalization in cats. *Experimental Neurology, 29*, 281–297.

Todisco, T., Maurizi, M., Paludetti, G., Dottorini, M., & Merante, F. (1984). Laryngeal cancer: Long-term follow-up of respiratory functions after laryngectomy. *Respiration, 45*, 303–315.

Togawa, K., Konno, A., & Hoshino, T. (1980). A physiologic study on respiratory handicap of the laryngectomized. *Archives of Oto-Rhino-Laryngology, 229*, 69–79.

Tolep, K., & Kelsen, S. G. (1993). Effect of aging on respiratory skeletal muscles. *Clinics in Chest Medicine, 14*, 363–378.

Usui, N. (1979). Ventilatory function in laryngectomized patients. *Auris Nasus Larynx, 6*, 87–96.

von Euler, C. (1997). Neural organization and rhythm generation. In R. G. Crystal, J. B. West, E. R. Weibel, & P. J. Barnes (Eds.), *The lung: Scientific foundations* (2nd ed., pp. 1710–1724). Baltimore, MD: Lippincott-Raven.

Ward, E. C., Hartwig, P., Scott, J., Trickey, M., Cahill, L., & Hancock, K. (2007). Speech breathing patterns during tracheoesophageal speech. *Asia Pacific Journal of Speech, Language, and Hearing, 10*, 33–42.

Warren, D. W. (1996). Regulation of speech aerodynamics. In N. J. Lass (Ed.), *Principles of experimental phonetics* (pp. 46–92). Saint Louis, MO: Mosby-Year Book, Inc.

Weinberg, B., Horii, Y., Blom, E., & Singer, M. (1982). Airway resistance during esophageal phonation. *Journal of Speech and Hearing Disorders, 47*, 194–199.

Weinberg, B., & Moon, J. (1982). Airway resistance characteristics of Blom-Singer tracheoesophageal puncture prostheses. *Journal of Speech and Hearing Disorders, 47*, 441–442.

Weinberg, B., & Moon, J. B. (1986). Impact of tracheoesophageal puncture prosthesis airway resistance on in-vivo phonatory performance. *Journal of Speech and Hearing Disorders, 51*(1), 88–91.

Wessendorf, T. E., Teschler, H., Wang, Y.-M., Konietzko, N., & Thilman, A. F. (2000). Sleep-disordered breathing among patients with first-ever stroke. *Journal of Neurology, 247*, 41–47.

West, J. B. (2013). *Pulmonary pathophysiology: The essentials* (8th ed.). Baltimore, MD: Wolters Kluwer – Lippincott Williams & Wilkins.

Wilder, C. N. (1983). Chest wall preparation for phonation in female speakers. In D. M. Bless & J. H. Abbs (Eds.), *Vocal fold physiology: Contemporary research and clinical issues* (pp. 109–123). San Diego, CA: College Hill Press.

Winkworth, A. L., Davis, P. J., Adams, R. D., & Ellis, E. (1995). Breathing patterns during spontaneous speech. *Journal or Speech and Hearing Research, 38*(1), 124–144.

Winkworth, A. L., Davis, P. J., Ellis, E., & Adams, R. D. (1994). Variability and consistency in speech breathing during reading: Lung volumes, speech intensity, and linguistic factors. *Journal of Speech and Hearing Research, 37*, 535–556.

Wyke, B. (1983). Neuromuscular control systems in voice production. In D. M. Bless & J. H. Abbs (Eds.), *Vocal fold physiology* (pp. 71–76). San Diego, CA: College-Hill.

Clinical Intervention for Airway Improvement: Establishing a New Nose

8

W. J. Bryan Lewis

Clinical Intervention for Airway Improvement: Establishing a New Nose

As discussed in Chap. 7, the pulmonary environment before and after total laryngectomy is significantly different, both anatomically and physiologically. Total laryngectomy results in a permanent, anatomical disconnection between the upper and lower airways. As the airway is now contingent on a tracheostoma versus the mouth and nose, humidification, warming, filtration, and resistance are significantly impacted.

This chapter presents information on the pulmonary environment before and after laryngectomy, specifically relating to the need for compensatory strategies and prostheses to combat the lost functions within the upper airway. Additionally, the importance of pulmonary protection after laryngectomy is examined, which includes the physical properties, effects, and benefits of heat and moisture exchange devices.

The Pulmonary Environment Before Laryngectomy

When considering the changes associated with total laryngectomy, it is important for clinicians to understand the value of the closed respiratory system that exists prior to laryngectomy. At rest, the nasal passages provide the main pathway through which air flows during breathing; for adults, it has been estimated that 10,000 liters of air travel these passageways daily (Kerr, 1997). In a normal respiratory system, inhalation and exhalation have but two options – through the nose and through the mouth. Primarily via the nose, resting inhalation conditions the ambient air creating an optimal pulmonary environment. That is, relative humidity increases to 95% as inhaled air reaches the nasopharynx via vascular mucosa (Kerr, 1997), and as it reaches the level of the carina, it is 37 °C/98.6 °F with 100% relative humidity (Keck, Leiacker, Heinrich, Kuhnemann, & Rettinger, 2000; Scheenstra, Muller, & Hilgers, 2011; Williams, Rankin, Smith, Galler, & Seakins, 1996). Humidification of air allows the body to maintain ciliary activity and mucosal integrity. The nasal passages also function as a valve, which in turn creates resistance to both inspiratory and expiratory air. This valving allows for adequate time as respiratory gases are exchanged at the level of the alveoli (Hairfield, Warren, Hinton, & Seaton, 1987).

W. J. Bryan Lewis (✉)
Department of Surgery, Walter Reed National Military Medical Center, Bethesda, MD, USA

Uniformed Services University of the Health Sciences, Bethesda, MD, USA

© Springer Nature Switzerland AG 2019
P. C. Doyle (ed.), *Clinical Care and Rehabilitation in Head and Neck Cancer*,
https://doi.org/10.1007/978-3-030-04702-3_8

Perhaps, the most well-known function of the nose is its critical role in filtrating inhaled debris and microbes, such as viruses, bacteria, and fungi. The thicker hairs of the nasal vibrissae are visible, but it is the smaller, fine hairlike structures, the cilia, that line the epithelium of the airway and provide the continuous, rhythmic highways for mucus to move as they transport smaller particles out of the airway. As Vareille, Kieninger, Edwards, and Regamey (2011) review aptly summarized, taking over "the first line of defense, the airway epithelium can be considered a soldier in the fight against airborne pathogens" (p. 211). After laryngectomy the pulmonary environment changes significantly as it is no longer a closed system. These changes not only impact the cilia but result in changes to the conditioning of inhaled air, filtration, and pulmonary pressures.

Pulmonary Environment After Laryngectomy

Following total laryngectomy, the upper airway (nasal passages, pharynx, and larynx above the vocal folds) and lower airway (larynx below the vocal folds, trachea, primary bronchi, and lungs) are permanently separated. Subsequently, air no longer actively passes through the nose or mouth during breathing. The upper airway is now void of actions associated with normal respiration. In addition to the loss of voicing, air no longer actively passes through the nasopharynx preventing odorant molecules from reaching and stimulating olfactory epithelium. This significantly diminishes the olfactory system, taste included and results in hyposomia and in some cases anosmia (Santos, Bergman, Coca, Garcia, & Valente, 2016). As those who are laryngectomized breathe, air now enters and exits the respiratory system directly through the tracheostoma which is located at the level of the sternal notch. Thus, conditioning, or warming and humidification, filtration, and pulmonary pressures are considerably impacted. This change is directly due to the loss of access to functions provided by structures of the upper airway as a result of surgery. At the level of the trachea, room air via the tracheostoma measures approximately 28 °C with a relative humidity of 50% (Scheenstra et al., 2009). Additionally, the cilia in the trachea become impaired, and mucous production increases, resulting in overproduction, crusting, and irritation. This increased mucous production is a direct result of the separation of the upper and lower airways, which results from inhalation of unconditioned air. This is the body's response to decreased heat and moisture exchange and lack of filtration of small airborne particles. As a result, a majority of laryngectomees report an increase in the production of sputum and associated coughing, as well as experiencing shortness of breath (Hilgers, Ackerstaff, Aaronson, Schouwenburg, & Van Zandwijk, 1990).

Respiratory Symptoms The impact of respiratory changes following total laryngectomy is well documented (Ackerstaff, Hilgers, Aaronson, & Balm, 1994; Hilgers et al., 1990; Mohide, Archibald, Tew, Young, & Haines, 1992; and others). These changes result in direct increases of involuntary coughing and sputum/phlegm production, as well as decreased alaryngeal voice quality for tracheoesophageal prosthetic users or esophageal speakers. These respiratory-related alterations also have second-order effects to include increased fatigue, anxiety and depression, difficulty sleeping, and social avoidance (Ackerstaff et al., 1994; Hilgers et al., 1990). Additionally, most laryngectomized patients often have preexisting, respiratory impairments not solely related to the separation of upper and lower airways. For example, chronic obstructive lung disease (COPD) is common given that many of these patients have a history of smoking (Brady et al., 2017). Further, Hess, Schwenk, Frank, and Loddenkemper (1999) have reported that 81% of laryngectomees also may suffer from pulmonary airway obstruction which creates additional respiratory challenges.

Impact on QOL The impact on perceived quality of life (QOL) in those with laryngeal cancer as a clinical population cannot be overstated regardless of the modality of treatment undertaken. The QOL of laryngectomees is of obvious concern, and as demonstrated by Batıoğlu-Karaaltın, Binbay, Yiğit, and Dönmez (2017), patients who have undergone a total laryngectomy are more often observed to have problems with depression, anxiety, self-esteem, and sexual functions when compared to patients with partial laryngectomy. Specific pulmonary changes as a result of laryngectomy may impact QOL. Increased sputum production, coughing, and forced expectoration impact energy levels, sleep, and social interactions (Ackerstaff et al., 1994; Hilgers et al., 1990). Additionally, olfactory and taste impairments may result in decreased appetite, weight loss, and poor nutritional status (Risberg-Berlin, Ylitalo, & Finizia, 2006). Therefore, preservation of the best possible QOL outcomes for laryngectomees includes rehabilitation and compensation of pulmonary functions lost or impaired due to laryngectomy. When considering these multiple areas of functioning, the clinician can directly and positively impact many areas through the application of clinical tools and education.

Pulmonary Protection After Laryngectomy: Addressing Heat, Moisture, Resistance, and Filtration

Across the last few decades, much information has been generated in an effort to further clinical understanding about the importance of post-laryngectomy pulmonary rehabilitation. In fact, based on the literature, it plays a significant role for improving a patient's quality of life as does voice restoration (Ackerstaff, Hilgers, Balm, & Tan, 1998; Hilgers, Aaronson, Ackerstaff, Schouwenburg, & van Zandwikj, 1991; Ackerstaff, Hilgers, Aaronson, Balm, & Zandwijk, 1993). When the larynx is removed, 100% of these individuals will have profound communication difficulties due to the loss of one's larynx. At the same time, 98% of laryngectomees will suffer from excessive sputum production, with a majority reporting significant coughing and frequent forced expectoration (Hilgers et al., 1990). Therefore, focusing on pul-

monary changes in these patients is fundamental to patient-centered care and crucial for improving quality of life for laryngectomees. It is worth noting that recent research has demonstrated reproducible methods for evaluating pulmonary function in laryngectomees (Castro, Dedivitis, & Macedo, 2011; Hess et al., 1999; Van den Boer et al., 2013; Vasquez de la Inglesia & Fernandez Gonzalez, 2006). Given the prevalence of lung conditions and associated respiratory difficulties, it is recommended that routine pulmonary evaluation occurs in this population. More directly, the clinical evaluation of pulmonary, olfactory, vocal, and swallowing functions should be completed for all who undergo total laryngectomy. Evaluation and treatment of changes in the pulmonary environment begin immediately following total laryngectomy; that is, as soon as the airways have been separated in the operating room, heat and moisture exchange, filtration, and conditioning of the airway by other means begin.

HME: The Three-Letter Answer

An essential treatment option for establishing a "new nose" in laryngectomees is the application of heat and moisture exchangers (HMEs). These devices target lost nasal functions, with a direct impact on air humidification, warming, resistance, and filtration post-laryngectomy. Routine use of HMEs has significant, positive effects on pulmonary changes and quality of life for laryngectomees (Ackerstaff et al., 1993; Hilgers et al., 1991). Clinical efforts directed toward restoring this function should begin immediately following surgery (Foreman, De Santis, Sultanov, Enepekides, & Higgins, 2016; Merol et al., 2011). As the tool to address pulmonary changes following laryngectomy, HMEs have unique physical qualities and well-documented effects and benefits.

Physical Properties of HMEs

HME devices are placed on the tracheostoma and possess three physical properties: air filtra-

a

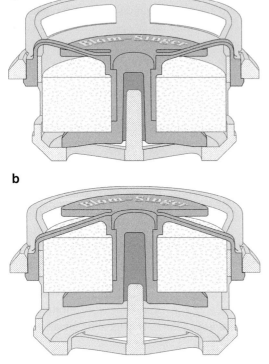

b

Fig. 8.1 HME cross section HME (**a**) (closed) and (**b**) (open). (*Image courtesy of InHealth Technologies©*)

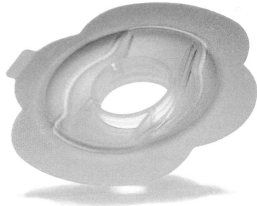

Fig. 8.2 Provox® StabiliBase™ OptiDerm adhesive. (*With permission of Atos Medical AB© and Chris Edghill*)

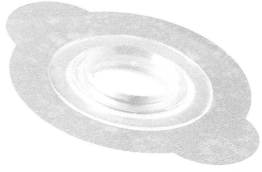

Fig. 8.3 Blom-Singer® TruSeal® Contour Low Profile Oval Adhesive Housing. (*Image courtesy of InHealth Technologies©*)

tion, heat and moisture exchanging capacity, and the addition of resistance to inspiratory airflow (Zuur, Muller, de Jongh, van Zandwijk, & Hilgers, 2006). All HMEs, regardless of manufacturer, are composed of foam, paper, or similar substances designed to absorb moisture and maintain condensation during the breathing cycle; a cross-sectional representation is provided in Fig. 8.1. Hygroscopic salts are used in many HMEs (e.g., Kapitex® Trachinaze®, Provox® XtraMoist™ HME, Blom-Singer® HumidiFilter®), a design feature that serves to increase water retention as respiration occurs. Additional options in some HMEs, such as the Blom-Singer® HumidiFilter®, include the device being impregnated with bactericide solution to combat bacterial colonization (Brusasco et al., 2013; Grolman, Blom, Granson, Schouwenburg, & Hamaker, 1997). Thus, these types of features provide an extra level of protection to the post-laryngectomy airway.

Heat and moisture exchangers utilize housings, or baseplates, to create an airtight seal at the level of the stoma (external and anterior). Successful use is aided with custom fitting as baseplates are available in a sundry of shapes, sizes, and materials (see Figs. 8.2 and 8.3). Additional options include trach tubes and buttons (e.g., Andreas Fahl Laryngotec® Kombi Laryngectomy Tubes, Provox® LaryButton™) which help support the stoma, as well as house HMEs.

Effects of HMEs

Though not as effective as the normal upper airway system, HMEs benefit laryngectomees in three primary ways: (1) by preserving moisture and heat within the lower respiratory track; (2) by providing resistance to inspiratory airflow, thus improving lung ventilation; and (3) by filtering large particles, such as dust, that may threaten the lungs.

Conditioning As previously stated, the upper airways condition (warm and humidify) and filter inspired air – such conditioning and filtering are significantly impacted when the upper and lower respiratory tracts are separated during laryngectomy. Humidification plays an important role in maintaining moisture and mucociliary clearance, which the respiratory cilia and epithelium depend upon (Wanner, Salathé, & O'Riordan, 1996). As Zuur et al. (2006) summarized so well, the impact of HMEs on conditioning the air of laryngectomees is substantial and is not to be ignored when treating patients post-laryngectomy. Zuur et al. (2006) demonstrated that inspired air without HME at 22 °C/40% relative humidity (RH) is naturally conditioned to 27–28 °C with 50% RH at the upper trachea. When an HME is used, this increases to 29–30 °C/70% RH. This does not replicate the same level of conditioning that occurs pre-laryngectomy (32 °C/90–100% RH), but demonstrates enough improvement to warrant immediate application and continual use post-laryngectomy. That is, any change in both temperature and RH is of benefit to the open, post-laryngectomy airway. Additionally, approximately 500 ml of moisture is lost daily during simple post-laryngectomy expiration, which is double the amount lost during nasal breathing pre-laryngectomy. This moisture loss in laryngectomees can be reduced to approximately 250–300 ml per day with routine HME use (Toremalm, 1960).

A 2013 study by Van den Boer et al. evaluated and compared the heat and moisture exchange performance of 23 commercially available HMEs, and their findings demonstrated a wide range of variance in "water exchange performance." As HMEs work to establish a new nose in laryngectomees, they must possess the ability to accumulate and liberate heat. Additionally, they must do so in enough quantities to optimize water exchange as air is inhaled and exhaled, especially given the direct correlation between water exchange and absolute humidity at end inhalation. Van den Boer et al. (2013) demonstrated that HMEs with hygroscopic salts performed best given that they generate a layer of water, which has a high heat capacity, improving HME performance. The sundry results obtained across the HMEs tested in the Van den Boer et al. study provide clinicians with multiple options for their patients. This is important given that the level of water retention in HMEs can directly impact resistance during inhalation and exhalation, and tolerance for this will vary patient to patient.

Resistance The nasal passages have three mechanisms that assist with respiratory resistance: the nasal vestibule, nasal valve, and nasal cavum; these structures account for more than 50% of the total airway resistance (Bailey, 1998). Resistance in non-laryngectomees provides prolonged opportunity for blood-gas exchange in the lungs, thus increasing tissue oxygenation. This upper airway resistance by the nose is lost when the lower and upper airways are separated as a result of laryngectomy.

It is widely understood that HMEs add resistance to the respiratory system, but how much and to what impact resistance affords is still unknown (Verkerke, Geertsema, & Schutte, 2002). One study by McRae, Young, Hamilton, and Jones (1996) found that an HME with increased resistance directly impacted tissue oxygenation. The measurement techniques used in their study, however, have been debated since. For example, Zuur, Muller, Sinaasappel, Hart, Van, and Hilgers (2007) found that tissue oxygenation did not increase in laryngectomees who used HMEs with a higher device resistance. Additionally, higher-resistance HMEs can cause resistance-related discomfort for patients, and given the well-established positive impact that HMEs have on the overall pulmonary environment, clinicians should focus on comfortable and consistent HME use as a primary importance. Low-resistance HMEs, for example, may benefit patients dur-

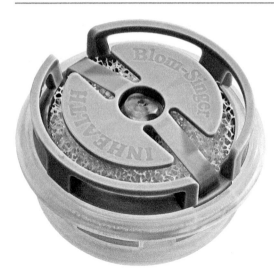

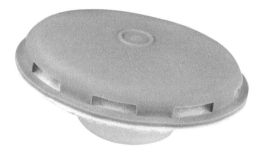

Fig. 8.5 Provox® Micron HME™. (*With permission of Atos Medical AB© and Chris Edghill*)

Fig. 8.4 Blom-Singer® EasyFlow® HME. (*Image courtesy of InHealth Technologies©*)

ing increased activity. Patients who were aerobically active before their laryngectomy have reported better tolerance of low-resistance HMEs as they attempt to maintain higher levels of aerobic activity after laryngectomy (Fig. 8.4). Consequently, changes in the rate of breathing and the volumes of inhaled and exhaled air should be considered when evaluating HMEs for patients. In summary, despite the mixed findings regarding resistance and HMEs, tidal volumes are positively impacted by HME use; when combined with improvements in temperature and humidity, this results in an improved tracheal climate compared to no HME use (Scheenstra et al., 2009).

Filtration Approximately 10,000 liters of air passes through the nose daily, and this is why the American Academy of Otolaryngology – Head and Neck Surgery rightfully calls the nose "the Guardian of Your Lungs." Airborne particles filtered by the nose include bacteria and viruses, pollen, allergens, and dust (Schwab & Zenkel, 1998). Because the nose is bypassed, those who are laryngectomees and tracheostomees are at greater risk of inhaling airborne particles putting them at greater risk for respiratory infections.

At first glance, the physical properties of an HME (housing and foam) demonstrate how large particles may be filtered by the device. However, the pores of HME filters are too large to capture smaller microparticles like viruses and bacteria (Zuur et al., 2006). Therefore, a balance must be maintained between the pore size of the filter and its breathability (resistance), as well as between antimicrobial filters and effective filters for heat and moisture exchange (Hedley & Allt-Graham, 1992; Shelly, Bethune, & Latimer, 1986). For example, some HMEs have the addition of an electrostatic filter designed to trap smaller particles with one device being the Provox® Micron HME (Atos Medical Inc., West Allis, WI) which is displayed in Fig. 8.5. These types of filters have been shown to capture microorganisms, water droplets, and pollen with a > 99% efficiency in bacterial and virus filtration (Nystrand, 2007). In their 2010 study, Sheenstra, Muller, Vincent, Ackerstaff, Jacobi, and Hilgers (2010) found that HMEs without an electrostatic filter are better at moistening inspired air and HMEs with electrostatic filters have better heating capacity. These properties allow the clinician flexibility as they may find value in electrostatic filters for patients in dusty environments or those patients who are at increased risk for community-acquired respiratory infections. Anecdotally, these types of HMEs have benefited patients with increased sputum production and those who frequently work in dusty environments such as woodshops. Overall, the clinician has a sundry of HME options for their patients, allowing for the balance of condition, resistance, and filtration to optimize benefits.

Benefits of HME Devices

The psychosocial consequences of total laryngectomy are well documented and include concerns such as fatigue, psychosocial distress, difficulties sleeping, and social disruption (Hilgers et al., 1990). Additionally, those who are diagnosed and treated for head and neck cancers often struggle with depression, anxiety, and fear of the unknown and of recurrence, as well as issues with changes in appearance and increased financial burdens (Doyle, 2005). Clinicians have many tools to aid laryngectomees, and an HME is one that improves a patient's life by positively impacting and reducing their respiratory symptoms.

HMEs benefit laryngectomees directly, and this is achieved primarily by helping replace lost functions of the nose. Subsequently, the quality of life for laryngectomees is significantly improved with long-term, consistent HME use (Ackerstaff et al., 1993, 1998, 2003; Bien, Okla, van As-Brooks, & Ackerstaff, 2009; Hilgers et al., 1991). A prime case is witnessed in increased sputum production, which is a common and primary complaint in as many as 98% of laryngectomees (Hilgers et al., 1990). With increased sputum production comes increased coughing (second highest reported complaint) which may then lead to fatigue and sleeping difficulties. Excessive sputum/phlegm production also may result in greater frequency of force expectoration, crusting at or within the stoma, shortness of breath, bronchorrhea, and decreased alaryngeal voice quality. Additionally, these problems may negatively impact a patient's desire for social interactions. Long-term, daily HME use has been shown to result in reduction of forced expectoration, stoma cleaning, and mean daily frequency of sputum production and subsequently results in improvements in malaise and fatigue, social anxiety, depression, ease of speech, and sleeping difficulties (Ackerstaff et al., 1993, 1995; Bien et al., 2009). Other benefits of HME use have included easier stoma occlusion, greater maximum phonation time in prosthetic speakers, and more fluent speech in prosthetic speakers (Bien et al., 2009; van As, Hilgers, Koopmans-van Beinum, & Ackerstaff, 1998).

Enhancements in psychosocial functioning via HME use are directly related to compliance (Ackerstaff et al., 1993, 1998; Bien et al., 2009). That is, consistent HME use may result in significant improvement with sleep disturbance, fatigue, shortness of breath, anxiety levels, and perceived voice quality. Education and support to laryngectomees are crucial, and clinicians play a fundamental role in helping these patients overcome difficulties related to the use of an HME and its tolerance by the user. Examples of difficulties include skin irritation from baseplate adhesives, irregularly shaped and/or deep stomas, or placement limitations due to manual dexterity restrictions. All of these issues can be overcome with careful consultation with an experienced speech-language pathologist, especially given the number of options available today (e.g., varying adhesive styles/materials, trach tubes). In their 2013 study, Pedemonte-Sarrias, Villatoro-Sologaistoa, Ale-Inostroza, Lopez-Vilas, Leon-Vintro, and Quer-Agusti analyzed the reasons patients abandoned HME use. In their prospective study, a total of 115 patients were included; 90 were habitual users and 25 stopped using HMEs. Of those who abandoned HME use, 72% stopped as a result of problems that were experienced with the adhesive. Perhaps, the most interesting finding in this study was compliance rates in relation to timing of education and application of HMEs. For patients where an HME was introduced secondarily (during a follow-up visit), continued HME use was found in 63% of the patients compared to >91% in patients where an HME was introduced during the immediate postoperative period. Thus, the factor of when an HME is introduced to those who undergo laryngectomy is critical to longer-term successful use and the associated respiratory benefits.

Additional benefits of immediate postoperative exposure and HME use have also been reported. Merol et al. (2011) compared the use of an HME with humidification and the use of an external humidifier in patients following total laryngectomy. With HME use, they found better compliance and greater patient satisfaction, as well as improvement in nursing time required and nursing preference and satisfaction. A similar comparison by Foreman et al. (2016) found that when compared to external humidification, HME use reduced episodes of mucus plugging and reduced the number of days physiotherapy was required. Foreman et al. (2016) conclude that an additional benefit of HME use is also noted in relation to a reduction in overall healthcare costs given its use reduced in-hospital complications. Though more study is warranted, Brook, Bogaardt, and van As-Brooks (2013) found through questionnaires that frequent (>20 h/day) HME users reported better pulmonary status and lower healthcare costs and that the use of external humidifiers was required less regularly.

Summary

Following a total laryngectomy, one will experience significant changes and lost functions as the upper airway is permanently separated from the lower airway. One of the most significant changes is the forfeiture of nasal functions and contributions to pulmonary health, primarily the conditioning, filtering, and resistance as part of breathing. This anatomical and physiological loss creates significant deficits in how breathing occurs. As a result, increased sputum/phlegm production, daily forced expectoration, and increased involuntary coughing commonly result and may then bring secondary effects such as malaise, fatigue, anxiety, social avoidance, and difficulty sleeping. Consequently, laryngectomees report significant loss in their overall quality of life with a majority rating of the pulmonary changes they experience as being more challenging than their loss of normal voice. Fortunately, compensation for these functional losses is available through the application of heat and moisture exchangers. The use of HMEs has demonstrated the positive influence such devices have on the post-laryngectomy airway and the resultant influence on quality of life. These external devices are composed of paper, foam, or similar substances that are designed to absorb moisture and maintain condensation. Water retention is increased through the application of hygroscopic salts, and some HMEs use bactericide solutions to prevent colonization of bacteria during the respiratory process. Utilizing a sundry of housings, baseplates, tracheostomy tubes, and buttons, HMEs can be fitted to most patients. Regardless of HME device, all possess three primary properties: heat and moisture exchanging capacity, filtration, and the capacity to add resistance to respiratory airflow.

As effective devices in the fight for pulmonary recovery in laryngectomees, HMEs require proper application and education by clinicians, and experienced speech-language pathologists are often best suited to fill this role. The importance of daily, long-term HME use is often not realized by the patient without continued training and education. Early introduction (immediately following surgery) of an HME increases the likelihood of its regular and routine use. Successful use of HMEs is especially important given the significant functional gains and improved quality of life that results. HMEs must be a primary tool for clinicians working with laryngectomees, and when applied appropriately, it builds the foundation for pulmonary improvement which serves to facilitate the best possible post-laryngectomy rehabilitation outcomes.

Acknowledgments I would like to acknowledge Marlene Lesnoff, the first laryngectomee I ever met and my mother-in-law. She taught me long before I entered this profession that life does not end post-laryngectomy, but it does change in ways that many do not appreciate. Her larynx was removed but not her joy, which was evident when she used her electrolarynx to tell inquisitive children she was Darth Vader's mother. Passing before I became a speech pathologist, it is her memory and passion that goes with me as I've had the privilege of helping these patients.

I am also deeply grateful for the incredible gift Marlene gave me in her daughter, who, along with my children, tolerated late nights of me with my nose buried in texts. I am forever grateful for their support, patience, and love.

References

Ackerstaff, A. H., Fuller, D., Irvin, M., Maccracken, E., Gaziano, J., & Stachowiak, I. (2003). Multicenter study assessing effects of heat and moisture exchanger use on respiratory symptoms and voice quality in laryngectomized individuals. *Otolaryngology and Head and Neck Surgery, 129*(6), 705–712.

Ackerstaff, A. H., Hilgers, F. J., Balm, A. J., & van Zandwijk, N. (1995). Long-term pulmonary function after total laryngectomy. *Clinical Otolaryngology, 20*(6), 547–551.

Ackerstaff, A. H., Hilgers, F. J. M., Aaronson, N. K., Balm, A. J., & van Zandwijk, N. (1993). Improvements in respiratory and psychosocial functioning following total laryngectomy by the use of a heat and moisture exchanger. *Annals of Otology, Rhinology, and Laryngology, 102*(11), 878–883.

Ackerstaff, A. H., Hilgers, F. J. M., Aaronson, N. K., & Balm, A. J. M. (1994). Communication, functional disorders and lifestyle changes after total laryngectomy. *Clinical Otolaryngology, 19*, 295–300.

Ackerstaff, A. H., Hilgers, F. J. M., Aaronson, N. K., De Boer, M. F., Meeuwis, C. A., Knegt, P. P., … Balm, A. J. (1995). Heat and moisture exchangers as a treatment option in the post-operative rehabilitation of laryngectomized patients. *Clinical Otolaryngology, 20*, 504–509.

Ackerstaff, A. H., Hilgers, F. J. M., Balm, A. J., & Tan, I. B. (1998). Long-term compliance of laryngectomized patients with a specialized pulmonary rehabilitation device: Provox Stomafilter. *Laryngoscopy, 108*, 257–260.

Bailey, B. (Ed.). (1998). *Head and neck surgery: otolaryngology* (2nd ed.). New York: Lippincott-Raven.

Batıoğlu-Karaaltın, A., Binbay, Z., Yiğit, Ö., & Dönmez, Z. (2017). Evaluation of life quality, self-confidence and sexual functions in patients with total and partial laryngectomy. *Auris Nasus Larynx, 44*, 188–194. [Epub ahead of print].

Bien, S., Okla, S., van As-Brooks, C. J., & Ackerstaff, A. H. (2009). The effect of a heat and moisture exchanger (Provox HME) on pulmonary protection after total laryngectomy: a randomized controlled study. *European Archives of Oto-Rhino-Laryngology, 267*(3), 429–435.

Brady, J. S., Crippen, M. M., Filimonov, A., Eloy, J. A., Baredes, S., & Park, R. C. W. (2017). *Laryngectomy and smoking: an analysis of postoperative risk. The laryngoscope*. https://doi.org/10.1002/lary.26615

Brook, I., Bogaardt, H., & van As-Brooks, C. (2013). Long-term use of heat and moisture exchangers among laryngectomees: medical, social, and psychological patterns. *Annals of Otology, Rhinology, and Laryngology, 122*(6), 358–363.

Brusasco, C., Corradi, F., Vargas, M., Bona, M., Bruno, F., Marsili, M., … Pelosi, P. (2013). In vitro evaluation of heat and moisture exchangers designed for spontaneously breathing tracheostomized patients. *Respiratory Care, 58*(11), 1878–1885.

Castro, M. A., Dedivitis, R. A., & Macedo, A. G. (2011). Evaluation of a method for assessing pulmonary function in Laryngectomees. *Acta Otorhinolaryngologica Italica, 31*, 243–247.

Doyle, P. C. (2005). Rehabilitation in head and neck cancer. In P. C. Doyle & R. L. Keith (Eds.), *Rehabilitation following treatment for head and neck cancer: voice, speech, and swallowing*. Austin: Pro-Ed Publishers.

Foreman, A., De Santis, R. J., Sultanov, F., Enepekides, D. J., & Higgins, K. M. (2016). Heat and moisture exchanger use reduces in-hospital complications following total laryngectomy: a case-control study. *Journal of Otolaryngology - Head & Neck Surgery, 45*(1), 40–45.

Grolman, W., Blom, E. D., Granson, R. D., Schouwenburg, P. F., & Hamaker, R. C. (1997). An efficiency comparison of four heat and moisture exchangers used in the laryngectomized patient. *Laryngoscope, 107*(6), 814–820.

Hairfield, W. M., Warren, D. W., Hinton, V. A., & Seaton, D. L. (1987). Inspiratory and expiratory effects of nasal breathing. *The Cleft Palate Journal, 24*, 183–189.

Hedley, R. M., & Allt-Graham, J. A. (1992). A comparison of the filtration properties of heat and moisture exchangers. *Anaesthesia, 47*, 414–420.

Hess, M. M., Schwenk, R. A., Frank, W., & Loddenkemper, R. (1999). Pulmonary function after total laryngectomy. *Laryngoscope, 109*, 988–994.

Hilgers, F. J. M., Aaronson, N. K., Ackerstaff, A. H., Schouwenburg, P. F., & van Zandwikj, N. (1991). The influence of a heat and moisture exchanger (HME) on the respiratory symptoms after total laryngectomy. *Clinical Otolaryngology & Allied Sciences, 16(2)*, 152–156.

Hilgers, F. J. M., Ackerstaff, A. H., Aaronson, N. K., Schouwenburg, P. F., & Van Zandwijk, N. (1990). Physical and psychosocial consequences of total laryngectomy. *Clinical Otolaryngology, 15*, 421–425.

Keck, T., Leiacker, R., Heinrich, A., Kuhnemann, S., & Rettinger, G. (2000). Humidity and temperature profile in the nasal cavity. *Rhinology, 38*, 167–171.

Kerr, A. (Ed.). (1997). *Scott-Brown's otolaryngology* (Vol. 4, 6th ed.). Oxford: Butterworth-Heinemann.

Mcrae, D., Young, P., Hamilton, J., & Jones, A. (1996). Raising airway resistance in laryngectomees increases tissue oxygen saturation. *Clinical Otolaryngology, 21*(4), 366–368.

Merol, J., Charpiot, A., Langagne, T., Hemar, P., Ackerstaff, A. H., & Hilgers, F. J. M. (2011). Randomized controlled trial on postoperative pulmonary humidification after total laryngectomy: external humidification versus heat and moisture exchanger. *Laryngoscope, 122*, 275–281.

Mohide, E. A., Archibald, S. D., Tew, M., Young, J. E., & Haines, T. (1992). Postlaryngectomy quality-of-life dimensions identified by patients and health care professionals. *American Journal of Surgery, 164*, 619–622.

Nystrand, R. (2007). Test summary Atos Medical HME Micron (Report no. AM 071024). Bio-TeQ Nystrand Consulting.

Pedemonte-Sarrias, G., Villatoro-Sologaistoa, J. C., Ale-Inostroza, P., Lopez-Vilas, M., Leon-Vintro, X., & Quer-Agusti, M. (2013). Chronic adherence to heat and moisture exchanger use in laryngectomized patients. *ACTA Otorhinolaryngology Espanola, 64*(4), 247–252.

Risberg-Berlin, B., Ylitano, R., & Finizia, C. (2006). Screening and rehabilitation of olfaction after total laryngectomy in Swedish patients: Results from an intervention study using Nasal Airflow-Induing Manuever. *Archives of Otolaryngology-Head and Neck Surgery, 132*, 301–306.

Santos, C. G., Bergmann, A., Coca, K. L., Garcia, A. A., & Valente, T. C. (2016). Olfactory function and quality of life after olfaction rehabilitation in total laryngectomies. *Codas, 28*(6), 669–677.

Scheenstra, R. J., Muller, S. H., & Hilgers, F. J. (2011). Endotracheal temperature and humidity in laryngectomized patients in a warm and dry environment and the effect of a heat and moisture exchanger. *Head & Neck, 33*, 1285–1293.

Scheenstra, R. J., Muller, S. H., Vincent, A., Annemieke, H., Ackerstaff, A. H., Jacobi, I., & Hilgers, F. J. M. (2010). Short-term endotracheal climate changes and clinical effects of a h and moisture exchanger with an integrated electrostatic virus and bacterial filter developed for laryngectomized individuals. *Acta Oto-Laryngologica, 130*, 739–746.

Scheenstra, R. J., Muller, S. H., Vincent, A., Sinaasappel, M., Zuur, J. K., & Hilgers, F. J. M. (2009). Endotracheal temperature and humidity measurements in laryngectomized patients: intra- and inter-patient variability. *Medical & Biological Engineering & Computing, 47*(7), 773–782.

Schwab, J. A., & Zenkel, M. (1998). Filtration of particulates in the human nose. *Laryngoscope, 108*(1), 120–124.

Shelly, M., Bethune, D. W., & Latimer, R. D. (1986). A comparison of five heat and moisture exchangers. *Anaesthesia, 41*, 527–532.

Toremalm, N. G. (1960). A heat-and-moisture exchanger for posttracheotomy care. An experimental study. *Acta Oto-Laryngologica, 52*, 461–472.

van As, C. J., Hilgers, F. J. M., Koopmans-van Beinum, F. J., & Ackerstaff, A. H. (1998). The influence of stoma occlusion on aspects of tracheoesophageal voice. *Acta Oto-Laryngologica, 118*, 732–738.

Van den Boer, C., Muller, S. H., Vincent, A. D., Zuchner, K., Van den Brekel, M. W. M., & Hilgers, F. J. M. (2013). A novel, simplified ex-vivo method for measuring performance of heat and moisture exchangers for postlaryngectomy pulmonary rehabilitation. *Respiratory Care, 58*, 1449–1458.

Vareille, M., Kieninger, E., Edwards, M. R., & Regamey, N. (2011). The airway epithelium: soldier in the fight against respiratory viruses. *Clinical Microbiology Reviews, 24*, 210–229.

Vasquez de la Inglesia, F., & Fernandez Gonzalez, S. (2006). Method for the study of pulmonary function in laryngectomized patients. *ACTA Otorhinolaryngology Espanola, 57*, 275–278.

Verkerke, G. J., Geertsema, A. A., & Schutte, H. K. (2002). Airflow resistance of heat and moisture exchange filters with and without a tracheostoma valve. *Annals of Otology, Rhinology, and Laryngology, 111*(4), 333–337.

Wanner, A., Salathé, M., & O'Riordan, T. G. (1996). Mucociliary clearance in the airways. *American Journal of Respiratory and Critical Care Medicine, 154*(6), 1868–1902.

Williams, R., Rankin, N., Smith, T., Galler, D., & Seakins, P. (1996). Relationship between the humidity and temperature of inspired gas and the function of the airway mucosa. *Critical Care Medicine, 24*, 1920–1929.

Zuur, J. K., Muller, S. H., de Jongh, F. H., van Zandwijk, N., & Hilgers, F. J. (2006). The physiological rationale of heat and moisture exchangers in post-laryngectomy pulmonary rehabilitation: a review. *European Archives of Oto-Rhino-Laryngology, 263*(1), 1–8.

Zuur, J. K., Muller, S. H., Sinaasappel, M., Hart, G. A., Van, Z. N., & Hilgers, F. J. M. (2007). Influence of heat and moisture exchanger respiratory load on transcutaneous oxygenation in laryngectomized individuals: a randomized crossover study. *Head & Neck, 29*(12), 1102–1110.

Elements of Clinical Training with the Electrolarynx

9

Kathleen F. Nagle

Elements of Clinical Training with the Electrolarynx

Laryngectomees have three main options for postsurgery speech communication: esophageal speech (ES) and tracheoesophageal (TE) speech, which have internal sound sources, and artificial speech produced using an external sound source. ES is a hands-free mode of postlaryngectomy speech that requires no prosthesis, device, additional surgery, or any particular maintenance. Successful ES speakers inject air into the esophagus and then control its release to create a "pseudo-voice" through vibration of pharyngoesophageal tissue (Globlek, Štajner-Katušić, Mušura, Horga, & Liker, 2004; Robbins, Fisher, Blom, & Singer, 1984; Štajner-Katušić, Horga, Mušura, & Globlek, 2006). TE speech, which is driven by pulmonary air, requires the creation of a fistula in the common tracheoesophageal wall, either at the time of laryngectomy or after the site of laryngeal reconstruction has healed (Brown, Hilgers, Irish, & Balm, 2003; Singer & Blom, 1980). A small, valved TE puncture prosthesis is then placed into the puncture site to maintain the link between the trachea and esophagus. This TE prosthesis provides unidirectional airflow from the lungs to the vocal tract. By most accounts, TE speech is judged by listeners to be more acceptable and intelligible than other types of alaryngeal speech (Hillman, Walsh, Wolf, Fisher, & Hong, 1998; Most, Tobin, & Mimran, 2000; Pindzola & Cain, 1988; Williams & Watson, 1987). It is not uncommon, however, for laryngectomees to abandon TE speech in favor of an artificial larynx, presumably due to complications related to leaking or repeated extrusion of the prosthesis (Mendenhall et al., 2002; Singer et al., 2013).

The artificial larynx is an external sound source driven by pneumatic or electromechanical vibration. Pneumatic, reed-based devices (e.g., "Tokyo" larynx) provide an external alaryngeal voice source via a vibrating reed similar to that used in wind instruments (Nelson, Parkin, & Potter, 1975). Pulmonary air is directed into the oral cavity via a small-diameter tube that is coupled to a housing placed on the tracheostoma. Users can therefore use preoperative respiratory speech patterns to create natural-sounding durational speech characteristics (Weinberg & Riekena, 1973). The sound produced by the reed-based devices is also quite similar to the human voice because the reed vibrates in the same way as the vocal folds. Most importantly, reed-based devices lack the radiated noise that is an integral component of electronic sound sources. Pneumatic devices are rarely used in the United States today, presumably because coupling the device to the tracheostoma and managing the oral tube can be

K. F. Nagle (✉)
Department of Speech-Language Pathology, Seton Hall University, South Orange, NJ, USA
e-mail: naglekat@shu.edu

© Springer Nature Switzerland AG 2019
P. C. Doyle (ed.), *Clinical Care and Rehabilitation in Head and Neck Cancer*,
https://doi.org/10.1007/978-3-030-04702-3_9

awkward and unacceptably unsanitary for the user (Barney, 1958; Blom, 2000; Nelson et al., 1975).

The electrolarynx (EL) is an electromechanically driven device that supplies an entirely external, electronic sound source; no pulmonary driving air pressure is required. Because EL devices are comparatively simple and easy to use, they are used both in the early stages of postoperative care and ultimately chosen as the primary, backup, or emergency mode of speech by most laryngectomees (Doyle, 2005; Graham, 2006; Hillman et al., 1998; Meltzner & Hillman, 2005). This chapter will focus on EL devices and training in their optimal use.

Electromechanical Speech

EL devices provide a "voice" source with a range of potential options. The location and method of sound source transmission is a major determinant of these options (Meltzner et al., 2005). Transcervical or *neck-type* devices produce an external sound source that is transmitted to the oral cavity via vibration of neck, chin, or cheek tissue. The neck-type EL is the most commonly used artificial larynx among those who have a choice (Koike, Kobayashi, Hirose, & Hara, 2002). The neck-type EL contains a vibrating element and an electromagnetically driven vibrating membrane housed within a plastic or metal cylinder; several examples are shown in Fig. 9.1. Vibration of the EL membrane is initiated using a power button controlled by thumb pressure, with

the amplitude of vibration controlled via a second button or dial. Successful use of this type of EL requires adequate coupling of the vibrating head of the device with the skin of the neck, chin, or cheek at what has been referred to clinically as the "sweet spot." The tissue in the sweet spot(s) must retain sufficient elasticity to transmit the maximum amount of vibratory energy to the oropharyngeal cavity for speech production.

Transoral or *oral-type* ELs deliver acoustic energy directly to the oral cavity via a small-diameter plastic tube inserted into the mouth. The Cooper-Rand Electronic Speech Aid is the best known oral-type device made specifically for this purpose (Fig. 9.2); however, most neck-type ELs can easily be converted into oral-type devices using an oral adaptor that can be attached to the vibrating head of the EL. Because oral-type devices bypass radiated or reconstructed neck tissue, they are particularly attractive in certain contexts. For example, immediately following laryngectomy, tenderness in the healing pharyngoesophageal segment makes ES and TE speech difficult and painful. Effects of neck dissection or radiation may reduce the vibratory capability of tissue typically used in neck-type EL speech production; similarly, placement of the vibrating head of the neck-type EL directly

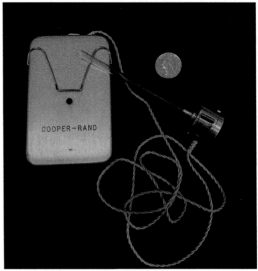

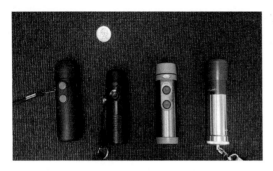

Fig. 9.1 Electrolarynges with quarter for scale. From left: (**a**) NuVois III Digital™; (**b**) TruTone™; (**c**) Servox® Inton; (**d**) Romet® R210. (Photo by K.F. Nagle)

Fig. 9.2 Cooper-Rand Electronic Speech Aid. (Photo by K.F. Nagle)

on neck tissue may also cause substantial discomfort. Oral-type ELs are, therefore, a good choice for alaryngeal speech if adequate and comfortable coupling of the vibrating head of a neck-type EL cannot be achieved in the long term (Doyle, 2005; Hillman et al., 1998; Ward, Koh, Frisby, & Hodge, 2003).

As noted, most neck-type ELs are sold with an oral adaptor, which can be fitted over the vibrating head to provide the benefits of an oral-type EL. New laryngectomees who plan to use a neck-type EL may acclimate to EL use in the postsurgery period by using an oral adaptor while they heal. If the effects of radiation or surgery prohibit identification of an adequate sweet spot, they may choose to use the oral adaptor for the longer term. The adaptor consists of a rubber, plastic, or silicone cover for the head of the EL, with an opening in the center (shown fitted to an EL in Fig. 9.3a), and a small-diameter plastic or silicone tube, often with a fitted tip at one end, as in Fig. 9.3b. One end of the tube is placed into the EL cover opening, and the tip, which acts as a filter for saliva and food particles, is placed in the mouth.

Use of an oral adaptor requires learning to control the placement of the tube within the oral cavity. The tip of the long-tubed adaptor is ide-

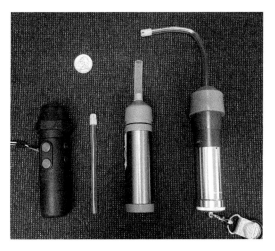

Fig. 9.3 Neck-type electrolarynges, with quarter for scale. From left: (**a**) NuVois III Digital™ fitted with head cover; (**b**) long oral tube; (**c**) Servox® Inton™ fitted with short-tube adaptor; (**d**) Romet® R210 fitted with long-tube adaptor. (Photo by K.F. Nagle)

ally placed off of midline by the upper teeth and inside of the cheek, with the open end facing the roof of the mouth. Figure 9.3d shows an EL fitted with long-tubed oral adaptor. Placement high in the mouth reduces interference from the tongue during articulation. High placement may also keep the tube cleaner for longer by reducing direct contact with the saliva that pools in the lower mouth. The open end of the short-tubed adaptor, shown fitted to an EL in Fig. 9.3c, is also placed between the teeth and cheek.

The hygiene issues related to constant use of a tube while speaking may be unpleasant and unacceptable for some users, and the presence of the tube can affect the user's intelligibility (Weinberg & Riekena, 1973). The voice produced with oral-type ELs also obviously lacks some of the spectral qualities of voice produced with the normal voice at the glottis (i.e., pharyngeal and nasal resonance); this further reduces the naturalness and intelligibility of speech already affected by the presence of the oral tube and its artificial source (Barney, 1958). Therefore, if they can use neck-type ELs, most laryngectomees opt for them over the oral-type (Koike et al., 2002).

Intraoral devices (also referred to as "palate devices") are variants of the oral-type EL. These devices mount to a dental plate or orthodontic retainer, generating a sound source directly within the oral cavity (e.g., Ultra Voice™). Vibration onset is controlled by the user with a remote switch that may be held in the hand, worn on the body, or kept in a pocket. Intraoral devices must be fitted to the individual user, making them comparatively expensive; however, once fitted, they are reportedly easy to use (Takahashi, Nakao, Kikuchi, & Kaga, 2005). There is limited empirical evidence of the popularity of intraoral ELs, but their use is likely restricted to laryngectomees who are unable to generate intelligible speech using other EL devices.

Users of EL devices must become physically and psychologically comfortable with the sound and feeling of the device, and the choice to make it a primary mode of communication depends on several factors. That is, not all laryngectomees are physically or cognitively able to use an EL. Surgery, chemotherapy, and radiation may impose temporary or permanent physiological and anatomical limitations that will affect successful use of the EL (e.g., fibrosis of neck tissue). For example, pain and impaired range of motion in the shoulder may lead to difficulty raising the arm or maintaining the position necessary for manual EL use (Doyle, 1994, 2005). Unlike ES and TE speech, EL speech has limited hands-free options.[1] Manual operation is generally required to initiate voice and adjust the amplitude of vibration for even the most advanced ELs currently available. Gripping the device while simultaneously manipulating one or more of its buttons may be particularly challenging. For some individuals, the need to operate an EL manually may make it an option of last resort, but most EL users are able to overcome this limitation.

Additional considerations may also create substantial challenges for some speakers. Some may initially reject the use of an EL because of the uniquely robotic, "buzzing" sound and the radiated noise associated with electromechanical speech (Doyle, 2005; Espy-Wilson, Chari, MacAuslan, Huang, & Walsh, 1998; Meltzner & Hillman, 2005; Qi & Weinberg, 1991). Artificial speech of any type is distracting, and even perfect coupling between EL and skin tissue cannot eliminate all non-speech noise radiated by the device. Moreover, most EL speech notoriously lacks the prosodic characteristics that make speech interesting and intelligible (Bien et al., 2008; Gandour & Weinberg, 1983; Gandour, Weinberg, & Garzione, 1983; Hillman et al., 1998). The sound of EL speech is especially problematic for female laryngectomees, who may be socially penalized for the perceived low pitch of their EL voices (Cox, Theurer, Spaulding, & Doyle, 2015; Nagle, Eadie, Wright, & Sumida, 2012). The monopitch quality of most ELs may also affect women to a greater degree than men, as women tend to have greater speaking fundamental frequency (f_0) ranges (Goy, Fernandes,

Pichora-Fuller, & van Lieshout, 2013; Pepiot, 2014). The consequence for female laryngectomees is frequent misidentification as male when listeners lack visual information (e.g., when speaking on the telephone; Smithwick, Davis, Dancer, Hicks, & Montague, 2002). Anecdotally, some EL users have reported that they or their family members or friends just do not like the sound of the EL (Eadie et al., 2016).

Given that all laryngectomees are likely to use an EL at some point, it is essential for SLPs to be aware of the basic and advanced features of ELs. The choice of a particular EL model depends on several design factors described in the next section.

Design Features of the Electrolarynx

The "perfect" artificial larynx would mimic a natural voice source. It would be unobtrusive, reliable, hygienically acceptable to the user, inexpensive, and simple to operate; its output would match that of a natural voice in volume, quality, and pitch inflection (Barney, 1958; pp. 558–559). To varying degrees, most of these criteria have been met by currently available ELs. The size and shape of ELs has changed over time so that some neck-type ELs can now be nearly hidden in a man's fist as he speaks. Technological advances have increased the EL's reliability, ease of use, and range of options for mimicking natural laryngeal speech (Searl, 2006; Meltzner et al., 2005). The relative cost has concurrently dropped. For users who are uncomfortable with the hygienic drawbacks of using an oral adaptor or intraoral device, neck-type ELs provide a relatively clean and user-friendly alternative. A discussion of ongoing developments in EL technology is beyond this chapter, but the current focus is on energy-efficient, wireless, hands-free activation and dynamic pitch modulation as a means of refining the naturalness of EL speech (Guo, Nagle, & Heaton, 2016; Heaton, Robertson, & Griffin, 2011; Matsui, Kimura, Nakatoh, & Kato, 2013; Nakamura, Toda, Saruwatari, & Shikano, 2012; Stepp, Heaton, Rolland, & Hillman, 2009;

---

[1]The HandsFree™ Electrolarynx Holder (Griffin Labs, Temecula, CA) is worn around the neck and activated with a chin press; it is not appropriate for all users, however, as optimal use may occur only within a specific and limited area of the user's neck space.

Wan, Wu, Wu, Wang, & Wan, 2012; Wu, Wan, Xiao, Wang, & Wan, 2014).

All ELs are designed with three features that the user can control directly: activation of vibration, volume adjustment, and base pitch setting. Even a basic analog EL model allows the user to control activation and amplitude of vibration using a button, dial, or "rocker switch." Volume range is preset by the manufacturer and intuitive for the user. Volume is usually adjusted by rotating a small thumb dial. The volume dial is frequently placed next to the activation button, allowing users to adjust the loudness of the device with the thumb as well. Despite the proximity of these mechanisms, however, two fingers would be needed to permit simultaneous control of activation and amplitude of vibration. Typically, thumb-button users have to stop "vocalizing," at least momentarily, in an effort to effectively adjust the amplitude of vibration. In such circumstances, one may subsequently observe limitations in real-time prosodic variation of loudness by the user.

Pitch capabilities vary significantly from device to device, and base pitch settings can be complicated to alter. Most ELs offer a range of potential base pitch settings. Users can adjust the EL to suit their preference as a base "speaking" pitch, but it will vibrate at a single f_0. For newer digital devices, pitch adjustments can be accomplished electronically, but analog ELs require manual adjustment. Adjusting the base pitch of an analog device may be as simple as dialing a wheel on the side of the device, or it may require opening the device to access its mechanical workings. For individuals with reduced dexterity or visual acuity, these adjustments may be an intractable challenge.

Several EL models offer two base pitch settings, with one button assigned to each. The advantage of two settings is that two preset f_0s can be achieved; each button produces its own pitch. The user is, therefore, able to alternate monotone base pitches. This ability to change pitch as a signal of paralinguistic features (e.g., "yelling" at the higher pitch, using the lower pitch only to sound authoritative, etc.) may be attractive to some users despite the monotone

quality of speech output. In some models, speech volume can also be adjusted separately for each pitch setting, which offers further flexibility of use, particularly across communication settings.

Dynamic (real-time) pitch modulation is currently available in a single EL model (TruTone™, Griffin Labs, Temecula, CA). This device allows users to produce more natural prosody by adjusting the degree of finger pressure placed on the activation button/tone sensor. Once the pitch range is set, users can modify pitch while speaking by altering finger or thumb pressure on the activation button located on the exterior of the device. Increased finger or thumb pressure on the activation button results in increased pitch; as the button is released, pitch drops to the baseline level. Setting a relatively wide pitch range accommodates more natural-sounding changes in prosody; however, as the set pitch range increases, it becomes more difficult to control pitch with finger pressure. It is relatively easy to maintain the maximum pitch with maximal thumb pressure. It can be difficult to sustain the minimum pitch, however, because of the necessity of keeping thumb pressure at a level that is "just detectible" by the device. Before operating such a device, users must set its pitch range by adjusting two tiny actuating dials inside the device housing. Very small adjustments to these dials can lead to rather large changes in fundamental frequency, so the process of setting a pitch range can be time-consuming and a bit frustrating, particularly if dexterity or visual problems exist.

In practice, many TruTone™ users do not take advantage of pitch variability inherent to the device (Nagle & Heaton, 2016, 2017). Clinical observation of EL users' behaviors with the device suggests three related reasons for this. First, there is not an intuitive link between subconscious prelaryngectomy pitch regulation (i.e., using laryngeal musculature) and conscious postlaryngectomy pitch modulation using the thumb. Attempting to execute real-time pitch changes may require an unusual degree of attention to speech output. Practically speaking, the cognitive load connected with using dynamic, thumb-button pitch modulation may be too much for many users. Second, the quick, precise muscular changes associated with intonation in laryngeal speech are quite difficult to match with thumb pressure alone. The dexterity needed to capitalize on thumb-button pitch modulation also may be too great for some EL users. Recent work by Al-Zanoon, Parsa, Lin, and Doyle (2017) has revealed that despite the mechanical capacity of an EL device to produce pitch changes, the ability for the user to effectively convey such changes is challenging. Third, although the thumb is used to control activation and adjustment of vibration in the TruTone™, it also may be needed to stabilize placement of the device against the skin for optimized signal transmission. That is, when maintaining coupling of the EL with the sweet spot, it is easier to apply consistent thumb pressure, than to attempt to vary it. In terms of intelligibility, it is arguably better to produce some pitch variability than none at all (Bunton, Kent, Kent, & Duffy, 2001). Nonetheless, both intelligibility and naturalness could likely be improved if TruTone™ users manipulated the device to match natural pitch contours (Watson & Schlauch, 2009). Ultimately, most TruTone™ users seem to produce speech that is perceived as nearly monopitch, despite the capability of the device to do more.

Using the Artificial Electrolarynx

It is rare for individuals to pick up an EL for the first time and immediately produce intelligible speech with it. To reduce the amount of radiated noise from the device, users must first be instructed to identify the location at which the device couples best to the tissue. In addition to finding the sweet spot, it is necessary to master the features of the device itself and to modulate the articulators to accommodate and maximize the quality of the artificial voice. With good instruction, most who are laryngectomized can learn to use either the neck-type or intraoral EL effectively.

Basic Operation of the Electrolarynx

When providing options to the new user, the SLP should be able to model the use of any ELs being considered, and familiarity with several EL mod-

els/types is advisable. If possible, users should initially be trained to hold and activate the device with their non-dominant hand. Although a simple button push activates the EL, most users need to be trained in how best to manage it during connected speech (Doyle, 1994, 2005). For example, many users' instinct is to deactivate the vibration between each word, producing a staccato-sounding speech quality that may reduce the intelligibility and naturalness of their speech. Modifying this behavior may require a discussion about pausing, phrasing, and the voicing characteristics of running speech. Conversely, new users may initially fail to deactivate vibration between utterances, producing one long buzz of noise. Fortunately, this latter tendency is easy to correct once it is pointed out and instructions for modification provided.

Laryngectomees need guidance as they find their electrolaryngeal "voice"; once they have identified and begun to use it, they are unlikely to want to make changes. Adaptability of in different communication contexts is a particular strength of ELs, and SLPs are uniquely qualified to instruct users in how to exploit this flexibility. For example, when setting the habitual volume for their devices, users may benefit from the practiced ear of the SLP to guide them. Some users set EL volume to a lower than optimal level in an apparent attempt to reduce its noise, unnaturalness, or robotic sound. These users can be trained to adjust the volume to suit their environment, including considering the effects of EL speech on potential communication partners with hearing loss. (Older EL users may also benefit from evaluation of their own hearing acuity as they contemplate maximizing communicative effectiveness.)

Clinical observation likewise suggests that new users may need assistance in choosing a base pitch setting. There are several rules of thumb regarding the pitch of EL speech. Although typical male laryngeal speaking f_0 ranges between 100 and 146 Hz (Baken & Orlikoff, 2000), evidence suggests that setting the EL below 100 Hz may provide a better outcome for most men, as intelligibility is relatively enhanced at lower speaking f_0 (Nagle et al., 2012; Watson &

Schlauch, 2008). The gender-neutral range of alaryngeal speech seems to be wider than that of laryngeal speech (roughly 145–165 Hz; Gelfer & Bennett, 2013); that is, there appears to be a bias toward perceiving EL speech at even higher f_0s as male (Nagle et al., 2012). In fact, setting the EL within the typical female speaking f_0 range of 188–221 Hz may be counterproductive (Baken & Orlikoff, 2000; Nagle et al., 2012). It is clear that female laryngectomees may have to choose between intelligibility and sounding female. This is a potential trade-off that must be considered by individual users, and SLPs are uniquely qualified to provide education and counseling to new laryngectomees.

Optimizing Electromechanical Speech

SLPs training new users should help them become comfortable with EL features, but they may also need to boost the user's knowledge of the features of speech that contribute most to comprehensibility and naturalness. Successful EL users have the metalinguistic awareness to maximize intelligibility and minimize distractions to communication partners that accompany the use of an artificial larynx.

One way for new EL users to think about their speech output is to imagine how it is perceived by potential communication partners. The sound of EL speech affects not only the user's comfort with the device but also the ability of listeners to understand what is said. Specifically, the speech signal should be perceptually separable from the accompanying non-speech noise emitted by an EL. Listeners may have trouble parsing signal from noise, however, if the user fails to couple the device properly to neck or cheek tissue or is unable to filter the EL voice source appropriately within the oral cavity. Likewise, paralinguistic aspects of speech such as pitch and loudness contours are lost in typical EL speech (Gandour & Weinberg, 1983; Gandour et al., 1983). These reductions in the complexity of signal quality can affect speech intelligibility (Doyle, 2012). Speech *intelligibility* is the degree to which the acoustic

signal is understood, without context. *Comprehensibility*, in contrast, encompasses acoustic, visual, gestural, and proxemic information, along with other contextual factors. Comprehensibility is the extent to which a listener understands utterances produced by a speaker in a communication context (Yorkston, Strand, & Kennedy, 1996). Speakers can improve their comprehensibility by improving their intelligibility and by making the most of gestural and other nonverbal cues to communication. Enhanced EL communication is aided by considering multiple factors that improve comprehensibility for which SLPs have particular expertise. These include optimizing perceptual quality, emphasizing salient suprasegmental cues, and attending to nonverbal communicative signals.

Perceptual aspects of voice quality beyond comprehensibility are particularly important for alaryngeal speech because of the potential effects of its atypical sound source on the success of communicative interactions (Doyle & Eadie, 2005; Meltzner & Hillman, 2005). Despite the similarity of electromechanical sources, the quality of EL speech can vary quite a bit among users, given the unique characteristics of an individual's oronasopharyngeal cavity (i.e., the speech filter) before and after laryngectomy. Dynamic aspects of speech production may be affected by additional medical or surgical procedures (e.g., glossectomy, radiation), reducing the accuracy of speech sound production for some laryngectomees. To compensate for a reduction in segmental accuracy, EL users must attend to suprasegmental factors such as pitch, duration, and loudness. Although they may not increase intelligibility per se, adjustments to suprasegmental aspects of EL speech may improve communicative success by enhancing speech and voice quality.

Alaryngeal voices are frequently described on the basis of their speech *acceptability* or perceived *naturalness* (Bennett & Weinberg, 1973; Eadie & Doyle, 2002, 2005). Speech acceptability is a multidimensional descriptor including naturalness, pleasantness, and the degree to which the voice is not distracting (Bennett & Weinberg, 1973; Most et al., 2000). Perceived naturalness typically addresses the degree to which the rate, intonation, rhythm, and stress pattern of disordered speech resemble normal speech (Eadie & Doyle, 2002; Meltzner & Hillman, 2005). Pitch, loudness, rate, and rhythm changes may affect not only comprehensibility but also overall communicative success if communication partners are "put off" by the sound of speech or feel that they have to expend too much effort to listen to it. Ultimately, if speech sounds unnatural enough, the EL user's quality of life may suffer (Eadie et al., 2016; Law, Ma, & Yiu, 2009).

Training Goals

Because of the unusual sound sources, alaryngeal speech provokes different perceptual expectations from other types of disordered speech or voice. ES and TE speeches are characterized by highly aperiodic sources of relatively low signal amplitude, whereas EL speech generally features flat or near flat intonation accompanied by radiated noise. EL speech introduces an external noise source that competes with the very speech signal it is designed to enhance. For example, differences between voiced and voiceless speech sounds are generally not perceptible in connected EL speech given the necessarily constant vibration of the device source. Overall goals of maximizing user comfort, comprehensibility, and naturalness depend heavily on minimizing the effects of radiated noise (Doyle, 1994; Graham, 2006). Finding a sweet spot where the EL produces the least rattle and the most oral resonance is the first goal of learning how to use a neck-type EL. The sweet spot should be a location where the tissue is most elastic and close enough to the oral cavity to maximally amplify the vibration of this tissue. If contact between the head of the EL and the skin is incomplete or lost, noise will radiate directly from the EL, and the capacity to produce speech will be lost until adequate contact is regained. Placement of the EL head must be also comfortable enough for the user to maintain during speech and reachable by the user every time he/she wants to speak. Likewise, when using an

intraoral-type EL, the optimal placement of the oral tube must be maintained.

As mentioned above, another way to improve the perceived naturalness of EL speech is to exaggerate its prosodic characteristics. For example, lexical and prosodic stresses are generally marked in normal laryngeal speech by longer duration, higher pitch, and increased volume. In contrast, EL users tend to intuitively mark lexical or syntactic stress using duration and by making stressed syllables relatively longer than unstressed syllables (Gandour & Weinberg, 1984). If they do not make such adjustments, instructing them to do so may increase the naturalness (and potentially comprehensibility) of their connected speech.

Maximizing intelligibility often increases comprehensibility and naturalness. As mentioned previously, perception and distinction of speech sounds that differ only in voicing are affected for EL speech because when the device is activated, its "voice" is always on. Turning off the EL during production of unvoiced cognate sounds (e.g., /p, t, k, s/) is not feasible during running speech and not advisable even for short phrases as a rule. Although on-off control serves as an important EL skill to enhance communication, the onset or termination of the signal must fall at points within a given utterance where such changes would also appear for a normal speaker. During speech, the EL should be silenced only at grammatically appropriate points in an utterance (i.e., between breath groups). Repeatedly turning the device on and off at very brief intervals creates an unpleasant staccato effect that is likely to negate any intelligibility gained by producing voiceless consonants without a voice. Simply put, the phonetic features of running speech change too quickly for this type of adjustment.

A more top-down approach that may maximize intelligibility for EL speech involves *clear speech* (Cox, 2016). Clear speech is a speaking style adopted to increase intelligibility in difficult listening situations (Krause & Braida, 2003). Speakers instructed to use clear speech make subconscious changes to enhance speech clarity. Initially it may be helpful to simply instruct the user to imagine speaking to someone who is hard of hearing, as this often prompts intuitive use of clear speech. Clear speech has specific properties that maximize intelligibility, such as over-articulation (Smiljanić & Bradlow, 2009). Using clear speech tends to cause individuals to reduce speech rate as well, often by taking longer and more frequent pauses (Smiljanić & Bradlow, 2009). Although reducing speech rate by too much can decrease its naturalness, existing data suggests that reducing speech rate is generally beneficial to intelligibility (Yorkston, Hammen, Beukelman, & Traynor, 1990).

Comprehensibility is also increased by capitalizing on nonverbal cues, and it may be necessary for SLPs to attend specifically to gesture, body language, and proxemics when training an EL user. Reduced paralinguistic information in EL speech heightens the relevance of these nonverbal communicative cues. Visual cues in particular can reinforce the delivery of an intended message to a communication partner. Because most ELs require manual voice activation, however, at least one of the user's hands may not be free for simultaneous gestural communication. Users of oral-type ELs may display unusual facial expressions while attempting to manage the oral tube. In addition to the potentially decreased intelligibility caused by the articulatory limitations of the EL, the user's comprehensibility may be further limited by reduced access to these types of nonverbal cues. Consequently, the next section outlines several specific tasks that can be used to train laryngectomees in the successful use of EL devices.

Training Targets

Certain speech tasks are difficult for all laryngectomees, but EL users face particular challenges. Because EL speech is continuously voiced and lacks driving air pressure, voicing and manner cues may be lost unless specific attention is paid to emphasizing them. Fortunately, phonetic cues such as duration can be exaggerated to influence what listeners perceive. Therefore, EL users should learn to make the most of segmental, suprasegmental, and nonverbal features that

complement what they are initially able to produce with an EL.

Production of specific segments Speech production is similar for all types of ELs, although the oral tube may complicate articulation of certain segments. For example, placement of the tube may interfere with lip closure and tongue movement for labial and lingual consonants. New users may want to take a hierarchical approach to learning to use the EL. That is, they might begin to practice by producing simple consonant-vowel or vowel-consonant syllable and then move to multisyllable words, phrases, and beyond (Graham, 2006). Given relatively intact articulators, EL users who have located their sweet spot should be able to produce vowels with little training. It may be most instructive to new EL users to start with production of diphthongs. Placing the EL at the sweet spot and producing oversized vowel combinations such as "ow" and "aye" will immediately give the user a sense of what to expect from EL speech. It may also be necessary at first to make big oral gestures for both consonants and vowels to compensate for the abnormal acoustic qualities of EL speech (Wu, Wan, Wang, & Wan, 2013). A trial-and-error approach is generally adequate for learning to differentiate vowels.

Skilled EL users can capitalize on the redundancy of speech cues, such as the influence of vowel features on the consonant perception. Duration can be strategically modified to hint at consonant features not fully articulated in alaryngeal speech. Vowels preceding voiceless consonants are perceived as shorter in duration than those preceding voiced consonants (Peterson & Lehiste, 1960). To create a voicing distinction in the absence of voicing cues, vowels preceding voiced consonants should be strategically lengthened (Weiss & Basili, 1985; Weiss, Yeni-Komshian, & Heinz, 1979). Likewise, vowels following /h/ may be perceived as longer than syllable-initial vowels. As an unvoiced glottal fricative, /h/ is problematic for EL speakers who lack access to pulmonary air or a glottis. Even if it were feasible to turn off an EL during running speech to produce /h/, laryngectomees would have difficulty generating adequate frication for the sound. To influence the listener to perceive /h/, a speaker can strategically lengthen vowels meant to follow /h/.

To differentiate consonant segments, EL users should be instructed exaggerate the phonetic features that remain available to them. Without voicing contrasts, they must over-articulate both place and manner characteristics. To the degree possible, EL users should approximate the burst "plosion" that accompanies stop consonants. Laryngectomees lacking a TE puncture cannot build up high intraoral pressures using pulmonary air. If the tongue, lips, and velum are intact and functioning, however, they can exploit ambient air pressure to overdo the release of stop consonants. Some refer to this as "popping" a consonant, a maneuver that is common to traditional esophageal speech training (Doyle, 1994). Similarly, with guidance, laryngectomees should work to lengthen the duration of fricative and nasal consonants, to exaggerate both their manner and place of articulation. They may also choose to produce voiceless targets for a relatively shorter duration than their voiced cognates.

For users of oral-type ELs, lingual consonants (e.g., /t, d, s, z/) can also be challenging because the oral tube may impede natural tongue movements. Individuals will have to experiment with the device to find the most practical way to produce these sounds clearly. For these and all speech sounds, it is critical that the user keep the oral tube relatively high and out of the way of the tongue. The use of a short-tubed adaptor may in some instances alleviate the interference of the tube with lingual movements, but because the EL itself must consequently be placed closer to the mouth, the tube adaptor may get in the way of labial movements. Thus, careful monitoring of a larger set of speech behaviors is essential in the treatment process.

Production of suprasegmentals Although the lack of a voicing distinction can affect the intelligibility of EL speech, the absence of prosodic features arguably affects it even more (Watson & Schlauch, 2008). The markers of stressed sylla-

bles, a major feature of prosody, are increased loudness, duration, and pitch. Because few users actually manipulate ELs with dynamic pitch and amplitude modulation to align with natural speech contours, the only prosodic feature available to most EL users is duration. Research suggests EL users tend to lengthen syllables to signal stress; they also lengthen pauses following a final stressed syllable or preceding an initial stressed syllable (Gandour & Weinberg, 1984). Those users who do not automatically differentiate stressed from unstressed syllables with duration differences may need to be instructed to do so. A directive to use clear speech may instigate an immediate change (Smiljanić & Bradlow, 2009).

As with the production of single segments and syllables, inter-syllable duration can be used strategically to modulate EL speech. For example, EL users can strategically lengthen the pause preceding or following a stressed syllable. Depending on the device, they may be able to adjust pitch or volume in real time as well (although no currently available EL device offers the option of adjusting both of them simultaneously). If pitch modulation is offered, it is sensible for the EL user to take advantage of it. At the very least, exploration of pitch modulation may provide the speaker with a better understanding of the complexity of speech. The two general options for pitch modulation are described in the following section.

Optimizing two-button pitch modulation As described previously, a few EL models allow the user access to two base pitches. The differences come down to the simplicity of pitch adjustment and the ease of button and switch activation. In addition to volume control, two-pitch-button ELs have upper and lower buttons on the upper side of the external casing. For example, the Servox® Inton™ (Servona, Troisdorf, Germany) has what the manufacturer calls a "base tone" button and an "accentuation tone" button (see Fig. 9.1c). The user is directed to use the upper button to produce a base pitch while speaking. To emphasize certain words, the user must press both buttons at the same time. Although the accentuation button is directly under the tone button, it is necessary for most speakers to use two fingers (rather than a thumb) to accomplish this task. As an option, the Inton™ EL can also be programmed by the SLP to drop slightly in pitch as the base pitch button is released. This pitch drop is meant to replicate the natural pitch drop at the end of declarative utterances. Because it must be adjusted via computer, this feature cannot be toggled on and off during use. Although the Inton™ is digital, pitch must be adjusted manually, by opening the device and toggling the "dip switch" for the given button.[2]

The NuVois III Digital™ (NuVois, Meridian, ID) has two pitch buttons and two volume buttons (Fig. 9.1a). Pitch is adjusted by toggling one of the pitch buttons and pressing the volume buttons until a pitch is chosen. Pitch can be changed without opening the device, but not in real time; the user must stop and make adjustments to the device each time he/she wishes to change its pitch. As with the Inton™, this device can produce two distinct pitches, one of which can be used to indicate emphasis. The pitch and volume buttons are roughly on the same horizontal plane, but the volume buttons are smaller; users can learn to differentiate them by their size.

The bottom line for two-button pitch modulation is that a maximum of two base pitches are available to the user. The user cannot produce the full range of pitch between the two settings and can only hint at intonation with the second pitch button. It is, therefore, important to decide how and when the second button will be used. If the pitch difference between the button settings is too great, any use of it will suggest great excitement or anger. If it is too small, it may not be registered to the listener as a linguistic difference. The user must also decide how frequently to use the second pitch. For example, will it indicate any stressed syllable or just the stressed syllable in the word with the most prominence in the utterance? Will it be used only to indicate a question? Once prosodic patterns have been used for a period of time, they will become part of the user's new voice identity. Attempts to modify how an

individual uses the EL, even in the interest of increasing comprehensibility or naturalness, may confuse listeners who have become used to the user's postlaryngectomy EL voice. Again the SLP can play an important role in identifying targets and providing practice for these changes.

Optimizing dynamic pitch modulation The TruTone™ EL has a single button for activation and pitch modulation, along with a volume wheel that must be operated separately. As described previously, modulating pitch for this device requires the user to gauge the degree to which the button is depressed using haptic feedback. There are limits to the range that can be accurately distinguished using thumb pressure. Assuming that an appropriate pitch range has been set, users will need to figure out their aptitude by experimenting with the device – an experimental approach is appropriate. Targeting natural pitch contours requires recognition of the characteristics of normal intonation; that is, users of ELs with dynamic pitch modulation may need to spend time just listening to natural laryngeal speech. Specifically, they will have to learn to where the greatest stress is placed in an utterance. Unlike users of two-button type ELs, however, they will have the ability to produce gradations of pitch change. To make the most of this feature, users will have to think about aspects of intonation beyond emphasizing the word with the most stress in an utterance. SLPs, who are trained to attend to and identify perceptual characteristics that increase intelligibility, can be invaluable during this phase.

Optimal use of dynamic pitch requires some attention to the role of prosody in laryngeal speech. One fairly easy way to capitalize on dynamic pitch modulation is to mark "WH" questions with a rising/falling set of terminal tones. Yes/no questions are similarly marked by rising terminal tones in North American English. A skilled EL user will drop the pitch slightly at the end of a declarative sentence. An even more skilled user will use pitch shifts when listing items, providing a string of numbers, or maintaining a turn before pausing within an utterance. Users should listen to themselves and decide what sounds most natural to them. They should

---

[2] There are videos online (e.g., https://www.youtube.com/watch?v=iV3rP%2D%2DrcTA) that demonstrate this process.

also get feedback not only from a SLP but also from familiar conversation partners. A systematic and integrated approach to enhancing communication is of extreme importance clinically. Such an approach necessarily includes attending to nonverbal communication.

Nonverbal Communication

Nonverbal communicative cues include vocal non-speech sounds, gesture, and body language. The loss of natural non-speech vocalizations can have a dramatic effect on the quality of communication interactions. Laughter, for example, is a spontaneous vocal reaction. EL users have to decide whether their new laugh will be silent or artificial or coded through respiratory sounds (Doyle, 2008). Some adopt a strategy of smiling and saying "ah-ah-ah" with the EL. It is similarly worth the effort for EL users to come up with replacements for conversational fillers, such as the grunting assent or the heavy sigh. Some EL users choose the silent nod or head shake to move conversation along; others may choose to activate the EL briefly. Appropriate decisions about these aspects of speech pay dividends in naturalness and overall comprehensibility, even if overall intelligibility may have been compromised.

As a rule, it is easy enough to raise the volume on most devices if the user wants to communicate anger or excitement. Similarly, speaking in short bursts of one or two words may signify that the user is upset. EL speech is currently incapable of conveying much else in the way of emotion, however, and EL users may have to rely on facial expressions or gesture to get their feelings across. Likewise, beyond lengthening its duration, the ability to emphasize a given word or utterance is lost to many EL users. To maximize comprehensibility in the absence of pitch modulation, EL users may want to use or exaggerate facial expressions or gestures that complement their speech. Even with only one hand available, the options listed in Table 9.1 can provide valuable paralinguistic cues.

Table 9.1 Gestures and facial expressions that complement EL speech

Communicative intent	Action
Questions	Upturned hand Raised eyebrows Tilted head
Emphasis	Raised, open hand Widened eyes
Approval/Disapproval	Thumbs up/thumbs down
Impatience	Closed eyes Pressing lips together

The specific nonverbal cues that an EL user provides, intentionally or otherwise, may vary, but the topic of nonverbal communication is important for SLPs to discuss with EL users. Comprehensibility may not seem like an issue for some EL users until they find themselves in a noisy environment or on the telephone, where nonverbal cues are not available. The comprehensibility and naturalness of EL speech may decrease if nonverbal cues are not intuitive to the user but may increase if these cues can be exploited appropriately. SLPs can help by role-playing situations in which nonverbal communication makes a difference.

Conclusions

This chapter has addressed optimal use of currently available ELs. Although EL use is not appropriate for all laryngectomees, most use it as a primary or backup mode of communication. SLPs should be familiar with the variety of EL features available and should be able to model appropriate use of numerous devices. Beyond choosing the suitable EL, the role of the SLP is to maximize the user's comfort with the chosen device and to assist in making EL speech as natural and comprehensible as possible. Specific EL training targets should target segmental, suprasegmental, and nonverbal aspects of communication unique to EL speech production. In particular, this means capitalizing on redundant phonetic cues that aid in perception of EL speech; attending to available options for dynamic pitch modulation; and heightening awareness of nonverbal communicative cues. Clinical attention to factors such as these will boost communicative success for EL users.

References

Al-Zanoon, N., Parsa, V., Lin, X., & Doyle, P.C. (2017, November). Using visual feedback to enhance intonation control of electrolarynx speakers. Paper presented at the Annual Convention of the American Speech-Language-Hearing Association, Los Angeles, CA.

Baken, R., & Orlikoff, R. (2000). *Clinical measurement of speech and voice* (2nd ed.). San Diego, CA: Singular Pub. Group.

Barney, H. L. (1958). A discussion of some technical aspects of speech aids for post-laryngectomized patients. *The Annals of Otology, Rhinology, and Laryngology, 67*(2), 558–570.

Bennett, S., & Weinberg, B. (1973). Acceptability ratings of normal, esophageal, and artificial larynx speech. *Journal of Speech and Hearing Research, 16,* 608–615.

Bien, S., Rinaldo, A., Silver, C. E., Fagan, J., Pratt, L., Tarnowska, C., … Ferlito, A. (2008). History of voice rehabilitation following laryngectomy. *The Laryngoscope, 118*(3), 453–458. https://doi.org/10.1097/MLG.0b013e31815db4a2

Blom, E. C. (2000). Current status of voice restoration following total laryngectomy...including commentary by Shah, J.P. *Oncology (08909091), 14*(6), 915–931.

Brown, D. H., Hilgers, F. J. M., Irish, J. C., & Balm, A. J. M. (2003). Postlaryngectomy voice rehabilitation: State of the art at the millennium. *World Journal of Surgery, 27*(7), 824–831. https://doi.org/10.1007/s00268-003-7107-4

Bunton, K., Kent, R. D., Kent, J. F., & Duffy, J. R. (2001). The effects of flattening fundamental frequency contours on sentence intelligibility in speakers with dysarthria. *Clinical Linguistics & Phonetics, 15*(3), 181–193.

Cox, S. R. (2016). *The application of clear speech in electrolaryngeal speakers* (Dissertation). The University of Western Ontario, London, Ontario.

Cox, S. R., Theurer, J., Spaulding, S., & Doyle, P. C. (2015). The multidimensional impact of total laryngectomy on women. *Journal of Communication Disorders, 56,* 59–75. https://doi.org/10.1016/j.jcomdis.2015.06.008

Doyle, P. C. (1994). *Foundations of voice and speech rehabilitation following laryngeal cancer*. San Diego, CA: Singular Pub. Group.

Doyle, P. C. (2005). Clinical procedures for training use of the electronic artificial larynx. In *Contemporary considerations in the treatment and rehabilitation of head and neck Cancer* (pp. 545–570). Austin, TX: Pro-Ed.

Doyle, P. C. (2008). Conveyance of emotion in postlaryngectomy communication. In K. Izdebski (Ed.), *Emotions in the Human Voice, Volume II: Clinical Evidence* (Vol. 2, pp. 49–67). San Diego, CA: Plural Publishing.

Doyle, P. C. (2012). Seeking to better understand factors that influence postlaryngectomy speech rehabilitation. *Perspectives on Voice and Voice Disorders, 22*(1), 45–51. https://doi.org/10.1044/vvd22.1.45

Doyle, P. C., & Eadie, T. L. (2005). The perceptual nature of alaryngeal voice and speech. In *Contemporary considerations in the treatment and rehabilitation of head and neck cancer: Voice, speech, and swallowing* (pp. 113–140). Austin, TX: Pro-Ed.

Eadie, T. L., & Doyle, P. C. (2002). Direct magnitude estimation and interval scaling of naturalness and severity in tracheoesophageal (TE) speakers. *Journal of Speech, Language, and Hearing Research, 45*(6), 1088–1096. https://doi.org/10.1044/1092-4388(2002/087

Eadie, T. L., & Doyle, P. C. (2005). Scaling of voice pleasantness and acceptability in tracheoesophageal speakers. *Journal of Voice, 19*(3), 373–383. https://doi.org/S0892-1997(04)00071-2 [pii]. https://doi.org/10.1016/j.jvoice.2004.04.004

Eadie, T. L., Otero, D., Cox, S., Johnson, J., Baylor, C. R., Yorkston, K. M., & Doyle, P. C. (2016). The relationship between communicative participation and postlaryngectomy speech outcomes. *Head & Neck, 38*(Suppl 1), E1955–E1961. https://doi.org/10.1002/hed.24353

Espy-Wilson, C. Y., Chari, V. R., MacAuslan, J. M., Huang, C. B., & Walsh, M. J. (1998). Enhancement of electrolaryngeal speech by adaptive filtering. *Journal of Speech, Language & Hearing Research, 41*(6), 1253–1264.

Gandour, J., & Weinberg, B. (1983). Perception of intonational contrasts in alaryngeal speech. *Journal of Speech and Hearing Research, 26,* 142–148.

Gandour, J., & Weinberg, B. (1984). Production of intonation and contrastive stress in electrolaryngeal speech. *Journal of Speech and Hearing Research, 27,* 605–612.

Gandour, J., Weinberg, B., & Garzione, B. (1983). Perception of lexical stress in alaryngeal speech. *Journal of Speech and Hearing Research, 26,* 418–424.

Gelfer, M. P., & Bennett, Q. E. (2013). Speaking fundamental frequency and vowel formant frequencies: effects on perception of gender. *Journal of Voice, 27*(5), 556–566. https://doi.org/10.1016/j.jvoice.2012.11.008.

Globlek, D., Štajner-Katušić, S., Mušura, M., Horga, D., & Liker, M. (2004). Comparison of alaryngeal voice and speech. *Logopedics Phoniatrics Vocology, 29*(2), 87–91.

Goy, H., Fernandes, D. N., Pichora-Fuller, M. K., & van Lieshout, P. (2013). Normative voice data for younger and older adults. *Journal of Voice: Official Journal of the Voice Foundation, 27*(5), 545–555. https://doi.org/10.1016/j.jvoice.2013.03.002

Graham, M. S. (2006). Strategies for excelling with alaryngeal speech methods. *SIG 3 Perspectives on Voice and Voice Disorders, 16*(2), 25–32. https://doi.org/10.1044/vvd16.2.25

Guo, L., Nagle, K. F., & Heaton, J. T. (2016). Generating tonal distinctions in Mandarin Chinese using an electrolarynx with preprogrammed tone patterns. *Speech*

Communication, 78, 34–41. https://doi.org/10.1016/j. specom.2016.01.002

Heaton, J. T., Robertson, M., & Griffin, C. (2011). Development of a wireless electromyographically controlled electrolarynx voice prosthesis. In *Proceedings of the Annual International Conference of the IEEE Engineering in Medicine and Biology Society, EMBS* (pp. 5352–5355).

Hillman, R. E., Walsh, M. J., Wolf, G. T., Fisher, S. G., & Hong, W. K. (1998). Functional outcomes following treatment for advanced laryngeal cancer. Part I – voice preservation in advanced laryngeal cancer. Part II – laryngectomy rehabilitation: The state of the art in the VA system. Research speech-language pathologists. Department of Veterans Affairs Laryngeal Cancer Study Group. *Annals of Otology, Rhinology & Laryngology, Supplement, 172,* 1–27.

Koike, M., Kobayashi, N., Hirose, H., & Hara, Y. (2002). Speech rehabilitation after total laryngectomy. *Acta Oto-Laryngologica, 122*(4), 107–112. https://doi.org/10.1080/000164802760057716

Krause, J. C., & Braida, L. D. (2003). Investigating alternative forms of clear speech: The effects of speaking rate and speaking mode on intelligibility. *Journal of the Acoustical Society of America, 112*(5), 2165–2172. https://doi.org/10.1121/1.1509432

Law, I., Ma, E. P.-M., & Yiu, E. M.-L. (2009). Speech intelligibility, acceptability, and communication-related quality of life in Chinese alaryngeal speakers. *Archives of Otolaryngology - Head and Neck Surgery, 135*(7), 704–711.

Matsui, K., Kimura, K., Nakatoh, Y., & Kato, Y. (2013). Development of electrolarynx with hands-free prosody control. In *Proceedings of the 8th ISCA Speech Synthesis Workshop* (pp. 273–278). Barcelona, Spain: International Speech Communication Association.

Meltzner, G. S., & Hillman, R. E. (2005). Impact of aberrant acoustic properties on the perception of sound quality in electrolarynx speech. *Journal of Speech, Language & Hearing Research, 48*(4), 766–779.

Meltzner, G. S., Hillman, R. E., Heaton, J. T., Houston, K. M., Kobler, J. B., & Qi, Y. (2005). Electrolaryngeal speech: The state of the art and future directions for development. In *Contemporary considerations in the treatment and rehabilitation of head and neck cancer: Voice, speech, and swallowing* (pp. 571–590). Austin, TX: Pro-Ed.

Mendenhall, W. M., Morris, C. G., Stringer, S. P., Amdur, R. J., Hinerman, R. W., Villaret, D. B., & Robbins, K. T. (2002). Voice rehabilitation after total laryngectomy and postoperative radiation therapy. *Journal of Clinical Oncology, 20*(10), 2500–2505. https://doi.org/10.1200/JCO.2002.07.047

Most, T., Tobin, Y., & Mimran, R. C. (2000). Acoustic and perceptual characteristics of esophageal and tracheoesophageal speech production. *Journal of Communication Disorders, 33*(2), 165–181. https://doi.org/10.1016/S0021-9924(99)00030-1

Nagle, K., & Heaton, J. (2016). Perceived naturalness of electrolaryngeal speech produced using sEMG controlled vs. manual pitch modulation. In *Proceedings of the 17th Annual Conference of the International Speech Communication Association* (pp. 238–242). San Francisco, CA. https://doi.org/10.21437/Interspeech.2016-1476

Nagle, K. F., Eadie, T. L., Wright, D. R., & Sumida, Y. A. (2012). Effect of fundamental frequency on judgments of electrolaryngeal speech. *American Journal of Speech-Language Pathology, 21*(2), 154–166. https://doi.org/10.1044/1058-0360(2012/11-0050

Nagle, K. F., & Heaton, J. T. (2017). Comparison of thumb-pressure vs. electromyographic modes of frequency modulation for electrolaryngeal speech. Poster presented at the 173rd Meeting of the Acoustical Society of America, Boston.

Nakamura, K., Toda, T., Saruwatari, H., & Shikano, K. (2012). Speaking-aid systems using GMM-based voice conversion for electrolaryngeal speech. *Speech Communication, 54,* 134–146. https://doi.org/10.1016/j.specom.2011.07.007

Nelson, I., Parkin, J. L., & Potter, J. F. (1975). The modified Tokyo larynx: An improved pneumatic speech aid. *Archives of Otolaryngology, 101*(2), 107–108. https://doi.org/10.1001/archotol.1975.00780310029008

Pepiot, E. (2014). Male and female speech: A study of mean f0, f0 range, phonation type and speech rate in Parisian French and American English speakers. In *Speech Prosody 2014* (pp. 305–309). Dublin, Ireland. https://doi.org/<halshs-00999332>

Peterson, G. E., & Lehiste, I. (1960). Duration of syllable nuclei in English. *J Acoust Soc Am, 32,* 693–703. https://doi.org/10.1121/1.1908183

Pindzola, R., & Cain, B. (1988). Acceptability ratings of tracheoesophageal speech. *Laryngoscope, 98*(4), 394–397.

Qi, Y. Y., & Weinberg, B. (1991). Low-frequency energy deficit in electrolaryngeal speech. *Journal of Speech & Hearing Research, 34*(6), 1250–1256.

Robbins, J., Fisher, H. B., Blom, E. C., & Singer, M. I. (1984). Acoustic differentiation of laryngeal, esophageal, and tracheoesophageal speech. *Journal of Speech & Hearing Research, 27*(4), 577–585.

Searl, J. (2006). Technological advances in alaryngeal speech rehabilitation. *SIG 3 Perspectives on Voice and Voice Disorders, 16*(July), 12–18. https://doi.org/10.1044/vvd16.2.12

Singer, M. I., & Blom, E. D. (1980). An endoscopic technique for restoration of voice after laryngectomy. *Annals of Otology, Rhinology & Laryngology, 89*(6), 529–533. https://doi.org/10.1177/000348948008900608

Singer, S., Wollbrück, D., Dietz, A., Schock, J., Pabst, F., Vogel, H.-J., … Meuret, S. (2013). Speech rehabilitation during the first year after total laryngectomy. *Head & Neck, 35*(11), 1583–1590. https://doi.org/10.1002/hed.23183

Smiljanić, R., & Bradlow, A. R. (2009). Speaking and hearing clearly: Talker and listener factors in speaking style changes. *Language and*

Linguistics Compass, 3(1), 236–264. https://doi.org/10.1111/j.1749-818X.2008.00112.x

Smithwick, L., Davis, P., Dancer, J., Hicks, G., & Montague, J. (2002). Female laryngectomees' satisfaction with communication methods and speech-language pathology services. *Perceptual and Motor Skills, 94*(1), 204–206.

Štajner-Katušić, S., Horga, D., Mušura, M., & Globlek, D. (2006). Voice and speech after laryngectomy. *Clinical Linguistics & Phonetics, 20*(2–3), 195–203. https://doi.org/10.1080/02699200400026975

Stepp, C. E., Heaton, J. T., Rolland, R. G., & Hillman, R. E. (2009). Neck and face surface electromyography for prosthetic voice control after total laryngectomy. *IEEE Transactions on Neural Systems and Rehabilitation Engineering, 17*(2), 146–155. https://doi.org/10.1109/TNSRE.2009.2017805

Takahashi, H., Nakao, M., Kikuchi, Y., & Kaga, K. (2005). Alaryngeal speech aid using an intra-oral electrolarynx and a miniature fingertip switch. *Auris, Nasus, Larynx, 32*(2), 157–162. https://doi.org/10.1016/j.anl.2005.01.007

Wan, C., Wu, L., Wu, H., Wang, S., & Wan, M. (2012). Assessment of a method for the automatic on/off control of an electrolarynx via lip deformation. *Journal of Voice, 26*(5), 674.e21–674.e30. https://doi.org/10.1016/j.jvoice.2012.03.002

Ward, E. C., Koh, S. K., Frisby, J., & Hodge, R. (2003). Differential modes of alaryngeal communication and long-term voice outcomes following pharyngolaryngectomy and laryngectomy. *Folia Phoniatrica et Logopaedica, 55*(1), 39–49.

Watson, P. J., & Schlauch, R. S. (2008). The effect of fundamental frequency on the intelligibility of speech with flattened intonation contours. *American Journal of Speech-Language Pathology, 17*(4), 348–355. https://doi.org/1058–0360_2008_07-0048 [pii] 10.1044/1058-0360(2008/07-0048).

Watson, P. J., & Schlauch, R. S. (2009). Fundamental frequency variation with an electrolarynx improves speech understanding: A case study. *American Journal of Speech-Language Pathology, 18*(2), 162–167.

Weinberg, B., & Riekena, A. (1973). Speech produced with the Tokyo artificial larynx. *Journal of Speech and Hearing Disorders, 38*(3), 383–389.

Weiss, M. S., & Basili, A. G. (1985). Electrolaryngeal speech produced by laryngectomized subjects: Perceptual characteristics. *Journal of Speech & Hearing Research, 28*(2), 294–300.

Weiss, M. S., Yeni-Komshian, G. H., & Heinz, J. M. (1979). Acoustical and perceptual characteristics of speech produced with an electronic artificial larynx. *The Journal of the Acoustical Society of America, 65*(5), 1298–1308. https://doi.org/10.1121/1.382697

Williams, S. E., & Watson, J. B. (1987). Speaking proficiency variations according to method of alaryngeal voicing. *Laryngoscope, 97*(6), 737-739.

Wu, L., Wan, C., Wang, S., & Wan, M. (2013). Improvement of electrolaryngeal speech quality using a supraglottal voice source with compensation of vocal tract characteristics. *IEEE Transactions on Biomedical Engineering, 60*(7), 1965–1974. https://doi.org/10.1109/TBME.2013.2246789

Wu, L., Wan, C., Xiao, K., Wang, S., & Wan, M. (2014). Evaluation of a method for vowel-specific voice source control of an electrolarynx using visual information. *Speech Communication, 57*, 39–49. https://doi.org/10.1016/j.specom.2013.09.006

Yorkston, K., Strand, E., & Kennedy, M. R. T. (1996). Comprehensibility of dysarthric speech: Implications for assessment and treatment planning. *American Journal of Speech-Language Pathology, 5*(1), 55–66.

Yorkston, K. M., Hammen, V. L., Beukelman, D. R., & Traynor, C. D. (1990). The effect of rate control on the intelligibility and naturalness of dysarthric speech. *Journal of Speech and Hearing Disorders, 55*(3), 550–560. https://doi.org/10.1044/jshd.5503.550

Teaching Esophageal Speech: A Process of Collaborative Instruction

10

Philip C. Doyle and Elizabeth A. Finchem

Introduction

Esophageal speech (ES) has a long history in the postlaryngectomy literature as a method of alaryngeal voice and speech rehabilitation. When the historical literature is assessed, results on the acquisition of ES demonstrate substantially varied rates of success. It is likely not unreasonable to suggest that these variable "acquisition" data may have been influenced by multiple factors. Additionally, terminology used in association with success, such as the term "functional" ES, also suffers the same limitations in definition. Thus, the identification of what characteristics define that group of individuals who undergo laryngectomy and ultimately acquire "successful" ES is unknown.

It is, however, our belief that ES currently remains an extremely viable option for postlaryngectomy rehabilitation. In fact, we believe that ES is an increasingly viable method of rehabilitation in the current era. Consequently, the purpose

of this chapter focuses on a discussion of ES and its training. This discussion will initially address the structures necessary and the general mechanism of ES with an initial focus on the pharyngoesophageal segment. Next, a brief historical perspective on ES will be provided, but the larger premise seeks to contextualize this method of postlaryngectomy voice and speech rehabilitation in the current era. Finally, this chapter advocates for collaboration between the speech-language pathologist (SLP) and qualified lay instructors of ES (Duguay, 1980). Such collaborative teaching efforts may further enhance the acquisition and refinement of ES by those who undergo total laryngectomy.

The Anatomical Basis of ES: The Pharyngoesophageal Segment

In his excellent review on the mechanism of ES, Diedrich (1968) used the term "pharyngoesophageal" to describe the anatomical region that may be used for the generation of a postlaryngectomy voicing source. The term pharyngoesophageal segment (PES) appears to have considerable merit in that it specifies a region or zone of function. It is essential to realize that alaryngeal voice generation may be a product of multiple sources of vibration (Diedrich & Youngstrom, 1966) and that the structures involved may vary between individuals.

P. C. Doyle (✉)
Voice Production and Perception Laboratory & Laboratory for Well-Being and Quality of Life, Department of Otolaryngology – Head and Neck Surgery and School of Communication Sciences and Disorders, Western University, Elborn College, London, ON, Canada
e-mail: pdoyle@uwo.ca

E. A. Finchem
Alaryngeal Speech Instructor, Tucson, AZ, USA

© Springer Nature Switzerland AG 2019
P. C. Doyle (ed.), *Clinical Care and Rehabilitation in Head and Neck Cancer*,
https://doi.org/10.1007/978-3-030-04702-3_10

145

Negus (1929) was one of the first authors to suggest that the "pseudoglottis" in those who were laryngectomized and used ES was formed by the cricopharyngeus muscle. Ten years later, Jackson and Jackson (1939) also suggested that this muscular structure served as the vicarious voicing source in esophageal speakers. The cricopharyngeus muscle is best described as the band of muscle located in the transitional region between the lower pharynx and the upper esophagus. But, while these authors suggested that the cricopharyngeus was likely to comprise the primary structure(s) involved in esophageal voice production, they offered a caveat that it might be best to identify this generalized region to be of importance.

Several authors have suggested that the source of esophageal phonation is primarily derived through an aerodynamic response of this muscle (Damste, 1958; Levin, 1962; Robe, Moore, Andrews, & Holinger, 1956; van den Berg & Moolenaar-Bijl, 1959; Vrticka & Svoboda, 1961). While some controversy exists regarding whether or not the cricopharyngeus is a distinct muscular structure, as opposed to a structurally distinct segment of another anatomical structure (e.g., the inferior pharyngeal constrictor muscle), it is clear that muscular fibers are present in this transitional anatomical region (Zemlin, 1988, p.274). Since the reports of Negus (1929) and Jackson and Jackson (1939), the term PES gained more widespread usage in the literature on postlaryngectomy voice, and the term was popularized in the clinical literature by Diedrich and Youngstrom (1966).

The Alaryngeal Voice Source

Over the years, considerable interest has been directed toward the use of an intrinsic, postsurgical voicing source for individuals who undergo laryngectomy. The term intrinsic refers to the fact that the speaker can utilize some internal, anatomically based structure(s) for alaryngeal voice (and speech) generation. Although three intrinsic methods of postsurgical alaryngeal communication have been reported in the literature, namely,

esophageal, buccal, and pharyngeal speech, only ES meets essential requirements for speech communication (see Weinberg & Westerhouse, 1971, 1973).

Use of the esophagus as a new postlaryngectomy vibratory source can provide greater utility to the speaker when compared to the other two methods, most specifically relative to listener assessments of speech acceptability and intelligibility[1] (Bennett & Weinberg, 1973; Doyle, Danhauer, & Reed, 1988; Sleeth & Doyle, Chap. 14; Weinberg & Westerhouse, 1971, 1973). In ES, the esophagus serves as an air chamber that provides the aerodynamic driving source that will oscillate the PES. The variable nature of this new voicing source and the tissues that comprise it has been recognized over the years (Brewer, Gould, & Casper, 1975; Daou, Shultz, Remy, Chan, & Attia, 1984). Thus, a more regionally oriented terminology which included tissues of both the pharynx and esophagus emerged, and this terminology will be used in the remainder of this chapter.

Variability of the PE Segment When the PE segment is considered, it is important to understand that total laryngectomy will not only create a large surgical physical defect due to the removal of the larynx, but it will also include discontinuous tissues such as the pharyngeal constrictor muscles that must be opposed and sutured together during surgical closure. Consequently, the true esophageal sound source will be comprised of multiple muscular structures including the cricopharyngeus, upper esophagus, and lower pharynx. Care in the preservation of essential tissues, those which may serve as an intrinsic alaryngeal voicing source, has been both implied and explicitly outlined by many (Damste, 1979; Finkbeiner, 1978, p. 67; Negus, 1929). But, individual variability is a characteristic of this newly reconstructed system.

---

[1] This reflects a simple issue of air volume available in the esophagus. Access to a greater amount of air carries with it an advantage relative to speech rate which is inherent to acceptability ratings, as well as for the generation of the sounds of speech that ultimately influence intelligibility.

The literature also suggests that the vibratory segment may be found in a variety of anatomical locations (Diedrich & Youngstrom, 1966). These findings indicate that the alaryngeal voice source associated with esophageal voice and speech may vary across a variety of "internal" structural dimensions, namely, size, length, and configuration.[2] It may also vary in regard to where the primary structure exists anatomically and the anatomical structures or regions most closely associated with it. Damste and Lerman (1969) have stated that the anatomical structure and form of the pharyngoesophageal junction may vary considerably and that these differences may be accounted for by multiple variables. The most intriguing variable is that which may occur over time, with practice, and which may result in "selective activation" of the musculature associated with esophageal voice. Specifically, Damste and Lerman (1969, p. 348) state: "The fact that pharyngeal voice can be reeducated into esophageal voice is proof that individuals can learn to differentiate constriction at various levels." This observation suggests that similar to its anatomy, the physiology of the PE segment is not invariant. However, in relation to its function, concerns specific to the neural control of this mechanism cannot be disregarded.

Control of the PE Segment While the statement offered by Damste and Lerman (1969, p. 348) may in fact be true and have relevance to the ES learning process (Torgerson & Martin, 1980), it assumes that normal afferent (sensory) feedback from the structures that comprise the new alaryngeal source is available to the learner. More explicitly, this suggestion may have limited our ability to consider "control" issues in a more comprehensive manner. The neurophysiology underlying use of the esophageal reservoir as an air supply and the PES as a voice source will be altered secondary to laryngectomy. Disruptions

to either motor or sensory aspects of the system cannot be discounted as contributors to the ease of ES acquisition. Thus, potential changes in afferent feedback secondary to laryngectomy and reconstruction remain a significant factor today, and further research can provide valuable information relative to understanding the mechanism of esophageal voice (Doyle & Eadie, 2005).

Damste (1979, 1986) addressed anatomical differences to the PES that occur postsurgery; he also raised concerns related to a potential relationship of its structure to problems in acquiring esophageal voice. He specifically noted that the outcome of voice rehabilitation may hinge on both the extent of surgical reconstruction and the "wound healing" process. In relation to the extent of surgical reconstruction, Damste was quite explicit regarding the anatomical form of the pseudoglottis. He states that the vibratory segment "…can vary from wide to narrow, from long to short, and its shape can be flat, round, and prominent…" (Damste, 1979, p. 55). Thus, neurological control (both efferent and afferent) may be equally variable, a factor that may contribute to the ease (or lack thereof) of learning ES. Diedrich and Youngstrom (1966, p. 21) have also noted "tremendous individual differences" of the pseudoglottis. Interestingly, they go on to state that individual differences were not only observed between different speakers who participated in their investigation but may also have been observed in relationship to specific tasks (e.g., swallowing, phonating, blowing, etc.). This information further supports the notion that the process of learning ES may be mediated at many levels.

Damste has considered the evolving nature of the reconstructed upper aerodigestive pathway from the point of laryngectomy until healing is complete. This information should be contemplated collectively with information on the rate of acquisition for esophageal voice and speech skills (Berlin, 1963, 1964, 1965; Ryan, Gates, Cantu, & Hearne, 1982). Does the possibility exist that changes in the development and/or refinement of particular ES skills over the early postoperative period are influenced by aspects of

---

[2] This suggestion is consistent with research findings that document a range of lowered fundamental frequency levels associated with ES. Mass characteristics of the PES, in concert with the vocal tract, will influence such measures.

tissue healing (e.g., the development of scar tissue, etc.)? These questions largely remain unanswered.

The Value of Learning ES

As one method of postlaryngectomy alaryngeal communication, ES has the following advantages, it: (1) uses a natural, biological source; (2) is highly functional when mastered; (3) requires no additional surgical procedure (secondary TE puncture) or prosthesis; (4) offers much less danger of aspiration; (5) has some pitch and volume control, although at times somewhat limited; (6) can offer speech on demand when one is proficient; and (7) eliminates emergency voice loss for delayed prosthesis appointments or equipment changes, repairs, and urgent problem-solving. We believe that it is important to acknowledge the relative advantages and disadvantages of all alaryngeal methods in order to facilitate an informed choice by the individual.

One's success (or failure) in acquiring usable ES may be related to multiple factors (Salmon, 1986; Schaefer & Johns, 1982). For example, postsurgical anatomical and physiological deficits; changes in the postlaryngectomy neurological control of the new vibratory source, namely, the PES; the quality of instruction; the extensiveness of instruction; inadequate definitions of what defines success; as well as many other variables may exist. However, as is often the case with hindsight and a willingness to reconsider past data with more acuteness, the cause of the much of the reported historic failure may in fact have been due to an anatomic-physiologic-neurologic cause (Salmon, 1986). Yet, historical literature has provided considerable insights into what defines a proficient esophageal speaker (Shames, Font, & Matthews, 1963; Snidecor, 1975).

Since the mid-twentieth century, several authors have provided information on particular physical attributes of ES and voice (frequency, intensity, and speech rate) and based on those data have offered defining characteristics of a "superior" esophageal speaker (Horii &

Weinberg, 1975: Snidecor, 1978; Snidecor & Curry, 1959, 1960) and data reported by others on specific characteristics of the ES signal (Angermeier & Weinberg, 1981). Although many years have passed, these reference points do serve as a valuable basis of comparison today.[3] Berlin (1963) provided very important data on ES, a verification that offered perhaps the best picture of the trajectory specific to the initial period of ES acquisition; it also provided the first index of acquisition parameters for comparison across speakers at similar stages of speech training. These findings provide valuable guidance to the training process. This may influence decisions on what ultimately constitutes successful ES acquisition in the earliest stages of training, to that which may be observed in later, more advanced stages of speech refinement.

Although objective measures do not constitute the sole measure of ES success (see Doyle, Chap. 17; Eadie, Chap. 29; Evitts, Chap. 28), they do provide a general framework from which the clinician may infer comparative performance. Further, Weinberg and his colleagues have also offered clinicians and researchers alike a considerable body of descriptive, comparative, and experimental data related to alaryngeal speakers, including those who used ES. This body of careful and well-focused work still provides a solid framework for understanding ES in the current era. Given current advances in the treatment for laryngeal carcinoma, as well as the changes in treatment protocols (REF), further extensions specific to the acquisition of ES are recommended.

Teaching Esophageal Speech

Methods of Air Insufflation Information from the literature on ES indicates that two general classes of air insufflation for voicing purposes

---

[3]These data may be of even greater pertinence today as opportunities for learning ES may be increasing. In the intervening period since the introduction of the tracheo-esophageal (TE) puncture voice restoration procedure by Singer and Blom in 1980, the option of learning ES as an alaryngeal option decreased considerably.

Fig. 10.1 Illustration of normal anatomy (left) and postlaryngectomy anatomy (right) with a representation of changes in respiration and location of the PES used for esophageal speech. (Courtesy of Dr. Philip Doyle)

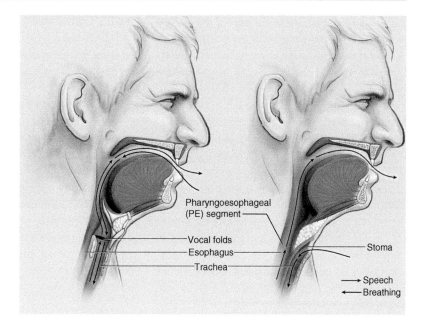

Pharyngoesophageal (PE) segment

Vocal folds
Esophagus
Trachea

Stoma

→ Speech
← Breathing

may be used. These two classes are defined by the primary physical principle that underlies the process. These processes are best classified as (1) positive pressure approaches and (2) a negative pressure approach. Regardless of which method is utilized, the speaker must effect a change in pressures between the oropharynx and the esophagus. By accomplishing this goal, natural physical laws come into play to equalize differences between these air pressures. An illustration depicting the relationship between anatomical structures pre- and postlaryngectomy is provided in Fig. 10.1.

The primary methods of positive pressure manipulations between the oropharynx and esophagus include the glossal or glossopharyngeal press (Weinberg & Bosma, 1970), stop consonant injection (Moolenaar-Bijl, 1953), and what may be best described as a "modified swallow" maneuver (Diedrich & Youngstrom, 1966) with other variations provided in the literature (c.f., Gately, 1976). To produce ES using a positive pressure approach, several prerequisite capacities must be met. Using a sequential model, the individual must be able to (1) trap and compress air in the oral cavity, (2) volitionally create an increase in air pressure above the pseudoglottal

sphincter (i.e., the PES), (3) create an increase in oral-pharyngeal pressure which is sufficient to overcome the resistance of the sphincter, (4) volitionally compress the contents of the esophageal reservoir, and (5) overcome the resistance of the PES in an outgoing manner for voice and speech production.

Negative or Passive Pressure Methods of Air Insufflation

All steps of esophageal air insufflation described in the previous section require an active process. That is, the individual needs to actively manipulate oral air in order to overcome the resistance of the PES, in order to charge the esophagus with air (Shipp, 1970). There is, however, an optional method of air insufflation that is termed the "inhalation" method. While this method also requires a volitional process, the movement of air into the esophagus results from a passive event. In order to understand this process, some additional details are necessary.

The insufflation method relies on the anatomical relationship between the trachea and the esophagus. This relationship is characterized by the esophagus sitting immediately behind the trachea. Because the posterior part of the trachea is formed by a soft tissue wall, its interplay with the anterior wall of the esophagus which it abuts is fundamental to the process of the inhalation method. Consider the following. When a rapid breath (inhalation) is taken through the tracheostoma by a laryngectomee, a negative pressure is created within the trachea. Because of this negative pressure, the posterior wall of the esophagus will be pulled forward (anterior) for a brief period of time. When the esophageal wall moves forward, there is a change in volumetric capacity within the esophagus. This increase in the size of the reservoir in turn creates a negative pressure in the esophagus below the PES. Because air pressures always seek equalization, atmospheric air pressures in the pharynx and oral cavity located above the are now relatively greater to that in the reservoir. This change in pressures will facilitate the passive movement of air from above the PES into the esophagus. Thus, the event of rapid inhalation creates a pressure change that is then passively equalized by air being "sucked" into the esophagus from above. Keep in mind that the active maneuver of taking a quick inspiration results in passive airflows in adjacent regions, namely, from the pharynx and oral cavity into the esophagus.

From an instructional perspective, positive pressure approaches are used most often in ES training. These types of maneuvers provide the learner with various levels of feedback (movement of the oral cavity, change in tongue position, etc.). However, insufflation approaches are also exploited at times by well-versed instructors of ES. During ES training, the initial and most essential goal is to move air into the esophagus. If the esophageal reservoir cannot be "charged" with air, its movement back across the PES to generate voice cannot be achieved. In the ES training vernacular, individuals who rely on positive pressure approaches to insufflation are termed "pumpers," while those that rely on the inhalation method are referred to as "suckers." It is, however, widely agreed by those who are highly experienced in ES training that the most proficient speakers use both methods, often doing so in a rather seamless fashion.

The ES Training Sequence

While the simplified sequence of speech events described previously captures the basic elements necessary to achieve esophageal sound, this sequence is not invariant. Further, aspects related to what occurs between each successive stage, particularly in respect to temporal intervals, will offer substantial benefit to the speaker and the listener alike. Rapid insufflation and expulsion of air provide the most basic element of ES fluency (Duguay, 1977, Snidecor, 1978). But it is critical to note that the above sequence of events assumes an active maneuver by the individual to increase oral-pharyngeal air pressure as an initial step. However, the sequence may change if other methods of esophageal reservoir air insufflation are used by the speaker.

Duguay (1979) has suggested that the inability to successfully acquire postlaryngectomy oral communication may be due to multiple factors. This includes anatomic, physiologic, psychologic, and sociologic factors. Ultimately, however, the inability to acquire functional ES is the result of the individual's inability to achieve several critical behaviors. Although Duguay has identified four specific factors that may impact the individual's success in acquiring ES, all center around the functional capacity and control of the PES and the esophageal reservoir. In order to learn ES, the individual must be able to (1) inject air into the reservoir, (2) maintain this injected air for at least a brief period of time, (3) eject air from the esophagus, and, finally, (4) exert some volitional control over the PES.

While some might view the four behaviors cited above as "physiologic" in nature, the combined act of moving air into and out of the esophagus is influenced by many factors. With this said, it is our opinion that the reduced rates of ES acquisition noted in the historical literature may lie more with postlaryngectomy anatomy, physiology, and associated neural control of the PE segment (Doyle, 1985; Gates et al., 1982; Gates, Ryan, Cantu, & Hearne, 1982). As a result, prediction of ES success has been challenging (Gates & Hearne, 1982). Interestingly, issues surrounding the functional capability of the PES as a postlaryngectomy voicing source gained more attention in the early 1980s, a change brought about by the introduction of the tracheoesophageal (TE) speech (Singer & Blom, 1980) and their observation of pharyngeal constrictor and cricopharyngeal spasm (Chodosh, Giancarlo, & Goldstein, 1984; Singer & Blom, 1981; Singer, Blom, & Hamaker, 1981, 1986). Of particular interest at that time was how the (tracheo)esophageal voicing source responds to air pressures and flows (Doyle & Eadie, 2005).

Evaluation and Clinical Expectations of ES

The beginning stages of ES rehabilitation must be structured in a manner for both the clinician and the learner to obtain direct feedback on performance. This feedback serves two distinct purposes. First, if a system of quantifying the learner's ability to acquire particular "base" skills for ES (or any other alaryngeal method) is utilized by the clinician, progress can be explicitly documented and provided to the learner. The ability of the ES learner to appreciate the fact that they are acquiring early skills, those essential to their long-term speech rehabilitation, can be very encouraging.

As it pertains to the acquisition of ES, a therapy program can be divided into two distinct training phases. The first provides the preliminary requirements for speech production in a reliable and consistent manner, and the second serves to refine and modify ES (Amster, 1986; and others). Details related to early tasks and objectives related to ES training are provided in Table 10.1. From a strict training perspective, the learner should be encouraged to increase the consistency of their ES production, to decrease the overall latency of voicing following insufflation (Berlin, 1963), and to achieve increasing levels of sustained voicing (typically on the order of 2.5–3.0 s in duration).

The first training phase initially focuses on the simple notion that each individual will most certainly have unique postsurgical anatomy and physiology (Shipp, 1970). The second deals with

Table 10.1 Tasks and objectives associated with initial stage of ES training

Task 1: Train air insufflation, injection, or inhalation
Objective: Successful "loading" or "charging" of esophageal reservoir
Task 2: Voice production on demand following insufflation
Objective: To achieve a level of reliability equal to 100%
Task 3: Repeated productions of voice following insufflation
Objective: Habituation of behavior
Task 4: Monitor development of detrimental behaviors during insufflation and/or sound production
Objective: Eliminate disruptive associated behaviors (grimacing, stoma blast, etc.)
Task 5: Reduce the degree of articulatory contact associated with insufflation and voice production
Objective: Facilitation of voicing control, refinement of speech production

Adapted from Weinberg (1983)

learning ES as a process. This process will likely ebb and flow as healing progresses and the individual demonstrates what he/she can and cannot do. While information in the literature suggests that acquisition patterns for those individuals who will likely learn serviceable ES may be quite rapid (Berlin, 1963, 1965), there is also information to suggest that esophageal "skills" may continue to develop over time (Palmer, 1970). But, it is also critical to note that the quality of instruction and the regularity and systematicity of training and practice comprise essential elements that may underlie the successful acquisition of ES. This must also be placed into the contemporary context where the postlaryngectomy PES may be appreciably different than it was 30 years ago.[4] For this reason, although the past data on ES acquisition are extremely important, current postlaryngectomy and reconstruction anatomy and physiology may be quite different. These differences may then provide for the increased likelihood that one can acquire ES.

---

[4]This change relates to current, proactive efforts at the time of laryngectomy surgery to optimize the reconstructed PES. This may include alterations in the method of surgical closure, myotomy, and/or neurectomy.

Table 10.2 Stages of esophageal speech development

1. Get air in; get air out
2. Produce plosive consonants, vowels, and diphthongs
3. Voice simple, useful, and monosyllabic words
4. Voice two-syllable words
(a) Initially with one air charge per syllable
(b) Terminally with both syllables on a single air charge
5. Voice simple phrases with a single air charge
6. Practice articulation and connected speech with emphasis on vowels, diphthongs, and consonants
7. Stress is achieved by changes in loudness, pitch, quality, and time
8. Use "active" conversation
9. The achievement of satisfactory rate usually results along with the mastery of the previous eight stages

Adapted from Snidecor (1978, pp. 183–193)

Snidecor (1978) suggested nine distinct stages of ES acquisition. These stages were deemed "levels of achievement rather than lessons as such" (Snidecor, 1978, p. 183). However, the elements which comprise the nine levels have direct consequences on how the ES learner progresses through therapy and what their proficiency level will be. A summary of these stages is presented in Table 10.2.

Initiating the ES Training Process

At the outset of developing an ES training program and designing its instruction, it is important to note what ES is and what it is not. More directly, ES is not gulping air and "burping" up a word. That is the way one of the authors (EAF) received instruction at the beginning of her post-laryngectomy speech therapy, an instruction that sent her down the wrong initial path of learning to use this method of alaryngeal speech. That gulping process often begins with too much air and quickly leads to an upper esophageal sphincter (sphincter used when swallowing) spasm.[5] The only potential benefit that can be derived from the "burp concept" is that it may provide the

learner with the feeling of the air pressure rising in esophagus and then timing it to say a word or two with that air. What is more important in that action is the slight tightening of the diaphragm, an action that keeps the air moving upwards through the PES instead of redirecting it into the stomach. Remember that it is called ES, not stomach speech.

Some instructors teach ES with a different approach. In fact, several very successful variations in instruction have been observed across master teachers of ES. However, the initial steps of learning ES are relatively invariant. After decades of training and the development of her own new voice by one of the authors (EAF), her experience of teaching others how to achieve ES may require approximately 8–10 weeks of training. Learning is a process, hence, the development of proficient skills that underlie ES will require a commitment of time and continuous education and practice. Recall that ES requires learning a new motor behavior, one that must sequence and manipulate multiple variables (tongue position, compression or oral, cavity, smooth control of voicing, etc.).

A Quick Review of the Three Methods of Air Intake for EES

Consonant injection This may be accomplished using any of the six stop consonants and the two affricates to send air backward in the mouth under pressure, which in turn may move past the sphincter formed by the PES and into the upper portion of the esophagus. While all of these sounds may be helpful in allowing air to be injected into the esophagus, the voiceless sounds (/p/, /t/, /k/, and /t∫/) are ideal sounds because they require the greatest oral pressures that may facilitate the movement of air into the esophagus.

Tongue (glossal) press The tongue tip is pressed just above the front teeth at the upper gum line to guide air along the roof of the mouth back into the esophagus. Tongue moves upward with lips apart or pressed together.

---

[5]The authors note that the upper esophageal sphincter (UES) is a complex structure that does include components of the PES.

Inhalation This method draws air into the esophagus as if yawning or gasping in surprise. The PES pops open breaking the vacuum (with the increasing volume of the esophagus when the common wall moves forward during inspiration creating a greater negative pressure) and draws enough air into the esophagus to say "ah." The tongue always remains down, and mouth is open. Example: opening a vacuum-packed jar and the air rushes in effortlessly.

Teaching the First Esophageal Sound

We begin ES instruction with the three basic methods of air intake: (1) consonant injection, (2) tongue press, and (3) inhalation. As noted in a prior section of this chapter, consonant injection and the tongue press are active maneuvers that require the learner go compress air in the oropha-ryngeal cavities. In contrast, "inhalation" is a passive insufflation process that occurs second-ary to active respiration; this process of changing pressures is merely a means of opening the PES (a structure that is generally believed to be con-tracted). When the inhalation maneuver occurs, movement of the common wall of the anterior esophagus and posterior trachea subsequently breaks the vacuum and allows air to passively enter the esophagus. For those who are laryngec-tomized, this is what you do when the ear, nose, and throat doctor asks you to say "ah" during an examination. You open this sphincter enough for examination of the esophagus. You should hear a little "click" sound as the wet tissue opens, and then you note that you have taken in enough air to say "ah." To further distinguish positive vs. pas-sive methods of insufflation, the tongue is always raised up in the mouth for "tongue press," and the tongue is always flattened down in the mouth for "inhalation."

As ES training progresses, instead of focusing on lengthy word lists that begin with a variety of consonants to facilitate the injection of air into the esophagus (Moolenaar-Bijl, 1953), we begin more simply with the syllable/word stimuli, such as /pi/, /ti/, and /ki/ or similar stop consonant and vowel combinations. Using these three stop con-sonants, coupled with vowels like "ee," "ay," or "ooh," provides a better balance of air moving into the esophagus with sound moving out. After a few attempts at these target syllables, it is important to take a sip or two of water. A small drink of water may moisten the oral and pharyn-geal tissue (remember that air is moving through this system and it will evaporate moisture), and it will also keep the PES relaxed enough to let the consonant air back up without a huge "burp" and rush of words, only to find out that one is "out of air." Then what?

The next step in the training process is as fol-lows. We begin again with the /p/ sound, but without pairing it with a vowel. This is done to illustrate that this sound can be felt on the fingers when held out away from the mouth about 4 to 6 inches. The production of an isolated sound /p/ will generate an airflow. Per the basic laws of physics, "for every action there is an opposite and equal reaction." The same amount of air felt on the fingers is also going backward into the esoph-agus which will then emerge as a vowel follow-ing the pressurize /p/; thus, this task will often result in the production of the syllable "pah" or the word "puh." Because /p/ requires a pressure build up prior to what is term its "release," some of the air will move across the PES and charge the esophagus. Remember that the air between your tongue and the roof of your mouth is about a tablespoon. That is plenty of air because the learner is going to use it immediately so there is room for the next tablespoon of air approximately 15 cc as one speaks simultaneously using conso-nants and releasing the air for vowels in each ES training stimulus.

Next in our sequence comes a request to pro-duce the consonant /t/; this enables the learner to position the tongue against the back of the front teeth at the gum line (the upper alveolus). A more posterior consonant, the stop /k/ is often the last sound used in early ES training because it requires a contact between the back of the tongue and the posterior region of the palate. Sometimes, this sound will introduce a lot of air into the esophagus, usually too much at first, an event which may result in a reduced outflow of air due to over-insufflation. One of the longstanding issues related to ES training relates to "what happens to extra air" in the esophagus? When excessive air fills the esophagus and cannot easily be moved out to initiate vibration of the PES, it has nowhere else to move other than into the lower esophagus. This transfer of air will not be available for ES. Rather, this air will pass across the lower esophageal sphincter and into the bowel. Thus, for those using ES, the equally longstanding assumption that the passing of gas is just "gas" is incorrect; the cause of gas in the bowel when learning ES is the result of not being able to move esophageal air across the PES. Often, this is the result of too much effort during the process of either injecting or expelling air for ES.

For several reasons, velar stops /k/ and /g/ may need to be softened or modified a bit for the right balance of air injected. Aggressive effort in moving air into the system should be avoided as it may not only be tiring to the learner, but it may introduce more global muscular force which may restrict the flow of air in and out of the system. Do you see grimacing, tension in the neck and shoulders, or a lot of struggling to manage all the excess air when they reload with air for each word … delivering a very choppy staccato way of speaking, or have they mastered speaking with a natural phrasing speech? ES is best when its production is easy and relaxed, as if speaking in the same manner that you did prior to the laryngectomy. It should be noted, however, that it is not unusual for a laryngectomee who vigorously over-articulates, often while mouthing words with the hope of being heard along with lip reading, to strike both a /k/ and /g/ with more aggressive contacts than occurs when using ES. This type of change with /k/ and /g/ is sometimes observed in those who use the electrolarynx. In either case, an excessive level of effort should be avoided during the ES learning process.

As part of the early, "first esophageal sound" training process, the learner should be relaxed and allow sound to emerge with as little effort as possible. We encourage the learner to "just let the sounds come out" like /p/ or /t/ or fricative or affricates "sh" and "j" and" ch," respectively. Because these sounds are of higher oral pressure,

they will furnish air to the esophagus, and in doing so, some words may also be produced (e.g., "pie" or "toe," or "Chuck"). As a related item, many teachers of ES have had the experience of observing the learner, or having one of them report, that they have at some point uttered a single word of profanity out loud but had no idea how they did it. Ask them what the word was without embarrassment and then explain to them why it happened. This is an excellent example of instruction in that the ES teacher can educate the learner "why" and "how" the sound could be produced. This type of report from the ES learner is an excellent example of how effortless ES can be when you're not trying so hard.

As soon as we can move onto multiple syllables, we begin working on short phrases that can be used daily. One simple task is to determine phrases that may be useful on a more regular basis during communication with others. For example, practicing the words "please" and "thank you" has wide application and is also meaningful to the learner. Rather than using extensive and potentially seldom used lists of "practice" words, we focus on using ES for simple questions and responses. Pet commands such as "sit", "stay", "come", and "down", along with the pet's name, are often highly functional, and these words can be used often each day. Family names and a few other phrases such as "car keys" and "get gas" and many others can be tailored for homework that will have value and meaning for the learner. Finally, learning the "wh" interrogatives – who, what, when, where, and why, as well as how – can keep a chat going while one uses their ES. We want these simple responses to become spontaneous. Again, as the ES learner progresses, meaningful stimuli will allow practice time to be much more productive.

In summary, other aspects of speech communication should be pointed out and encouraged. For example, it is important to be aware that expecting people to read lips is not helpful to learning ES. Doing so places burden on the listener, and it increases the chance that they will miss the intended message. Similarly, the ES speaker should encourage the listener to ask for a repetition when something is not understood. The obligation here is on the speaker to increase the likelihood that their message will be heard and understood. In this situation, one also needs to be reminded that ES is much lower in its intensity than normal speech. So, if the listener has a hearing loss (Clark, 1985), or communication takes place in situations of background noise (Horii & Weinberg, 1975), the demands of the communication process are increased substantially. The speaker and the listener must work together. Efforts to reduce the speaker's apprehension will foster better communication (Byles, Forner, & Stemple, 1985).

The ultimate goal of ES is closely tied to learning how to produce the vowel sounds that are now missing due to the loss of the normal sound generator: the voice box. We know that it is possible to learn to produce esophageal vowel sounds by injecting enough air into the esophagus and then moving it through the PES via contraction of the diaphragm and esophageal muscles; this process will serve to achieve the new source of ES. People are always surprised to learn that some proficient ES speakers do not breath when they speak. Instead they have learned to inhale, exhale, inject, and then speak. If this process is not controlled, we hear a good deal of "stoma blast" during the process of exhalation. Stoma blast may actually mask ES which makes the listener's work more difficult (Till, England, & Law-Till, 1987). As a fundamental objective when training ES, we aim for intelligibility, as well as effortless speech (see Table 10.1).

Some Additional Considerations and Caveats

Learning ES can be tiring for some, particularly early on in the training process. Instruction and expectations must also be individualized because everyone is different. It is unrealistic to expect that if Learner A acquired ES in 3 weeks, 3 months, or 3 years that you can too. One person's learning curve does not mean that is how it will go for you, because every case will be different. Individual differences are due to factors such as previous treatment such as radiation or chemoradiation therapy, the type and extent of surgery, the need for flap reconstruction, complicated recoveries, early or late side effects of treatment, and lack of qualified

instruction or support, and then there may be cost concerns – some insurance coverage for ES instruction may be quite limited (e.g., six sessions only). This limitation is of concern even though the successful acquisition of ES would likely reduce future costs associated with other alaryngeal methods (TE speech or use of the electrolarynx). However, the clear message that must be conveyed to all laryngectomees who seek to learn ES is that different patterns exist for everyone at all stages of training.

As an interesting observation, sometimes those who are learning ES but currently use an electrolarynx will demonstrate an esophageal sound while using an EL. This is the result of the movement of air during the act of speaking. Remember that ambient air is always in the oral cavity and pharynx and as EL speech is produced and sound "targets" hit, air may move into the esophagus. Clinicians should carefully listen for esophageal voice that overrides the usual EL voice in these circumstances. This phenomenon is called "double phonating." This type of voicing also may occur with some individuals when they are mouthing or whispering to communicate.

Neither mouthing or whispering is viable or useful communication methods for those who are laryngectomized, and it should be discouraged. However, during both of these behaviors, air pressures will change, and esophageal insufflation will occur. When ES voice is heard, it indicates candidacy for ES development. It should be reiterated that ES is a function of ongoing changes in air pressures within the oral, pharyngeal, and esophageal spaces. Pre-loading is not always necessary. Thus, any behavior that potentially changes pressure gradients in these regions also holds the potential for the generation of ES. While speaking with an EL, the consonants will move air into the esophagus to produce an ES word or phrase. This may be particularly noticeable in words such as "teak," "peak," "tool," or "pool."

How to know air is in there? Use a mirror for easy biofeedback; watch the air inflate the ES learner's neck in the area of your esophagus. To illustrate this to the learner, ask them to do the following. When you say "p-ah," how quickly does the "p" fill the esophagus with air? Visual cues are helpful. Similarly, instruct the learner to lightly place a finger across their neck just above the stoma to feel the esophagus inflate. Next, once the air is there, ask them to generate the ES target while placing their finger across the neck to feel when and where the vibration begins.

A balanced air supply from multiple methods of air intake will maintain sufficient air for fluent ES. This occurs as the result of frequent, rapid injections of small amounts of air by the speaker, something which in turn powers the vowel sound, allowing it to emerge and become intelligible. Too much air injected at once will be heard as a "klunk." "Double pumping," as if to prime a pump, also provides too much air. The learner who states that "I ran out of air" is usually a result of excessive air in the esophagus, subsequently causing the PES sphincter to grab tightly; some call this spasm. As noted previously, a pause to sip water and to inhale/exhale is the quickest way to off-load excess air with a "burp" or two. Finally, linking air from a final consonant of a single word to that of the next word may facilitate smoother ES. For example, as practice, begin with a target that allows for one to blend a phrase – "thank you" becomes "than-que" without injecting air between "thank" and "you."

Troubleshooting ES Careful observation by the clinician or teacher and self-awareness and acknowledgement by the ES learner are critical components of the training process. Practice often leads to hammering away at word lists with only consonant injection and no vowel sounds which leads to too much air. This will lock up the swallow sphincter (a grabbing, or spasm) and stop all voicing temporarily.

It is not always necessary to pre-load with one or more tongue presses before beginning with a consonant. This becomes an unmanageable amount of air in your esophagus. As noted, a sip of water will immediately relax the tightening and allowing the air to escape. Take time to swallow a couple of times to clear the esophagus. Lastly, speaking loudly will impair the fluency of ES. Loudness is always related to the volume and speed of airflow; if you have a reduced volume of air (the esophagus) and you expel it rapidly for increase loudness, the duration will be reduced (Blood, 1981; Isshiki, 1964; Isshiki & Snidecor, 1965; Sleeth & Doyle, Chap. 14; Shanks, 1979; Snidecor, 1978; Snidecor & Isshiki, 1965). You can use the air for volume or vowel duration, but you cannot do both at the same time.

How Much Practice Is Required?

In the beginning, ES training may be tiring to the learner as it is a physical activity that requires considerable concentration and patterning. Thus, we recommend that it is best if you plan to practice 5–10 min out of every hour until you can use ES in words and short phrases spontaneously. Always try to work in a quiet area so you can hear your first sounds; turn off extraneous or distracting noise so you can be easily heard by others if someone is present. A significant listener that knows what your ES goals are can be very helpful during practice. If you are working with a knowledgeable instructor, allow them to reinstruct and to provide feedback in real time. Both the ES learner and the ES teacher wish to achieve the same objective, but at times, providing feedback on what is not be done correctly can be very valuable. Additionally, in many situations what may be perceived as "negative" feedback early on in ES training is necessary. This type of early feedback serves as the first step in eliminating habits that will be detrimental to ES. If such a behavior continues, it will negatively influence communication and become more difficult to eliminate at a later time (Doyle, 1994). Feedback should be instructive and supportive, not punitive. Finally, tape record and date practices, and from time to time, allow the learner to listen carefully for ways to improve; recordings also provide an excellent way to hear progress which is always beneficial to the learner.

What to practice The following tasks provide excellent practice and the opportunity to observe improvements in ES: (1) use tongue press injection to say "ah" for consistency and duration; (2) interrupt the "ah" several times, or try changing the pitch of the sound up and down with "ah" on one tongue press; (3) use consonant injection with stop consonants followed by a long vowel, for example, the words pie, tea, bow, day, etc.; (4) count the number of times you can say "tie" sequentially with a goal of ten times without a misfire (each will be produced with an separate insufflation) – this is called "speech on demand"; (5) keep a record of the learner's progress; and (6). say the names of objects in the room (coffee cup, carpet, curtain, cupboard, picture, bookcase, etc.). These types of practice tasks are objective which allow for the tracking of progress, and they are easier than attempts at conversation in the beginning.

Once ES is increasingly acquired and the learner is able to exert greater control of the insufflation and speech output process, tasks may involve reading aloud (a newspaper is a good source of material because the language used is not too advanced) and/or recite rhymes from memory. When ES skills continue to improve, ask the learner to sing lyrics from songs; this type of task permits the speaker to manipulate their speech which will serve as a means for vowel duration practice. Finally, as a consistent requirement when the ES learner is working with an SLP, they should be asked to read aloud the Rainbow Passage (Fairbanks, 1960); the clinician should then monitor the pacing of the reading, the overall intelligibly, variation in pitch range and expression (Curry & Snidecor, 1961; McHenry, Reich, & Minifie, 1982) the ultimate goal. Effortless ES is the objective of this ongoing learning process.

Monitoring of progress Careful monitoring of progress can indicate whether or not a given learner is acquiring essential behaviors that form the foundation of ES development and refinement. If progress is not being made, the expert clinician can observe this directly and modify the program accordingly. However, the treatment program can be modified in two ways dependent upon the data obtained.

In the case where ES progress is slow, or more importantly when the acquisition of basic skills is not occurring, the clinician is posed with two options. The logical first step is for the clinician to assess whether or not a modification in the program (e.g., changing the air insufflation technique, modifying instructions, etc.) will result in better performance. Obviously, ES instruction essentially seeks to train the same basic introductory skills; however, the approach used may vary from teacher-to-teacher and when certain starting points are achieved, from learner-to-learner. Thus, the clinician must assess whether minor adjustments will facilitate the learner's ability to acquire a particular skill or whether large-scale changes in the program must be undertaken.

The other potential scenario that may emerge pertains to those who cannot acquire basic skills, even once modifications are undertaken and exhausted. While this outcome is unfortunate, it does at times happen. Remember that all ES learners come to training with unique histories relative to their cancer treatment and recovery and some may exhibit factors that will not allow them to progress sufficiently. The clinician should never have this occur unknowingly. That is, if simple, yet careful data are collected on a session-by-session basis, and the instruction has been of high quality, the clinician should always be able to assess how their learner is performing over the course of initial treatment. If ES progress does not occur, it will be apparent early on. In such instances, the clinician/teacher should prepare sessions to include ongoing counseling that redirects the learner to an artificial laryngeal device. However, with that said, it is our opinion that all of those who undergo laryngectomy should be exposed to and receive basic instruction regarding use of the EL in the early postlaryngectomy period.

According to Weinberg (1983), the initial emphasis of any alaryngeal voice reacquisition program should involve three goals: (1) the production of alaryngeal voice both quickly and reliably, (2) the ability to sustain the duration of alaryngeal voicing so that short phrases can be produced, and (3) the ability to sustain voicing for production of all voiced phonemes (vowels

Table 10.3 Advanced objectives associated with reacquisition and refinement of alaryngeal speech production

Goal 1: Seek to maintain voicing throughout progressively more lengthy utterances
Goal 2: Maintain levels of high intelligibility
Goal 3: Work to minimize the presence of any associated noises or behaviors that may interfere with communication
Goal 4: Seek to maintain an adequate rate of speech during productions of increasing length
Goal 5: Seek to acquire ability to signal linguistic contrasts and prosodic features of speech (e.g., lexical stress, intonation, junctures, etc.)

Adapted from Weinberg (1983)

and voiced consonants). These basic goals have clear implications for the development of proficient alaryngeal speech that can fully support functional communication purposes. The generic therapy program outlined by Weinberg (1983) also addressed several additional areas that are essential components of advancing ES skills so as to achieve proficient esophageal communication (see Table 10.3). This includes the development and refinement of skills in the areas of (1) speech rate and temporal patterning, (2) articulatory function and associated speech intelligibility, (3) the overall reduction of extraneous behaviors that may coexist with voice and speech output, and (4) the speaker's ability to realize and successfully produce prosodic and linguistic contrasts (see Evitts, Chap. 28).

In regard to the initial capacity to produce ES, extended goals require that the learner is able to exert some degree of control over both ingoing and outgoing air. That is, they must demonstrate the capacity to "load" the esophagus with air in order to supply the power source for oscillation of the PE segment (see Sleeth & Doyle, Chap. 14). As noted by Snidecor (1978), an essential goal of any esophageal voice and speech treatment program is to "get air in" and then to "get air out." If insufflation of the esophageal reservoir cannot be done efficiently, the individual is unlikely to be able to meet the general goal pertaining to rapid production of esophageal voice. A major component of goals provided by Weinberg (1983) focus on the efficient generation and maintenance of esophageal voicing at a variety of levels (single

sounds through short phrases). Therefore, the ultimate success in acquiring ES rests with the learner's ability to carefully manipulate air in the system in order to facilitate esophageal insufflation, followed by controlled airflow for speech production (Connor, Hamlet, & Joyce, 1985).

Advanced Esophageal Voice and Speech Training

The refinement of esophageal voice and further developing ES proficiency is a long-term process. The continued use of ES will in many cases serve to improve the individual's ability to make such changes. However, the primary influence upon one's ability to acquire advanced skill centers on what has occurred early on in the rehabilitative process. Inappropriate behaviors, or those that interfere with communication (e.g., stoma noise, facial grimaces, etc.), must be identified and reduced or eliminated before they become habitual (Shanks, 1986; Weinberg, 1983). Thus, the SLP must be vigilant in identifying such negative behaviors.

Numerous approaches to the development of advanced ES skills have been provided previously in the literature (Amster, 1986; Doyle, 1994; Gardner, 1971; Lauder, 1989; Martin, 1986; Snidecor, 1978; and others). The current authors encourage both SLPs and lay teachers who will work collaboratively on ES training to consult these sources as they provide a rich and important resource to the ES teaching process. The recommendations by such authors may appear to differ somewhat in the general composition of tasks; however, they do share one specific component. Regardless of the materials or tasks employed, all programs follow an organized, systematic approach to training. Treatment is structured so that learners can acquire skills that are progressively more challenging.

The skills to be developed in the intermediate or advanced stages of ES training are seen to cross many discrete areas of performance. Yet overall assessment of how proficient the speaker has become must also be evaluated in a combined manner. That is, specific dimensions of speech performance and proficiency may be objectively assessed to determine changes that occur over time. For example, acoustic and temporal attributes, intelligibility, etc. can be monitored on a regular basis (Hoops & Noll, 1969). This focus on discrete elements of ES should not replace global judgments of performance as this is what the nonprofessional listener will encounter. However, the identification of problem areas will serve to direct the clinician toward establishing more advanced methods of training to remediate the perceived deficit.

Conclusions

ES as a method of postlaryngectomy alaryngeal speech has been recognized for decades in the laryngectomy rehabilitation literature. Currently, it is our belief that ES remains an excellent voice and speech option for postlaryngectomy rehabilitation. In fact, we believe that ES is an increasingly viable method of rehabilitation in the current era of postlaryngectomy speech rehabilitation. This chapter has provided a discussion of the anatomical basis for and physiologic mechanism of ES. Detailed aspects related to a structured and highly systematic approach to the training of ES, from point of first sound production to more advanced training, have been outlined. Finally, this chapter has sought to provide support and advocacy for continued collaboration between the SLP and qualified lay instructors of ES; this type of collaboration is viewed to be critical component of comprehensive postlaryngectomy rehabilitation programs. Consequently, voice and speech rehabilitation efforts that involve collaborative teaching may further enhance the opportunity for the acquisition and refinement of ES by those who have undergone total laryngectomy.

Authors' Note Elizabeth Finchem underwent a total laryngectomy at the Mayo Clinic, Rochester, MN, on October 2, 1978. She has been listed in the IAL Directory of Alaryngeal Speech Instructors since 1984. In 2009, Elizabeth began teaching ES via Skype to laryngectomees from many countries. Since that time, there has been a steadily increasing interest in ES, enough to start a support group focused on ES only. On January 19, 2019 Esophageal Speech Support was launched on FB; as of June 2018, the group has 554 members. https://www.facebook.com/groups/elizabethfinchem/

References

Amster, W. W. (1986). Advanced stage of teaching alaryngeal speech. In R. L. Keith & F. L. Darley (Eds.), *Laryngectomee rehabilitation* (pp. 177–192). San Diego: College-Hill Press.

Angermeier, C. B., & Weinberg, B. (1981). Some aspects of fundamental frequency control by esophageal speakers. *Journal of Speech and Hearing Research, 46,* 85–91.

Bennett, S., & Weinberg, B. (1973). Acceptability ratings of normal, esophageal, and artificial larynx speech. *Journal of Speech and Hearing Research, 16,* 608–615.

Berlin, C. I. (1963). Clinical measurement of esophageal speech: I. Methodology and curves of skill acquisition. *Journal of Speech and Hearing Disorders, 28,* 42–51.

Berlin, C. I. (1964). Hearing loss, palatal function, and other factors in post-laryngectomy rehabilitation. *Journal of Chronic Diseases, 17,* 677–684.

Berlin, C. I. (1965). Clinical measurement of esophageal speech: III. Performance of non-biased groups. *Journal of Speech and Hearing Disorders, 30,* 174–183.

Blood, G. W. (1981). The interaction of amplitude and phonetic quality in esophageal speech. *Journal of Speech and Hearing Research, 24,* 308–312.

Brewer, D. W., Gould, L. V., & Casper, J. (1975). Fiberoptic video study of the post-laryngectomized voice. *The Laryngoscope, 85*(4), 666–670.

Byles, P. L., Forner, L. L., & Stemple, J. C. (1985). Communication apprehension in esophageal and tracheoesophageal speakers. *Journal of Speech and Hearing Disorders, 50,* 114–119.

Chodosh, P. L., Giancarlo, H. R., & Goldstein, J. (1984). Pharyngeal myotomy for vocal rehabilitation postlaryngectomy. *Laryngoscope, 94,* 52–57.

Clark, J. G. (1985). Alaryngeal speech intelligibility and the older listener. *Journal of Speech and Hearing Disorders, 50,* 60–65.

Connor, N. P., Hamlet, S. L., & Joyce, J. C. (1985). Acoustic and physiologic correlates of the voicing distinction in esophageal speech. *Journal of Speech and Hearing Disorders, 50,* 378–384.

Curry, E. T., & Snidecor, J. C. (1961). Physical measurement and pitch perception in esophageal speech. *Laryngoscope, 71,* 415–424.

Damste, P. H. (1958). *Oesophageal speech after laryngectomy.* Groningen, Netherlands: Boedrukkefif Voorheen Grbroeders Hoitsema.

Damste, P. H. (1979). Some obstacles in learning esophageal speech. In R. L. Keith & F. L. Darley (Eds.), *Laryngectomee rehabilitation* (pp. 49–61). San Diego: College-Hill Press.

Damste, P. H. (1986). Some obstacles to learning esoph-ageal speech. In R. L. Keith & F. L. Darley (Eds.), *Laryngectomee rehabilitation* (2nd ed., pp. 85–92). San Diego: College-Hill Press.

Damste, P. H., & Lerman, J. W. (1969). Configuration of the neoglottis: An x-ray study. *Folia Phoniatrica, 21*, 347–358.

Daou, R. A., Shultz, J. R., Remy, H., Chan, N. T., & Attia, E. L. (1984). Laryngectomee study: Clinical and radio-logic correlates of esophageal voice. *Otolaryngology - Head and Neck Surgery, 92*, 628–634.

Diedrich, W. M. (1968). The mechanism of esophageal speech. *Annals of the New York Academy of Sciences, 155*, 303–317.

Diedrich, W. M., & Youngstrom, K. A. (1966). *Alaryngeal speech.* Springfield, IL: Charles C. Thomas.

Doyle, P. C. (1985). Another perspective on esophageal insufflation testing. *Journal of Speech and Hearing Disorders, 50*, 408–409.

Doyle, P. C. (1994). *Foundations of voice and speech rehabilitation following laryngeal cancer.* San Diego, CA: Singular Publishing Group.

Doyle, P. C., & Eadie, T. L. (2005). The pharyngo-esophageal segment as an alaryngeal voicing source: A review and reconsideration. In P. C. Doyle & R. L. Keith (Eds.), *Rehabilitation following treatment for head and neck cancer: Voice, speech, and swallowing.* Austin, TX: Pro-Ed Publishers.

Doyle, P. C., Danhauer, J. L., & Reed, C. G. (1988). Listeners' perceptions of consonants produced by esophageal and tracheoesophageal talkers. *Journal of Speech and Hearing Disorders, 53*, 400–407.

Duguay, M. J. (1977). Esophageal speech. In M. Cooper & M. H. Cooper (Eds.), *Approaches to vocal reha-bilitation* (pp. 346–381). Springfield, IL: Charles C. Thomas.

Duguay, M. (1979). Special problems of the alaryn-geal speaker. In R. L. Keith & F. L. Darley (Eds.), *Laryngectomee rehabilitation* (pp. 423–444). San Diego, CA: College-Hill Press.

Duguay, M. J. (1980). The speech-language pathologist and the laryngectomized lay teacher in alaryngeal speech rehabilitation. *ASHA, 22*, 965–966.

Fairbanks, G. (1960). *Voice and articulation drillbook.* New York: Harper & Row.

Finkbeiner, E. R. (1978). Surgery and speech, the pseudo-glottis and respiration in total standard laryngectomee. In J. C. Snidecor (Ed.), *Speech rehabilitation of the laryngectomized* (pp. 58–85). Springfield, IL: Charles C. Thomas.

Gardner, W. H. (1971). *Laryngectomee speech and reha-bilitation.* Springfield, IL: Charles C. Thomas.

Gately, G. (1976). Another technique for teaching the lar-yngectomized person to inject air for the production of esophageal tone. *Journal of Speech and Hearing Disorders, 42*, 311.

Gates, G. A., & Hearne, E. M. (1982). Predicting esoph-ageal speech. *Annals of Otology, Rhinology and Laryngology, 3*, 454–457.

Gates, G. A., Ryan, W., Cantu, E., & Hearne, E. (1982). Current status of laryngectomee rehabili-tation: II. Causes of failure. *American Journal of Otolaryngology, 3*, 8–14.

Gates, G. A., Ryan, W., Cooper, J. C., Jr., Lawlis, G. F., Cantu, E., Lauder, E., … Hearne, E. (1982). Current status of laryngectomee rehabilitation: I. Results of therapy. *American Journal of Otolaryngology, 3*(1), 1–7.

Hoops, H. R., & Noll, J. D. (1969). Relationship of selected acoustic variables to judgments of esopha-geal speech. *Journal of Communication Disorders, 2*, 1–13.

Horii, Y., & Weinberg, B. (1975). Intelligibility character-istics of superior esophageal speech presented under various levels of masking noise. *Journal of Speech and Hearing Research, 18*, 413–419.

Isshiki, N. (1964). Regulatory mechanism of voice intensity variation. *Journal of Speech and Hearing Research, 7*, 17–29.

Isshiki, N., & Snidecor, J. C. (1965). Air intake and usage in esophageal speech. *Acta Oto-Laryngologica, 59*, 559–574.

Jackson, C., & Jackson, C. L. (1939). *Cancer of the lar-ynx.* Philadelphia, PA: W.B. Saunders.

Lauder, E. (1989). *Self-help for the laryngectomee.* San Antonio, TX: Lauder Publishing.

Levin, N. M. (1962). *Voice and speech disorders: Medical aspects.* Springfield, IL: Charles C. Thomas.

Martin, D. E. (1986). Pre-and post-op anatomical and physiological observations in laryngectomy. In R. L. Keith & F. L. Darley (Eds.), *Laryngectomy rehabilita-tion* (2nd ed., pp. 221–225). California: College-Hill Press.

McHenry, M., Reich, A., & Minifie, F. (1982). Acoustical characteristics of intended syllabic stress in excellent esophageal speakers. *Journal of Speech and Hearing Research, 25*, 554–564.

Moolenaar-Bijl, A. (1953). Connection between conso-nant articulation and the intake of air in oesophageal speech. *Folia Phoniatrica, 5*, 212–216.

Palmer, J. M. (1970). Clinical expectations in esophageal speech. *Journal of Speech and Hearing Disorders, 35*, 160–169.

Robe, E. Y., Moore, P., Andrews, A. H., Jr., & Holinger, P. H. (1956). A study of the role of certain factors in the development of speech after laryngectomy: 1. Type of operation; 2. Site of pseudoglottis; 3. Coordination of speech with respiration. *The Laryngoscope, 66*(5), 481–499.

Ryan, W., Gates, G. W., Cantu, E., & Hearne, E. (1982). Current status of laryngectomee rehabilitation: III. Understanding esophageal speech. *American Journal of Otolaryngology, 3*, 91–96.

Salmon, S. J. (1986). Factors that may interfere with acquiring esophageal speech. In R. L. Keith & F. L. Darley (Eds.), *Laryngectomy rehabilitation* (2nd ed., pp. 357–363). San Diego, CA: College-Hill Press.

Schaefer, S., & Johns, D. F. (1982). Attaining function esophageal speech. *Archives of Otolaryngology, 108,* 647–650.

Shames, G. H., Font, J., & Matthews, J. (1963). Factors related to speech proficiency of the laryngectomized. *Journal of Speech and Hearing Disorders, 28,* 273–287.

Shanks, J. C. (1979). Essentials for alaryngeal speech: Psychology and physiology. In R. L. Keith & F. L. Darley (Eds.), *Laryngectomee rehabilitation* (pp. 469–489). San Diego, CA: College-Hill.

Shanks, J. C. (1986). Development of the feminine voice and refinement of esophageal voice. In R. L. Keith & F. L. Darley (Eds.), *Laryngectomy rehabilitation, 2nd* (pp. 269–276). San Diego, CA: College-Hill Press.

Shipp, T. (1970). EMG of pharygoesophageal musculature during alaryngeal voice production. *Journal of Speech and Hearing Research, 13,* 184–192.

Singer, M. I., & Blom, E. D. (1980). An endoscopic technique for restoration of voice after laryngectomy. *Annals of Otology, Rhinology and Laryngology, 89,* 529–533.

Singer, M. I., & Blom, E. D. (1981). Selective myotomy for voice restoration after total laryngectomy. *Archives of Otolaryngology, 107,* 670–673.

Singer, M. I., Blom, E. D., & Hamaker, R. C. (1981). Further experience with voice restoration after total laryngectomy. *Annals of Otology, Rhinology and Laryngology, 90*(5), 498–502.

Singer, M. I., Blom, E. D., & Hamaker, R. C. (1986). Pharyngeal plexus neurectomy for alaryngeal speech rehabilitation. *Laryngoscope, 96*(1), 50–54.

Snidecor, J. C. (1975). Some scientific foundations for voice restoration. *Laryngoscope, 85,* 640–648.

Snidecor, J. C. (1978). *Speech rehabilitation and the laryngectomized* (2nd ed.). Springfield, IL: Charles C. Thomas.

Snidecor, J. C., & Curry, E. T. (1959). Temporal and pitch aspects of superior esophageal speech. *Annals of Otology, Rhinology and Laryngology, 68,* 1–14.

Snidecor, J. C., & Curry, E. T. (1960). How effectively can the laryngectomee expect to speak? *Laryngoscope, 70,* 62–67.

Snidecor, J. C., & Isshiki, N. (1965). Air volume and air flow relationships of six esophageal speakers. *Journal of Speech and Hearing Disorders, 30,* 205–216.

Till, J. A., England, K. E., & Law-Till, C. B. (1987). Effects of auditory feedback and phonetic context on stomal noise in laryngectomized speakers. *Journal of Speech and Hearing Disorders, 52,* 243–250.

Torgerson, J. K., & Martin, D. E. (1980). Acoustic and temporal analysis of esophageal speech produced by alaryngeal and laryngeal talkers. *Folia Phoniatrica et Logopaedica, 32*(4), 315–322.

van den Berg, J., & Moolenaar-Bijl, A. J. (1959). Cricopharyngeal sphincter, pitch, intensity, and fluency in esophageal speech. *Practical Otorhinolaryngology, 21,* 298–315.

Vrticka, K., & Svoboda, M. (1961). A clinical and x-ray study of 100 laryngectomized speakers. *Folia Phoniatrica, 13,* 174–186.

Weinberg, B. (1983). Voice and speech restoration following total laryngectomy. In W. H. Perkins (Ed.), *Voice disorders* (pp. 109–125). New York: Thieme-Stratton.

Weinberg, B., & Bosma, J. F. (1970). Similarities between glossopharyngeal breathing and injection methods of air intake for esophageal speech. *Journal of Speech and Hearing Disorders, 35,* 25–32.

Weinberg, B., & Westerhouse, J. (1971). A study of buccal speech. *Journal of Speech and Hearing Research, 14,* 652–658.

Weinberg, B., & Westerhouse, J. (1973). A study of pharyngeal speech. *Journal of Speech and Hearing Disorders, 38,* 111–118.

Zemlin, W. R. (1988). *Speech and hearing science: Anatomy and physiology* (2nd ed.). Englewood Cliffs, NJ: Prentice Hall.

Voice Restoration with the Tracheoesophageal Voice Prosthesis: The Current State of the Art

11

Donna J. Graville, Andrew D. Palmer, and Rachel K. Bolognone

Introduction

Tracheoesophageal (TE) puncture voice restoration method has been shown to be a viable and effective method of speech rehabilitation after laryngectomy since the introduction of the Blom-Singer TE voice prosthesis. Drs. Mark Singer and Eric Blom (1980) were the first to describe and operationalize a method for surgically creating a midline puncture between the trachea and esophagus into which a small, one-way silicone valve could be placed to keep the puncture patent and allow for voicing while at the same time preventing aspiration. The small surgically created tract between the trachea and the esophagus is known as a *tracheoesophageal puncture*, while the one-way valve is referred to as a *tracheoesophageal voice prosthesis.*[1] Subsequent studies by the developers demonstrated that the surgical techniques and equipment that they pioneered could be consistently and effectively used as a method of postlaryngectomy voice restoration (Blom, Singer, & Hamaker, 1986; Singer, 1983; Singer, Blom, & Hamaker, 1981; Singer, Blom, Hamaker, & Yoshida, 1989). More importantly, these techniques were then replicated at other facilities, demonstrating the reliability of this technique (Johns & Cantrell, 1981; Lavertu et al., 1989; McConnel & Duck, 1986; Stiernberg, Bailey, Calhoun, & Perez, 1987; Westmore, Johns, & Baker, 1981; Wood, Rusnov, Tucker, & Levine, 1981).

TE voice production occurs when pulmonary air is redirected via the voice prosthesis (VP) into the esophagus, putting the musculature of the pharyngoesophageal segment into vibration. Once in vibration, this air is resonated by the vocal tract and

---

[1]A note on terminology: Some authors prefer to use the abbreviation TEP or TEF to refer to the tracheoesophageal puncture or fistula tract and use the abbreviation VP to refer to the voice prosthesis. Commonly, however, the term TEP is also used to refer to the voice prosthesis, and this is true of the research literature, as well as clinical and commercial parlance. There can also be confusion between a surgically created and intentional "fistula" and one which occurs spontaneously and delays recovery. For clarity, therefore, we have used the term "VP" to refer to the voice prosthesis throughout this chapter. We have used "TE puncture" to refer to the surgically created tract in which the TEP sits and the term "fistula" is used only to refer to a wound breakdown resulting in an unwanted opening in the tissues of the head or neck.

D. J. Graville (✉) · A. D. Palmer · R. K. Bolognone
Northwest Center for Voice and Swallowing,
Department of Otolaryngology – Head & Neck
Surgery, Oregon Health and Science University,
Portland, OR, USA
e-mail: graville@ohsu.edu

© Springer Nature Switzerland AG 2019
P. C. Doyle (ed.), *Clinical Care and Rehabilitation in Head and Neck Cancer*,
https://doi.org/10.1007/978-3-030-04702-3_11

Fig. 11.1 The tracheoesophageal voice prosthesis. (Image courtesy of InHealth Technologies©)

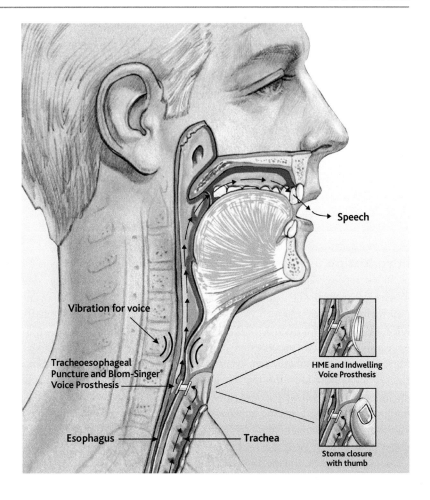

shaped into speech by the articulators. Respiration is unchanged as the individual continues to breathe through the tracheostoma in the neck, but, when the tracheostoma is occluded, the air is redirected through the VP into the cervical esophagus. The purpose of the TE puncture, therefore, is to partially undo one of the major anatomic changes of a total laryngectomy, namely, the total separation of the airway from the aerodigestive tract, by reestablishing a pathway for pulmonary air to reach the vocal tract (see Searl, Chap. 13).

The purpose of the VP itself is twofold: first, to prevent the newly created surgical puncture from closing, and, second, to prevent the aspiration of foods and liquids from the esophagus into the trachea. There are a variety of VP devices, all of which have a one-way valving mechanism. The valve is designed to easily open, allowing air to flow from the trachea into the esophagus when the stoma is occluded, in order to enable speech.

Additionally, when swallowing, the one-way valve should remain closed to prevent aspiration (Fig. 11.1). The VP can be placed at the time of the patient's initial total laryngectomy surgery (*primary placement*) or at a later date once healing from the laryngectomy surgery is complete (*secondary placement*). VP devices come in two different styles, one of which is patient-maintained (a *non-indwelling* or *patient-maintained device*) and one of which must be placed by an otolaryngologist or speech-language pathologist (SLP) with specialty training (an *indwelling device*).

TE Puncture Surgery

As originally described by Singer and his colleagues, it is technically feasible to create a primary TE puncture at the time of total laryngectomy as long as the surgeon is attentive to a number of key surgical considerations, including (a) the creation of the tracheostoma and the TE puncture itself, (b) the performance of a pharyngeal constrictor myotomy or pharyngeal plexus neurectomy, and (c) the nature of the surgical closure (Hamaker, Singer, Blom, & Daniels, 1985; Yoshida, Hamaker, Singer, Blom, & Charles, 1989). Attention to all of these elements will increase the likelihood of successful voice restoration. The creation of an adequately sized tracheostoma is fundamentally important. The tracheostoma must be large enough for the patient to be able to breathe adequately and minimize the risk of tracheostomal stenosis, but not so large or irregularly shaped that the tracheostoma cannot be easily occluded for voicing (Blom, 1995). Further, the anatomical placement of the TE puncture within the trachea is critical. The puncture must be placed in a location that can be easily visualized and accessed for routine care, management, and the insertion and replacement of the VP.

It is also important to address the *pharyngoesophageal (PE) segment* surgically in order to reduce the tonicity of the musculature in this area to facilitate successful voice rehabilitation (Singer & Blom, 1981; Singer, Blom, & Hamaker, 1986). The "PE segment" is a descriptive term used to refer to the musculature at the level of the cervical spine from C4 to C7, comprising the inferior pharyngeal constrictor, the cricopharyngeus, and the upper esophageal segment. Collectively these muscles form the vibratory sound source for TE speech (Blom, Singer, & Hamaker, 1985). With regard to the nature of the closure, it is important

to close the pharyngeal defect in three layers to decrease the risk of a postoperative wound healing problems such as a *pharyngocutaneous fistula,* namely, a wound breakdown resulting in an opening between the pharynx and the external neck. Should this occur, a pharyngocutaneous fistula may result in delayed resumption of an oral diet and the inability to initiate voicing trials with the VP and may require additional surgery for closure (see Damrose & Doyle, Chap. 3).

Prevalence of TE Speech Usage

Although TE voice restoration has gained ground as a method of alaryngeal voice rehabilitation, it is not universally available. In one of the most comprehensive studies published to date, the rehabilitation of 166 individuals receiving rehabilitation after laryngectomy was described for patients treated at multiple Veterans Affairs hospitals in the United States (Hillman, Walsh, Wolf, Fisher, & Hong, 1998). As can be seen in Fig. 11.2, rates of TE speech use rose steadily, while rates of electrolarynx use declined over the period of the study, but by 24 months postoperatively, only 31% of the participants had become TE speakers. These statistics highlight the fact that although many medical facilities are able to perform a total laryngectomy, not all patients are appropriate candidates for TE speech rehabilitation. Surveys of laryngectomy support group members in North America have reported rates of TE speech use ranging from 17% to 55% (Palmer, Childes,

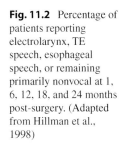

Fig. 11.2 Percentage of patients reporting electrolarynx, TE speech, esophageal speech, or remaining primarily nonvocal at 1, 6, 12, 18, and 24 months post-surgery. (Adapted from Hillman et al., 1998)

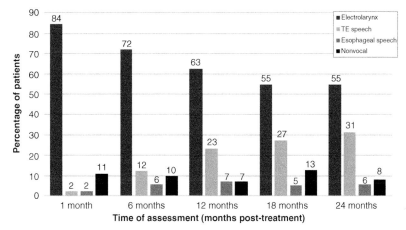

Fried-Oken, & Graville, 2016; Palmer & Graham, 2004). In contrast, while some recent studies have reported that 89% of patients who undergo total laryngectomy will receive a TE puncture (Moon et al., 2014), statistics from multisite studies in Europe as well as specialty medical centers in North America report lower TE puncture rates of around 60% (Gitomer et al., 2016; Singer et al., 2013). Thus, discrepancies exist regarding the frequency of TE puncture and its long term use by those who undergo total laryngectomy.

The Importance of Access to Specialty Care

A number of nonsurgical factors may be the strongest predictors of long-term TE success. These factors include appropriate patient education, the availability of knowledgeable clinicians for management, and access to healthcare resources for ongoing care. Although many studies from centers with specialty expertise have reported success rates of 90% or more (Graville, Gross, Andersen, Everts, & Cohen, 1999; Izdebski, Reed, Ross, & Hilsinger, 1994; Kao, Mohr, Kimmel, Getch, & Silverman, 1994; Op de Coul et al., 2000; Singer et al., 1981; Wood et al., 1981), several studies have demonstrated that in those who receive a TE puncture, success is far from assured. In some studies, the percentage of patients who continue to use the VP long term has been reported to be considerably lower, ranging from 58% to 85% (Gitomer et al., 2016; Lavertu et al., 1996; Moon et al., 2014; Singer et al., 2013). The importance of knowledgeable care was underscored by one study of Australian patients in which only 26% were successfully using their VP a year after it was placed (Frowen & Perry, 2001). These authors emphasized a number of key factors for successful long-term rehabilitation, including (a) the importance of specialty centers of expertise for TE speech rehabilitation, (b) a team approach between surgeons and speech pathologists with specialty training, and (c) the need for ongoing follow-up for the management of complications (Messing, Ward & Lazarus, Chap. 6). For individuals in the United States, the relative roles and responsibilities of the

surgeon and SLP are outlined in a position statement by the American Speech-Language-Hearing Association (American Speech-Language-Hearing Association, 2004a) which states:

> Ideally, the surgeon and the SLP work as a team when a TE prosthesis is used, beginning with the preoperative patient selection and assessment of the capacity for the patient to generate fluent voicing via the pharyngoesophageal segment. It is primarily the responsibility of the SLP to participate in the selection and fitting of the TE prosthesis, to teach the care and use of the TE prosthesis, and to identify and facilitate resolution of problems related to sound generation, the effective use of the prosthesis for speaking, and the TE puncture site. The SLP is also primarily responsible for evaluating and training the patient to use a tracheostomal valve for hands-free speech.

More detailed information about the procedures involved and knowledge and skills required for appropriate management are available (American Speech-Language-Hearing Association, 2004b, 2004c), and similar types of policy statements are available for clinicians in other countries as well (e.g., Royal College of Speech and Language Therapists, 2010; Speech Pathology Australia, 2013). Internationally there are issues relating to the availability of training resources for safe and knowledgeable management of TE speakers (Beaudin, Godes, Gowan, & Minuk, 2003; Bradley, Counter, Hurren, & Cocks, 2013; Hancock et al., 2017; Melvin, Frank, & Robinson, 2001).

TE Voice Restoration in the "Organ Preservation" Era

The importance of specialty expertise has become all the more important in recent years due to a significant change in the nature of the laryngectomy population. Following the development of TE voice restoration as one method of alaryngeal speech, there was a fundamental change in the nature of the laryngectomy population. After landmark studies by the Veterans Affairs Laryngeal Study Group demonstrated that radiation and chemotherapy could treat laryngeal cancer as effectively as surgery with radiation, the treatment algorithm for individuals with advanced laryngeal cancer shifted dramatically (Forastiere et al., 2003; Wolf et al., 1991). With the advent of "organ preservation" protocols as a primary treatment method, total laryngectomy has become a procedure that tends to be reserved for those with more advanced cancer, persistent or recurrent disease, and those with a "dysfunctional larynx" after chemoradiation (Holsinger, Funk, Roberts, & Diaz, 2006; Theunissen et al., 2012). As a result, there has been a decline in the number of laryngectomy surgeries performed. Maddox and Davies (2012) reported that the number of total laryngectomies performed in the United States decreased by almost half between 1997 and 2008 and that surgery was performed more often in large medical centers or teaching hospitals, with an increased length of postsurgical stay and fewer patients discharged directly home. Owen and Paleri (2013) reported similar findings in a survey of national trends in the United Kingdom. Despite a reduction in the number of surgeries, total laryngectomy was more frequently performed after failed chemoradiation. Surgical voice restoration continued to be the most common method of communication rehabilitation (76%), but centralized delivery of head and neck cancer and SLP services in the United Kingdom were identified as barriers to the timely provision of knowledgeable care for TE speakers. In addition, in the United States, reduced reimbursement and coverage by Medicare for VP devices has increased patient out-of-pocket costs and reduced the availability of TE services for many patients nationwide (Kaufman & Searl, 2014).

Compared to those who undergo primary total laryngectomy, those who experience cancer recurrence and undergo total laryngectomy after previously receiving radiation or chemoradiation, a procedure referred to as *salvage laryngectomy*, tend to have higher rates of complications, delayed recovery, and poorer long-term functional outcomes (Agrawal & Goldenberg, 2008; Hasan et al., 2017; Weber et al., 2003). Because of the difficulty of performing such an extensive surgery in tissue that has been previously irradi-

ated, more complex surgical techniques may be required to avoid wound breakdown (Hanasono, Lin, Wax, & Rosenthal, 2012). Postoperative complications are more common as a result and may delay both speech and swallowing rehabilitation (Ganly et al., 2005; Weber et al., 2003).

Salvage laryngectomy and a previous history of radiation are not necessarily a contraindication to TE speech, as it has been reported that as many as 77% of individuals can be successful VP users (Sandulache et al., 2016). However, individuals who undergo more extensive surgery at the time of their salvage laryngectomy may be poorer candidates for a TE puncture, as well as being at greater risk for more negative long-term communication and associated problems (Hutcheson, Lewin, Sturgis, & Risser, 2012; Starmer et al., 2009; Ward, Koh, Frisby, & Hodge, 2003). Following the development of the first generation of indwelling VP devices in appropriately selected patients, complications were typically managed relatively easily, and the average device lifetime of the VP was typically 3–6 months (Graville et al., 1999; Leder & Erskine, 1997; Op de Coul et al., 2000). It has recently been estimated that the average VP life for most TE speakers is now significantly less than that reported historically, and, in the salvage laryngectomy era, it appears that patients should now be counseled that the indwelling VP may need to be replaced as frequently as every 2 to 3 months (Lewin, Baumgart, Barrow, & Hutcheson, 2017).

Advantages and Disadvantages of Tracheoesophageal Speech

As a result of the factors described previously, it is more important than ever that judgments about who is an appropriate candidate for a VP should be conducted by experienced healthcare professionals. Implications of the TE puncture should include a full discussion of all of the potential risks and benefits to allow for informed decision-making, with particular attention to the long-term costs, need for follow-up, and likelihood of success (Abemayor, 2017). In comparison to the two other methods of alaryngeal communication

Table 11.1 Advantages and disadvantages of tracheo-esophageal speech

Advantages	Disadvantages
1. Uses patient's own pulmonary air supply	1. May require an additional small surgery for secondary TE puncture
2. More natural voice and speech characteristics compared to other methods (e.g., longer phrase length, increased speech rate, pitch and loudness, and improved prosody)	2. Requires the use of one hand for voicing or the use of a tracheostoma attachment in order to be hands-free
3. Proficiency may be achieved more quickly and easily compared to other methods	3. Daily care and maintenance of VP
	4. Potential lifelong cost of VP replacement and other devices
	5. May require lifelong access to clinic for routine VP care or management of complications
4. High success rate in carefully chosen patients	6. Risk for aspiration of foods, liquids, secretions, and/or the VP itself

Adapted from Graham (1997)

(i.e., esophageal speech and use of an electrolarynx), there are a number of relative advantages and disadvantages associated with TE speech (Table 11.1). The advantages include the potential for a more natural quality of speech, particularly in respect to speech rate, as well as the relative ease of skill acquisition and proficiency for the VP user, compared to the artificial larynx or esophageal speech. The disadvantages relate to issues of caring for the VP itself and the need for periodic replacement and the associated costs. After thorough consideration of both the advantages and disadvantages of TE speech, the SLP, surgeon, or patient may decide that this method of alaryngeal communication is not suitable and thus may choose to explore other speech rehabilitation options. As such, assessing candidacy is an essential part of clinical care.

Determining Candidacy for Tracheoesophageal Puncture Voice Restoration

When deciding if a patient is an appropriate candidate for a VP, it is important to consider a number of important factors that may influence success (Table 11.2). The patient must demonstrate appropriate cognition to understand and

Table 11.2 TE selection criteria when assessing patient for primary or secondary TE puncture

Characteristic	Primary TE puncture	Secondary TE puncture
Pt wishes to have TE puncture based on personal motivation and not external pressure from others (e.g., family, medical team, and other patients) and understands long-term implications	✓	✓
Pt is aware of the need for ongoing follow-up for replacement (for indwelling) or training and management in case of difficulties (for non-indwelling), has adequate transportation to return for follow-up as needed, and has insurance coverage/finances to cover cost of care	✓	✓
Pt has adequate cognition to follow instructions for use and care	✓	✓
Pt has adequate vision and manual dexterity for care and cleaning of the tracheostoma and VP and manual occlusion of the tracheostoma for voicing	✓	✓
Pt has adequate pulmonary support for TE speech production	✓	✓
Stoma of adequate size (at least ½″ or 12.5 mm in diameter)		✓
Tolerating an oral diet without significant difficulty (stricture, if present, is amenable to dilation)		✓
GERD and/or esophageal dysmotility, if present, is well managed. Pt compliant with medical and/or behavioral management, as appropriate		✓
No evidence of active cancer/recurrence or other medical conditions which would interfere with ongoing use		✓
Successful self-insufflation test. If voice not achieved or only achieved with lidocaine block, prepare for possible necessity of management of CP hypertonicity, if needed		✓

Adapted from Bosone (1986); Graham (1997)

learn the skills critical for care of the tracheostoma and VP (Bosone, 1986). Visual acuity and manual dexterity are also important for daily VP maintenance and for manual occlusion of the stoma for voicing. Negative factors include visual impairment, arthritis, and neuropathy of the hands at baseline assessment (Graham, 1997), as well as postoperative arm or hand weakness, such as can occur with spinal accessory nerve injury after neck dissection and following radial forearm free tissue transfer (Boulougouris & Doyle, Chap. 23; Salerno et al., 2002; Skoner, Bascom, Cohen, Andersen, & Wax, 2003). The patient should understand the other available alaryngeal communication options and choose to pursue TE speech only after receiving education on the relative strengths and weakness of each speech option. Given the costs associated with the devices and accessories, it is equally important to consider whether the patient has adequate medical insurance coverage and/or sufficient finances to cover the supplies, devices, and materials necessary for successful long-term laryngectomee rehabilitation. The patient must also understand that should they have an indwelling device, they must be willing and able to get to a knowledgeable clinician (typically an SLP or an otolaryngologist with appropriate expertise) for routine VP replacement in the clinic every several months (Frowen & Perry, 2001). Alternatively, if they have a non-indwelling device, they must be relatively independent with self-care after initial training, but may also require appropriate follow-up if there are any problems with the VP.

Ideally, the patient should not have significant oropharyngeal or esophageal dysphagia, poorly managed esophageal dysmotility, or significant gastroesophageal reflux (GERD). These factors have been shown to be associated with a shorter VP lifespan, granulation tissue around the TE tract, and increased risk for aspiration due to leakage through or around the VP (Cocuzza, Bonfiglio, Chiaramonte, & Serra, 2014; Gerwin, Culton, & Gerwin, 1997; Pattani, Morgan, & Nathan, 2009). Similarly, the presence of stricture or stenosis at the level of the PE segment can result in poorer voice outcomes, as well as frequent device failure (Lavertu et al., 1996). If a myotomy is not performed at the time of surgery, hypertonicity of the PE segment can result in strained, effortful voice quality or even a total inability to voice (Singer & Blom, 1980; Singer et al., 1986). Hypertonicity can be addressed by dilation, cricopharyngeal myotomy, pharyngeal plexus block or neurectomy, or more conservatively with Botox injections to the PE segment (Doyle, 1994; Hamaker & Blom, 2003; Zormeier et al., 1999). It has been shown that Botox injections as an intervention in TE voice restoration may be successful in the majority of cases (Khemani, Govender, Arora, O'Flynn, & Vaz, 2009). Lastly, the patient should have adequate pulmonary function and a tracheostoma that is adequate in size for care and maintenance of the VP (see Bohnenkamp, Chap. 7; Blom, 1995).

Assuming the patient is judged to be a suitable candidate, deciding when to perform the TE puncture is the next consideration. A primary puncture may be considered in a patient undergoing a total laryngectomy without extensive reconstruction or other negative risk factors for delayed recovery. Some surgeons prefer to decide whether to perform a primary puncture intraoperatively, once they have directly evaluated whether there is adequate tissue to close the surgical defect without risk of stenosis. Although historically there have been concerns raised about whether a primary TE puncture might increase the risk of pharyngocutaneous fistula, the majority of studies have reported that this does not appear to be the case (Cheng et al., 2006; Trudeau, Schuller, & Hall, 1988; Wenig, Levy, Mullooly, & Abramson, 1989). Primary TE puncture can be safely performed in previously irradiated patients (Cheng et al., 2006; Kao et al., 1994) and in those undergoing microvascular free flap reconstruction (see Sahovaler, Yeh, and Fung, Chap. 1; Scharpf & Esclamado, 2003; Sinclair et al., 2011). In general, however, if there are doubts about a patient's candidacy, it may be more prudent to perform a secondary TE puncture after the patient has healed postoperatively and undergone a complete postlaryngectomy work-up.

Secondary TE puncture is often preferable in patients who are perceived to be at higher risk for wound complications, such as those with significant radiation-related changes, those who will require extensive pharyngeal resection and reconstruction with free flap (e.g., total laryngopharyngectomy with circumferential flap and/or esophagectomy), and also those with significant medical comorbidities (Yeh, Sahovaler & Yoo, Chap. 2; Gitomer et al., 2016). Some research has reported higher success rates in those who have undergone primary placement (Cheng et al., 2006), a finding which may indicate that there are also some benefits to early speech rehabilitation. In those who require free flap reconstruction, however, higher long-term success rates have been found in those who undergo secondary TE puncture, perhaps because secondary placement affords more time for preoperative work-up, counseling, and shared decision-making (Gitomer et al., 2016). The advantages and disadvantages of primary and secondary placements are summarized in Table 11.3.

Preoperative work-up for a secondary TE puncture involves consideration of all candidacy characteristics described previously in this chapter. In individuals with complaints of dysphagia, radiographic evaluations can allow the clinician to better visualize the postoperative anatomy and physiology. These types of studies also allow the identification of factors that may negatively impact TE voice such as dysphagia, stricture, stenosis, esophageal dysmotility, or GERD (Arrese & Schieve, Chap. 19; Starmer, Chap. 18). Similarly, in patients with a VP who are experiencing voicing difficulties, radiographic work-up can also be used to help identify properties of the PE segment that are potentially interfering with TE phonation (Blom, 1995; McIvor, Evans, Perry, & Cheesman, 1990; van As, Op de Coul, van den Hoogen, Koopmans–van Beinum, & Hilgers, 2001).

Self-insufflation testing is a valuable part of the work-up prior to creating the TE puncture for two reasons. First, it may allow the clinician and the patient to identify how compliant the PE segment may be for voicing and potentially identify whether additional intervention is likely to be required to achieve TE voice (Lewin, Baugh, & Baker, 1987). In addition, this test may allow the patient to "hear for themselves" what the TE voice might sound like in order to judge its adequacy and acceptability. During self-insufflation testing, the clinician inserts a rubber catheter transnasally and advances the tip past the level of the PE segment (Blom et al., 1985). Using an adhesive housing, the external portion of the

Table 11.3 Advantages and disadvantages of primary and secondary TE puncture

Type	Advantages	Disadvantages
Primary	One operation	Pt may be overwhelmed while recovering from laryngectomy surgery
	Psychological benefits of early resumption of speech[1]	If VP malfunctions during radiation, it could result in treatment break
	Associated with better long-term success in those who undergo laryngectomy with primary closure[2]	Tracheostoma may be incompletely healed, swollen, or painful, which may interfere with digital occlusion
Secondary	Healing complete	Two operations
	Allows extra time for discussion of pros and cons of VP and assessment of candidacy	Delayed resumption of speech
	Pt has additional time to trial electrolarynx and/ or esophageal speech before deciding to pursue VP	
	Associated with better long-term success in those who undergo laryngectomy with free flap reconstruction[3]	

Adapted from Elmiyeh et al. (2010). Additional references: [1]Yoshida et al. (1989); [2]Cheng et al. (2006); [3]Gitomer et al. (2016)

catheter is attached to the patient's tracheostoma, and the patient is instructed to inhale (Fig. 11.3). The clinician then digitally occludes the tracheostoma prior to expiration, and the patient is asked to phonate. This method results in insufflation of the esophagus with pulmonary air and, ideally, as the air passes up through the PE segment via the catheter, vibration suitable for voicing. Absent voice; a high-pitched, strained, weak, or significantly wet vocal quality; and poor

Fig. 11.3 The insufflation test for determining TE prosthesis candidacy. (Image courtesy of InHealth Technologies©)

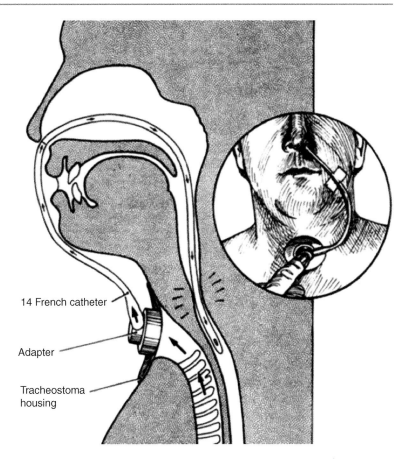

14 French catheter

Adapter

Tracheostoma housing

speech fluency would all be considered negative outcomes (Blom, 1995). Optimally, the patient should be able to sustain phonation for 10 s or more and count to 15 on a single breath without significant phonatory effort. Lewin et al. (1987) found that measurements of intraesophageal pressure could be used to predict the likelihood of successful TE speech outcomes. Fluent speakers, nonfluent speakers, and nonspeakers demonstrated low (<20 mmHg), intermediate (20–40 mmHg), and high intraesophageal pressures (>40 mmHg), respectively. Patients with intermediate and high preoperative pressures were not able to achieve fluent TE speech without a myotomy. When hypertonicity was suspected, a lidocaine block was performed during the self-insufflation test to cause temporary relaxation of the PE segment and assess the impact on voice to further assess candidacy for myotomy.

The final consideration in determining candidacy relates to selecting the optimal type of VP for each patient. As noted, there are two types of TE voice prostheses: the non-indwelling (or patient-directed) device and the indwelling (or clinician-directed) device. When first introduced by Singer and Blom (1980), the only VP available was a non-indwelling device that had to be changed independently by the patient. As a result, the candidacy criteria for TE voice restoration were much more stringent because users had to be able to manage the VP on their own. In the 1990s, the second generation of indwelling TE prostheses was developed (Hilgers & Schouwenburg, 1990). These indwelling devices were designed for extended wear without the need for replacement by the individual at home. This development allowed a wider group of patients to use TE speech successfully, since the ability to self-change was no longer required (Graville et al., 1999). As a result, visual acuity and manual dexterity play a lesser role in self-care of the indwelling VP today; the patient only needs to be able to clean the device daily with a brush or flushing device.

Indwelling VPs require periodic replacement by specially trained clinicians, so access to care remains a significant factor in determining candidacy for TE voice restoration.

Properties of TE Voice Prostheses and Insertion Methods

There are a large number of TE prostheses currently on the market. The devices are manufactured in a variety of diameters, lengths, and styles to provide the clinician with a range of options that can more specifically meet the unique needs of each patient. In choosing the best VP for a particular patient, the clinician must weigh the properties of the available devices in order to achieve the best outcome for the patient, namely, a balance between providing the optimal voice, with the easiest care, and the longest device life.

Design of the VP: Although there are many variations, there are a number of commonalities in the design of most voice prostheses (Figs. 11.4 and 11.5). Typically, the VP consists of a silicone tube with a one-way valve assembly housed within it. The tracheal and esophageal flanges act as retention collars to keep the prosthesis snugly within the TE party wall. The safety straps allow

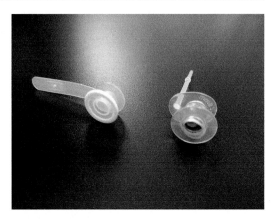

Fig. 11.5 The InHealth Classic Indwelling (left) and ATOS Medical Provox3 (right) VPs with detachable tabs, which are removed after insertion

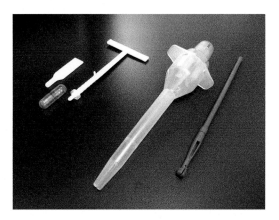

Fig. 11.6 The InHealth indwelling VP insertion system with gelatin cap placement device (left) and the ATOS Provox3 indwelling VP insertion system with loading tool (right) both of which are used to contain the esophageal flange prior to insertion

for the device to be fastened to the insertion stick and may be kept in place after insertion to allow for ease of removal of the device.

VP Placement: The VP is placed using the insertion tool and procedures outlined by the manufacturer (Fig. 11.6). Additional tools may include a sizer and dilator for use during replacement (Figs. 11.7 and 11.8). After proper sizing and dilation of the TE tract, the VP is placed within the tract using the inserter tool. Confirmation of placement is achieved via 360° rotation of the

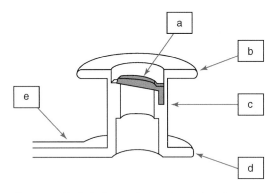

Fig. 11.4 Typical characteristics of a VP include a one-way silicone valve (a), an esophageal retention flange (b), a body that holds the valve assembly (c), a tracheal retention flange (d), and a neck strap (e) that is removed after insertion of the device. Note: letters and arrows added. (Image courtesy of InHealth Technologies©)

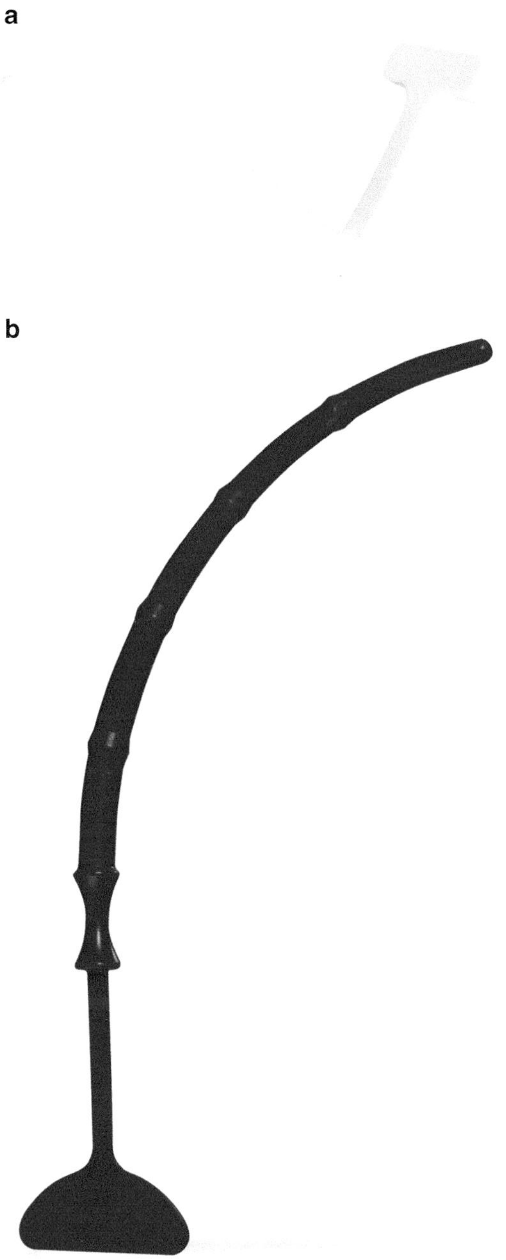

a

b

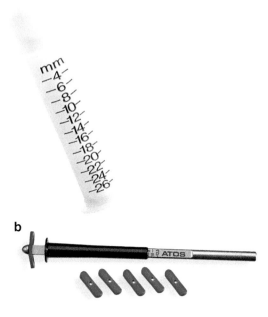

a

b

Fig. 11.8 Tracheoesophageal sizers manufactured by (**a**) InHealth and (**b**) ATOS medical for measuring the length of the TE tract during VP replacement. ((**a**) Courtesy of InHealth Technologies©, (**b**) With permission of ©Atos Medical AB and Chris Edghill)

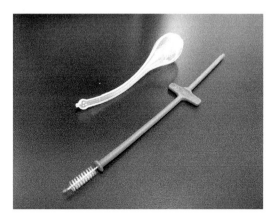

Fig. 11.9 A flushing pipette and cleaning brush, which can be used with either system to remove debris within the VP to ensure correct opening of the valve for voicing and closing of the valve to prevent aspiration

Fig. 11.7 Tracheoesophageal dilators manufactured by (**a**) InHealth and (**b**) ATOS medical for stenting the tract during VP replacement. ((**a**) Courtesy of InHealth Technologies©, (**b**) With permission of ©Atos Medical AB and Chris Edghill)

prosthesis by the clinician within the TE tract; a gentle tug on the safety strap is also performed to ensure that the esophageal flange has deployed.

After insertion, the VP is briefly cleaned with a small brush or pipette (Fig. 11.9), just as the patient is instructed to do at home, in order to (a) remove any material from the one-way valve and

(b) to make sure the one-way valve is in place (valves can be inverted during the insertion process). The clinician then typically asks the patient to perform two tasks in order to ensure that the VP is functioning correctly. First, the patient's voice is first evaluated to make sure it has returned to baseline. Second, the patient is then given 2–4 oz. of water or a colored liquid to drink while the clinician carefully observes the VP with a flashlight. Should normal voicing not be achieved or should leakage through or around the VP occur, the clinician must ascertain why the device is not functioning properly. It is possible that the valve of the VP is inverted, the VP is not in place, or the VP is incorrectly sized for the TE tract. If cleaning the VP in place does not resolve the issue, the SLP will typically remove the VP and attempt to assess the reason for malfunction. The SLP may then attempt reinsertion of the VP after appropriate dilation and sizing of the TE tract, obtain confirmation of VP placement endoscopically or radiographically, and perform additional troubleshooting as required.

Stoma Buttons, Laryngectomy Tubes, Heat and Moisture Exchangers, and Hands-Free Speech

The respiratory symptoms experienced by patients after laryngectomy can have a profoundly negative influence on daily life (Natvig, 1984). Daily sputum production is one of the most frequent postop-

erative complaints, as is coughing and the need for frequent stoma cleaning (Hilgers, Ackerstaff, Aaronson, Schouwenburg, & Zandwijk, 1990). The consistent use of a *heat-and-moisture exchanger* (HME) has been shown to have a positive impact with regard to both physical and psychosocial complaints (Lewis, Chap. 8). An HME is a device that reduces the amount of moisture and heat lost by the lungs during expiration and filters the air during inspiration. With such a device, it appears possible to reduce the amount of excess moisture lost due to stoma breathing by approximately 60% (Myer, 1987). The benefits of consistent use include better respiratory function, improved sleep, and enhanced psychological well-being (Ackerstaff, Hilgers, Balm, Aaronson, & van Zandwuk, 1993).

In TE speakers, the use of an HME has also been shown to have a number of benefits with regard to voicing. Benefits reported include improved self-perceived vocal quality, easier digital occlusion of the stoma, longer maximum phonation time, and increased dynamic range (Hilgers, Ackerstaff, Balm, & Gregor, 1996; van As, Hilgers, Koopmans-Van Beinum, & Ackerstaff, 1998; Searl, Chap. 13). The HME can be worn with a peristomal adhesive housing that is replaced daily or with an intraluminal device such as a laryngectomy tube or a laryngectomy button (Figs. 11.10 and 11.11). The advantages to intraluminal devices (such as a Barton-Mayo Button or LaryButton) are that they can be used to prevent stomal stenosis and, if the patient has a

Fig. 11.10 Examples of a laryngectomy buttons (**a**) and a laryngectomy tubes (**b**) which can be used to stent the tracheostoma to prevent stenosis and can also be used to contain an HME filter cassette. (With permission of ©Atos Medical AB and Chris Edghill)

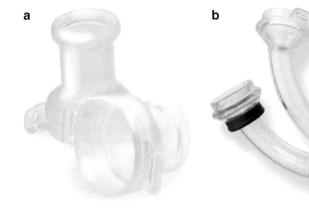

360° circumferential lip around the stoma, can be used to achieve an airtight seal for voicing without the need for an adhesive housing. Given the cost of adhesive housings, this can result in a significant cost saving to patients long term. In some institutions, customization of these devices by a prosthodontist has been used for the successful rehabilitation of TE speakers using a hands-free tracheostoma valve (Lewin et al., 2000; Lewin, Montgomery, Hutcheson, & Chambers, 2009).

Hands-Free Speech: TE speech typically utilizes one hand for voicing; however, a hands-free tracheostoma valve eliminates the need to seal the tracheostoma digitally (Fig. 11.12). The hands-free tracheostoma valve is typically attached externally with an adhesive housing and also contains an HME filter within it for pulmonary rehabilitation. To voice, the patient must exhale more forcefully than during normal respiration. The quick change in pulmonary pressure engages the hands-free tracheostoma valve, causing it to close and redirect the air through the VP. It was estimated at one time that only 30% of TE speakers were daily long-term users of the hands-free tracheostoma valves due, primarily, to difficulty attaching the valve to the peristomal skin (Doyle, Grantmyre, & Myers, 1989; van den Hoogen, Meeuwis, Oudes, Janssen, & Manni, 1996). Other factors limiting the use of these valves include increased resistance during breathing, inadvertent closure of the valve during physical exertion, an inconvenient cough-relief mechanism, and the amount of maintenance required for daily use. Poor pulmonary function and excessive mucous production can interfere and prevent successful use of a hands-free valve (Bohnenkamp, Chap. 7; Bosone, 1986; Gilmore, 1994). The newer generation of hands-free devices was developed to address some of these issues (Hilgers, Ackerstaff, van As, et al., 2003; Lorenz, Groll, Ackerstaff, Hilgers, & Maier, 2007). TE speakers with a weak vocal quality, however, may find that they are able to achieve stronger voice using digital pressure with an HME cassette (Lewis, Chap. 8; Op de Coul et al., 2005).

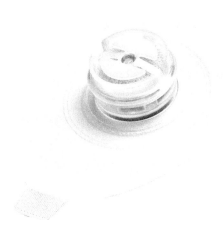
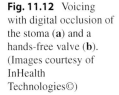

Fig. 11.11 An HME cassette with an adhesive housing. (Image courtesy of InHealth Technologies©)

Fig. 11.12 Voicing with digital occlusion of the stoma (**a**) and a hands-free valve (**b**). (Images courtesy of InHealth Technologies©)

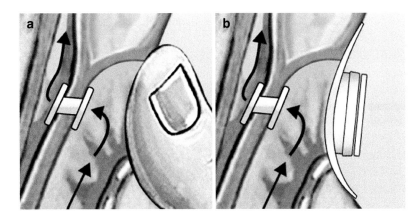

Rehabilitation
of the Tracheoesophageal Speaker

Once oral intake is established and tissue healing is complete, voice rehabilitation can typically begin. Some surgeons may use a catheter intraoperatively when the TE tract is created, while others may place a VP at the time of surgery. If a catheter is in place or if the VP fits poorly or is nonfunctional, a new VP of the appropriate diameter and length may need to be placed at the first visit (Blom, 1995). The patient is then taught proper digital occlusion techniques. The coordination of breath, tracheostoma occlusion, and voicing can be difficult to master initially. Frequent modeling and clinical practice with tracheostoma occlusion techniques are often helpful. In addition to voice rehabilitation, the patient must also be trained in self-care of the VP.

For an indwelling VP, the patient must be taught how to clean the VP in place using a specially designed flushing pipette or brush (see Fig. 11.9). Precautions for accidental extrusion of the VP and signs that the VP needs to be reevaluated (such as change in voice quality, change in the appearance of the TE tract, or leakage while drinking) should be reviewed extensively, and emergency procedures should be given in written form (Casper & Colton, 1998). For a non-indwelling device, self-change procedures will need to be taught. Initially, frequent follow-ups with the patient and continued home practice are critical for successful rehabilitation. It is not uncommon for the patient to need the VP downsized after the initial placement and the tract should be resized during subsequent replacements as there can be changes in the length of the TE tract over time (Jiang, Kearney, & Damrose, 2016). Placement of a VP of the appropriate length is always important for proper function. If the VP is too long, it should be downsized to decrease irritation due to pistoning of the VP within the TE tract and also to prevent leakage around the VP. If the VP is too short, frequent leakage, loss of voice, and potentially closure of the TE tract and extrusion of the VP can occur (Blom, 1995); thus, appropriate prosthesis length must be ensured.

Graham (1997) has described a hierarchical approach to the teaching of TE speech. She describes five target behaviors that are essential to proficiency, namely, valving, articulation, rate, phrasing, and attention to nonverbal behaviors. With regard to the first of these behaviors, valving refers to the ability to achieve an airtight seal at the level of the tracheostoma in order to redirect pulmonary air from the trachea through the VP into the esophagus. Valving can be achieved either digitally using manual occlusion of the tracheostoma or with an external hands-free tracheostoma valve; sometimes, a mirror may be useful for practice. For individuals with an overlarge or irregularly shaped tracheostoma, the use of an HME with an adhesive housing or a laryngectomy button or tube may facilitate occlusion, as well as be beneficial for pulmonary rehabilitation (Ackerstaff et al., 1993; Hilgers, Aaronson, Schouwenburg, & Zandwijk, 1991). Care must be taken to not occlude the tracheostoma too forcefully in order to facilitate easy voicing.

Articulation refers to the appropriate shaping of the vibration from the TE voice into intelligible speech. Initially, the individual may need to "overarticulate" (i.e., use greater precision than normal) in order to compensate for differences in voice quality, as with the other methods of alaryngeal speech (Hyman, 1986). If necessary, dentition and hearing may need to be addressed in order to facilitate speech production. Again, as with other methods of alaryngeal speech, there is no voiced/voiceless contrast between consonants which can produce perceptual confusions between cognates such as plosives, fricatives, and affricates (Doyle, Danhauer, & Reed, 1988). TE speakers seem to demonstrate a "voicing advantage" with fewer voiced-voiceless perceptual errors than esophageal speakers, perhaps due to the availability of a larger pulmonary air supply for emphasizing these distinctions (Doyle et al., 1988). In therapy, intelligibility can be improved by practicing voiced-voiceless distinctions through drill with cognate pairs and also shaping an approximation for the glottal fricative /h/ (Graham, 1997). Finally, a wet vocal quality is another common problem, and thus, dry swallowing several times before speaking may be beneficial.

Phrasing refers to the ability to produce natural prosody and break sentences into shorter, meaningful units in order to improve intelligibility. Some individuals produce extended run-on sentences before taking a breath, resulting in inadequate loudness and shortness of breath. Others produce single words at a time on each breath, resulting in staccato, effortful, and unnatural speech. During therapy, more natural rate and improved intelligibility can be achieved by encouraging speakers to use phrasal breaks while speaking which may also reduce the amount of vocal effort required for speaking (Doyle, 1994).

Speech rate is directly related to phrasing. The rate of TE speech is slower than that of laryngeal speakers, but faster than that of esophageal speakers due to the easier method of "recharging" the PE segment with air (Pindzola & Cain, 1989; Robbins, Fisher, Blom, & Singer, 1984). In one comparison of laryngeal, esophageal, and TE speech, the values obtained for TE speech were closer to laryngeal speech for all measures collected (Robbins et al., 1984), and these data are provided in Table 11.4. In general, values of 128–192 words per minute

(wpm) have been reported for TE speech during oral reading tasks which are comparable to rates of 150–196 wpm for laryngeal speakers (Hillman et al., 1998; Pindzola & Cain, 1989; Robbins et al., 1984). The optimal speech rate is difficult to define and is typically a combination of individual factors including adequate articulation and phrasing, together with regional and personality characteristics, in order to maximize intelligibility and naturalness (Graham, 1997).

Finally, attention to nonverbal behaviors must be undertaken. It is important to address extraneous factors that hinder the ease and naturalness of the speaker, such as facial grimaces, excessive tension, failure to make eye contact, and other appropriate pragmatic behaviors (Amster, 1986). Failure to pay attention to nonverbal behaviors may cause the speaker to be perceived more negatively by naïve listeners (Hartman & Scott, 1974).

Measuring TE Speech Outcomes

As shown in Table 11.4, compared to esophageal speech, TE speech is closer to laryngeal speech with regard to measures of pitch, loudness, and speech rate. This finding is consistent across studies (Doyle & Eadie, 2005). It is also commonly reported that the quality and intelligibility of TE speech evolves over time. Singer et al. (2013) described their findings from a multicenter, prospective cohort study of 225 individuals who used a variety of alaryngeal speech methods. Both objective and subjective speech intelligibility improved between 6 months and 1 year after laryngectomy, with TE speakers demonstrating significantly better intelligibility outcomes at both time points. There do appear to be differences in outcomes by gender, however, with male TE speakers perceived as having more natural and pleasant voices by naïve listeners than females (Eadie & Doyle, 2004).

With regard to tracking patient outcomes, a number of published scales have been used (Hurren & Miller, 2017; see Eadie, Chap. 29). Published dysphonia scales have been used with TE speakers, including the Voice Handicap Index (Jacobson et al., 1997) and Voice-Related Quality of Life

Table 11.4 Acoustic characteristics of laryngeal, tracheoesophageal, and esophageal speech for sustained phonation and reading tasks

	Laryngeal speech	TE speech	Esophageal speech
Sustained phonation			
F_0 (Hz)	103.4 (±23.7)	82.8 (±42.8)	65.3 (±30.5)
Jitter (Hz)	0.1 (±0.1)	0.7 (±0.6)	4.1 (±5.2)
Intensity (dB)	76.9 (±4.8)	88.1 (±3.9)	73.8 (±5.0)
Shimmer (dB)	0.3 (±0.1)	0.8 (±0.5)	1.9 (±0.7)
Maximum phonation time (s)	21.8 (±9.1)	12.2 (±5.2)	1.9 (±0.7)
Paragraph reading task			
Intensity (dB)	69.3 (±2.9)	79.4 (±2.1)	59.3 (±4.8)
Words per minute	172.8 (±23.3)	127.5 (±21.1)	99.1 (±24.8)
Total duration (s)	34.0 (±7.0)	47.3 (±7.9)	62.5 (14.0)
Total pause time (s)	6.3 (±3.8)	11.6 (±4.0)	22.9 (±8.6)

Adapted from Robbins et al. (1984)

Note: All values are mean (± standard deviation)

(Hogikyan & Sethuraman, 1999) survey, as have general head and neck cancer-related instruments such as the *University of Washington Quality of Life* scale (Hassan & Weymuller, 1993), the *Performance Status Scale for Head and Neck Cancer* (List, Ritter-Sterr, & Lansky, 1990), and the *University of Michigan Head and Neck Quality of Life* instrument (Terrell et al., 1997). Two measures specifically for VP users have also been published, and, although they have not gained widespread use, they provide good examples of the types of characteristics that can be used to track outcomes. For non-indwelling VP users, the *Harrison-Robillard Shultz Tracheoesophageal Puncture Rating Scale* (Shultz & Harrison, 1992) is a clinician-rated instrument for three parameters of successful TE speech relating to (a) use, i.e., the frequency of use of TE speech; (b) quality, i.e., the ease of production and intelligibility of TE speech as determined by fluency and the ability to occlude the tracheostoma; and (c) care, i.e., the patient's ability to independently maintain the

device with regard to insertion, cleaning, ordering supplies, and seeking help when appropriate. The *Patient Satisfaction Questionnaire* (PSQ) developed by Silverman and Black (1994) is a 15-item survey designed to measure patient perception and satisfaction with TE speech. Part A relates to emotional response to laryngectomy, level of verbal communication, listener reactions, and comparison to other speech methods. Part B covers four dimensions of TE voice production and how disturbing or acceptable they are to the speaker.

VP Troubleshooting, Device Selection, and Management of Complications

For the most part, complications that occur with the VP can be easily managed, if they are identified and addressed early (Table 11.5). The reasons typically attributed to the need for a

Table 11.5 Long-term tracheoesophageal prosthesis problems and solutions

Problem	Cause	Solution
Leakage through VP	1. Valve deterioration	1. Replace VP
	2. Biofilm deposits on or in valve mechanism	2. Replace VP, begin antifungal protocol
	3. Pooling of liquid or food at or above prosthesis	3. Alternate liquids and solids, avoid talking while eating, and consider esophageal dilation
Leakage around VP	1. VP too long, resulting in piston-like action	1. Downsize VP so that anterior and posterior flanges are flush to party wall
	2. TE tract larger in diameter than VP	2. Change VP type (different style or larger diameter) or use large esophageal flange (LEF) or Xtra Flange
Granulation tissue formation	1. Irritation caused by VP that is too short	1. Upsize VP so that anterior and posterior flanges are flush to party wall
	2. Irritation caused by VP that is too long	2. Downsize VP so that anterior and posterior flanges are flush to party wall
Immediate post-fitting aphonia	1. VP valve stuck closed	1. Use cleaning brush to release valve
	2. Excessive pressure during tracheostoma occlusion	2. Light finger pressure over tracheostoma
	3. Cricopharyngeal spasm	3. Assess "open tract" voicing without VP in place, insufflation under fluoroscopy, pharyngeal plexus nerve block with lidocaine to assess candidacy for Botox or cricopharyngeal myotomy
Delayed post-fitting aphonia	1. VP valve stuck closed	1. Use cleaning brush to release valve and/or remove debris
	2. Posterior end of tract closing because of inadequate VP length	2. Resize TE tract and insert appropriately sized VP and confirm placement via nasoendoscopy
	3. Failure to fully insert VP	3. Resize TE tract and reinsert VP and confirm placement via nasoendoscopy

Adapted from Blom (1995); Graville et al. (1999)

prosthesis change are leakage through the voice prosthesis, leakage around it, and poor or absent voice quality. Management often merely involves changing the TEP to a more suitable length, size, or style. If biofilm buildup on the valve is a problem and the cause of frequent VP replacement, daily use of an antifungal agent may improve VP life (Izdebski, Ross, & Lee, 1987; Mahieu, van Saene, den Besten, & van Saene, 1986) or the use of a specialty VP manufactured of biofilm-resistant material (Hilgers, Ackerstaff, Balm, et al., 2003; Leder, Acton, Kmiecik, Ganz, & Blom, 2005). It is critical to note, however, that delays in care and management of initially simple difficulties can create more serious complications including aspiration pneumonia, VP extrusion, closure of the TE tract, airway compromise, and even death due to aspiration and subsequent pneumonia. A wide range of medical problems have been associated with the failure to develop successful TE speech including pharyngocutaneous fistula, stomal stenosis, persistent aspiration, false tract creation, stricture, and PE spasm (Hillman, Walsh, & Heaton, 2005). Patient- and VP-related characteristics associated with poorer outcomes include lack of motivation, problems with VP size/fit, and problems with self-care/maintenance (Hillman et al., 2005; Singer et al., 2013).

A number of complications deserve special consideration. The most common long-term complications associated with TE speech are (1) early failure of the VP requiring frequent replacement and (2) problems with the size of the TE tract, which include frequent granulation tissue (causing displacement of the VP), as well as enlargement of the TE tract causing leakage around VP and extrusion. These problems can be interrelated and sometimes share a common cause, such as esophageal stricture, stenosis, dysmotility, GERD, cricopharyngeal spasm, and the health of the TE party wall. Collectively these problems, if not appropriately managed, may result in significantly reduced chances of successful long-term TE outcomes (Hillman et al., 2005).

Esophageal dysmotility or delayed transit of food or liquids due to poor peristalsis, stenosis, or stricture can result in early device failure and poor voice quality. For chronic early device failure, an esophageal work-up is often beneficial. Esophageal stricture or stenosis can often be dilated to alleviate poor transit. Poor esophageal peristalsis and GERD can be managed behaviorally and medically, often reducing the incidence of granulation tissue around the TE tract (Cocuzza et al., 2014). In addition to esophageal mobility deficits, the integrity of the TE party wall also can be associated with VP-related complications. A systematic review of the literature demonstrates that enlargement of the TE puncture occurs in approximately 7% of TE speakers, often more than a year after surgery (Hutcheson et al., 2012). The clinician may be able to manage some of the symptoms of an enlarging TE tract by placing a larger diameter device or using periprosthetic flanges to hold the device in place (Lewin et al., 2012). Other solutions include temporary VP removal, use of an electrocautery, TEP site injections with a variety of injectable materials (such as collagen, autologous fat, or Cymetra®), and purse-string sutures around the TEP (Hutcheson, Lewin, Sturgis, Kapadia, & Risser, 2011). However, most of these techniques provide only temporary solutions to the problem and need to be repeated over time (Hutcheson et al., 2011). It is essential that the clinician also ensures that the patient receives appropriate medical evaluation for the possible causes of this problem. An enlarging TE tract can be caused by low levels of thyroid hormones, low calcium levels, poorly managed diabetes, delayed effects of radiation, and also cancer recurrence (Hutcheson et al., 2012).

In some cases, the VP may no longer be functional, or the patient may choose not to continue to use TE speech for a variety of reasons. In this situation, one option is to plug the TE tract using specially designed devices, such as a *total occluder* (i.e., a dummy VP) or an adjustable bi-flanged fistula prosthesis, both of which are available from InHealth Technologies. Another option is to allow the TE tract to close which requires removal of the VP and temporary placement of a feeding tube to prevent aspiration. If the TE tract does not close spontaneously, surgery may be required for definitive closure.

TE Voice Restoration After Laryngopharyngectomy and Reconstruction

In many individuals, sufficient healthy tissue for primary closure after total laryngectomy is not available. After laryngectomy, defects can be classified into three general categories, namely, (a) those with sufficient mucosa to close primarily; (b) those with mucosa present but insufficient to close, thus requiring "patch" reconstruction with tissue from another part of the body to reinforce the surgical closure; and (c) those requiring total laryngopharyngectomy with a "tubed" reconstruction where tissue from another part of the body is used to replace the entire pharynx (Hanasono et al., 2012; Yeh, Sahovaler & Yoo, Chap. 2). There are a variety of reconstructive options for surgical wound closure after laryngectomy, such as the radial forearm, pectoralis major, anterolateral thigh, and ulnar and musculocutaneous flaps (Deschler & Gray, 2004; Patel et al., 2013; Yeh, Sahovaler & Yoo, Chap. 2). The use of nonirradiated, vascularized tissue has been shown to reduce the incidence of and duration of fistula after salvage total laryngectomy (Patel et al., 2013). Consequently, the use of vascularized muscle flaps is now advocated for the closure of radiation-compromised pharyngectomy defects (Genden, 2013), and it has been recommended that reconstructive flaps should be considered all previously irradiated individuals, even in those in whom primary closure is technically possible (Hanasono, 2013).

A number of studies have shown that functional TE speech can be attained in individuals who have undergone reconstruction after total laryngectomy with partial pharyngectomy or total laryngopharyngectomy (Deschler, Herr, Kmiecik, Sethi, & Bunting, 2015; Fung et al., 2007; Graville et al., 2017; Iwai et al., 2002; Revenaugh, Knott, Alam, Kmiecik, & Fritz, 2014; Withrow et al., 2007). In general, however, long-term outcomes are worse after laryngopharyngectomy than laryngectomy alone, and VP users are at greater risk for more negative long-term communication and associated problems (Hutcheson et al., 2012; Starmer et al., 2009; Ward et al., 2003). The properties of the recon-structed segment may affect both the timing and candidacy for a TE puncture and the likelihood of long-term success (Table 11.6).

Differences in TE voice are due to differences in the properties of the vibratory segment. For example, after laryngopharyngectomy, the vibratory sound source is created by motion of the reconstructed segment (Haughey, Fredrickson, Sessions, & Fuller, 1995). In contrast, after TL with partial pharyngectomy and reconstruction, the remnant of pharyngeal mucosa may provide an alternative sound source (Iwai et al., 2002). In general, when the TE voice is compared between those who have had a primary laryngectomy to those who have had reconstruction, the reconstructed voice is poorer in terms of both acoustic and perceptual characteristics (Cavalot et al., 2001; Deschler & Gray, 2004; McAuliffe, Ward, Bassett, & Perkins, 2000; Mendelsohn, Morris, & Gallagher, 1993). However, work by Doyle and colleagues has suggested that when evaluated using robust psychophysical methods for auditory-perceptual evaluation, categorical differences between those with flaps and those without do not exist (Doyle et al., 2014). Deschler et al. (2015) reported that TE speakers who had undergone reconstruction were rated more negatively by listeners and had lower self-rated scores relating to voice, speech, and communication than those who had undergone primary closure. Similarly, McAuliffe and colleagues (2000) reported poorer TE voice quality and reduced levels of speech intelligibility after total laryngopharyngectomy with jejunal interposition compared to those in a non-reconstructed group. Despite these negative findings, however, the reconstructed group was satisfied with their speech rehabilitation and reported levels of handicap and well-being/distress that were comparable to those in the non-reconstructed group. Consequently, it appears that despite differences in voice quality, many individuals who undergo TE puncture after reconstruction can still be classified as "successful" VP users (Graville, Palmer, Wax, & Andersen, 2009).

Judgments about who is an appropriate candidate for a VP should be conducted by experienced healthcare professionals with full

Table 11.6 Voice outcomes, timing, and candidacy after total laryngectomy and reconstruction

Type of reconstruction	Voice outcomes	Timing, candidacy, and additional considerations
Tubed pectoralis major myocutaneous flap	Poorer than primary closure without reconstruction but superior to jejunal interposition	Typically secondary
Tubed radial forearm free tissue transfer (RFFTT)	Poorer than primary closure without reconstruction; comparable to jejunal interposition[1]	Typically secondary
Tubed anterolateral thigh flap (ALT)	Poorer than primary closure without reconstruction but superior to jejunal interposition[2]	Typically secondary
Jejunal interposition	Wet, low-pitched, sometimes strained, or dysfluent. Voice may be associated with peristaltic activity of flap. Poorer than tubed ALT[2]	Secondary. Presence of significant dysphagia may be a contraindication. Voice quality may not be acceptable to some patients, particularly women
Gastric pull-up	Highly variable voice outcomes, ranging from tight and strained to loose and wet	Secondary. Candidacy should be assessed after all treatment is completed. The presence of significant dysphagia and/or reflux may be a contraindication
Total laryngectomy and total glossectomy	Acceptable outcomes achieved very rarely and only in exceptional patients[3]	Secondary. Candidacy should be assessed after all treatment is completed. Adequate oral bulk to replace glossectomy defect essential and may require a combination of reconstruction, prosthetic tongue, and/or palatal drop. Dysarthria expected. Functional speech achieved in very rare cases after significant rehabilitation

Adapted from Casper and Colton (1998); Deschler and Gray (2004). Additional references: [1]Deschler et al. (2015); [2]Lewin et al. (2005); [3]Meeker, Lavertu, & Hicks (1997)

discussion of the potential risks and benefits to allow for informed decision-making. A recent editorial by Dr. Elliot Abemayor (2017) on the current state of TE speech restoration in the era of salvage total laryngectomy provides a strong endorsement for knowledgeable care and management of a population that is more prone to complications:

> Care for patients who have undergone [total laryngectomy], particularly following organ preservation attempts, is a complicated enterprise and I believe should be performed at high-volume centers that include on-site integrated teams well-versed in TL rehabilitation. It does no patient a service to operate and then refer out for rehabilitative care. Judgments as to whether a patient is even a candidate for TEP placement should be done with experienced healthcare professionals in a deliberate fashion with adequate discussion of risk, benefit, device life, and patient preferences so as to allow for informed decision-making. Recommendations for TEP placement should not be an afterthought. (p.72)

Conclusions

Since its introduction in 1980, techniques for surgical voice restoration using the VP have been operationalized and standardized, thus, demonstrating their efficacy across a wide variety of patients. The development of newer VP devices in addition to tracheostoma buttons and laryngectomy tubes to use with hands-free devices has further expanded the range of options available to the clinician for voice rehabilitation. Over the same period, however, the laryngectomy population has changed dramatically. With the advent of organ preservation protocols as a treatment method for advanced laryngeal cancer, many individuals may now undergo salvage laryngectomy as a secondary, curative procedure. The combined effects of chemoradiation and surgery, often in combination with reconstruction, mean that postoperative complications are common and may delay speech and swallowing rehabilitation. Further, those who undergo complex surgical reconstruction may be poorer candidates for a VP. Increasingly, TE voice restoration is an area that is best managed by centers with specialty expertise in this clinical practice area. The availability of long-term, knowledgeable professional care and access to resources is essential for long-term success. Ensuring the availability of these resources will minimize the possibility of negative sequelae, such as aspiration pneumonia, hospitalization, and the need for surgical closure of the tract. These observations reinforce the need for careful and comprehensive evaluation of patient candidacy with full discussion of risks, benefits, device life, and complications, in order to allow for informed decision-making. Challenges for the future include ensuring the availability of services and minimizing patient-related costs.

References

Abemayor, E. (2017). Prosthetic voice rehabilitation following laryngectomy: It's the archer not the arrow. *JAMA Otolaryngology. Head & Neck Surgery, 143*(1), 72.

Ackerstaff, A. H., Hilgers, F. J., Balm, A. J., Aaronson, N. K., & van Zandwijk, N. (1993). Improvements in respiratory and psychosocial functioning following total laryngectomy by the use of a heat and moisture exchanger. *The Annals of Otology, Rhinology, and Laryngology, 102*(11), 878–883.

Agrawal, N., & Goldenberg, D. (2008). Primary and salvage total laryngectomy. *Otolaryngologic Clinics of North America, 41*, 771–780.

American Speech-Language-Hearing Association. (2004a). *Roles and responsibilities of speech-language pathologists with respect to evaluation and treatment for tracheoesophageal puncture and prosthesis [Position Statement]*. Available from www.asha.org/policy.

American Speech-Language-Hearing Association. (2004b). *Evaluation and treatment for tracheoesophageal puncture and prosthesis: Technical report [Technical Report]*. Available from www.asha.org/policy.

American Speech-Language-Hearing Association. (2004c). *Knowledge and skills for speech-language pathologists with respect to evaluation and treatment for tracheoesophageal puncture and prosthesis [Knowledge and Skills]*. Available from www.asha.org/policy.

Amster, W. W. (1986). Advanced stage of teaching alaryngeal speech. In R. L. Keith & F. L. Darley (Eds.), *Laryngectomee rehabilitation* (2nd ed., pp. 177–192). San Diego, CA: College-Hill Press.

Beaudin, P. G., Godes, J. R., Gowan, A. C., & Minuk, J. L. (2003). An education and training survey of speech-language pathologists working with individuals with cancer of the larynx. *Journal of Speech-Language Pathology and Audiology, 27*(3), 144–157.

Blom, E. D. (1995). Tracheoesophageal speech. *Seminars in Speech and Language, 16*(3), 191–204.

Blom, E. D., Singer, M. I., & Hamaker, R. C. (1985). An improved esophageal insufflation test. *Archives of Otolaryngology, 111*(4), 211–212.

Blom, E. D., Singer, M. I., & Hamaker, R. C. (1986). A prospective study of tracheoesophageal speech. *Archives of Otolaryngology – Head & Neck Surgery, 112*(4), 440–447.

Bosone, Z. T. (1986). Tracheoesophageal fistulization for voice restoration: Presurgical considerations and troubleshooting procedures. In R. L. Keith & F. L. Darley (Eds.), *Laryngectomee rehabilitation* (2nd ed., pp. 193–209). San Diego, CA: College-Hill Press.

Bradley, P. J., Counter, P., Hurren, A., & Cocks, H. C. (2013). Provision of surgical voice restoration in England: Questionnaire survey of speech and language therapists. *The Journal of Laryngology and Otology, 127*(8), 760–767.

Casper, J. K., & Colton, R. H. (1998). *Clinical manual for laryngectomy and head/neck cancer rehabilitation* (2nd ed.). San Diego, CA: Singular Publishing.

Cavalot, A. L., Palonta, F., Preti, G., Nazionale, G., Ricci, E., Vione, N., ... Cortesina, G. (2001). Qualitative and quantitative evaluation of some vocal function parameters following fitting of a prosthesis. *Journal of Voice, 15*, 587–591.

Cheng, E., Ho, M., Ganz, C., Shaha, A., Boyle, J. O., Singh, B., ... Kraus, D. H. (2006). Outcomes of primary and secondary tracheoesophageal puncture: A 16-year retrospective analysis. *Ear, Nose, & Throat Journal, 85*(4), 262–267.

Cocuzza, S., Bonfiglio, M., Chiaramonte, R., & Serra, A. (2014). Relationship between radiotherapy and gastroesophageal reflux disease in causing tracheoesophageal voice rehabilitation failure. *Journal of Voice, 28*(2), 245–249.

Deschler, D. G., & Gray, S. T. (2004). Tracheoesophageal speech following laryngopharyngectomy and pharyngeal reconstruction. *Otolaryngologic Clinics of North America, 37*, 567–583.

Deschler, D. G., Herr, M. W., Kmiecik, J. R., Sethi, R., & Bunting, G. (2015). Tracheoesophageal voice after total laryngopharyngectomy reconstruction: Jejunum versus radial forearm free flap. *Laryngoscope, 125*(12), 2715–2721.

Doyle, P., Cox, S. R., Scott, G. M., Nash, M. M., Theurer, J., Khalili, S., ... Fung, K. (2014, July). *The influence of flap reconstruction on auditory-perceptual evaluation of voice acceptability for tracheoesophageal speakers*. Paper presented at the 5th World Congress of the International Federation of Head and Neck Oncology Society, New York, NY.

Doyle, P. C. (1994). *Foundations of voice and speech rehabilitation following laryngeal cancer*. San Diego, CA: Singular Publishing.

Doyle, P. C., Danhauer, J. L., & Reed, C. G. (1988). Listener' perceptions of consonants produced by esophageal and tracheoesophageal talkers. *The Journal of Speech and Hearing Disorders, 53*(4), 400–407.

Doyle, P. C., & Eadie, T. L. (2005). The perceptual nature of alaryngeal voice and speech. In P. C. Doyle & R. L. Keith (Eds.), *Contemporary considerations in the treatment and rehabilitation of head and neck cancer: Voice, speech, and swallowing* (pp. 113–140). Austin, TX: Pro-Ed.

Doyle, P. C., Grantmyre, A., & Myers, C. (1989). Clinical modification of the tracheostoma breathing valve for voice restoration. *The Journal of Speech and Hearing Disorders, 54*, 189–192.

Eadie, T. L., & Doyle, P. C. (2004). Auditory-perceptual scaling and quality of life in tracheoesophageal speakers. *Laryngoscope, 114*(4), 753–759.

Elmiyeh, B., Dwivedi, R. C., Jallali, N., Chisholm, E. J., Kazi, R., Clarke, P. M., & Rhys-Evans, P. H. (2010). Surgical voice restoration after total laryngectomy: An overview. *Indian Journal of Cancer, 47*(3), 239–247.

Forastiere, A. A., Goepfert, H., Maor, M., Pajak, T. F., Weber, R., Morrison, W., … Peters, G. (2003). Concurrent chemotherapy and radiotherapy for organ preservation in advanced laryngeal cancer. *The New England Journal of Medicine, 349*(22), 2091–2098.

Frowen, J., & Perry, A. (2001). Reasons for success or failure in surgical voice restoration after total laryngectomy: An Australian study. *The Journal of Laryngology and Otology, 115*, 393–399.

Fung, K., Teknos, T. N., Vandenberg, C. D., Lyden, T. H., Bradford, C. R., Hogikyan, N. D., … Chepeha, D. B. (2007). Prevention of wound complications following salvage laryngectomy using free vascularized tissue. *Head & Neck, 27*, 425–430.

Ganly, I., Patel, S., Matsuo, J., Singh, B., Kraus, D., Boyle, J., … Shah, J. (2005). Postoperative complications of salvage total laryngectomy. *Cancer, 103*, 2073–2081.

Genden, E. M. (2013). Use of vascularized muscle flaps in the healing of compromised wounds. *JAMA Otolaryngology. Head & Neck Surgery, 139*(11), 1162–1162.

Gerwin, J. M., Culton, G. L., & Gerwin, K. S. (1997). Hiatal hernia and reflux complicating prosthetic speech. *American Journal of Otolaryngology, 18*, 66–68.

Gilmore, S. I. (1994). The physical, social, occupational, and psychological concomitants of laryngectomy. In R. L. Keith & F. L. Darley (Eds.), *Laryngectomee rehabilitation* (3rd ed., pp. 395–486). Austin, TX: Pro-Ed.

Gitomer, S. A., Hutcheson, K. A., Christianson, B. L., Samuelson, M. B., Barringer, D. A., Roberts, D. B., … Zafereo, M. E. (2016). Influence of timing, radiation, and reconstruction on complications and speech outcomes with tracheoesophageal puncture. *Head & Neck, 38*, 1765–1771.

Graham, M. S. (1997). *The clinician's guide to alaryngeal speech therapy*. Boston, MA: Butterworth-Heinemann.

Graville, D., Gross, N., Andersen, P., Everts, E., & Cohen, J. (1999). The long-term indwelling tracheoesophageal prosthesis for alaryngeal voice rehabilitation. *Archives of Otolaryngology – Head & Neck Surgery, 125*, 288–292.

Graville, D. J., Palmer, A. D., Chambers, C. M., Ottenstein, L., Whalen, B., Andersen, P. E., … Cohen, J. I. (2017). Functional outcomes and quality of life after total laryngectomy with noncircumferential radial forearm free tissue transfer. *Head & Neck, 39*(11), 2319–2328.

Graville, D. J., Palmer, A. D., Wax, M. K., & Andersen, P. E. (2009). Tracheoesophageal voice restoration after salvage total laryngectomy. American Speech Language Hearing Association, Rockville, MD, Special Interest Group 3. *Perspectives on Voice and Voice Disorders, 19*(2), 58–65.

Hamaker, R. C., & Blom, E. D. (2003). Botulinum neurotoxin for pharyngeal constrictor muscle spasm in tracheoesophageal voice restoration. *Laryngoscope, 113*(9), 1479–1482.

Hamaker, R. C., Singer, M. I., Blom, E. D., & Daniels, H. A. (1985). Primary voice restoration at laryngectomy. *Archives of Otolaryngology, 111*(3), 182–186.

Hanasono, M. M. (2013). Use of reconstructive flaps following total laryngectomy. *JAMA Otolaryngology. Head & Neck Surgery, 139*(11), 1163–1163.

Hanasono, M. M., Lin, D., Wax, M. K., & Rosenthal, E. L. (2012). Closure of laryngectomy defects in the age of chemoradiation therapy. *Head & Neck, 34*, 580–588.

Hancock, K., Ward, E. C., Burnett, R., Edwards, P., Lenne, P., Maclean, J., & Megee, F. (2017). Tracheoesophageal speech restoration: Issues for training and clinical support. *Speech, Language and Hearing, 21*(2), 117–122.

Hartman, D. E., & Scott, D. A. (1974). Overt responses of listeners to alaryngeal speech. *Laryngoscope, 84*(3), 410–416.

Hasan, Z., Dwivedi, R. C., Gunaratne, D. A., Virk, S. A., Palme, C. E., & Riffat, F. (2017). Systematic review and meta-analysis of the complications of salvage total laryngectomy. *European Journal of Surgical Oncology, 43*(1), 42–51. https://doi.org/10.1016/j.ejso.2016.05.017

Hassan, S. J., & Weymuller, E. A. (1993). Assessment of quality of life in head and neck cancer patients. *Head & Neck, 15*(6), 485–496.

Haughey, B. H., Fredrickson, J. M., Sessions, D. G., & Fuller, D. (1995). Vibratory segment function after free flap reconstruction of the pharyngoesophagus. *Laryngoscope, 105*, 487–490.

Hilgers, F. J., Aaronson, N. K., Schouwenburg, P. F., & Zandwijk, N. (1991). The influence of a heat and moisture exchanger (HME) on the respiratory symptoms after total laryngectomy. *Clinical Otolaryngology, 16*(2), 152–156.

Hilgers, F. J., Ackerstaff, A. H., Aaronson, N. K., Schouwenburg, P. F., & Zandwijk, N. (1990). Physical and psychosocial consequences of total laryngectomy. *Clinical Otolaryngology, 15*(5), 421–425.

Hilgers, F. J., Ackerstaff, A. H., Balm, A. J., Van Den Brekel, M. W., Bing Tan, I., & Persson, J. O. (2003). A new problem-solving indwelling voice prosthesis, eliminating the need for frequent Candida- and "underpressure"-related replacements: Provox ActiValve. *Acta Oto-Laryngologica, 123*(8), 972–979.

Hilgers, F. J., Ackerstaff, A. H., van As, C. J., Balm, A. J., van Den Brekel, M. W., & Tan, I. B. (2003). Development and clinical assessment of a heat and moisture exchanger with a multi-magnet automatic tracheostoma valve (Provox FreeHands HME) for vocal and pulmonary rehabilitation after total laryngectomy. *Acta Oto-Laryngologica, 123*(1), 91–99.

Hilgers, F. J., & Schouwenburg, P. F. (1990). A new low-resistance, self-retaining prosthesis (Provox™) for voice rehabilitation after total laryngectomy. *Laryngoscope, 100*(11), 1202–1207.

Hilgers, F. J. M., Ackerstaff, A. H., Balm, A. J. M., & Gregor, R. T. (1996). A new heat and moisture exchanger with speech valve (Provox® Stomafilter). *Clinical Otolaryngology, 21*(5), 414–418.

Hillman, R. E., Walsh, M. J., & Heaton, J. T. (2005). Laryngectomy speech rehabilitation: A review of outcomes. In P. C. Doyle & R. L. Keith (Eds.), *Contemporary considerations in the treatment and rehabilitation of head and neck cancer: Voice, speech, and swallowing* (pp. 75–90). Austin, TX: Pro-Ed.

Hillman, R. E., Walsh, M. J., Wolf, G. T., Fisher, S. G., & Hong, W. K. (1998). Functional outcomes following treatment for advanced laryngeal cancer. Part I--Voice preservation in advanced laryngeal cancer. Part II--Laryngectomy rehabilitation: The state of the art in the VA System. Research Speech-Language Pathologists. Department of Veterans Affairs Laryngeal Cancer Study Group. *The Annals of Otology, Rhinology & Laryngology. Supplement, 172*, 1–27.

Hogikyan, N. D., & Sethuraman, G. (1999). Validation of an instrument to measure voice-related quality of life (VRQOL). *Journal of Voice, 13*(4), 557–569.

Holsinger, F. C., Funk, E., Roberts, D. B., & Diaz, E. M. (2006). Conservation laryngeal surgery versus total laryngectomy for radiation failure in laryngeal cancer. *Head & Neck, 28*, 779–784.

Hurren, A., & Miller, N. (2017). Voice outcomes post total laryngectomy. *Current Opinion in Otolaryngology & Head and Neck Surgery, 25*(3), 205–210.

Hutcheson, K. A., Lewin, J. S., Sturgis, E. M., Kapadia, A., & Risser, J. (2011). Enlarged tracheoesophageal puncture after total laryngectomy: A systematic review and meta-analysis. *Head & Neck, 33*(1), 20–30.

Hutcheson, K. A., Lewin, J. S., Sturgis, E. M., & Risser, J. (2012). Multivariable analysis of risk factors for enlargement of the tracheoesophageal puncture after total laryngectomy. *Head & Neck, 34*, 557–567.

Hyman, M. (1986). Factors influencing the intelligibility of alaryngeal speech. In R. L. Keith & F. L. Darley (Eds.), *Laryngectomee rehabilitation* (2nd ed., pp. 165–172). San Diego, CA: College-Hill Press.

Iwai, H., Tsuji, H., Tachikawa, T., Inoue, T., Izumikawa, M., Yamamichi, K., & Yamashita, T. (2002). Neoglottic formation from posterior pharyngeal wall conserved in surgery for hypopharyngeal cancer. *Auris Nasus Larynx, 29*, 153–157.

Izdebski, K., Reed, C. G., Ross, J. C., & Hilsinger, R. L. (1994). Problems with tracheoesophageal fistula voice restoration in totally laryngectomized patients: A review of 95 cases. *Archives of Otolaryngology – Head & Neck Surgery, 120*(8), 840–845.

Izdebski, K., Ross, J. C., & Lee, S. (1987). Fungal colonization of tracheoesophageal voice prosthesis. *Laryngoscope, 97*(5), 594-597.

Jacobson, B. H., Johnson, A., Grywalski, C., Silbergleit, A., Jacobson, G., Benninger, M. S., & Newman, C. W. (1997). The voice handicap index (VHI): Development and validation. *American Journal of Speech-Language Pathology, 6*(3), 66–70.

Jiang, N., Kearney, A., & Damrose, E. J. (2016). Tracheoesophageal fistula length decreases over time. *European Archives of Oto-Rhino-Laryngology, 273*(7), 1819–1824.

Johns, M. E., & Cantrell, R. W. (1981). Voice restoration of the total laryngectomy patient: The Singer-Blom technique. *Otolaryngology and Head and Neck Surgery, 89*(1), 82–86.

Kao, W. W., Mohr, R. M., Kimmel, C. A., Getch, C., & Silverman, C. (1994). The outcome and techniques of primary and secondary tracheoesophageal puncture. *Archives of Otolaryngology – Head & Neck Surgery, 120*(3), 301–307.

Kaufman, M., & Searl, J. (2014, September 1). Medicare TEP policy hurts providers, patients. *ASHA Leader*. Rockville, MD: American Speech Language Hearing Association.

Khemani, S., Govender, R., Arora, A., O'Flynn, P. E., & Vaz, F. M. (2009). Use of botulinum toxin in voice restoration after laryngectomy. *The Journal of Laryngology and Otology, 123*(12), 1308–1313.

Lavertu, P., Guay, M. E., Meeker, S. S., Kmiecik, J. R., Secic, M., Wanamaker, J. R., … Wood, B. G. (1996). Secondary tracheoesophageal puncture: Factors predictive of voice quality and prosthesis use. *Head & Neck, 18*, 393–398.

Lavertu, P., Scott, S. E., Finnegan, E. M., Levine, H. L., Tucker, H. M., & Wood, B. G. (1989). Secondary tracheoesophageal puncture for voice rehabilitation after laryngectomy. *Archives of Otolaryngology – Head & Neck Surgery, 115*(3), 350–355.

Leder, S. B., Acton, L. M., Kmiecik, J., Ganz, C., & Blom, E. D. (2005). Voice restoration with the advantage tracheoesophageal voice prosthesis. *Otolaryngology and Head and Neck Surgery, 133*(5), 681–684.

Leder, S. B., & Erskine, M. C. (1997). Voice restoration after laryngectomy: Experience with the Blom–Singer extended-wear indwelling tracheoesophageal voice prosthesis. *Head & Neck, 19*(6), 487–493.

Lewin, J. S., Barringer, D. A., May, A. H., Gillenwater, A. M., Arnold, K. A., Roberts, D. B., & Yu, P. (2005). Functional outcomes after circumferential pharyngoesophageal reconstruction. *Laryngoscope, 115*(7), 1266–1271.

Lewin, J. S., Baugh, R. F., & Baker, S. R. (1987). An objective method for prediction of tracheoesophageal speech production. *The Journal of Speech and Hearing Disorders, 52*(3), 212–217.

Lewin, J. S., Baumgart, L. M., Barrow, M. P., & Hutcheson, K. A. (2017). Device life of the tracheoesophageal voice prosthesis revisited. *JAMA Otolaryngology. Head & Neck Surgery, 143*(1), 65–71.

Lewin, J. S., Hutcheson, K. A., Barringer, D. A., Croegaert, L. E., Lisec, A., & Chambers, M. S. (2012). Customization of the voice prosthesis to prevent leakage from the enlarged tracheoesophageal puncture: Results of a prospective trial. *Laryngoscope, 122*(8), 1767–1772.

Lewin, J. S., Lemon, J., Bishop-Leone, J. K., Leyk, S., Martin, J. W., & Gillenwater, A. M. (2000). Experience with Barton button and peristomal breathing valve attachments for hands-free tracheoesophageal speech. *Head & Neck, 22*(2), 142–148.

Lewin, J. S., Montgomery, P. C., Hutcheson, K. A., & Chambers, M. S. (2009). Further experience with modification of an intraluminal button for hands-free tracheoesophageal speech after. *The Journal of Prosthetic Dentistry, 102*(5), 328–331.

List, M. A., Ritter-Sterr, C., & Lansky, S. B. (1990). A performance status scale for head and neck cancer patients. *Cancer, 66*(3), 564–569.

Lorenz, K. J., Groll, K., Ackerstaff, A. H., Hilgers, F. J. M., & Maier, H. (2007). Hands-free speech after surgical voice rehabilitation with a Provox® voice prosthesis: Experience with the Provox FreeHands HME tracheostoma valve® system. *European Archives of Oto-Rhino-Laryngology, 264*(2), 151–157.

Maddox, P. T., & Davies, L. (2012). Trends in total laryngectomy in the era of organ preservation: A population-based study. *Otolaryngology and Head and Neck Surgery, 147*, 85–90.

Mahieu, H. F., van Saene, J. J., den Besten, J., & van Saene, H. K. (1986). Oropharynx decontamination preventing *Candida* vegetation on voice prostheses. *Archives of Otolaryngology – Head & Neck Surgery, 112*(10), 1090–1092.

McAuliffe, M. J., Ward, E. C., Bassett, L., & Perkins, K. (2000). Functional speech outcomes after laryngectomy and pharyngolaryngectomy. *Archives of Otolaryngology – Head & Neck Surgery, 126*, 705–709.

McConnel, F., & Duck, S. W. (1986). Indications for tracheoesophageal puncture speech rehabilitation. *Laryngoscope, 96*(10), 1065–1068.

McIvor, J., Evans, P. F., Perry, A., & Cheesman, A. D. (1990). Radiological assessment of post laryngectomy speech. *Clinical Radiology, 41*(5), 312–316.

Meeker, S. S., Lavertu, P., & Hicks, D. M. (1997). Successful tracheoesophageal puncture voice restoration in a patient with total glossectomy. *Otolaryngology and Head and Neck Surgery, 116*(1), 113–115.

Melvin, C., Frank, E. M., & Robinson, M. S. R. (2001). Speech-language pathologist preparation for evalu-ation and treatment of patients with tracheoesophageal puncture. *Journal of Medical Speech-Language Pathology, 9*(2), 129–140.

Mendelsohn, M., Morris, M., & Gallagher, R. (1993). A comparative study of speech after total laryngectomy and total laryngopharyngectomy. *Archives of Otolaryngology – Head & Neck Surgery, 119*, 508–510.

Moon, S., Raffa, F., Ojo, R., Landera, M. A., Weed, D. T., Sargi, Z., & Lundy, D. (2014). Changing trends of speech outcomes after total laryngectomy in the 21st century: A single-center study. *Laryngoscope, 124*(11), 2508–2512.

Myer, C. M., III. (1987). The heat and moisture exchanger in post-tracheotomy care. *Otolaryngology and Head and Neck Surgery, 96*(2), 209–210.

Natvig, K. (1984). Laryngectomees in Norway. Study no. 5: Problems of everyday life. *The Journal of Otolaryngology, 13*(1), 15–22.

Op de Coul, B., Hilgers, F. J. M., Balm, A. J. M., Tan, I. B., van den Hoogen, F. J. A., & van Tinteren, H. (2000). A decade of postlaryngectomy vocal rehabilitation in 318 patients: A single institution's experience with consistent application of provox indwelling voice prostheses. *Archives of Otolaryngology – Head & Neck Surgery, 126*(11), 1320–1328.

Op de Coul, B. M. R., Ackerstaff, A. H., van As-Brooks, C. J., van den Hoogen, F. J. A., Meeuwis, C. A., Manni, J. J., & Hilgers, F. J. M. (2005). Compliance, quality of life and quantitative voice quality aspects of hands-free speech. *Acta Oto-Laryngologica, 125*(6), 629–637.

Owen, S., & Paleri, V. (2013). Laryngectomy rehabilitation in the United Kingdom. *Current Opinion in Otolaryngology & Head and Neck Surgery, 21*(3), 186–191.

Palmer, A. D., Childes, J. M., Fried-Oken, M., & Graville, D. J. (2016). *Predictors of communication effectiveness after total laryngectomy.* Presented at the American Head and Neck Society, 9th International Conference on Head and Neck Cancer, Seattle, WA.

Palmer, A. D., & Graham, M. S. (2004). The relationship between communication and quality of life in alaryngeal speakers. *Journal of Speech Language Pathology & Audiology, 28*, 6–24.

Patel, U. A., Moore, B. A., Wax, M., Rosenthal, E., Sweeny, L., Militsakh, O. N., ... Flohr, J. (2013). Impact of pharyngeal closure technique on fistula after salvage laryngectomy. *JAMA Otolaryngology. Head & Neck Surgery, 139*(11), 1156–1162.

Pattani, K. M., Morgan, M., & Nathan, C. A. O. (2009). Reflux as a cause of tracheoesophageal puncture failure. *Laryngoscope, 119*(1), 121–125.

Pindzola, R. H., & Cain, B. H. (1989). Duration and frequency characteristics of tracheoesophageal speech. *The Annals of Otology, Rhinology, and Laryngology, 98*(12), 960–964.

Revenaugh, P. C., Knott, P. D., Alam, D. S., Kmiecik, J., & Fritz, M. A. (2014). Voice outcomes following reconstruction of laryngopharyngectomy defects using the radial forearm free flap and the anterolateral thigh free flap. *Laryngoscope, 124*(2), 397–400.

Robbins, J., Fisher, H. B., Blom, E. C., & Singer, M. I. (1984). A comparative acoustic study of normal, esophageal, and tracheoesophageal speech production. *The Journal of Speech and Hearing Disorders, 49*(2), 202–210.

Royal College of Speech and Language Therapists. (2010). *Prosthetic surgical voice restoration (SVR): The role of the speech and language therapist [Policy Statement 2010]*. Available from: www.rcslt.org/speech_and_language_therapy/rcslt_position_papers.

Salerno, G., Cavaliere, M., Foglia, A., Pellicoro, D. P., Mottola, G., Nardone, M., & Galli, V. (2002). The 11th nerve syndrome in functional neck dissection. *Laryngoscope, 112*(7), 1299–1307.

Sandulache, V. C., Vandelaar, L. J., Skinner, H. D., Cata, J., Fuller, C. D., Phan, J., … Zafereo, M. E. (2016). Salvage total laryngectomy after external-beam radiotherapy: A 20-year experience. *Head & Neck, 38*, E1962–E1968.

Scharpf, J., & Esclamado, R. M. (2003). Reconstruction with radial forearm flaps after ablative surgery for hypopharyngeal cancer. *Head & Neck, 25*(4), 261–266.

Shultz, J. R., & Harrison, J. (1992). Defining and predicting tracheoesophageal puncture success. *Archives of Otolaryngology – Head & Neck Surgery, 118*, 811–816.

Silverman, A. H., & Black, M. J. (1994). Efficacy of primary tracheoesophageal puncture in laryngectomy rehabilitation. *The Journal of Otolaryngology, 23*, 370–377.

Sinclair, C. F., Rosenthal, E. L., McColloch, N. L., Magnuson, J. S., Desmond, R. A., Peters, G. E., & Carroll, W. R. (2011). Primary versus delayed tracheoesophageal puncture for laryngopharyngectomy with free flap reconstruction. *Laryngoscope, 121*(7), 1436–1440.

Singer, M. I. (1983). Tracheoesophageal speech: Vocal rehabilitation after total laryngectomy. *Laryngoscope, 93*(11), 1454–1465.

Singer, M. I., & Blom, E. D. (1980). An endoscopic technique for restoration of voice after laryngectomy. *The Annals of Otology, Rhinology, and Laryngology, 89*(6), 529–533.

Singer, M. I., & Blom, E. D. (1981). Selective myotomy for voice restoration after total laryngectomy. *Archives of Otolaryngology, 107*(11), 670–673.

Singer, M. I., Blom, E. D., & Hamaker, R. C. (1981). Further experience with voice restoration after total laryngectomy. *The Annals of Otology, Rhinology, and Laryngology, 90*(5), 498–502.

Singer, M. I., Blom, E. D., & Hamaker, R. C. (1986). Pharyngeal plexus neurectomy for alaryngeal speech rehabilitation. *Laryngoscope, 96*(1), 50–54.

Singer, M. I., Blom, E. D., Hamaker, R. C., & Yoshida, G. Y. (1989). Applications of the voice prosthesis during laryngectomy. *The Annals of Otology, Rhinology, and Laryngology, 98*(12), 921–925.

Singer, S., Wollbrück, D., Dietz, A., Schock, J., Pabst, F., Vogel, H. J., … Breitenstein, K. (2013). Speech rehabilitation during the first year after total laryngectomy. *Head & Neck, 35*, 1583–1590.

Skoner, J. M., Bascom, D. A., Cohen, J. I., Andersen, P. E., & Wax, M. K. (2003). Short-term functional donor site morbidity after radial forearm fasciocutaneous free flap harvest. *Laryngoscope, 113*, 2091–2094.

Speech Pathology Australia. (2013). *Clinical guideline: Laryngectomy*. Melbourne: The Speech Pathology Association of Australia Ltd.

Starmer, H. M., Ishman, S. L., Flint, P. W., Bhatti, N. I., Richmon, J., Koch, W., … Gourin, C. G. (2009). Complications that affect postlaryngectomy voice restoration: Primary surgery vs salvage surgery. *Archives of Otolaryngology – Head & Neck Surgery, 135*, 1165–1169.

Stiernberg, C. M., Bailey, B. J., Calhoun, K. H., & Perez, D. G. (1987). Primary tracheoesophageal fistula procedure for voice restoration: The University of Texas medical branch experience. *Laryngoscope, 97*(7), 820–824.

Terrell, J. E., Nanavati, K. A., Esclamado, R. M., Bishop, J. K., Bradford, C. R., & Wolf, G. T. (1997). Head and neck cancer—specific quality of life: Instrument validation. *Archives of Otolaryngology – Head & Neck Surgery, 123*(10), 1125–1132.

Theunissen, E. A., Timmermans, A. J., Zuur, C. L., Hamming-Vrieze, O., de Boer, J. P., Hilgers, F. J., & van den Brekel, M. W. (2012). Total laryngectomy for a dysfunctional larynx after (chemo) radiotherapy. *Archives of Otolaryngology – Head & Neck Surgery, 138*, 548–555.

Trudeau, M. D., Schuller, D. E., & Hall, D. A. (1988). Timing of tracheoesophageal puncture for voice restoration: Primary vs. secondary. *Head & Neck, 10*, 130–134.

van As, C. J., Hilgers, F. J., Koopmans-Van Beinum, F. J., & Ackerstaff, A. H. (1998). The influence of stoma occlusion on aspects of tracheoesophageal voice. *Acta Oto-Laryngologica, 118*(5), 732–738.

van As, C. J., Op de Coul, B. M., van den Hoogen, F. J., Koopmans–van Beinum, F. J., & Hilgers, F. J. (2001). Quantitative videofluoroscopy: A new evaluation tool for tracheoesophageal voice production. *Archives of Otolaryngology – Head & Neck Surgery, 127*(2), 161–169.

van den Hoogen, F. J. A., Meeuwis, C., Oudes, M. J., Janssen, P., & Manni, J. J. (1996). The Blom-Singer tracheostoma valve as a valuable addition in the rehabilitation of the laryngectomized patient. *European Archives of Oto-Rhino-Laryngology, 253*, 126–129.

Ward, E. C., Koh, S. K., Frisby, J., & Hodge, R. (2003). Differential modes of alaryngeal communication and long-term voice outcomes following pharyngolaryngectomy and laryngectomy. *Folia Phoniatrica et Logopaedica, 55*, 39–49.

Weber, R. S., Berkey, B. A., Forastiere, A., Cooper, J., Maor, M., Goepfert, H., … Chao, K. C. (2003). Outcome of salvage total laryngectomy following organ preservation therapy: The Radiation Therapy Oncology Group trial 91-11. *Archives of Otolaryngology – Head & Neck Surgery, 129*, 44–49.

Wenig, B. L., Levy, J., Mullooly, V., & Abramson, A. L. (1989). Voice restoration following laryngectomy: The role of primary versus secondary tracheoesophageal puncture. *The Annals of Otology, Rhinology, and Laryngology, 98*(1), 70–73.

Westmore, S. J., Johns, M. E., & Baker, S. R. (1981). The Singer-Blom voice restoration procedure. *Archives of Otolaryngology – Head & Neck Surgery, 107*(11), 674–676.

Withrow, K. P., Rosenthal, E. L., Gourin, C. G., Peters, G. E., Magnuson, J. S., Terris, D. J., & Carroll, W. W. (2007). Free tissue transfer to manage salvage laryngectomy defects after organ preservation failure. *Laryngoscope, 117*(5), 781–784.

Wolf, G. T., Hong, W. K., Fisher, S. G., Urba, S., Endicott, J. W., Close, L., … Cheung, N. K. (1991). Induction chemotherapy plus radiation compared with surgery plus radiation in patients with advanced laryngeal cancer. *The New England Journal of Medicine, 324*, 1685–1690.

Wood, B. G., Rusnov, M. G., Tucker, H. M., & Levine, H. L. (1981). Tracheoesophageal puncture for alaryngeal voice restoration. *The Annals of Otology, Rhinology, and Laryngology, 90*(5), 492–494.

Yoshida, G. Y., Hamaker, R. C., Singer, M. I., Blom, E. D., & Charles, G. A. (1989). Primary voice restoration at laryngectomy: 1989 update. *Laryngoscope, 99*, 1093–1095.

Zormeier, M. M., Meleca, R. J., Simpson, M. L., Dworkin, J. P., Klein, R., Gross, M., & Mathog, R. H. (1999). Botulinum toxin injection to improve tracheoesophageal speech after total laryngectomy. *Otolaryngology and Head and Neck Surgery, 120*(3), 314–319.

Clinical Problem-Solving in Tracheoesophageal Puncture Voice Restoration

12

Jodi Knott

Introduction

Based on current statistics within the United States, there are approximately 1.7 million cases of cancer diagnosed yearly (Noone et al., 2018). Of all cancers, head and neck cancer (HNCa) is the 12th most commonly diagnosed malignancy (https://seer.cancer.gov/statfacts/html/laryn. html). Thus, HNCa is considered to comprise a relatively small subgroup of cancers, encompassing approximately 3–5% of all cancer diagnoses. Of those in this population, 50% of diagnoses are identified in the region of the oral cavity, and approximately 3% are located in the larynx (Noone et al., 2018) with approximately 13,000 new cases of laryngeal cancer diagnosed yearly in the United States (SEER, Statistics and Facts, 2018). For the larger group of these cancers, squamous cell carcinoma (SCC) is the most commonly identified cell type associated with HNC. Although recent research indicates an overall increase in the incidence of HNC as a result of the human papilloma virus (HPV), the majority are oropharyngeal cancers (see Theurer, Chap. 4). However, for those diagnosed with laryngeal cancer, a larger percentage will report a significant history of smoking and alcohol use

(Noone et al., 2018). Thus, while details related to cancer itself are essential, additional personal and lifestyle factors must always be considered in relation to treatment planning and rehabilitation.

In the "era of organ preservation," the incidence of total laryngectomy has decreased more than the incidence of laryngeal cancer itself. This observation is a data-driven conclusion that is consistent with the trend toward nonsurgical treatment as the first course of action (Maddox & Davies, 2012). When total laryngectomy is required, these procedures are often performed in larger centers or in teaching hospitals. Because of this trend, if a laryngectomy is performed in a smaller center, there may be less, if any access to an experienced Speech-Language Pathologist (SLP) who is formally trained in the evaluation and treatment of individuals who undergo total laryngectomy. For SLPs, a large part of their responsibilities with those who have undergone total laryngectomy will relate to voice and speech rehabilitation. Although several methods of postlaryngectomy "alaryngeal" methods of speech rehabilitation exist (i.e., esophageal speech, artificial larynx speech, and tracheoesophageal puncture voice restoration), use of these methods may vary by center and experience. In the contemporary era, tracheoesophageal (TE) speech is widely used as a method of postlaryngectomy speech rehabilitation (Graville, Palmer, & Bolognone, Chap. 11).

Over the past 10–15 years, those who are diagnosed with advanced laryngeal cancer and

J. Knott (✉)
Department of Speech Pathology and Audiology, University of Texas, MD Anderson Cancer Center, Houston, TX, USA
e-mail: Jknott@mdanderson.org

© Springer Nature Switzerland AG 2019
P. C. Doyle (ed.), *Clinical Care and Rehabilitation in Head and Neck Cancer*,
https://doi.org/10.1007/978-3-030-04702-3_12

will undergo a total laryngectomy are frequently better informed of their postoperative status and, as a result, may have higher expectations. When all postlaryngectomy speech rehabilitation options are considered, those who undergo TE puncture voice restoration will require that SLPs have extensive knowledge of the procedure, the range of voice prostheses available, as well as related prosthetic devices that will aid the rehabilitation process. For this reason, the importance of having an experienced clinician who demonstrates broad and comprehensive knowledge related to laryngectomy rehabilitation following TE puncture voice restoration is paramount.

Since the introduction of TE puncture voice restoration (Singer & Blom, 1980), considerable knowledge has been gained relative to this alaryngeal speech method. In the previous chapter, Graville et al. (Chap. 11) have provided details related to the process of TE voice and speech rehabilitation, including its history and evolution. However, as noted by Graville et al., TE voice restoration is not free of challenges and significant problems may emerge. Some of these problems are rare and unique. The purpose of this chapter seeks to address the issue of clinical problem-solving with those who undergo TE puncture voice restoration. A further objective seeks to systematically address approaches to management in situations where a specific problem occurs. A fundamental concern that drives successful problem-solving associated with TE voice restoration is built on a sound and comprehensive level of knowledge and the emergent experience of the clinician. This chapter focuses on clinical problems that may impact successful use of a TE voice prosthesis. The topics will primarily address approaches to evaluation, management, and resolution of problems when TE puncture voice restoration fails or is met with challenges.

Understanding Treatment Options

When working with those individuals diagnosed with advanced laryngeal tumors (i.e., T3 or T4 lesions), the standard treatment will likely involve radiation treatment either with or without concomitant chemotherapy (Noone et al., 2018). However, if a patient is diagnosed with a return of previously treated disease following a failed course of treatment (recurrent cancer), the treatment plan will likely involve a total laryngectomy (Noone et al., 2018). Those individuals who have failed nonsurgical organ preservation treatment(s) and then go on to require surgery may confront additional problems secondary to salvage laryngectomy.

Further, the ever-changing reimbursement restrictions introduced by programs such as Medicare in the United States, as well as those of third-party payers, further complicates management of the TE voice and speech and patients' access to care. As a result, it is critical to set realistic expectations for postlaryngectomy voice rehabilitation for healthcare providers and their patients. Additionally, the reported median device life of a TE voice prosthesis may only be 2–3 months, and the cost associated with its replacement may be an added obstacle to successful voice restoration (Lewin, Baumgart, Barrow, & Hutcheson, 2017).

Based on the above cited issues, the SLP must be able to effectively and efficiently manage these patients in order to justify services and provide the patient with optimal rehabilitation care. This becomes an even greater challenge when faced with those who present with more extensive and complex health histories, as well as those who experience short- and long-term complications or side effects of treatment. As such, the ability to systematically problem-solve a variety of issues related to TE puncture voice restoration is essential.

Because some individuals requiring a total laryngectomy may have had previous radiation, it is not uncommon for them to require pedicled or free-flap reconstruction (Yeh, Sahovaler, & Yoo, Chap. 2). While flap reconstruction is not a contraindication for TE puncture voice restoration, the potential for problems to arise is increased to some extent; this is true whether the puncture was performed as a primary or secondary procedure (Graville et al., Chap. 11). More directly, and as previously noted, patients today are much more likely to present with more complicated medical histories. In such cases, patients may exhibit extensive comorbidities that may not only influence the integrity of the TE puncture but the likelihood of longer-term success with speech rehabilitation. Extended resections necessitating free-flap reconstruction (Yeh et al, Chap. 2) are increasingly common in the era of salvage laryngectomy following failure of conservative treatment approaches such as radiation or chemoradiation. These added factors demand that advanced clinical skills are acquired by the SLP.

Preoperative Evaluation and Counselling

Patient interaction that involves the clinician's ability to both provide and interpret information related to laryngectomy and voice and speech rehabilitation is an important part of the clinical process (Doyle, 1994). The SLP should meet with patients who are going to undergo a total laryngectomy prior to surgery. During this preoperative counselling session, the clinician should seek to confirm the patient's understanding of the plan of care. That is, how much does the patient know and understand about what lies ahead for their medical treatment? In addition, the SLP can acknowledge the patient's worries while also seeking to reassure the patient. Such reassurance may serve to increase the patient's potential success of returning to a normal lifestyle postoperatively. Thus, evaluation and counselling should be viewed as an ongoing process that provides a valuable foundation to the patient and members of their family; this in turn may further facilitate the goals that will underlie one's successful rehabilitation.

In all cases where a laryngectomy is planned, preoperative contacts for evaluation and counselling are highly valuable. As part of this session, the patient should be made aware of the most significant anatomical changes following a total laryngectomy. This should include discussion of changes in the airway, including changes in inspiration and expiration, in additional to providing information on the presence of a permanent tracheostoma postlaryngectomy (Boehnenkamp,

Chap. 7; Lewis, Chap. 8; Searl, Chap. 13). If a primary puncture is planned (i.e., the puncture will be performed at the time of laryngectomy), information on what the patient should expect immediately postoperatively should be presented. This would include a basic discussion of information related to the presence of an oxygen mask on the neck (tracheostoma), a catheter in the puncture site, and similar expectations. Knowing this information in advance will help to reduce any unexpected concerns in the early postoperative period (see Damrose & Doyle, Chap. 3; Doyle, 1994).

Inpatient Postoperative Recovery

Patients will attend their initial outpatient speech pathology consult with a 14 French catheter in situ, stenting the TE puncture. If the patient has not undergone previous radiation, this initial outpatient visit occurs approximately 7–10 days following surgery. If the patient has undergone prior radiation and/or has required an extended resection with reconstruction, the initial visit typically will occur between 2 and 6 weeks following surgery. During this consult, the SLP will remove the catheter and size the length of the puncture. Sizing the length of the TE tract is considered to be one of the most important aspects of management. The sizing tool must be fully inserted into the esophageal lumen, and the clinician should be mindful not to forcibly pull anteriorly on the sizing tool, as this can result in undersizing and placement of a prosthesis that is too short. A sizing device is shown in Fig. 12.1. Once the length of the TE puncture tract has been determined, options related to the type and size of voice prosthesis[1] can be considered.

Following determination of length, the initial fitting of a voice prosthesis into the puncture will be performed (Graville et al, Chap. 11). As a general rule at our center, the patient will require five

---

[1] The reader should be aware that many varieties of TE puncture voice prostheses are commercially available, many of which have been designed with particular patient needs in mind.

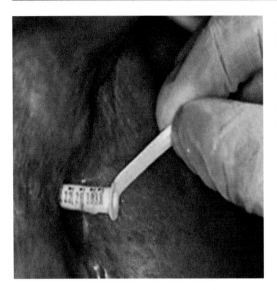

Fig. 12.1 Prosthesis sizer inserted within the TE puncture site. (Lengths in mm are provided on the sizing device).

total visits in the immediate postoperative period – the first for the initial placement of the voice prosthesis, with four additional speech pathology sessions for education and speech rehabilitation. During the subsequent treatment sessions, the prosthesis will require downsizing. As reduced edema of the TE tract is noted, the length of the prosthesis will likely need to be decreased.

When considering the type of prosthesis to be placed (indwelling or low pressure), characteristics such as the size of the tracheostoma, diameter of the esophageal lumen, and the patient's ease of access to a trained SLP are important factors. Regardless of prostheses selection, the average prosthesis life may typically be less than 3 months (Lewin et al., 2017); thus, the need for regular changes when devices fail must be emphasized to the patient.

Essentials in Educating the Patient About TE Voice Prosthesis Use

As noted in the previous chapter (Graville et al., Chap. 11), TE voice prostheses are made by various manufacturers; they are available as standard or low-pressure devices, or in either patient changeable or indwelling formats. The standard low-pressure prosthesis is available in various diameters (e.g., 16, 17, 20 French sizing); the length varies from 4 to 28 millimeters. All TE voice prostheses have a posterior and anterior retention collar, as well as a strap. While most prostheses have a one-way valve located within the cylinder of the prosthesis, the duckbill prosthesis does not. The low-pressure prosthesis is traditionally managed by the patient or the patient's caregiver; it is also generally considered to be less expensive than an indwelling-type voice prosthesis. The indwelling, patient-managed voice prosthesis may be considered for selected patients who do not have easy access to a trained SLP or healthcare facility knowledgeable in TE voice restoration. If the SLP deems the patient to be a good candidate to change their own voice prosthesis, several outpatient speech pathology sessions will usually be necessary in order to provide adequate education on use and maintenance.

The ultimate goal of these outpatient sessions seeks to ensure the patient's success with device placement, as well as instructing them relative to "self-troubleshooting" should problems occur with TE prosthesis use. Reports on the long-term use of TE speech have revealed a considerable range of success that varies between 50% and 95% (Op de Coul et al., 2000; Ramírez, Doménech, Durbán, Llatas, Ferriol, & Martínez, 2001; Mendenhall et al., 2002, and others). Therefore, TE speakers must be provided with clear and understandable details regarding their TE puncture and prosthesis safety and, most importantly, when to seek medical attention. Providing information to patients is essential in that knowledge about the TE puncture, the prosthesis, and what is normal and what is not will assist them in seeking professional assistance in order to reduce serious complications. In this regard, the first part of educating the patient begins at the time of initial postsurgical evaluation and the observations made during that visit.

Several essential issues must be addressed and emphasized with all patients who undergo a TE puncture. First, the clinician should instruct the patient regarding daily care and cleaning of the voice prosthesis in situ. Cleaning includes flushing water through the prosthesis, as well as placing the appropriate cleaning brush through the center of the prosthesis. They must also be trained in the correct use of tweezers to remove any dried mucus on the prosthesis and, in doing so, avoid damaging the device. The clinician also should instruct the patient regarding potential problems that may arise in the future, including the inability to achieve TE speech and/or leakage through or around the prosthesis. It is essential for the patient to understand issues related to the TE puncture itself, the prosthesis and its expected functioning, and accordingly, the ability to identify when a problem may be emerging. In the sections to follow, issues related to the evaluation of TE speech, baseline assessment of speech, and a review of common problems encountered and solutions to remedy these problems will be provided.

Evaluation of Tracheoesophageal Speech

Clinicians and patients usually anticipate the production of fluent and good quality TE speech after initial placement of the voice prosthesis. Unfortunately, this anticipation may at times meet with failure. When the patient is not successful at easily acquiring speech, the clinician should be knowledgeable about the types of problems that may occur and the necessary assessments and clinical solutions necessary to remedy the problem and facilitate TE speech. As part of this process, a number of clinical and instrumental evaluation procedures are available to assist the clinician with alaryngeal voice restoration. Thus, a systematic and structured approach to assessment is recommended, and this sequence will be presented in the subsequent section.

The Initial Baseline Assessment

Prior to the fitting and placement of the initial TE voice prosthesis, it is imperative that the clinician carefully assess the patient's baseline capacity for "open tract" TE voice production. That is, the patient must be able to produce voice through an open (no prosthesis inserted) TE puncture tract, once the stenting catheter is withdrawn. This is performed by asking the patient to swallow several times and then removing the catheter which has been inserted into the TE puncture. The request for swallowing is done to clear saliva secretions from the pharynx to avoid leakage of secretions into the airway through the unstented (open) TE puncture.

Once the catheter is removed, the patient is asked to inhale, and then the clinician will typically provide digital occlusion over the tracheostoma; an easy exhalation is then requested. The clinician will request the patient to exhale in order to initiate TE "voice" production. Digital occlusion of the tracheostoma will seal the airway and permit pulmonary air to move through the open puncture into the esophageal reservoir. The clinician should then instruct the patient to produce a vowel (typically /a/) and to sustain this TE phonation for as long as possible at a relatively normal level of loudness. The clinician may then ask the patient to count from one to ten or request production of simple sentences, etc. TE speech is considered "fluent" if the patient can sustain consistent TE voicing for greater than 10 s and achieve 10–15 syllables per breath; typically, fluent TE speech will be characterized by intraesophageal peak pressures that are less than 20 mmHg during objective esophageal insufflation (Lewin, Baugh, & Baker, 1987).

During these trials of initial voicing, the clinician should evaluate the overall "quality" and acceptability of TE voice production (Eadie & Doyle, 2004), as well as observe the amount of effort required for the patient to generate and maintain TE speech during exhalation. Once voicing is successfully achieved, then the next step in evaluation is the sizing of the TE tract. This is done by inserting a sizing device fully into the puncture and then withdrawing it anteriorly until the intraluminal collar on the sizing device is in contact with the anterior esophageal wall (Graville et al., Chap. 11). This will allow the clinician to identify the length of the tract from the sizing device.[2] Once the TE tract has been sized,

---

[2] As shown in Fig. 12.1, lengths in mm, are provided on the sizing device.

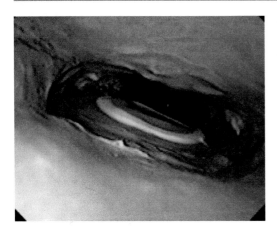

Fig. 12.2 Endoscopic view of an indwelling TE puncture voice prosthesis

the clinician will determine the type and diameter of voice prosthesis to be inserted (Graville et al., Chap. 11). The next step in the fitting process is to insert the selected TE voice prosthesis into the puncture site. However, the most critical component of the clinician's fitting is ensuring that the esophageal retention collar (regardless of prosthesis type or the manufacturer) is fully deployed within the esophageal lumen (Fig. 12.2). Blom, Singer, and Hamaker (1998) have provided considerable details on the procedural process of correct sizing and fitting of the TE voice prosthesis.

Following sizing and initial placement of the TE prosthesis, the clinician will next instruct the patient to occlude the tracheostoma. This will be achieved by using the pad of the patient's thumb, index finger, or middle finger, depending on the diameter of the tracheostoma. In seeking to achieve manual closure of the airway, the clinician should consider general mobility issues given potential limitations in upper extremity dexterity following laryngectomy (see Boulougouris & Doyle, Chap. 23). If the patient has difficulty with occluding the tracheostoma, the clinician may choose to do this for them in order to assess voicing with the prosthesis in place. As was done during the baseline open tract assessment, the clinician should listen to and assess the fluency and overall quality of TE speech, as well as identify how much effort is required to generate speech. At

the time of the initial TE prosthesis fitting, TE speech should closely mimic that which the patient achieved with open tract phonation. It is, however, important to note that speech produced with a prosthesis in place will require additional respiratory effort due to the increase resistance provided by the device relative to open tract voicing, and minor changes in quality will occur (Bunting, 2004).

Following placement of the voice prosthesis, if TE speech does not closely approximate open tract speech, the clinician should begin to systematically move through a series of problem-solving tasks. The first of these tasks seeks to confirm that the prosthesis has been properly inserted into the TE tract. If the prosthesis has not been completely inserted, voicing will be difficult to produce; in such instances the prosthesis may need to be removed and reinserted, resized, and potentially replaced entirely. Nonfluency or the complete absence of TE speech production will require further evaluation.

Nonfluency of TE Speech or Aphonia

If the patient demonstrates nonfluency or immediate post-fitting aphonia following initial prosthesis placement, the clinician should consider the following possibilities to identify the cause and alleviate the problem.

1. If the patient has also reported dysphagia, the clinician should consider an objective evaluation of swallowing (i.e., modified barium swallow). If the patient demonstrates an esophageal stricture, a narrow esophageal lumen, or other anatomical abnormality of the esophagus, the fluency of TE speech can be impacted.

2. If the prosthesis was placed using a gel cap, a portion of the cap could remain attached to the posterior portion of the prosthesis. If this occurs, the ability to move air through the prosthesis will be restricted. To further determine if some residual gel cap may be present,

the clinician should gently attempt to manually open the voice prosthesis valve by inserting a cotton-tipped applicator or brush into the prosthesis. Care must be taken to ensure that the applicator tip or cleaning brush is not aggressively inserted too far into the prosthesis; the goal of this task is to confirm that the internal value within the prosthesis is functional (i.e., not stuck as a by-product the gel cap or due to manufacturing).

3. The clinician should then evaluate the amount of force that the patient is applying to the tracheostoma during digital occlusion. If too much force is applied, the posterior portion of the prosthesis may contact the posterior esophageal wall, which may then impede efficient airflow through the prosthesis which is required to insufflate the esophagus. The clinician should reinforce the concept of light digital occlusion from the very first session. While such concerns may exist in those who use digital closure for voicing, this type of problem may also be observed in those who use a heat and moisture exchange (HME) device (Lewis, Chap. 8). The clinician should consider trial use of various styles of the cassette filter. An HME that requires light finger occlusion (Figs. 12.3a, b) versus one that requires increased digital pressure to close it may alleviate force against the prosthesis, thus allowing easier airflow through the prosthesis.

4. Ensure that the patient is not immediately swallowing prior to the initiation of TE speech. Doing so may impede the flow of air through the esophagus. A period of brief rest between voicing trials is often helpful if this concern is suspected.

5. Anatomical changes secondary to surgery can result in nonfluent TE speech. For example, significant postoperative edema can result in either complete aphonia or various degrees of nonfluency. When this type of edema is observed or suspected, the clinician should cease TE voicing attempts and schedule the patient for reassessment in 5–7 days. In many instances, this brief period of deferral may allow for edema to resolve so that voicing can be achieved.

6. Finally, if the patient demonstrates persistent aphonia or nonfluency approximately 2 weeks following initial placement of the TE voice prosthesis, hypertonicity of the pharyngoesophageal segment should be suspected. The clinician should evaluate the patient through use of esophageal insufflation testing (Lewin et al., 1987). If pharyngoesophageal segment spasm is suspected (Doyle & Eadie, 2005), one approach to its remediation is through use of a Botox® injection (Lewin, Bishop-Leone, Forman, & Diaz, 2001). A brief summary of the protocol for this procedure is provided in the following section.

Evaluation for Hypertonicity or "Spasm" of the Pharyngoesophageal Segment

Hypertonicity is defined as excess tone of the pharyngeal constrictor muscles. It is widely agreed that the alaryngeal voice source used during TE speech is generated by tissues that comprise what is termed the pharyngoesophageal (PE) segment (Diedrich, 1968; Doyle, 1994; Doyle & Eadie,

Fig. 12.3 (**a**) Blom-Singer® Humidifilter holder and replacement foam filters (not pictured). (Images courtesy of InHealth Technologies©). (**b**) Provox® HME. (With permission of ©Atos Medical AB and Chris Edghill)

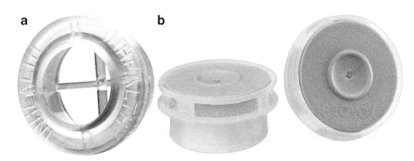

2005). Involuntary contraction or airflow-induced spasm of these muscles will interfere with the egress of air through the esophagus and pharynx, resulting in an effortful, strained, and nonfluent TE speech. In some instances, TE voice cannot be initiated at all. If PE spasm is suspected, performing an esophageal insufflation test will be necessary for the clinician to objectively identify and confirm this suspicion. In addition, esophageal insufflation testing may provide baseline measurements which could serve to predict outcomes of TE speech. In cases where a secondary TE puncture is being considered, insufflation testing allows both the patient and the clinician with the opportunity to hear TE speech before a puncture is performed.

Esophageal air insufflation testing can be performed using two methods: (1) objective esophageal air insufflation (Lewin et al., 1987) or (2) through self-insufflation testing (Blom, Singer, & Hamaker, 1985). Objective air insufflation can be performed in individuals who have undergone a total laryngectomy with primary closure. The evaluation can be performed as a *transnasal* procedure (through the nose) if the patient does not yet have a TE puncture (Fig. 12.4), or by using a *transtracheal* procedure if a TE puncture is present (Fig. 12.5).

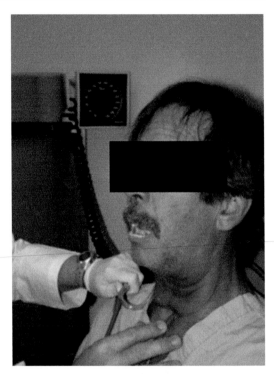

Fig. 12.5 Objective intraesophageal insufflation test, transtracheal approach through the TE puncture site

Objective Esophageal Insufflation

Objective esophageal insufflation testing involves several steps and a standard assessment procedure provided in the subsequent section is recommended.

1. Initially, a size 14 French rubber catheter is placed through the nares; it is then inserted to a distance of 23–25 cm from the tip of the nose. If the catheter is placed using a transtracheal approach through the puncture site, the catheter should be placed through the length of the TE tract and into the esophageal lumen. Regardless of method, the opposite end of the catheter is secured to a separate controllable air source. With the use of a "Y" connector, the additional port is secured to a pressure manometer.
2. Once the catheter is positioned, a three-liter volume of air is passed through the catheter.

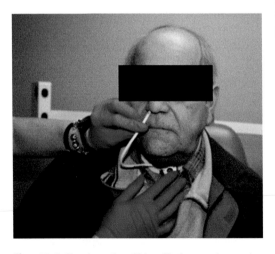

Fig. 12.4 Esophageal self-insufflation testing using Blom-Singer® insufflation test manufactured by InHealth® Technologies (Carpinteria, CA)

The patient is instructed to open their mouth and passively sustain TE phonation for approximately 10 s. The clinician must ensure that the patient understands what they are to do in this task. The patient must understand that voicing will be driven through the use of an external air source that will fill the esophageal reservoir. The clinician should then determine the peak intraesophageal pressure through a direct reading of the manometer when voicing is achieved. This assessment procedure should be performed three times, with measures noted for all trials.

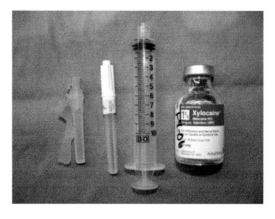

Fig. 12.6 Lidocaine, syringe, and needle for pharyngeal plexus block

Patients who demonstrate low intraesophageal peak pressure measurements, specifically those that are <20 mm Hg, have been shown to generate fluent TE speech (Lewin et al., 1987).

Self-Insufflation Testing

Self-insufflation testing also can be performed using the InHealth™ self-insufflation kit. Using this system, the catheter is placed transnasally and positioned at a distance of 23–25 cm from the tip of the nares. The opposite end of the catheter is secured over the patient's tracheostoma with use of a standard peristomal attachment. The patient is then instructed to digitally occlude the opening on the peristomal attachment during exhalation. In doing so, the sealing of the airway will shunt airflow through the catheter into the esophagus, and voicing can occur. Again, the patient must understand the task, as well as the sequence of TE voice production. Once voice production occurs, the clinician should perceptually evaluate the fluency and quality of TE voice and speech.

Based on the results of the esophageal insufflation test, and if the clinician suspects PE spasm, they should contact a physician to consider performing a lidocaine block of the pharyngeal plexus which serves muscles in this region (Hamaker & Blom, 2003a, 2003b; Terrell, Lewin, & Esclamado,

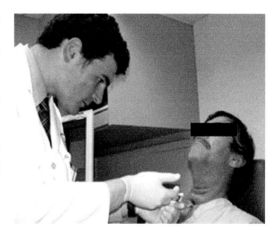

Fig. 12.7 Lidocaine block of pharyngeal plexus

1995). In this process, the physician injects 1% lidocaine into the tissue plane in the region of the pharyngeal constrictors. Each injection of lidocaine typically consists of a volume of 1–3 cc (Fig. 12.6). The injections are directed by the physician lateral and superior to the stoma in order to provide blockage of the neural signals (Fig. 12.7). Following the lidocaine injection, insufflation testing should be repeated. If the patient demonstrates improved fluency and if decreased peak intraesophageal pressures are noted, the clinician can assume that the patient exhibits PE spasm. This determination will then serve to identify the patient as a likely candidate for Botox® injection in order to facilitate fluent TE speech.

Botox Injection Protocol

If nonfluent TE speech is observed and other factors are ruled out, PE segment spasm may be present. In such circumstances, the following protocol may be pursued (Lewin, 2001). Initially, the patient should be evaluated under videofluoroscopy as part of a modified barium swallow (MBS) study. With the patient seated in the oblique view, they should be presented with stock barium to coat the neopharyngeal structures, as well as the posterior portion of the voice prosthesis. Next, the patient should be instructed to digitally occlude the stoma and attempt to initiate TE voicing during production of a sustained vowel. The clinician should be able to visualize the PE segment and the presence of potential spasm. The clinician will then mark both the inferior and superior borders of the anatomical region of the spasm on the image obtained (Fig. 12.8). It is often helpful to use radiology "nipple markers," as these markers are easily visualized under fluoroscopy and/or if the markings of the PE spasm need to be adjusted.

The SLP identification of the area of PE spasm will assist the physician during the Botox™ injection procedure. Increased accuracy of Botox® injection is attained when electromyography (EMG) is utilized during the procedure. Because of the nature of Botox® and its influence on muscle, the patient should follow up with speech pathology approximately 2 weeks after the injection for a repeated esophageal insufflation test. Following Botox® injec-

tion, peak intraesophageal pressures should be decreased, and the patient should demonstrate improved TE speech fluency. At the time of follow-up evaluation, it is possible that TE voicing will continue to be nonfluent; however, a noticeable improvement in voicing should be observed. Thus, careful pre-Botox® injection baseline measures are essential for comparative purposes.

Troubleshooting Fluent, but "Different" TE Speech

At times, some patients may present with fluent TE speech; however, their voice quality can be tight, effortful, wet, or breathy, all of which can impact one's ability to communicate effectively. In such circumstances, the following information may provide guidance on the assessment, identification, and potential remediation of these observed TE voice and speech characteristics. Results from the literature have noted that voice quality ratings range from fair to excellent in a majority of those who use TE speech (Eadie & Doyle, 2002, 2004; Op de Coul et al., 2000; and others).

Tight/Effortful TE Voice and Speech When a patient demonstrates fluent TE speech but the vocal quality is judged to be tight and/or there appears to be an excess amount of physical effort necessary to produce speech, the patient should be evaluated for a potential esophageal stricture or narrow esophageal lumen. In all instances where a stricture or narrowing is suspected, the evaluation should consist of an MBS study. During this evaluation the patient should be presented with stock barium, puréed, and solid consistencies. The patient should be seated in oblique view for the clinician to visualize the TE voice prosthesis and to confirm that the posterior portion of the prosthesis is fully positioned within the esophageal lumen. Patients should be instructed to attempt TE speech during this exam. The radiologist and SLP should attempt to rule out anatomical narrowing of the esophageal lumen. However, if the patient demonstrates an

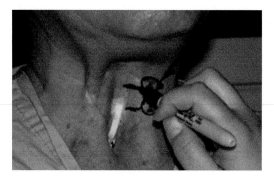

Fig. 12.8 Identifiation of hypertonic PE segment and marking with radiopaque nipple markers and pen

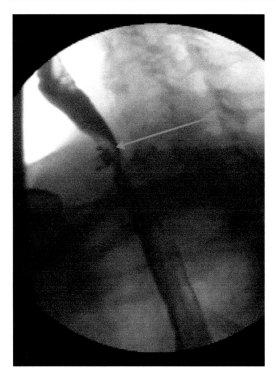

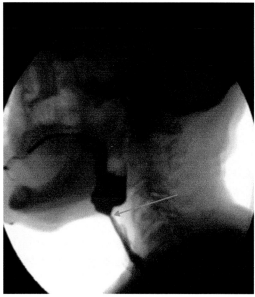

Fig. 12.10 Radiographic image of an esophageal stricture (arrow)

Fig. 12.9 Radiographic image of narrow esophageal lumen (arrow)

esophageal stricture and/or a narrow esophageal lumen (Fig. 12.9), the clinician will observe delayed bolus transit through the region of narrowing, as well as bolus residue located superior to the stricture/narrowing (Fig. 12.10). In most instances, the TE voice produced will sound wet and "gurgly" and may coexist with perceptual judgments of increased effort during voice production. Based on the MBS evaluation, if an esophageal stricture and/or narrowing of the lumen is observed, the patient should be referred to a gastroenterologist to consider candidacy for esophageal dilation.

Management Approaches for Esophageal Stricture or Narrowing

Several clinical options exist for managing the TE voice prosthesis and voice production in patients who have objectively demonstrated an esophageal stricture or narrow esophageal lumen.

If a stricture or esophageal narrowing is identified, the following approaches may be useful.

1. The clinician can increase the diameter of the voice prosthesis to a larger size, for example, upsizing the prosthesis to a 20 or 22.5 French device. Another prosthetic option would be for the clinician to consider a voice prosthesis that does not have a hood on the posterior flange. The presence of a hood may contribute to obstruction of the esophageal lumen, reducing airflow through this region.

2. The clinician may consider using a heat moisture exchange (HME) filter that does not require digital closure (pushing) of the HME to generate TE speech (see Lewis, Chap. 8). Excess amounts of pressure against the voice prosthesis secondary to airway closure through the HME can obstruct airflow into the esophageal lumen with a direct influence on voice and speech quality.

3. Similarly, the clinician should avoid the use of a TE voice prosthesis that has increased resistance to airflow as this will also increase the expiratory effort required for the production of TE speech (Searl, Chap. 13).

Hypotonic/Breathy TE Speech When a patient demonstrates fluent TE speech but their vocal quality sounds weak or "breathy," the patient is considered to demonstrate PE segment "hypotonicity." Hypotonicity is defined as a lack of or reduction in the tonicity of the PE segment which serves as the alaryngeal "neoglottis." Because of this limitation in muscular tonicity, there often will be poor contact between the mucosal walls of the esophagus (Hilgers, van As-Brooks, Polak, & Bing, 2006). A hypotonic PE segment *will not* provide adequate tissue approximation for generation of adequate TE speech.

Some patients who demonstrate a breathy TE vocal quality, most notably when it occurs early in the rehabilitation process, may improve with use over time. It is possible that with native pharyngeal muscle present, increased use of the muscular tube will result in increased tone and strength of the vibrating muscle itself, thus, improving TE speech. As an analogy, this is similar to the physical exercise that improves muscle tone of the biceps or triceps. However, in patients with reconstruction utilizing outside tissue that is not comprised of muscle, it is unlikely that tone will change; hence, the quality of TE voice may not improve despite extended practice. There may be improvement noted in the quality of TE speech in patients with or without reconstruction, simply as the patient becomes more familiar with the method of TE speech. Thus, understanding anatomy and physiology and the relationship of a variety of surgical factors is important to many clinical problem-solving procedures.

Breathy TE speech may be associated with reduced vocal volume. In those cases, the clinician should consider compensatory strategies to improve the overall quality and volume of TE speech. One clinical approach involves the use of a pressure band which is placed around the neck, superior to the tracheostoma. A pressure band is comprised of elastic material that is positioned around the patient's neck with a secondary object secured to the elastic to provide a focal "pressure point" (Fig. 12.11). Often, patients or clinicians will fabricate their own pressure band with the

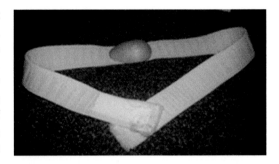

Fig. 12.11 Pressure band used for patients with hypotonic TE speech

use of objects including a small wooden bead, marble, etc. Regardless of structure, the pressure band is used to generate a relatively light degree of pressure to a specific region when attached to the neck, carefully avoiding over-constriction of the carotid arteries. The clinician and patient will need to work cooperatively to search for the best position for pressure to be applied, as well as to determine the level of pressure required. This often requires a trial and error approach that is not dissimilar to efforts used when seeking to identify the "sweet spot" for use of a transcervical electrolarynx (Doyle, 2005).

Finally, turning the patient's head to one side or another can improve the consistency of PE segment vibration. If that occurs, an improvement in the loudness of TE speech may also be observed. In either case, practice is essential so that the patient can be as consistent as possible in the use of this approach. However, it is also important to mention that when these types of maneuvers are used, they may also have indirect and potentially negative effects on the overall act of communication (Evitts, Chap. 28). Thus, the relative benefits/limitations of particular approaches to improving voice must always be considered. Similarly, excessive compensation by the speaker also may result in negative changes to TE voice quality.

In the case of perceived vocal strain and increased effort during the generation of TE voice, the patient may be seeking to overcome the lack of tonicity by increasing expiratory force as a compensation for the reduced loudness of the

TE voice signal. It is important to note, however, that the observed tightness/effort is compensatory as opposed to the patient exhibiting a structurally hypertonic PE segment. Although it does not occur in all cases, hypotonic TE speech is often associated with patients who have had an extended laryngectomy with the resection involving partial or circumferential reconstruction of the pharynx (see Yeh et al., Chap. 2).

Tracheoesophageal Puncture in Extended Laryngectomy with Reconstruction

Careful patient selection is necessary when considering potential candidates for a TE puncture, particularly in those who have undergone an extended laryngectomy with reconstruction (Sahovaler et al., Chap. 1). By description, an extended laryngectomy would include individuals who have undergone a partial or circumferential pha ryngeal reconstruction, laryngectomy with extension into the esophagus, and/or patients who have undergone a laryngopharyngectomy and/or glossectomy. While reconstruction of the tongue, oropharynx, and/or esophagus is not a uniform contraindication for consideration of a TE puncture, the patient should be educated regarding the potential risks associated with a primary or secondary puncture and potential issues that may negatively influence post-TE puncture outcomes. This would include discussion of reduced speech intelligibility and potential premature leakage around and/or through the voice prosthesis. Leakage through and/or around the voice prosthesis can result in chronic aspiration and require frequent appointments with an SLP to rectify such problems.

Issues related to speech intelligibility should also be carefully considered and discussed directly with the patient and family members (see Constantinescu & Rieger, Chap. 16; Doyle, Chap. 17). Similarly, if the patient did not receive a primary TE puncture and is considering one as a secondary procedure, the clinician should perform esophageal insufflation testing. This will allow the patient and family members to have the opportunity to hear what TE speech sounds like prior to undertaking the surgical procedure. Due to the potential for "amotility" of the neopharynx following reconstructive flap procedures and its potential impact on swallowing, TE speech may be characterized by a range of voice qualities. For example, in some instances following flap reconstruction, one may observe TE speech to be with a wet, aperiodic vocal quality. In contrast, in the presence of free-flap reconstruction of the pharynx and the variability of vibration of the flap, TE voice may also at times be characterized as having a breathy and/or somewhat inconsistent voice quality (Lewin et al., 2005).

A laryngectomy may include additional resection of structures that are critical to speech production. In cases when the patient has also undergone a total glossectomy in addition to laryngopharyngectomy, not only will the quality of TE voice be affected, but articulatory precision is also likely to be impacted. These postsurgical deficits may be persistent and substantially challenging not only to aspects of speech intelligibility, but also to one's overall well-being (Doyle, Chap. 26). In such instances, changes in both speech intelligibility and more variable changes in voice quality may be observed. In combination, deficits in these areas of voice and speech can create substantial challenges for the listener. These patients should be counselled preoperatively that their intelligibility will be impacted and that communication with others may be problematic.

In some cases, patients may find greater success in their attempts to communicate with family and familiar listeners; these listeners may not only "learn" how to listen, but they may also be more willing to seek repetitions and clarifications when they do not understand. Communication with an unknown listener would likely be perceived as less intelligible and that overall communication may be significantly disrupted. Although the clinician does not wish to provide information to the patient that is discouraging, the patient must understand the very real potential for changes in voice and speech and its larger impact on communication.

Leakage through and around the Voice Prosthesis

Premature leakage through and around the TE voice prosthesis is the most common challenge with this alaryngeal voice option. When leakage occurs, it can lead to a reduction in long-term patient satisfaction (Op de Coul et al., 2000). For that reason, several issues related to leakage will be addressed.

Leakage through the Prosthesis Due to Biofilm Early leakage through a voice prosthesis is a common problem for the laryngectomized individual. Although the average life of a voice prosthesis varies, most data suggest that patients should expect to achieve only 2–3 months of wear before the prosthesis begins to leak (Lewin et al., 2017; Op de Coul et al., 2000). Leakage can occur through the prosthesis due to the presence of microbial colonization or increased negative intraesophageal pressure during speech/swallowing. It is, therefore, necessary for the SLP to be aware of the potential cause of premature leakage in order to correctly identify this problem and appropriately manage the complication.

Gitomer et al. (2016) revealed that 83% of patients at MD Anderson Cancer Center who had undergone a total laryngectomy with TE puncture had experienced complications. The most commonly reported problem was the leakage of liquids through the voice prosthesis (28%), which in turn caused aspiration during swallowing. However, prosthesis device life was not found to differ in relation to the type of surgical closure, presence of free-flap reconstruction, or radiation, or the type, diameter, or length of the prosthesis (Lewin et al., 2017).

Biofilm (bacterial or fungal strains) can grow on the posterior portion of the voice prosthesis, preventing a complete seal of the valve within the prosthesis. Due to this incomplete seal, when the patient drinks, liquids may leak through the prosthesis. The development of biofilm is likely the result of contaminants in the oral cavity that are swallowed and/or reflux (Cardoso & Chambers, Chap. 21) and subsequently make contact along

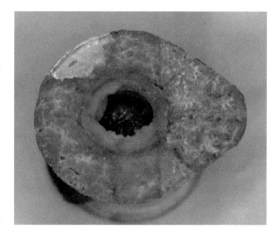

Fig. 12.12 Microbial colonization of TE voice prosthesis

the posterior portion of the prosthesis. Over time, colonization grows onto the prosthesis, and its lifespan may be reduced (van der Mei et al., 2014); an illustration of this type of biofilm formation is shown in Fig. 12.12.

Historically, clinicians have considered the presence of biofilm to be a result of "yeast" colonization. As a result, it was recommended that those with observed fungal colonization should begin an "…indefinite protocol of Nystatin oral suspension BID", being asked to "swish in the mouth for 3 min" (Leder & Erskine, 1997, p. 492). Within the last several years, the importance of determining the type of microbial species and strain by using culture and sensitivity testing has been realized. In the case of bacterial strains, it is critical to know which antibiotic will be effective against a particular pathogen causing the problem. Culture and sensitivity testing provides objective information to inhibit the growth of the pathogen. Results of biofilm analyses often indicate the presence of mixed contamination on the prosthesis, including both fungal and bacterial strains. Consequently, traditional antifungal rinses may no longer solely eradicate colonization on the prosthesis (Somogyi-Ganss, Chambers, Lewin, Tarrand, & Hutcheson, 2017).

Manufacturers currently provide a variety of antifungal and antimicrobial prostheses for patients. For example, modifying the physiochemical properties of the surface of the prosthesis has been undertaken in an effort to reduce the force of attraction between the microorganisms and the surface of the biomaterial. If microorganisms cannot easily attach to a prosthesis, the potential for a longer device life may result. Some prosthetic valves are coated with silver oxide to reduce this attraction (Kress, Schäfer, & Schwerdtfeger, 2006); however, not all microbes are susceptible to silver oxide. It is helpful to consider the type of colonization on the prosthesis prior to selecting a "specialty" prosthesis for the patient. The patient should be informed of the technique for proper cleaning of the prosthesis, as well as the tracheostoma and mouth; doing so may inhibit the growth of microorganisms in the airway and vocal tract that could adhere to the TE voice prosthesis and reduce its functional lifespan.

There has been longstanding clinical discussion about the use of probiotics with the goal of extending prosthesis life and preventing the growth of biofilm in those who use a TE voice prosthesis. Unfortunately, the evidence appears to be somewhat anecdotal without sufficient scientific support to confidently recommend use of supplemental probiotics for this purpose. Despite the lack of evidence, some patients may find the consumption of probiotics to be helpful. However, it is important to note that use of probiotics does not appear to have any detrimental effects on prosthesis life.

Finally, the presence of esophageal reflux has also been reported to be associated with decreased prosthetic life (Cocuzza et al., 2012). In some cases, reflux management may be beneficial.

Leakage through the Prosthesis Due to Increased Intraesophageal Pressure In recent years, there has been an increased focus on other factors that might contribute to early prosthesis failure, particularly in relation to increased intraesophageal pressures. Such increases in pressure have been suspected by some to cause inadvertent opening of the prosthetic valve during swallowing or upon inspiration (Hilgers et al., 2003). If this is the case, the suspicion is that higher esophageal pressures may place greater stresses on the prosthesis valve which may influence its valving capacity. If the internal valve is disrupted and loses the ability to "spring" back to a closed position, over

time this will limit its full closure resulting in leakage. Patients who demonstrate premature leakage through the prosthesis due to increased intraesophageal pressure will typically report intermittent leakage when drinking. The patient may also report bloating or gastric filling, an indication that intraesophageal pressures are excessive.

Other swallowing-related problems such as pharyngoesophageal stricture, structural abnormalities, or surgical consequences such as a pseudo-epiglottis or a narrow esophageal lumen, may also adversely impact pressure gradients in the pharyngoesophagus during swallowing. If this situation occurs, it may contribute to early leakage through the prosthesis because of increased negative pressures. As such, a modified barium swallow study is often indicated to determine the efficiency of the system. Leakage through the prosthesis, as a result of increased negative intraesophageal pressure, can be eliminated by fitting the patient with a prosthesis which has a higher valve opening resistance or what is termed "cracking" pressure. However, a prosthesis with higher resistance to airflow will likely increase the effort required for TE speech.

Leakage around the prosthesis Leakage around the prosthesis can be a more difficult problem to control. This may be a result of excessive prosthesis length (Fig. 12.13), but it can also be due to an enlarged TE puncture as shown in Fig. 12.14 (Hutcheson, Lewin, Sturgis, Kapadia, & Risser, 2011a). With the rising incidence of salvage laryngectomy after chemoradiation failure, there is an associated increase in leakage around the prosthesis (Starmer et al., 2009). Clinicians must understand the most current clinical research on etiologies of leakage in order to determine the most appropriate solutions for these challenges. The savvy clinician must take a systematic approach to determine which prosthetic option is best suited to each individual patient. Understanding prosthetic options will likely minimize costs, reduce complications and patient frustration, and ultimately, facilitate improved outcomes.

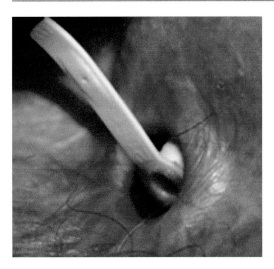

Fig. 12.13 TE voice prosthesis that has been overfitted relative to length

These factors include advanced nodal disease at time of diagnosis, postlaryngectomy stricture, locoregional recurrence, or distant metastasis following total laryngectomy, preoperative or postoperative radiation, extended surgical resection/reconstruction, total laryngopharyngectomy, and nutritional deficiencies (Hutcheson & Lewin, 2012). The literature reports several treatment options to eliminate leakage around the voice prosthesis.

For example, if leakage is observed, the patient may require (1) a special length prosthesis or use of a prosthesis with a larger posterior retention collar (Fig. 12.15) or (2) a custom, enlarged anterior and/or posterior retention collar (Fig. 12.16). Other types of specialty prostheses are also available for consideration (Figs. 12.17

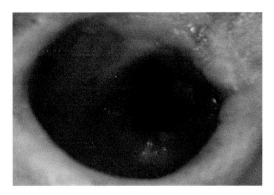

Fig. 12.14 Enlarged TE puncture site (note vertical orientation and expansion of tract)

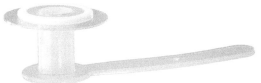

Fig. 12.15 Blom-Singer® large esophageal flange voice prosthesis. (Image courtesy of InHealth Technologies©)

Leakage around the prosthesis can be the result of an ill-fitting prosthesis (Blom et al., 1998) or as a result of the voice prosthesis being too long which allows "pistoning" of the device in the TE tract (Fig. 12.13). In these instances, the clinician should remove the voice prosthesis, resize the TE tract, and replace the original device with a shorter voice prosthesis.

The enlarged TEP can be very challenging for the SLP to manage. An enlarged puncture site may be the result of poor tissue integrity resulting in a poor seal around the voice prosthesis leading to leakage (Fig. 12.14). Research from MD Anderson has revealed several risk factors for enlargement of the TE puncture tract.

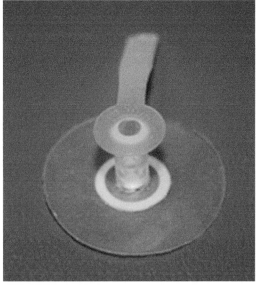

Fig. 12.16 Blom-Singer® classic indwelling voice prosthesis with custom enlarged esophageal flange. (Image courtesy of InHealth Technologies©)

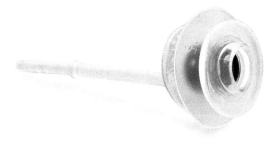

Fig. 12.17 Provox® Xtra Flange™ voice prosthesis. (With permission of ©Atos Medical AB and Chris Edghill)

Fig. 12.18 Provox® Vega™ XtraSeal™ voice prosthesis. (With permission of ©Atos Medical AB and Chris Edghill)

and 12.18). In some instances, particularly when leakage around the prosthesis is substantial, the surgeon may provide a local injection (i.e., Cymetra™, Radiesse™ gel, Prolaryn™) around the enlarged puncture tract in an effort to better seal the puncture site around the prosthesis.

If leakage occurs, the patient may benefit from consuming thickened liquids as they may be less likely to leak around the prosthesis. If leakage is substantial, the potential for airway risks may be increased, and the patient may require a temporary or permanent feeding tube. Lastly, if significant problems exist with leakage around the prosthesis, a combination of approaches may be necessary in order to eliminate the problem (Hutcheson, Lewin, Sturgis, & Risser, 2011b). However, the clinician should be cautious in placing a larger diameter prosthesis, as this may increase the risk for further enlargement of the TEP. Finally, underlying swallowing dysfunction should be evaluated and, if present, addressed for effective management of leakage around the prosthesis.

Conclusions

Tracheoesophageal (TE) puncture voice restoration is currently a widely used method of post-laryngectomy speech rehabilitation. The TE puncture voice restoration procedure has transformed rehabilitation for patients who undergo total laryngectomy by providing another communication option. Data from the literature show a range of successful long-term use of TE speech, but the likelihood of success is increased with comprehensive care and thorough education and instruction provided by the clinician to the patient. Data also suggest that TE voice quality, while not normal, is associated with acceptable ratings when evaluated by listeners. However, TE voice restoration and post-puncture management have become increasingly complex within the last decade. Contemporary patients commonly present with complicated medical histories and extensive comorbidities that may influence the integrity of the TE puncture and, ultimately, successful TE speech production. These medical complexities often contribute to premature prosthesis failure, enlargement of the TE puncture, or other associated problems. For this reason, it is essential that the SLP who works with patients who have undergone a total laryngectomy with TE puncture is familiar with the current literature, as well as alternative management strategies should problems arise. Clinical expertise and familiarity are the key elements to facilitate success in those who undergo TE puncture for post-laryngectomy speech rehabilitation.

References

Blom, E. D., Singer, M. I., & Hamaker, R. C. (1985). An improved esophageal insufflation test. *Archives of Otolaryngology, 111*(4), 211–212.

Blom, E. D., Singer, M. I., & Hamaker, R. (Eds.). (1998). *Tracheoesophageal voice restoration following total laryngectomy*. San Diego, CA: Singular.

Bunting, G. M. (2004). Voice following laryngeal cancer surgery: Troubleshooting common problems after tracheoesophageal voice restoration. *Otolaryngology Clinics of North America, 37*, 597–612.

Cocuzza, S., Bonfiglio, M., Chiaramonte, R., Aprile, G., Mistretta, A., Grosso, G., & Serra, A. (2012). Gastroesophageal reflux disease and postlaryngectomy tracheoesophageal fistula. *European Archives of Oto-Rhino-Laryngology, 269*(5), 1483–1488.

Diedrich, W. M. (1968). The mechanism of esophageal speech. *Annals of the New York Academy of Sciences, 155*(1), 303–317.

Doyle, P. C. (1994). *Foundations of voice and speech rehabilitation following laryngeal cancer*. San Diego, CA: Singular.

Doyle, P. C. (2005). Clinical procedures for training use of the electronic artificial larynx. In P. C. Doyle & R. L. Keith (Eds.), *Contemporary considerations following treatment for head and neck cancer: Voice, speech, and swallowing*. Austin, TX: Pro-Ed Publishers.

Doyle, P.C., & Eadie, T. L. (2005). Pharyngoesophageal segment function: A review and reconsideration. Contemporary considerations in the treatment and rehabilitation of head and neck cancer: Voice, speech, and swallowing, 521–544

Eadie, T. L., & Doyle, P. C. (2002). Direct magnitude estimation and interval scaling of naturalness and severity in tracheoesophageal (TE) speakers. *Journal of Speech, Language, and Hearing Research, 45*(6), 1088–1096.

Eadie, T. L., & Doyle, P. C. (2004). Auditory-perceptual scaling and quality of life in tracheoesophageal speakers. *Laryngoscope, 114*(4), 753–759.

Gitomer, S. A., Hutcheson, K. A., Christianson, B. L., Samuelson, M. B., Barringer, D. A., Roberts, D. B., … Zafereo, M. E. (2016). Influence of timing, radiation, and reconstruction on complications and speech outcomes with tracheoesophageal puncture. *Head & Neck, 38*(12), 1765–1771.

Hamaker, R. C., & Blom, E. D. (2003a). Botulinum neurotoxin for pharyngeal constrictor muscle spasm in tracheoesophageal voice restoration. *Laryngoscope, 113*(9), 1479–1482.

Hamaker, R. C., & Blom, E. D. (2003b). Botulinum neurotoxin for pharyngeal constrictor muscle spasm in tracheoesophageal voice restoration. *Laryngoscope, 113*(9), 1479–1482.

Hilgers, F. J., Ackerstaff, A. H., Balm, A. J., Van Den Brekel, M. W., Bing Tan, I., & Persson, J. O. (2003). A new problem-solving indwelling voice prosthesis, eliminating the need for frequent Candida- and "underpressure"-related replacements: Provox ActiValve. *Acta Oto-laryngologica, 123*(8), 972–979.

Hilgers, F. J., van As-Brooks, C. J., Polak, R. M., & Bing, T. I. (2006). Surgical improvement of hypotonicity in tracheoesophageal speech. *Laryngoscope, 116*(2), 345–348.

Hutcheson, K. A., & Lewin, J. S. (2012). Multivariable analysis of risk factors for enlarged tracheoesophageal puncture after total laryngectomy. *Head & Neck, 34*, 557–567.

Hutcheson, K. A., Lewin, J. S., Sturgis, E. M., Kapadia, A., & Risser, J. (2011a). Enlarged tracheoesophageal puncture after total laryngectomy: a systematic review and meta-analysis. *Head & Neck, 33*(1), 20–30.

Hutcheson, K. A., Lewin, J. S., Sturgis, E. M., & Risser, J. (2011b). Outcomes and adverse events of enlarged tracheoesophageal puncture after total laryngectomy. *Laryngoscope, 121*(7), 1455–1461.

Kress, P., Schäfer, P., & Schwerdtfeger, F. P. (2006). Clinical use of a voice prosthesis with a flap valve containing silver oxide (Blom-Singer Advantage), biofilm formation, in-situ lifetime and indication. *Laryngo-rhino-otologie, 85*(12), 893–896.

Leder, S. B., & Erskine, M. C. (1997). Voice restoration after laryngectomy: Experience with the Blom–Singer extended-wear indwelling tracheoesophageal voice prosthesis. *Head & Neck, 19*(6), 487–493.

Lewin, J. S., Barringer, D. A., May, A. H., Gillenwater, A. M., Arnold, K. A., Roberts, D. B., & Yu, P. (2005). Functional outcomes after circumferential pharyngoesophageal reconstruction. *Laryngoscope, 115*(7), 1266–1271.

Lewin, J. S., Bishop-Leone, J. K., Forman, A. D., & Diaz, E. M. (2001). Further experience with Botox injection for tracheoesophageal speech failure. *Head & Neck, 23*(6), 456–460.

Lewin, J. S., Baugh, R. F., & Baker, S. R. (1987). An objective method for prediction of tracheoesophageal speech production. *Journal of Speech and Hearing Disorders, 52*, 212–217.

Lewin, J. S., Baumgart, L. M., Barrow, M. P., & Hutcheson, K. A. (2017). Device life of the tracheoesophageal voice prosthesis revisited. *JAMA Otolaryngology–Head & Neck Surgery, 143*(1), 65–71.

Noone, A.M., Howlader, N., Krapcho, M., Miller, D., Brest, A., Yu, M., Ruhl, J., Tatalovich, Z., Mariotto, A., Lewis, D.R., Chen, H.S., Feuer, E.J., & Cronin, K.A. (2018). Surveillance, Epidemiology, and End Results (SEER) Program Cancer Statistics Review, 1975-2015, National Cancer Institute. Bethesda, MD, https://seer.cancer.gov/csr/1975_2015/, based on November 2017 SEER data submission, posted to the SEER web site, April 2018.

Maddox, P. T., & Davies, L. (2012). Trends in total laryngectomy in the era of organ preservation. A population-based study. *Otolaryngology–Head & Neck Surgery, 147*(1), 85–90.

Mendenhall, W. M., Morris, C. G., Stringer, S. P., Amdur, R. J., Hinerman, R. W., Villaret, D. B., & Robbins, K. T. (2002). Voice rehabilitation after total laryngectomy and postoperative radiation therapy. *Journal of Clinical Oncology, 20*(10), 2500–2505.

Op de Coul, B. O., Hilgers, F. J. M., Balm, A. J. M., Tan, I. B., Van den Hoogen, F. J. A., & Van Tinteren, H. (2000). A decade of postlaryngectomy vocal rehabilitation in 318 patients: a single Institution's experience with consistent application of Provox indwelling voice prostheses. *Archives of Otolaryngology–Head & Neck Surgery, 126*(11), 1320–1328.

Ramírez, M. F., Doménech, F. G., Durbán, S. B., Llatas, M. C., Ferriol, E. E., & Martínez, R. L. (2001).

Surgical voice restoration after total laryngectomy: Long-term results. *European Archives of Oto-Rhino-Laryngology, 258*(9), 463–466

Singer, M. I., & Blom, E. D. (1980). Selective myotomy for voice restoration after total laryngectomy. *Archives of Otolaryngology, 107*(11), 670–673.

Somogyi-Ganss, E., Chambers, M. S., Lewin, J. S., Tarrand, J. J., & Hutcheson, K. A. (2017). Biofilm on the tracheoesophageal voice prosthesis: considerations for oral decontamination. *European Archives of Oto-Rhino-Laryngology, 274*(1), 405–413.

Starmer, H. M., Ishman, S. L., Flint, P. W., Bhatti, N. I., Richmon, J., Koch, W., … Gourin, C. G. (2009). Complications that affect postlaryngectomy voice restoration: Primary surgery vs salvage surgery. *Archives of Otolaryngology–Head & Neck Surgery, 135*(11), 1165–1169.

Surveillance, Epidemiology, and End Results (SEER) Cancer Facts (2018). https://seer.cancer.gov/statfacts/html/laryn.html

Terrell, J. E., Lewin, J. S., & Esclamado, R. (1995). Botulinum toxin injection for postlaryngectomy tracheoesophageal speech failure. *Otolaryngology–Head and Neck Surgery, 113*(6), 788–791.

van der Mei, H. C., Buijssen, K. J., van der Laan, B. F., Ovchinnikova, E., Geertsema-Doornbusch, G. I., Atema-Smit, J., … Busscher, H. J. (2014). Voice prosthetic biofilm formation and Candida morphogenic conversions in absence and presence of different bacterial strains and species on silicone-rubber. *PLoS One, 9*(8), e104508.

Alaryngeal Speech Aerodynamics: Lower and Upper Airway Considerations

Jeff Searl

Speech aerodynamics that occur during alaryngeal speech are significantly different than those during laryngeal speech because of the separation of the lower from the upper airway. This chapter considers three factors that have the potential to impact alaryngeal speech aerodynamics. The first relates to alterations to the physiological function of the lower respiratory tract postlaryngectomy. The second set of factors to be addressed are those stemming from the alaryngeal voice source. The primary methods of alaryngeal voice and speech used after total laryngectomy, namely, esophageal (ES), tracheoesophageal (TE), and artificial larynx (AL) speech, have very distinct aerodynamic characteristics. Third, and finally, aerodynamic changes associated with production of consonants across the primary methods of alaryngeal speech options are reviewed.

J. Searl (✉)
Department of Communicative Sciences and Disorders, Michigan State University, East Lansing, MI, USA
e-mail: searljef@msu.edu

Function of the Lower Airway in People with a Laryngectomy

Histological and Physiological Changes After Laryngectomy

A wide range of changes in the lower respiratory tract are to be anticipated after total laryngectomy. These changes will occur at both histological and physiological levels. For many decades it has been known that the separation of the lower from the upper airway following total laryngectomy results in histological changes within the trachea that are indicative of chronic inflammation of the epithelium (Griffith & Friedberg, 1964; Rosso, Prgomet, Marjanović, Pušeljić, & Kraljik, 2015). Work by Hilgers and colleagues over many years has delineated the changes in the tracheal and lung environments that are induced by this disconnection between the upper and the lower airway (see Zuur, Muller, de Jongh, van Zandwijik, and Hilgers (2006) for a review; also see Bohnenkamp, Chap. 7, and Lewis, Chap. 8). Briefly, the epithelial irritation stems primarily from reduced warming and humidification of inspired air when breathing through an open tracheostoma. Reduced filtering of particles from the inspired air also can contribute to this tissue inflammation. As a result, irritation and drying of the epithelium results in increased mucus production (Rosso et al., 2015) and a diminished number and functioning of cilia in the tracheobronchial

© Springer Nature Switzerland AG 2019
P. C. Doyle (ed.), *Clinical Care and Rehabilitation in Head and Neck Cancer*,
https://doi.org/10.1007/978-3-030-04702-3_13

tree (Roessler, Grossenbacher, & Walt, 1988). If left unmanaged through the use of a HME, an increase in bacterial infections and bronchial obstruction that worsens over time may be expected to occur (Todisco, Maurizi, Paludetti, Dottorini, & Merante, 1984; van den Boer, van Harten, Hilgers, van den Brekel, & Retèl, 2014). These changes in the respiratory tract are the cause of a wide range of respiratory complaints that individuals with a laryngectomy self-report, such as a presence of excess phlegm and involuntary coughing (Hilgers, Ackerstaff, Aaronson, Schouwenburg, & Van Zandwijk, 1990).

Standard pulmonary measures obtained via spirometry have been used to quantify the physiological functioning of the respiratory system after total laryngectomy. Ackerstaff, Hilgers, Balm, and Van Zandwijk (1995) reported data for pulmonary measures in 58 individuals after total laryngectomy (median 2.9 years postsurgery). Total lung capacity, maximum vital capacity, forced expiratory volume, peak expiratory flow, and maximum expiratory flow at 50% were reduced relative to predicted values. The finding of reduced lung function by Ackerstaff et al. is consistent with reports in other studies of standard lung function after total laryngectomy (Harris & Jonson, 1974; Todisco et al., 1984).

In a subsequent study, Ackerstaff, Hilgers, Meeuwis, Knegt, and Weenink (1999) also found vital capacity and forced expiratory volumes were reduced when measured at 9 days after laryngectomy and again at 6 months postoperatively. The degree of pulmonary function reduction in this early time period was not as great as the reduction in pulmonary function that Ackerstaff et al. (1995) reported when data collection occurred much further out from the laryngectomy surgery (median of 2.9 years postsurgery). Ackerstaff et al. (1999) posited that respiratory changes after total laryngectomy may worsen as the time from surgery increases. Finally, the upper airway and in particular the nose and nasopharynx provide beneficial airway resistance that ultimately results in high arterial oxygen saturation as well as total lung volume (McRae, Young, Hamilton, & Jones, 1996). Several studies have reported that using a HME

results in an increase in tissue oxygen saturation levels (Ackerstaff et al., 2003; McRae et al., 1996; Jones et al., 2003). Overall, the literature supports the conclusion that there are substantial changes in the respiratory system after total laryngectomy.

Although the surgery itself may be a direct cause of pulmonary changes after total laryngectomy, it is also possible that lung function is degraded prior to the laryngectomy procedure. Smoking is a well-documented primary risk factor for laryngeal cancer (Sadri, McMahon, & Parker, 2006; Wynder, Bross, & Day, 1956; Wynder & Stellman, 1977). Approximately 80–85% of people who require total laryngectomy will either be former or current smokers (Achim et al., 2017; Goepfert et al., 2017). The percentage of people who continue to smoke after a total laryngectomy has ranged widely across studies from approximately 7% (Achim et al., 2017) to 30% (Goepfert et al., 2017). The large range of percentage of patients who continue to smoke that is reported across studies may be related to how far out from the surgery patients are queried. Eichler et al. (2016) reported that the percentage of people who continued to smoke immediately after surgery was approximately 22%, dropping to 7.5% at 3 months and eventually dropping to 3.8% at 3 years after surgery in a large German cohort study.

Regardless of whether a person was a former smoker or remains a smoker after total laryngectomy, the risk of respiratory disease is elevated. Chronic obstructive pulmonary disease (COPD) is known to be strongly associated with smoking (Centers for Disease Control and Prevention, 2017). Further, COPD in particular has been identified as a common condition among those who have had a total laryngectomy, occurring in about 80% of people who undergo the procedure (Hess, Schwenk, Frank, & Loddenkemper, 1999; Togawa, Konno, & Hoshino, 1980).

Even without respiratory disease, lung function is known to decline from approximately the fourth decade of life with a steeper slope of change presenting in the seventh decade (Zeleznik, 2003). Overall, the changes in pulmonary function that are observed after total laryngectomy are likely the sum of impacts from smoking prior to surgery, any associated lung disease that might have been caused by smoking, advancing age, and the direct impacts from surgery when the lower and upper airways are separated.

Impact of Lower Airway Changes on Alaryngeal Speech Aerodynamics

The impact that altered pulmonary function after total laryngectomy can have on an individual's quality of life is well documented (Dassonville et al., 2011; Hilgers, Aaronson, Ackerstaff, Schouwenburg, & van Zandwikj, 1991; Parrilla et al., 2015). The issue considered here is whether altered pulmonary health and baseline pulmonary functioning directly or indirectly impacts the aerodynamics of alaryngeal voice and speech production. Before discussing available literature on how lower airway function might directly impact the aerodynamics of ES, TE, and AL speech, a few indirect impacts from poor pulmonary health are presented in the subsequent section.

Indirect Impact of Pulmonary Status on Alaryngeal Speech

The indirect impacts that pulmonary disease might have on alaryngeal voice and speech are focused more broadly on the rehabilitation process rather than directly on alaryngeal speech aerodynamics. That is, the comorbidities of COPD, specifically fatigue, depression, and cognitive impairment, are of particular concern given that COPD occurs commonly in the total laryngectomy population (Hess et al., 1999). Fatigue has repeatedly been identified as a common complaint in people with COPD (Kentson et al., 2016; Stridsman, Mullerova, Skar, & Lindberg, 2013). In fact, fatigue has been described as the main extra pulmonary symptom of the disease (Antoniu & Ungureanu, 2015). In addition to possible fatigue associated with COPD, it is estimated that 40–90% of individuals with cancer who have been treated with chemoradiation experience cancer-related fatigue (CRF; Prue, Rankin, Allen, Gracey, & Cramp, 2006). Cancer-related fatigue is a complex of symptoms distinct from the fatigue that someone without cancer experiences because CRF usually lasts longer, does not improve with rest, results in significant distress, and is unpredictable relative to activity level (Gerber, 2017; Jereczek-Fossa et al., 2007; Medysky, Temesi, Culos-Reed, & Millet, 2017).

If the fatigue from COPD with or without CRF is substantial enough, rehabilitation attempts could be negatively impacted because a person is less able or willing to attend sessions or complete scheduled therapeutic activities. Thus, adherence to rehabilitation recommendations and demands may be influenced by the altered respiratory state (see Bohnenkamp, Chap. 7 and Lewis, Chap. 8). Indirectly, then, the ability to learn and use any of the alaryngeal communication methods could be reduced by the presence of fatigue from COPD, CRF, or both. For example, a person who only intermittently is able to keep scheduled treatment sessions with their therapist or who cannot practice with their new alaryngeal communication mode at home may show inconsistent, slow, or no progress in acquiring functional alaryngeal speech and voice. There could be a range of other potential impacts depending on the severity of the fatigue. In some cases, a person may not have the energy to perform the daily care of the stoma or the TE prosthesis, or they may lack the strength to maintain arm, shoulder, and head positions for practicing with an artificial larynx.

Depression among those who have had a total laryngectomy occurs at a rate higher than that of the general population (Batioğlu-Karaaltin, Binbay, Yiğit, & Dönmez, 2017; Perry, Casey, & Cotton, 2015). There are several factors that might cause depression in this patient population, including COPD (Lou et al., 2012; Ng, Niti, Fones, Yap, & Tan, 2009; Ng et al., 2007). Other factors associated with depression in people after laryngectomy include altered feelings regarding sex and sexuality (Batioğlu-Karaaltin et al., 2017), changes in physical appearance (Danker et al., 2010) and a shifting of family dynamics (Offerman, Pruyn, de Boer, Busschbach, &

Baatenburg de Jong, 2015). Depression, regardless of the cause(s), is known to reduce compliance with medical treatment regimens (DiMatteo, Lepper, & Croghan, 2000). A person who is depressed may have decreased motivation to attend treatment sessions, less energy to practice alaryngeal communication skills, and less desire to interact with others, thereby impacting the acquisition and improvement in using any alaryngeal communication method.

Aspects of cognitive function are known to decline as a person ages whether or not they have COPD. For example, age-related declines have been reported for attentional control, working memory, and cognitive processing speed (Edelstein, Pergolizzi, & Alici, 2016). A diagnosis of cancer appears to be associated with further risk of cognitive decline. Dubruille et al. (2015) reported that 46% of adults ≥65 years old who were diagnosed with cancer but had not started treatment demonstrated cognitive declines. Specific to people with head and neck cancer, Bond, Dietrich, and Murphy (2012) and Bond et al. (2016) reported neurocognitive impairment in 38–47% of patients prior to the start of cancer treatment. Furthermore, others have reported cognitive declines following chemoradiation treatments in people with head and neck cancer (e.g., Gan et al., 2011; Hsiao et al., 2010; Yuen et al., 2008). COPD is a further risk factor for cognitive decline to consider for a person with a laryngectomy. Individuals with COPD are now recognized as having a higher incidence of cognitive decline compared to their age-matched peers regardless of other medical diagnoses (Yohnnes, Chen, Moga, Leroi, & Connolly, 2017). Roncero et al. (2016) reported that 39% of 940 adults with COPD were determined to have cognitive impairment as documented on standardized testing. A meta-analysis by Zhang et al. (2016) concluded that those with COPD have a higher risk of cognitive decline compared to participants without COPD. Overall, these declines may not be the most debilitating aspect of a person's cancer treatment, but a clinician should be vigilant for potential impacts on the therapeutic process. For example, diminished working memory and speed of information processing might require that the

pace of providing instructions be altered and that information be provided in several formats (e.g., verbally, written, pictorial). Additional reminders may be needed to help the person complete practice at home. Assistance from others in the household might be needed to remember daily tasks such as charging of a backup AL battery, replacing an HME filter, and so forth. Of particular importance to the communication rehabilitation process are findings from Bond et al. (2012). They identified specific deficits in verbal learning and verbal memory in 99 head and neck cancer patients prior to treatment. In their follow-up study after the patients had undergone chemoradiation therapy (Bond et al., 2016), they reported that 13% had further declines in language domains of verbal fluency and verb retrieval. It is not known how severe those deficits were, but a treating SLP should be mindful that communication deficits could go beyond speech and voice. While language intervention may not take precedence over reestablishing alaryngeal voice and speech, the language deficits could manifest in communication exchanges or could require adjustments to account for reduced verbal memory skills.

Direct Impacts of Pulmonary Function on Alaryngeal Speech

Esophageal Speech

Esophageal speech production does not utilize pulmonary air to initiate voicing. As such, there is limited expectation of a mechanism by which poor pulmonary health or functioning will directly alter ES voice and speech aerodynamics. However, Ackerstaff et al. (2003) provide some data suggesting that improved pulmonary function through the use of an HME can positively influence dimensions of voice across ES, TE, and AL speech. Specifically, they reported that improvements occurred for the dimensions of loudness, intelligibility, and fluency in 59 patients with a laryngectomy who wore an HME regularly during the study. However, broad generalization to ES speech is tempered by the small proportion of the study population that used this method of speech (3 participants out of 59) and lack of description of outcomes per alaryngeal communication mode. However, as a general finding, the Ackerstaff et al. (2003) results indicated improvements in various dimensions of the voice for a heterogenous group of alaryngeal speakers, several for whom the voice source is not directly dependent on lung function, i.e., the 3 ES and 12 AL speech participants.

DiCarlo, Amster, and Herer (1955) investigated speech breathing during ES speech using kinematic measures of chest wall movements. Movements of the rib cage and abdomen were reduced in amplitude during ES speech, as was utterance length, compared to the laryngeal speaking participants. There was evidence that the ES participants judged to exhibit better speaking skills coordinated inspiration through the stoma with their attempt to insufflate the esophagus. Those who were less adept at ES speech demonstrated increased discoordination between these two events. It is difficult to definitively draw conclusions from the finding that ES speech skill level is related to how well a person coordinates inspiration with esophageal insufflation because details about the specific method of esophageal insufflation were not provided. A speculative conclusion is that those with more coordinated action between inspiration and insufflation were utilizing the "inhalation method" to get air into the esophagus. This method relies on respiratory movements to decrease air pressure in the esophagus (see Doyle & Finchem, Chap. 10). This would suggest that the inhalation method is associated with better ES speech skill and would be consistent with the following statement from Gardner (1971) regarding this insufflation method: "The speaker feels this as a sensation of sucking in air, as we all do with breathing. He naturally will believe that the inhalation method is the most natural and the easiest way of moving air into the esophagus" (p. 43). However, evidence from Deidrich and Youngstrom (1966) indicated that superior ES speech skill level is not dependent on the use of the insufflation method.

Additional information about respiratory activity during ES speech is limited. Stepp, Heaton, and Hillman (2008) provide the only other specific investigation of relevance. They investigated the pattern of speech breathing changes over several months and years in ES, TE, and AL speech. More specifically they were looking at the percentage of speaking time that occurred during the inspiratory portion of the breathing cycle. Larger percentages would suggest a dissociation occurring between talking and breathing relative to what happens in people without a laryngectomy for whom talking occurs almost exclusively on exhalation. One ES participant was included in Stepp et al. (2008) and that person's data were collapsed with data from the larger TE group for statistical purposes. However, Stepp et al. did include a figure that showed the ES speaker's data recorded at 5, 11, and 15 months postlaryngectomy. At 5 months postsurgery, this person had less than 5% of their total speaking time occurring during the inspiratory cycle. This increased to about 25% of speaking occurring during inspiration when the patient was seen at 10 months postsurgery and then 17% when last evaluated at the 15-month mark. Prudence dictates caution in over interpreting the results from one person. However, if there is a pattern of increased dissociation between speaking and breathing in ES speakers that occurs in the initial months after surgery, it will be important for researchers and clinicians to determine if this dissociation impacts ES speech proficiency. DiCarlo et al. (1955) suggest the possibility that retaining coordination between talking and breathing may be important for good ES speech, but the empirical literature is silent on the matter. At this point in time, there is not sufficient evidence to advocate for direct intervention to alter the relationship between breathing and ES talking unless within a given individual, the SLP can systematically observe and document how such intervention results in improved communication. When teaching the "inhalation method," it does make logical sense to insure respiratory-talking coordination. This is because the esophageal insufflation method relies on the inspiratory movement to assist in getting air to flow into the esophagus.

Tracheoesophageal Speech

Pulmonary air provides the power supply for TE voice production. It is therefore logical to consider whether poor pulmonary health impacts this method of alaryngeal voice production. One source of evidence which indicates that pulmonary status is influential in TE speech stems from outcome studies on the use of HMEs which are designed to improve pulmonary function. In Ackerstaff et al. (2003), for example, 75% of the participant pool were TE speakers. Not only did pulmonary symptoms improve after wearing an HME for several months, but voice related parameters also improved. Ackerstaff et al. noted that improvements in loudness, fluency, and intelligibility were most apparent when data from TE participants were evaluated without inclusion from the 1 ES and 12 AL speakers who were part of the study. One direct inference from these data is that if pulmonary status is improved in TE speakers, voice parameters are likely to improve. The authors attributed the improved TE voice function following several months of HME usage to a few factors: reduced mucus production that could diminish "bubbly" sounding voice, reduced mucus leading to less frequent obstruction of the prosthesis, increased humidity in the air diverted through the prosthesis resulting in less drying of esophageal mucosa, and improved distribution of stoma occlusion pressures (digital) in the peristomal region, thereby placing less pressure on the voice prosthesis, pharynx, and tracheostoma.

The Ackerstaff et al. (2003) results are consistent with those reported by Dassonville et al. (2011). The latter reported that 25 individuals who were TE speakers self-reported improvements in ease of TE voice production, intensity, and fluency after wearing an HME over a 3-month timeframe. Pulmonary function in terms of coughing, dyspnea, and forced expectoration also improved. The implication provided by the authors was that improved baseline pulmonary functioning was the likely basis for the self-rated improvements in TE voice parameters.

Ward et al. (2007) reported respiratory kinematic data in TE speakers compared to participants who have not had a total laryngectomy.

They found that the TE participants initiated speech at a higher percentage of vital capacity and terminated speech at a lower percentage of the vital capacity, than did laryngeal speakers. Bohnenkamp, Forrest, Klaben, and Stager (2011) reported rib cage and abdomen movements in TE speakers during spontaneous speech and while reading that were comparable to those of Ward et al. (2007). Additionally, Bohnenkamp et al. demonstrated an increase in their TE speakers' resting expiratory levels (REL) which resulted in them continuing to speak into their functional residual capacity. Adults with respiratory compromise are known to consistently terminate speech below their REL (Lee, Loudon, Jacobson, & Stuebing, 1993). Increased lung volume at speech initiation, stopping speech below REL, and producing shorter utterance lengths compared to laryngeal speakers suggest that TE speakers may have an increased respiratory effort to speak (Bohnenkamp, Forrest, Klaben, & Stager, 2012).

Finally, the Stepp et al. (2008) study cited above included two TE speakers tracked over several months and two others who were seen for a single evaluation of respiratory kinematics. The two who were tracked over several months demonstrated an increase in the percentage of their total speaking time that occurred during respiratory inhalation. For one TE speaker, about 5% of their speaking time was spent inhaling when they were evaluated 1.5 months postsurgery; when evaluated at 33 months postsurgery, the percentage had increased to 11%. The second TE speaker was tracked from 4 to 12 months and demonstrated an increase from approximately 15–33% in the amount of their speaking time spent inhaling. A percentage increase in total speaking time that is occurring during inhalation is interpreted as an increased dissociation between speaking and breathing. Overall, these studies suggest that the TE voice may improve as pulmonary function is improved by HME usage. There are changes in the lung volume levels at which TE speech is initiated and terminated, with speech extending below one's REL. Finally, for TE speakers there may be a dissociation in the temporal relationship between breathing and speaking that increases as a function of time postsurgery. That is, the percentage of the total time spent talking that occurs during inspiration may increase the further the TE speaker is from the time of their surgery.

Artificial Larynx Speech

Electrolaryngeal (EL) speech is not dependent on pulmonary air to produce voice. Therefore, there is perhaps a limited expectation that poor pulmonary function will impact EL speech. However, a few reports relevant to this topic are in the literature. Two studies support the conclusion that EL speakers are likely to talk during the inspiratory portion of the respiratory cycle. Stepp et al. (2008) included nine EL speakers, three of whom were tracked over several months and six who were seen one time at least 12 months postsurgery. Those tracked over time demonstrated a 27% increase, on average, in the total amount of their EL speaking time that occurred during inhalation when assessed 2–4 months after surgery compared to 8–12 months after surgery. This finding is in contrast to a 12% increase of speaking time happening during inspiration for TE/ES speakers in that same study (Stepp et al., 2008). Considering only the single time-point of evaluation that was done for six other EL participants, 33% of the EL talking occurred during inhalation compared to 19% for the TE/ES participants.

Similar to the findings reported by Stepp et al. (2008), Bohnenkamp, Stowell, Hesse, and Wright (2010) recorded chest and abdominal movements in six EL speakers while also recording their speech. The EL speakers started to talk with the EL before peak inspiration occurred (i.e., during inspiration) for 61% of spontaneous utterances and 58% of reading utterances from the Rainbow Passage. Findings from Stepp et al. and Bohnenkamp et al. support the conclusion that the relationship between EL speaking and the respiratory cycle is altered for a substantial portion of the time an EL speaker spends talking. The fact that the respiratory system is not integral

to the production of EL speech is speculated to result in this "decoupling" of respiration and speech production (Bohnenkamp et al., 2010), wherein EL talking often occurs during inspiration. However, the findings from Stepp et al. (2008) and Bohnenkamp et al. (2010) differ from those of Liu, Wan, Wang, and Niu (2004) who noted only 1 EL participant out of 12 who spoke on inspiration during sentence and poem reading. Four others in the Liu et al. study were noted to hold their breath, and the remaining were observed to speak during the expiratory phase of respiration. Of note was that breath holding occurred in those who had used the EL the longest, and further, these individuals also had better ratings of acceptability of the EL voice. The authors implied that those who were utilizing a pattern of expiring air during speaking would, or perhaps should, gravitate toward the breath hold pattern over time. Overall, these three studies offer varied data, but one consistent message is that as the time from surgery increases, there is an increased decoupling of EL talking and the respiratory cycle. The variation across studies is that two of them (Bohnenkamp et al., 2010; Stepp et al., 2008) indicate that the dissociation is toward an increased percentage of EL talk time that happens during inspiration, whereas Liu et al. (2004) reported that EL talking occurred during breath holding in speakers who were further out from surgery. From a practical standpoint, breath holding during EL talking imposes a physiological limit on how long the person can talk before needing to stop for breath. Although Liu et al. (2004) appear to encourage breath holding as a positive goal for EL speakers, further investigation of the issue is warranted to determine the benefit and drawbacks of breath holding. Anecdotal evidence suggests that breath holding is not necessary for functional or excellent EL usage.

Bohnenkamp et al. (2010) also provided information about respiratory behavior in EL communication beyond the temporal issues discussed in the previous section by also reporting on various measures of lung volume and respiratory kinematics. The lung volumes utilized by EL participants during speaking tasks were found to be comparable to those reported for adults without a laryngectomy, that is, approximately 60% of vital capacity at speech onset and 40% at termination (Hixon, 1973; Hixon, Mead, & Goldman, 1976). The REL was noted to increase in EL speakers, and they consistently continued to speak into their functional residual capacity. Taken together, the findings of Bohnenkamp et al. (2010) regarding the lung volume data indicate a respiratory system in the EL speaker that is being taxed more than what occurs in normal, non-laryngectomy speakers.

The studies to date on EL speakers indicate that a person becomes increasingly likely to spend more time talking during the inspiratory portion of the respiratory cycle or during breath holding, suggesting a dissociation between the usual pattern of speaking on exhalation. Additionally, the results from Bohnenkamp et al. (2010) further indicate that a person speaking with an EL may be stressing the respiratory system by talking further into their functional residual capacity.

In contrast to the electronic artificial larynx, the pneumatic artificial larynx requires a pulmonary air supply to create voice. It is, therefore, reasonable to speculate that altered pulmonary function after total laryngectomy might have an impact on this form of alaryngeal speech. However, there are no available descriptions of how reduced or altered pulmonary function impacts the use of a pneumatic artificial larynx.

Alaryngeal Voice Source Aerodynamics

The aerodynamics of alaryngeal voice production are altered because of two major changes to anatomy. The first is removal of the normal voice source, namely, the larynx and vocal folds. Alaryngeal voicing requires replacement of this vibratory source. Dependent on the method, the replacement alaryngeal voice source will impact the aerodynamics of sound production. The second anatomical change that alters alaryngeal voicing aerodynamics is the diversion of pulmonary air out of a stoma at the base of the midline neck. Pulmonary air cannot be used to initiate and sustain alaryngeal voice source vibration unless the airstream can be routed toward and through the replacement voice source. The aerodynamics of each method of alaryngeal communication are described separately given that the vibratory source, the air supply, or both can differ across alaryngeal options. As a basis for comparison to studies of alaryngeal speakers, Table 13.1 presents representative data on voice source aerodynamics for laryngeal speakers.

Table 13.1 Representative normative values for aerodynamic parameters involving the voice source in laryngeal speakers

Parameter	Speech sample	Range of mean values across studies	Reference(s)[a]
Subglottal air pressure (cmH_2O)	/pa/ syllable train	5.8–8.0	Holmberg, Hillman, and Perkell (1988) Higgins and Saxman (1993); Rosenthal, Lowell, and Colton (2014); Zraick, Smith-Olinde, and Shotts (2012); Gillespie, Slivka, Atwood, and Verdolini Abbott (2015)
Average flow rate (mL/s)	Vowel	112–182	Hirano (1981); Horii and Cooke (1978)
	Reading	177–191	Woo, Colton, and Shangold (1987); Zraick et al. (2012); Gillespie et al. (2015); Rosenthal et al. (2014)
Laryngeal resistance ($cmH_2O/L/s$)	/pa/ syllable train	50–79	Zraick et al. (2012); Gillespie et al. (2015); Rosenthal et al. (2014)

[a]Data included are extracted from studies of adults producing the speech sample in a "normal" or "comfortable" speaking task. Range of values across several studies is reported for each measure

Esophageal Voice

Esophageal voice is produced using the pharyngoesophageal segment (PES) as the vibratory source and air within the esophagus as the driving force that initiates and sustains vibration (see Doyle & Finchem Chap. 10, for details about this process). Briefly, air from the upper vocal tract (mouth, nose, throat) is compressed or drawn into the esophagus and then returned in a controlled fashion to set the PES into vibration. One clear aerodynamic difference between esophageal and laryngeal voice production is the total volume of air that is potentially available to power vibration of the voice source. The esophagus has the capacity to hold approximately 80 cc of air (Deidrich, 1968; Van den Berg & Moolenaar-Bijl, 1959) which is substantially less than the ~3000–5000 cc available in the lungs of adult men and women (Zemlin, 1997). Even though the esophagus may hold approximately 80 cc of air, the amount of air actually injected or drawn into the esophagus per insufflation attempt is substantially less. Stetson (1937) reported that about 3–5 cc of air was injected with each insufflation attempt during esophageal speech, while Snidecor and Isshiki (1965) reported values ranging from 5 to 16 cc. The reduction in the volume of air available or actually used for esophageal phonation can impact on parameters of ES speech production such as loudness, phrase length, syllables produced per esophageal insufflation, pause time, etc.

The use of the PES in ES speech also contributes to the aerodynamic changes reported for this form of alaryngeal communication. In laryngeal voice, air pressure beneath the vocal folds, referred to as subglottal air pressure, must be generated from the lungs to a magnitude that is sufficient to initiate and then sustain vocal fold vibration. The parallel to subglottal air pressure in ES speech is esophageal air pressure, i.e., sub-PES pressure, sometimes called subneoglottal air pressure. A summary of aerodynamic data related to the esophageal voice source is provided in Table 13.2.

Table 13.2 Values for aerodynamic parameters involving the voice source in esophageal speakers

Laryngeal parameter for comparison	Equivalent parameter for alaryngeal voice?	Speech sample	Male	Combined or unknown sex	Female	References
Subglottal air pressure (cmH$_2$O)	Sub-PE segment pressure (cmH$_2$O)	?		R: 10–70	–	Damsté (1958)
		VC train	M: 25 (R: 11–31)			Ng (2011)
		Vowel + CV trains		M: 2.9 (R: 0.5–12.5)		Schutte and Nieboer (2002)
Average flow rate (mL/s)	Average flow rate (mL/s)	Vowel	R: 47–49			Isshiki and Snidecor (1965)
			R: 27–72			Snidecor and Isshiki (1965)
			M: 71 (R: 17–153)			Motta et al. (2001)
			M: 75 (R: 62–84)			Ng (2011)
		Vowels + CV trains		M: 82 (R: 10–360)		Schutte and Nieboer (2002)
Laryngeal resistance (cmH$_2$O/L/s)	PE resistance (cmH$_2$O/L/s)	VC train	M: 345 (R: 153–497)			Ng (2011)

PE pharyngoesophageal, *VC* vowel consonant, *CV* consonant vowel, *M* mean, *R* range
[a]Data reporting in the original manuscripts varied resulting in the need to report results in various formats (ranges, means). Values from original reports were rounded to the nearest whole number

Based on existing data, sub-PES pressure has been shown to be higher in esophageal voice for two of three available studies. Both Damsté (1958) and Ng (2011) reported pressure values ranging from approximately 10–70 cmH$_2$O compared to 5–8 cmH$_2$O in studies of laryngeal speakers. The elevated sub-PES pressure is attributed to the fact that the PES has greater mass and resistance than the true vocal folds. Values from Schutte and Nieboer (2002), however, are much more consistent with laryngeal voice data. It is not clear if this discrepancy with Damsté (1958) and Ng (2011) is due to a sampling, methodological, or instrumentation difference. Schutte and Nieboer (2002) did use transnasal insertion of a pressure sensor that passed through the PES, and it seems possible that the tube could have prevented complete PES closure. If so, this might decrease the pressures measured. In total, the data generally suggest elevated sub-PES air pressure in those who are ES speakers relative to subglottal air pressure for normal speakers.

In addition to the importance of air pressure to ES voice, the rate of airflow through the vibratory source during esophageal phonation is markedly reduced compared to laryngeal voice (see Tables 13.1 and 13.2 for comparative values). Laryngeal voice is generated with about 100–200 mL/s of airflow, while mean flow values for esophageal voice have ranged from 27 to 82 mL/s across studies (Isshiki & Snidecor, 1965; Motta, Galli, & Di Rienzo, 2001; Ng, 2011; Schutte & Nieboer, 2002). A combination of the increased mass and resistance of the PES and substantial limits in overall esophageal air available for esophageal phonation are the presumed causes for the reduced airflow through the PE segment. Elevated pressure below the PE segment and limited trans-PES airflow are believed to have resulted in an elevation of PE voice source resistance as reported by Ng (2011). Voice source resistance values in that study were approximately half an order of magnitude higher than the values reported for laryngeal voice.

Overall, the volume of air available for esophageal voice production is limited for each air insufflation of the esophagus. However, individuals who are proficient at ES speech can consistently and rapidly reload the esophagus with small volumes of air to produce increasingly fluent speech. Additionally, the PES provides higher resistance to airflow than the vocal folds do, causing high sub-PES air pressure. As a result, the primary focus of learning and using ES often centers on producing voice with limited effort and tension. The assumption in such a clinical focus is that it will be easier to get air into the esophagus, as well as easier to return air to start and sustain PE segment vibration (Snidecor, 1969). Interestingly, Ng (2011) included only participants who were carefully selected for inclusion in their study because of their "superior" ES speech skill. High air pressure below the PE segment, restricted airflow through the PE segment, and high voice source resistance were characteristic of those superior speakers. This indicates that lower pressures and resistance, and increased airflow, are not a prerequisite for good ES.

Tracheoesophageal Voice

The PES serves as the voice source in TE speech, as it does for ES. However, the lungs serve as the air supply for TE speech (see Graville, Palmer, & Bolognone, Chap. 11). Briefly, air from the trachea is diverted through a one-way valved prosthesis that is placed in a fistula in the common wall between the trachea and esophagus. When the tracheostoma is sealed, pulmonary air is diverted into the esophagus; when air pressure is sufficient to overcome the resistance of the PES, vibration is initiated. Because the lungs serve as the air supply for TE speech, this alaryngeal mode does not operate under the same degree of air volume restriction that is present in ES speech. However, the need to channel the pulmonary air into the esophagus through a small-diameter prosthesis introduces a degree of airflow resistance. That is, the cross-sectional area and length of the TE prosthesis as well as the hinged valve within the prosthesis all offer resistance to airflow. This allows for the possibility that airflows, pressures, and resistances might be altered in TE speech.

Table 13.3 provides a summary of the available literature detailing the aerodynamics of PES voicing that occurs during TE speech. Studies have varied in terms of the speech sample utilized, but most of the data on sub-PES pressure in TE voice indicates expected values between 13 and 44 cmH$_2$O, on average. These pressures below the PES are higher than what occurs below the vocal folds in laryngeal speech. Two studies allow a comparison of TE to ES speech. Schutte and Nieboer (2002) assessed 18 participants who used TE speech, 5 of whom also used ES. Additionally, they included eight other participants who only used ES speech. The TE participants, excluding those who used both TE and ES speech, were found to use significantly higher sub-PES pressure than the ES speech participants when phonating on sustained vowels and CV syllable trains. For the within-speaker comparison of the five laryngectomees who could use both TE and ES speech, two exhibited significantly higher pressure below the PES when using TE speech, while the other three did not differ statistically between the two modes of alaryngeal voice. In contrast, Ng (2011) reported significantly higher sub-PES pressures for ES compared to TE speech. At present, there currently is not clear evidence of the existence of higher pressures required for voicing in one method over the other. Both TE and ES speech utilize higher sub-PES pressures compared to subglottal pressures in laryngeal voicing. Additionally, there are individual differences across TE speakers in terms of the pressures below the PE segment that are needed for voicing as exhibited in Schutte and Nieboer (2002).

With the exception of one study (Kotby, Hegazi, Kamal, Gamal El Dien, & Nassar, 2009), group mean values for average trans-PES flow rates in TE speech fall generally within the range of mean values for laryngeal speakers (see Table 13.1). Comparable flow rates between TE and laryngeal voice have most often been attributed to the use of the pulmonary air stream for both methods of voice production. When comparing TE and ES voice aerodynamics in Tables 13.2 and 13.3, the general trend which emerges is that trans-PES airflow rates in TE speakers are

about twice the rate reported for individuals using ES speech. Again, two studies directly compared TE and ES participants using the same stimuli, procedures, and instrumentation. Ng (2011) and Schutte and Nieboer (2002) reported significantly higher trans-PES flow for the TE group. Recall that Schutte and Nieboer (2002) also had five participants for whom they could do within-speaker comparisons across the two alaryngeal voicing methods. Four of their five participants had significantly higher flows when using TE voice. Based on these data, a broad conclusion is that TE voice is characterized by higher trans-PES airflow compared to ES voice, although a given individual may not show this difference.

Resistance to airflow in TE voicing can occur at two levels: the PES and the TE voice prosthesis. Several studies evaluating the in vitro aerodynamic characteristics of various TE prostheses have been published in the literature (Belforte, Carello, Miani, & Staffieri, 1998; Chung, Patel, Ter Keurs, Van Lith Bijl, & Mahieu, 1998; Heaton & Parker, 1994; Hilgers, Cornelissen, & Balm, 1993; Miani et al., 1998; Smith, 1986; Weinberg & Moon, 1982, 1984, 1986). These are not reviewed here other than in summary fashion. The set of studies have established that the aerodynamic characteristics of a TE prosthesis vary depending on a number of parameters such as the prosthesis diameter, prosthesis length, position of the valve within the length of the prosthesis, type of valve, and flow rate used for the testing. TE voice prostheses can be selected that have been specifically designed to have greater or lesser resistance to valve opening depending on the needs of a particular patient (see Graville, Palmer & Bolognone, Chap. 11 and Knott, Chap. 12). What is clear is that the prosthesis itself offers higher resistance to airflow than does the normal open glottis. It also is important to note that the resistance of a given prosthesis to airflow is likely to change over its lifetime when used in vivo. In vitro studies have generally concluded that biofilm development increases the prosthesis' resistance to airflow (Chung et al., 1998; Heaton & Parker, 1994; Heaton, Sanderson, Dunsmore, & Parker, 1996; Zijlstra, Mahieu, van Lith-Bijl, &

Table 13.3 Values for aerodynamic parameters involving the voice source in tracheoesophageal speakers

Laryngeal parameter for comparison	Tracheoesophageal voice[a]					
	Equivalent parameter for alaryngeal voice	Speech sample	Reported values			References
			Male	Combined or unknown sex	Female	
Subglottal air pressure (cmH₂O)	Sub-PE segment pressure (cmH₂O)	Vowel		M: 42 (SD: 22)		Aguiar-Ricz, Ricz, de Mello-Filho, Perdona, and Dantas (2010)
		Vowel		M: 22 (digital occlusion)		Grolman, Eerenstein, Tan, Tange, and Schouwenburg (2007)
		Vowel		M: 24 (hands-free occlusion)		Grolman et al. (2007)
		Vowel		M: 33 (R: 10–69)		Takeshita, Zozolotto, Ricz, Dantas, and Aguiar-Ricz (2010)
		Vowel		M: 28 (R: 20–35)		Weinberg, Horii, Blom, and Singer (1982)
		Vowel	M: 13 (SD: 11)			Kotby et al. (2009)
		VC train	M: 23 (R: 17–25)		–	Ng (2011)
		VC train		M: 36 (SD: 22)		Aguiar-Ricz et al. (2010)
		Sentence		M: 44 (SD: 24)		Aguiar-Ricz et al. (2010)
		Combination of samples		M: 5 (R: 1–11)		Schutte and Nieboer (2002)
Average flow rate (mL/s)	Average flow rate (mL/s)	Vowel	M: 138 (R: 78–240)			Motta et al. (2001)
		Vowel	M: 134 (R: 128–139)			Ng (2011)
		Vowel		M: 150 (digital occlusion)		Grolman et al. (2007)
				M: 167 (SD: 72; hands-free occlusion)		Grolman et al. (2007)
		Vowel	M: 53 (R: 34–74)		–	Kotby et al. (2009)
		Vowel		M: 170 (R: 74–336)		Moon and Weinberg (1987)
		Vowel		M: 133 (R: 104–182)		Weinberg et al. (1982)
		Vowels + CV trains		M: 131 (R: 20–800)		Schutte and Nieboer (2002)

Table 13.3 (continued)

Laryngeal parameter for comparison	Tracheoesophageal voice[a]						
	Equivalent parameter for alaryngeal voice	Speech sample	Reported values			References
			Male	Combined or unknown sex	Female	
Laryngeal resistance (cmH₂O/L/s)	PE resistance (cmH₂O/L/s)	Vowel	M: 237 (R: 102–403)			Kotby et al. (2009)
		Vowel		M: 210 (R: 154–270)		Weinberg et al. (1982)
		VC train	M: 171 (R: 119–200)		–	Ng (2011)
	PE + prosthesis resistance (cmH2O/L/s)	Vowel		M: 211 (R: 142–383)	–	Moon and Weinberg (1987)

PE pharyngoesophageal, *V* vowel, *C* consonant, *M* mean, *R* range, *SD* standard deviation
[a]Data reporting in the original manuscripts varied resulting in the need to report results in various formats (ranges, means, standard deviations). Values from original reports were rounded to the nearest whole number

Schutte, 1991). In contrast, Schwandt, Tjong-Ayong, van Weissenbruch, der Mei, and Albers (2006) evaluated prosthesis performance in vivo to compare new versus dysfunctional prostheses that had been influenced by the development of biofilm. They reported that biofilm development on the prosthesis created a reduction in airflow resistance. This might occur because of altered structural properties of the valve or changes in prosthesis opening and closing movements of the valve due to biofilm.

In summary, investigations of TE voice source aerodynamics indicate that air pressure below the PES is greater than subglottal pressures associated with laryngeal voice. The data are not clear, however, about whether air pressures below the PES are expected to be higher for TE compared to ES speech. A number of variables are likely to be influential on the pressures in these two speaker groups including speaker proficiency, speech stimuli utilized, the presence of PE tissue hypertonicity, as well as other factors. Average trans-PES airflow in TE speech is typically greater than what is documented in ES speech and similar to what occurs trans-glottally in laryngeal speech. Finally, resistance to airflow in TE voice production is increased compared to

laryngeal speech, and this increase is likely related to elevated resistance associated with both the PES and the structural properties of the TE puncture voice prosthesis.

Artificial Larynx Voice

The EL voice is generated via excitation of the static air within the upper vocal tract via transmission of vibration through tissues of the neck or face or alternatively via a small-diameter tube placed within the oral cavity (see Nagle, Chap. 9). The power supply for the EL voice is battery driven, and voice generation occurs via a small piston striking a plastic plate. As such, air pressures and airflows are not part of the EL voice production process like they are for ES and TE speech. However, the pneumatic artificial larynx (also referred to as the Tokyo device) does operate on principals that parallel laryngeal and PE segment voice production. That is, an air pressure differential must be established to create air flows between or across a voice source capable of vibrating. The pneumatic artificial larynx uses a reed or flexible diaphragm (natural, plastic, metal, or rubber) as a voice source. This diaphragm is housed within a chamber that is external to the body. A tube running from the stoma to the chamber allows pulmonary air to serve as the driving force that sets the diaphragm into vibration. A second tube exits the chamber and runs to the oral cavity to deliver the voice signal into the vocal tract. Over the last 10–15 years, there has been a resurgence of interest in pneumatic artificial larynges as evidenced by increasing study of this alaryngeal method (Liao, 2016; Ng & Chu, 2009; Ng, Liu, Zhao, & Lam, 2009; Xu, Chen, Lu, & Qiao, 2009). However, these studies have focused almost exclusively on auditory-perceptual and acoustic parameters to the exclusion of associated speech aerodynamics.

An emerging possibility related to the traditional pneumatic artificial larynx is the development of a TE puncture voice prosthesis with a built-in sound producing element. In this approach, a membrane that can be set into vibration is housed within the prosthesis; as such, it might be described as a pneumatic artificial larynx. Early versions of the approach have been described by van der Torn, de Vries, Festen, Verdonck-de Leeuw, and Mahieu (2001) and van der Torn et al. (2006). Second-generation versions are described by Tack, Verkerke, van der Houwen, Mahieu, and Schutte (2006) and Tack, Rakhorst, van der Houwen, Mahieu, and Verkerke (2007). These second-generation devices have a double membrane lying within the body of a TE prosthesis; this membrane is set into vibration when pulmonary airflows through the prosthesis. The use of the device is described as being potentially beneficial to females who have had a laryngectomy. This suggestion is made because the membrane-based voice-generating prosthesis can attain higher fundamental frequencies than is possible with PES vibration. A higher fundamental frequency may be more appropriate, acceptable, and desired for the female alaryngeal speaker. Additionally, the device could allow for a pulmonary-driven sound source in laryngectomees who have a hypotonic PES that is not capable of vibrating. Tack et al. (2008) reported aerodynamic data for this kind of voice prosthesis for 17 females who had a total laryngectomy; all but 3 had hypotonic or atonic PES vibration and resultant tone.

The voice-producing element was inserted into the lumen of a Groningen ultra-low resistance prosthesis, and tracheal pressure was measured (Tack et al., 2008). Tracheal pressure serves as the force that sets the voice-producing element within the prosthesis into vibration. The tracheal pressures in these 17 females averaged 32 cmH_2O on soft phonation attempts and 58 cmH_2O during loud phonation attempts. These pressure values were comparable to the tracheal pressures measured in the same participants when wearing the TE valve without the voice-producing element. Airflow values were markedly lower with the voice-producing element inserted in the prosthesis, averaging 43 mL/s during soft phonation vs. 154 mL/s with the standard TE prosthesis, and 78 mL/s during loud phonation vs. 314 mL/s with the standard TE prosthesis. The fundamental frequency produced with the voice-generating prosthesis averaged 234 and 313 Hz for soft and loud phonation, respectively. These fundamental frequencies were notably higher than those reported when using the standard TE prosthesis, which were 66 and 87 Hz for loud and soft phonation. Overall, these frequency-based data appear promising for such a device to serve as an improved postlaryngectomy voice source option, particularly for females.

Articulatory Aerodynamics in Alaryngeal Speech

The aerodynamics of articulatory events in alaryngeal speech could be altered from two sources: (1) separation of the lower from the upper airway limiting availability of air for creating plosive elements and frication and (2) alterations to how the articulators are used after the larynx is removed. There are limited empirical data related to articulatory aerodynamics after total laryngectomy for any of the alaryngeal methods of communication. As a general rule, and regardless of alaryngeal method, a person is instructed to be more careful with their articulation in order to maximize intelligibility (Salmon, 1999; Searl & Reeves, 2014; van As & Fuller, 2014). However, in doing so care also is taken to not make speech appear or sound more unnatural. Such clinical instruction could reasonably be expected to alter the aerodynamics of articulation with any of the three alaryngeal communication methods. The sections below provide a summary of the available literature on the articulatory aerodynamics for ES, TE, and EL speech.

Esophageal Speech

Three of the four studies presented in Table 13.4 have reported oral pressure values during esophageal speech to be elevated during consonant production when compared to expectations for normal speakers. The lone exception was provided by Connor, Hamlet, and Joyce (1985) who reported oral pressure values for /t/ and /d/ that were generally within the 3–7 cmH$_2$O range found in laryngeal speech. Two of three studies that included both voiced and voiceless consonants found that individuals using ES speech produced lower oral air pressures on the voiced cognates similar to what is evidenced in laryngeal speech (Connor et al., 1985; Gorham, Morris, Brown, & Huntley, 1996). Swisher (1980) was the exception, reporting comparable values across voicing feature. Overall, and despite some discrepancies, the preponderance of the data in the literature indicates that oral air pressure during pressure consonant production is elevated during ES compared to laryngeal speech. Additionally, and similar to normal speakers, an oral air pressure difference tends to be maintained between voiced and voiceless cognates.

There is some indication that oral air pressures may differ depending on ES speech proficiency level. Motta et al. (2001) divided their ES participants into a group judged perceptually to be "good" and another judged as "mediocre." The good speakers generated significantly less oral pressure (mean = 40.5 cmH$_2$O, SD = 5 cmH$_2$O) compared to the mediocre group (mean = 57 cmH$_2$O, SD = 16 cmH$_2$O). It should be noted, however, that the oral pressures for both groups are still substantially greater than what occurs during laryngeal speech. Connor et al.

(1985) compared oral pressure for /t/ and /d/ for one ES speaker with low intelligibility and another with high intelligibility. The high-intelligibility speaker demonstrated significantly lower oral air pressure. In contrast to Motta et al. (2001), however, both the low- and high-intelligibility participant in Connor et al. (1985) had mean pressure values that were well within the range expected of laryngeal speech.

Additional aerodynamic studies of articulation in ES speech are not readily available in the literature. Yet there is a suggestion from auditory-perceptual studies (Duguay, 1999) and cinefluoroscopic studies (Deidrich & Youngstrom, 1966; Struben & van Gelder, 1958) that nasals are more likely to be produced with the velopharyngeal port closed. This would result in no or limited nasal airflow on nasals. Deidrich and Youngstrom's (1966) cinefluoroscopic data further revealed that participants judged perceptually to be "good ES" speakers had more complete palatal closure during a Valsalva maneuver compared to participants judged to be poor ES speakers. The authors suggested that poor palatal closure impedes acquisition of higher level ES speech abilities. In a review of clinical cases as well as the literature available at the time, Berlin (1964) reiterated that palatal weakness is associated with poor ES speech. However, aerodynamic data related to velopharyngeal function in ES has not been reported.

Tracheoesophageal Speech

Several studies have reported high oral air pressure on the bilabial stop, /p/, spoken by individuals using TE speech (Motta et al., 2001; Ng, 2011; Saito, Kinishi, & Amatsu, 2000; Searl, 2002, 2007; Searl & Evitts, 2004). In most of these studies, the pressures ranged from approximately 15–40 cmH$_2$O, a value that is 3–8 times greater than expected in normal laryngeal speakers. Searl (2002) used an oral tube running in the buccogingival sulcus and around the last molar to allow measurement of oral air pressure on other consonants in addition to /p/; these included /t, d, s, z, ʃ, ʒ/. The measured pressures for the voiced

Table 13.4 Articulatory aerodynamics by alaryngeal speech mode

Speech mode	Speech sample	Sex	Oral air pressure (consonant) Mean (with SD or range) cmH$_2$O		Nasal airflow (cc/s)	References
			Voiceless: 5–7	Voiced: 3–5		
Laryngeal	Various consonants and constructions	M, F			/p/ <10	Arkebauer, Hixon, and Hardy (1967)
					/m/ 40–200	Bernthal and Beukelman (1978)
						Brown and McGlone (1969)
Esophageal	/p,b,t,d,s,f/ in CVC	M	/p/ 36 (no R or SD) /t/ 17 (no R or SD) /f/ 11 (no R or SD) /s/ 10 (no R or SD)	/b/ 33 (no R or SD) /d/ 17 (no R or SD)		Swisher (1980)
	/t,d/ in CV and VCV	M	/t/ 3–4 high intell. /t/ 5–11 low intell.	/d/ 1–2 high intell. /d/ 3–9 low intell.		Connor et al. (1985)
	/p,b,t,d,s,z/ in CV, VCV, VC	M, F	/p/ 21 (R: 14–27) /t/ 12 (R: 4–23) /s/ 17 (R: 7–26)	/b/ 9 (R: 3–17) /d/ 7 (R: 1–19) /z/ 10 (R: 2–19)		Gorham et al. (1996)
	/ipipi/	M	/p/ 25 (R: 10–31)			Ng (2011)
	/pipi/	M	/p/ 40–57 (R: 31–83) depending on intelligibility			Motta et al. (2001)
Tracheoesophageal	/ipipi/	M	/p/ 22 (R: 17–25)			Ng (2011)
	/pipi/	M	/p/ 39 (SD: 15)			Motta et al. (2001)
	/apa/, /aba/	M	/p/ 21–23 (R: 13–31)	/b/ 6–9 (R: 3–11)		Saito et al. (2000)[a]
	/mVCV/ with C=/p,b,t,d,f,v,s,z,sh,shz/	M, F	/p/ 16 (SD: 4) /t/ 17 (SD: 5) /f/ 14 (SD: 4) /s/ 14 (SD: 4) /sh/ 13 (SD: 4)	/b/ 7 (SD: 3) /d/ 7 (SD: 3) /v/ 6 (SD: 3) /z/ 8 (SD: 3) /zh/ 8 (SD: 4)		Searl (2002)
	/p,b,m/ in CV trains, sentences	M, F	/p/ 5 (SD: 2)	/b/ 6 (SD: 3) /m/ 6 (SD: 3)	/p/ 7 (SD: 8) /m/ 202 (SD: 68)	Searl (2007)[b]
	/p, m/ in CV trains	M, F	/p/ 20 (SD: 8)	/m/ 1 (SD: 0.5)		Searl and Evitts (2004)
Artificial larynx	–	–	–		–	–

R range, *SD* standard deviation, *C* consonant, *V* vowel

[a]Summary of values from Tables 1 and 2 in Saito et al. (2000)

[b]Summary of values for phonemes across all stimulus contexts in Searl (2007)

consonants ranged from 13 to 17 cmH$_2$O, while pressures on the voiceless counterparts ranged from 6 to 8 cmH$_2$O. Overall, these oral pressures were higher than what occurs in laryngeal speakers for this extended set of consonants, although measures for voiceless consonants are much closer to normal laryngeal speech.

Oral pressures also have been recorded for the nasal phoneme /m/ produced by TE speakers in two studies. Searl (2007) found that pressures on /m/ were elevated to approximately 6 cmH$_2$O, values comparable to the pressures on the oral phoneme /b/ from these same speakers. In laryngeal speakers, oral pressure on /m/ is expected to be quite low (1 cmH$_2$O or less) because the velopharyngeal port is open. The interpretation of these data was that TE speakers in the study may have maintained some greater degree of velopharyngeal closure resulting in the elevated pressure on the nasal phoneme. However, in an earlier study, Searl and Evitts (2004) reported a group mean pressure of 1 cmH$_2$O on /m/ in individuals using TE speech. This is equivalent to laryngeal speech and much lower than pressures recorded with the same instrumentation on different TE speakers in Searl (2007). It may be the case that there is variability across TE speakers regarding how they produce nasal phonemes.

The Searl and Evitts (2004) study is the sole report of nasal airflows in TE speech with data acquired for both consonants /m/ and /p/. Nasal flow values for /m/ were found to be at or above what has been reported for individuals without a laryngectomy, suggesting velopharyngeal opening by the TE speakers. There was essentially absent nasal airflow on the oral phoneme /p/ which parallels what occurs in laryngeal speech. Thus, the lone study of nasal airflow in TE speech during consonant production, which in this case is limited to /m/ and /p/, suggests that nasal airflow may not be substantially altered in TE speech.

Artificial Larynx Speech

There are no reports of articulatory aerodynamics for individuals using an artificial larynx in the peer-reviewed literature. Various textbooks make

reference to the need for individuals to compress air intraorally, usually following an instruction for exaggerated or precise speech. The presumed goal of this instruction is to generate a strong burst of air or frication noise. Clinical descriptions from those working with individuals using ALs also often include comments about this type of clinical focus (Doyle, 1994; Duguay, 1983). Quantitative measurements of how articulatory aerodynamics are altered, however, remain lacking in the literature.

Conclusions

Aerodynamic characteristics of ES, TE, and EL speech are impacted greatly by the total laryngectomy procedure which separates the lower from the upper airway and removes the normal voice source. Pulmonary function after total laryngectomy is expected to be altered because of changes that are induced by the surgery and the reaction of the body to the surgery when inspired air is not warmed, humidified, or filtered to the extent that it was presurgically. Additionally, baseline pulmonary functioning prior to surgery has a high likelihood of being reduced if the person was a long-time smoker. The pulmonary changes can have both direct and indirect impacts on the aerodynamics of alaryngeal speech. The aerodynamics of the alaryngeal voice source vary across ES, TE, and EL methods. For ES and TE speech, elevated voice source driving pressures are expected. Likewise, resistance to airflow for the voice source in ES and TE speech is increased. Airflow also is markedly reduced in ES yet may be minimally reduced in TE speech. Although EL voice is not dependent on airflow for production, pneumatic artificial larynx voice is. Unfortunately, however, little is known about the pneumatic artificial larynges that have been on the market for many decades. Emerging work is occurring on a pneumatically driven voice source that can be inserted into a TE voice prosthesis. In terms of aerodynamics involved in articulation, an elevation in oral air pressure is commonly reported for ES and TE speakers; no data are available for EL speech. Furthermore, individuals using ES or TE speech tend to retain an oral air pressure difference between voiced-voiceless cognates. There is very limited aerodynamic data available on other aspects of articulation in alaryngeal speech. Continued gathering of data regarding articulatory changes in ES, TE, and EL speech is important because that information can help researchers and clinicians know what articulatory parameters change, the manner in which they are different compared to presurgical articulation, and the variability to expect in an articulatory parameter within and across alaryngeal speakers. Additionally, more detailed information on articulatory changes is important for developing effective therapeutic approaches and for establishing reasonable treatment goals for alaryngeal speakers.

References

Achim, V., Bash, J., Mowery, A., Guimaraes, A. R., Schindler, J., Wax, M., ... Clayburgh, D. (2017). Prognostic indication of sarcopenia for wound complication after total laryngectomy. *JAMA Otolaryngology. Head & Neck Surgery, 4*, E1–E7.

Ackerstaff, A. H., Fuller, D., Irvin, M., Maccracken, E., Gaziano, J., & Stachowiak, L. (2003). Multicenter study assessing effects of heat and moisture exchanger use on respiratory symptoms and voice quality in laryngectomized individuals. *Otolaryngology and Head and Neck Surgery, 129*(6), 705–712.

Ackerstaff, A. H., Hilgers, F. J., Balm, A. J., & Van Zandwijk, N. (1995). Long-term pulmonary function after total laryngectomy. *Clinical Otolaryngology and Allied Sciences, 20*(6), 547–551.

Ackerstaff, A. H., Hilgers, F. J., Meeuwis, C. A., Knegt, P. P., & Weenink, C. (1999). Pulmonary function pre- and post-total laryngectomy. *Clinical Otolaryngology and Allied Sciences, 24*(6), 491–494.

Aguiar-Ricz, L., Ricz, H., de Mello-Filho, F. V., Perdona, G. C., & Dantas, R. O. (2010). Intraluminal esophageal pressures in speaking laryngectomees. *Annals of Otology, Rhinology and Laryngology, 119*(11), 729–735.

Antoniu, S. A., & Ungureanu, D. (2015). Measuring fatigue as a symptom in COPD: From descriptors and questionnaires to the importance of the problem. *Chronic Respiratory Disease, 12*(3), 179–188.

Arkebauer, H. J., Hixon, T. J., & Hardy, J. C. (1967). Peak intraoral air pressures during speech. *Journal of Speech and Hearing Research, 10*(2), 196–208.

Batioğlu-Karaaltin, A., Binbay, Z., YiBatioğlu-Karaaltin, Ait, Ö., & Dönmez, Z. (2017). Evaluation of life quality, self-confidence and sexual functions in patients with total and partial laryngectomy. *Auris Nasus Larynx, 44*(2), 188–194.

Belforte, G., Carello, M., Miani, C., & Staffieri, A. (1998). Staffieri tracheo-oesophageal prosthesis for voice rehabilitation after laryngectomy: An evaluation of characteristics. *Medical & Biological Engineering & Computing, 36*(6), 754–760.

Berlin, C. I. (1964). Hearing loss, palatal function, and other factors in post-laryngectomy rehabilitation. *Journal of Chronic Diseases, 17*, 677–684.

Bernthal, J. E., & Beukelman, D. R. (1978). Intraoral air pressure during the production of /p/ and /b/ by children, youths, and adults. *Journal of Speech and Hearing Research, 21*(2), 361–371.

Bohnenkamp, T. A., Forrest, K., Klaben, B. K., & Stager, J. (2012). Chest wall kinematics during speech breathing in tracheoesophageal speakers. *The Annals of Otology, Rhinology, and Laryngology, 121*(1), 28–37.

Bohnenkamp, T. A., Forrest, K. M., Klaben, B. K., & Stager, J. M. (2011). Lung volumes used during speech breathing in tracheoesophageal speakers. *The Annals of Otology, Rhinology, and Laryngology, 120*(8), 550–558.

Bohnenkamp, T. A., Stowell, T., Hesse, J., & Wright, S. (2010). Speech breathing in speakers who use an electrolarynx. *Journal of Communication Disorders, 43*(3), 199–211.

Bond, S. M., Dietrich, M., Gilbert, J., Ely, E. W., Jackson, J. C., & Murphy, B. A. (2016). Neurocognitive function in patients with head and neck cancer undergoing primary or adjuvant chemoradiation treatment. *Supportive Care in Cancer, 24*(10), 4433–4442.

Bond, S. M., Dietrich, M., & Murphy, B. A. (2012). Neurocognitive function in head and neck cancer patients prior to treatment. *Support Care Cancer, 20*(1), 149–157.

Brown, W. S., Jr., & McGlone, R. E. (1969). Constancy of intraoral air pressure. *Folia Phoniatrica, 21*(5), 332–339.

Centers for Disease Control and Prevention. (2017). *Smoking and tobacco use: Basic information.* www.cdc.gov/tobacco/basic_information/index.htm/. Accessed May 2, 2017.

Chung, R. P., Patel, P., Ter Keurs, M., Van Lith Bijl, J. T., & Mahieu, H. F. (1998). In vitro and in vivo comparison of the low-resistance Groningen and the Provox tracheosophageal voice prostheses. *Revue de Laryngologie Otologie Rhinologie, 119*(5), 301–306.

Connor, N. P., Hamlet, S. L., & Joyce, J. C. (1985). Acoustic and physiologic correlates of the voicing distinction in esophageal speech. *Journal of Speech and Hearing Disorders, 50*(4), 378–384.

Damsté, P. H. (1958). *Oesophageal speech after laryngectomy.* Groningen, The Netherlands: Gebroeders Hoitscma.

Danker, H., Wollbrück, D., Singer, S., Fuchs, M., Brähler, E., & Meyer, A. (2010). Social withdrawal after laryngectomy. *European Archives of Oto-Rhino-Laryngology, 267*, 593–600.

Dassonville, O., Merol, J. C., Bozec, A., Swierkosz, F., Santini, J., Chais, A., … Poissonnet, G. (2011). Randomised, multi-centre study of the usefulness of the heat and moisture exchanger (Provox HME(R)) in laryngectomised patients. *European Archives of Oto-Rhino-Laryngology, 268*(11), 1647–1654.

Deidrich, W. (1968). The mechanism of esophageal speech. *Annals of the New York Academy of Sciences, 155*, 303–317.

Deidrich, W., & Youngstrom, K. (1966). *Alaryngeal speech*. Springfield, IL: Thompson.

DiCarlo, L., Amster, W., & Herer, G. (1955). *Speech after laryngectomy*. Syracuse, NY: Syracuse University Press.

DiMatteo, M. R., Lepper, H. S., & Croghan, T. W. (2000). Depression is a risk factor for noncompliance with medical treatment: Meta-analysis of the effects of anxiety and depression on patient adherence. *Archives of Internal Medicine, 160*(14), 2101–2107.

Doyle, P. C. (1994). *Foundations of voice and speech rehabilitation following laryngeal cancer*. San Diego, CA: Singular Publishing Group, Inc.

Dubruille, S., Libert, Y., Merckaert, I., Reynaert, C., Vandenbossche, S., Roos, M., … Razavi, D. (2015). The prevalence and implications of elderly inpatients' desire for a formal psychological help at the start of cancer treatment. *Psychooncology, 24*(3), 294–301.

Duguay, M. (1983). Teaching use of an artificial larynx. In W. H. Perkins (Ed.), *Voice disorders* (pp. 127–135). New York: Thieme-Stratton.

Duguay, M. (1999). Esophageal speech training: The initial phase. In J. Salmon (Ed.), *Alaryngeal speech rehabilitation: For clinicians, by clinicians* (2nd ed., pp. 151–164). Austin, TX: Pro_Ed, Inc.

Edelstein, A., Pergolizzi, D., & Alici, Y. (2016). Cancer-related cognitive impairment in older adults. *Current Opinion in Supportive and Palliative Care, 11*(1), 60–69.

Eichler, M., Keszte, J., Meyer, A., Danker, H., Guntinas-Lichius, O., Oeken, J., … Singer, S. (2016). Tobacco and alcohol consumption after total laryngectomy and survival: A German multicenter prospective cohort study. *Head & Neck, 38*(9), 1324–1329.

Gan, H. K., Bernstein, L. J., Brown, J., Ringash, J., Vakilha, M., Wang, L., … Siu, L. L. (2011). Cognitive functioning after radiotherapy or chemotherapy for head-and-neck cancer. *International Journal of Radiation Oncology-Biology-Physiology, 81*(1), 126–134.

Gardner, W. H. (1971). *Laryngectomee speech and rehabilitation*. Springfield, IL: Charles C. Thomas.

Gerber, L. (2017). Cancer-related fatigue. *Physical Medicine and Rehabilitation Clinics of North America, 28*(1), 65–88.

Gillespie, A. I., Slivka, W., Atwood, C. W., Jr., & Verdolini Abbott, K. (2015). The effects of hyper- and hypocapnia on phonatory laryngeal airway resistance in women. *Journal of Speech, Language, and Hearing Research, 58*(3), 638–652.

Goepfert, R. P., Hutcheson, K. A., Lewin, J. S., Desai, N. G., Zafereo, M. E., Hessel, A. C., … Gross, N. D. (2017). Complications, hospital length of stay, and readmission after total laryngectomy. *Cancer, 15*(123), 1760–1767.

Gorham, N. M., Morris, R. J., Brown, W. S., & Huntley, R. A. (1996). Intraoral air pressure of alaryngeal speakers during a no-air insufflation maneuver. *Journal of Communication Disorders, 29*(2), 141–155.

Griffith, T. E., & Friedberg, S. A. (1964). Histologic changes in the trachea following laryngectomy. *Annals of Otology, Rhinology and Laryngology, 73*, 883–892.

Grolman, W., Eerenstein, S. E., Tan, F. M., Tange, R. A., & Schouwenburg, P. F. (2007). Aerodynamic and sound intensity measurements in tracheoesophageal voice. *ORL: Journal of Oto-Rhino-Laryngology and Its Related Specialties, 69*(2), 68–76.

Harris, S., & Jonson, B. (1974). Lung function before and after laryngectomy. *Acta Oto-Laryngologica, 78*(3–4), 287–294.

Heaton, J. M., & Parker, A. J. (1994). In vitro comparison of the Groningen high resistance, Groningen low resistance and Provox speaking valves. *The Journal of Laryngology and Otology, 108*(4), 321–324.

Heaton, J. M., Sanderson, D., Dunsmore, I. R., & Parker, A. J. (1996). In vivo measurements of indwelling tracheo-oesophageal prostheses in alaryngeal speech. *Clinical Otolaryngology and Allied Sciences, 21*(4), 292–296.

Hess, M. M., Schwenk, R. A., Frank, W., & Loddenkemper, R. (1999). Pulmonary function after total laryngectomy. *Laryngoscope, 109*(6), 988–994.

Higgins, M. B., & Saxman, J. H. (1993). Inverse-filtered airflow and EGG measures for sustained vowels and syllables. *Journal of Voice, 7*(1), 47–53.

Hilgers, F. J., Aaronson, N. K., Ackerstaff, A. H., Schouwenburg, P. F., & van Zandwikj, N. (1991). The influence of a heat and moisture exchanger (HME) on the respiratory symptoms after total laryngectomy. *Clinical Otolaryngology and Allied Sciences, 16*(2), 152–156.

Hilgers, F. J., Ackerstaff, A. H., Aaronson, N. K., Schouwenburg, P. F., & Van Zandwijk, N. (1990). Physical and psychosocial consequences of total laryngectomy. *Clinical Otolaryngology and Allied Sciences, 15*(5), 421–425.

Hilgers, F. J., Cornelissen, M. W., & Balm, A. J. (1993). Aerodynamic characteristics of the Provox low-resistance indwelling voice prosthesis. *European Archives of Oto-Rhino-Laryngology, 250*(7), 375–378.

Hirano, M. (1981). *Clinical examination of the voice*. Wien, Austria: Springer-Verlag.

Hixon, T. J. (1973). Kinematics of the chest wall during speech production: Volume displacements of the rib cage, abdomen, and lung. *Journal of Speech and Hearing Research, 16*(1), 78–115.

Hixon, T. J., Mead, J., & Goldman, M. D. (1976). Dynamics of the chest wall during speech production: Function of the thorax, rib cage, diaphragm, and abdomen. *Journal of Speech and Hearing Research, 19*(2), 297–356.

Holmberg, E. B., Hillman, R. E., & Perkell, J. S. (1988). Glottal airflow and transglottal air pressure measurements for male and female speakers in soft, normal, and loud voice. *The Journal of the Acoustical Society of America, 84*(2), 511–529.

Horii, Y., & Cooke, P. A. (1978). Some airflow, volume, and duration characteristics of oral reading. *Journal of Speech and Hearing Research, 21*(3), 470–481.

Hsiao, K., Yeh, S., Chih, C., Tsai, P., Wu, J., & Gau, J. (2010). Cognitive function before and after intensity-modulated radiation therapy in patients with nasopharyngeal carcinoma: A prospective study. *International Journal of Radiation Oncology-Biology-Physiology, 77*(3), 722–726.

Isshiki, N., & Snidecor, J. C. (1965). Air intake and usage in esophageal speech. *Acta Oto-Laryngologica, 59*, 559–574.

Jereczek-Fossa, B. A., Santoro, L., Alterio, D., Franchi, B., Rosaria, F., Fossati, P., … Orecchia, R. (2007). Fatigue during head-and-neck radiotherapy: Prospective study on 117 consecutive patients. *International Journal of Radiation Oncology, Biology, Physics, 68*(2), 403–415.

Jones, A. S., Young, P. E., Hanafi, Z. B., Makura, Z. G., Fenton, J. E., & Hughes, J. P. (2003). A study of the effect of a resistive heat moisture exchanger (Trachinaze) on pulmonary function and blood gas tensions in patients who have undergone a laryngectomy: A randomized control trial of 50 patients studied over a 6-month period. *Head & Neck, 25*(5), 361–367.

Kentson, M., Todt, K., Skargren, E., Jakobsson, P., Ernerudh, J., Unosson, M., & Theander, K. (2016). Factors associated with experience of fatigue, and functional limitations due to fatigue in patients with stable COPD. *Therapeutic Advances in Respiratory Disease, 10*(5), 410–424.

Kotby, M. N., Hegazi, M. A., Kamal, I., Gamal El Dien, N., & Nassar, J. (2009). Aerodynamics of the pseudo-glottis. *Folia Phoniatrica et Logopaedica, 61*(1), 24–28.

Lee, L., Loudon, R. G., Jacobson, B. H., & Stuebing, R. (1993). Speech breathing in patients with lung disease. *The American Review of Respiratory Disease, 147*(5), 1199–1206.

Liao, J. S. (2016). An acoustic study of vowels produced by alaryngeal speakers in Taiwan. *American Journal of Speech-Language Pathology, 25*(4), 481–492.

Liu, H., Wan, M., Wang, S., & Niu, H. (2004). Aerodynamic characteristics of laryngectomees breathing quietly and speaking with the electrolarynx. *Journal of Voice, 18*(4), 567–577.

Lou, P., Zhu, Y., Chen, P., Zhang, P., Yu, J., Zhang, N., … Zhao, J. (2012). Prevalence and correlations with depression, anxiety, and other features in outpatients with chronic obstructive pulmonary disease in China: A cross-sectional case control study. *BMC Pulmonary Medicine, 12*, 53.

McRae, D., Young, P., Hamilton, J., & Jones, A. (1996). Raising airway resistance in laryngectomees increases

tissue oxygen saturation. *Clinical Otolaryngology and Allied Sciences, 21*(4), 366–368.

Medysky, M., Temesi, S., Culos-Reed, S. N., & Millet, G. Y. (2017). Exercise, sleep and cancer-related fatigue: Are they related? *Neurophysiologie Clinique, 47*, 111–122. https://doi.org/10.1016/j.neucli.2017.03.001

Miani, C., Bellomo, A., Bertino, G., Staffieri, A., Carello, M., & Belforte, G. (1998). Dynamic behavior of the Provox and Staffieri prostheses for voice rehabilitation following total laryngectomy. *European Archives of Oto-Rhino-Laryngology, 255*(3), 143–148.

Moon, J. B., & Weinberg, B. (1987). Aerodynamic and myoelastic contributions to tracheoesophageal voice production. *Journal of Speech and Hearing Research, 30*(3), 387–395.

Motta, S., Galli, I., & Di Rienzo, L. (2001). Aerodynamic findings in esophageal voice. *Archives of Otolaryngology – Head & Neck Surgery, 127*(6), 700–704.

Ng, M. (2011). Aerodynamic characteristics associated with oesophageal and tracheoesophageal speech of Cantonese. *International Journal of Speech-Language Pathology, 13*(2), 137–144.

Ng, M. L., & Chu, R. (2009). An acoustical and perceptual study of vowels produced by alaryngeal speakers of Cantonese. *Folia Phoniatrica et Logopaedica, 61*(2), 97–104.

Ng, M. L., Liu, H., Zhao, Q., & Lam, P. K. (2009). Long-term average spectral characteristics of Cantonese alaryngeal speech. *Auris Nasus Larynx, 36*(5), 571–577.

Ng, T. P., Niti, M., Fones, C., Yap, K. B., & Tan, W. C. (2009). Co-morbid association of depression and COPD: A population-based study. *Respiratory Medicine, 103*(6), 895–901.

Ng, T. P., Niti, M., Tan, W. C., Cao, Z., Ong, K. C., & Eng, P. (2007). Depressive symptoms and chronic obstructive pulmonary disease: Effect on mortality, hospital readmission, symptom burden, functional status, and quality of life. *Archives of Internal Medicine, 167*(1), 60–67.

Offerman, M. P. J., Pruyn, J. F. A., de Boer, M. F., Busschbach, J. J. V., & Baatenburg de Jong, R. J. (2015). Psychosocial consequences for partners of patients after total laryngectomy and for the relationship between patients and partners. *Oral Oncology, 51*, 389–398.

Parrilla, C., Minni, A., Bogaardt, H., Macri, G. F., Battista, M., Roukos, R., … de Vincentiis, M. (2015). Pulmonary rehabilitation after total laryngectomy: A multicenter time-series clinical trial evaluating the Provox XtraHME in HME-naive patients. *Annals of Otology, Rhinology and Laryngology, 124*(9), 706–713.

Perry, A., Casey, E., & Cotton, S. (2015). Quality of life after total laryngectomy: Functioning, psychological well-being and self-efficacy. *International Journal of Language and Communication Disorders, 50*(4), 467–475.

Prue, G., Rankin, J., Allen, J., Gracey, J., & Cramp, F. (2006). Cancer-related fatigue: A critical appraisal. *European Journal of Cancer, 42*, 846–863.

Roessler, F., Grossenbacher, R., & Walt, H. (1988). Effects of tracheostomy on human tracheobronchial mucosa: A scanning electron microscopic study. *Laryngoscope, 98*(11), 1261–1267.

Roncero, C., Campuzano, A. I., Quintano, J. A., Molina, J., Perez, J., & Miravitlles, M. (2016). Cognitive status among patients with chronic obstructive pulmonary disease. *International Journal of Chronic Obstructive Pulmonary Disease, 11*, 543–551.

Rosenthal, A. L., Lowell, S. Y., & Colton, R. H. (2014). Aerodynamic and acoustic features of vocal effort. *Journal of Voice, 28*(2), 144–153.

Rosso, M., Prgomet, D., Marjanović, K., Pušeljić, S., & Kraljik, N. (2015). Pathohistological changes of tracheal epithelium in laryngectomized patients. *European Archives of Oto-Rhino-Laryngology, 272*(11), 3539–3544.

Sadri, M., McMahon, J., & Parker, A. (2006). Laryngeal dysplasia: Aetiology and molecular biology. *The Journal of Laryngology and Otology, 120*(3), 170–177.

Saito, M., Kinishi, M., & Amatsu, M. (2000). Acoustic analyses clarify voiced-voiceless distinction in tracheoesophageal speech. *Acta Oto-Laryngologica, 120*(6), 771–777.

Salmon, J. (1999). Artificial larynx devices and their use. In S. J. Salmon (Ed.), *Alaryngeal speech rehabilitation: For clinicians, by clinicians* (2nd ed., pp. 79–104). Austin, TX: Pro-Ed, Inc.

Schutte, H. K., & Nieboer, G. J. (2002). Aerodynamics of esophageal voice production with and without a Groningen voice prosthesis. *Folia Phoniatrica et Logopaedica, 54*(1), 8–18.

Schwandt, L. Q., Tjong-Ayong, H. J., van Weissenbruch, R., der Mei, H. C., & Albers, F. W. (2006). Differences in aerodynamic characteristics of new and dysfunctional Provox 2 voice prostheses in vivo. *European Archives of Oto-Rhino-Laryngology, 263*(6), 518–523.

Searl, J. (2002). Magnitude and variability of oral pressure in tracheoesophageal speech. *Folia Phoniatrica et Logopaedica, 54*(6), 312–328.

Searl, J. (2007). Bilabial contact pressure and oral air pressure during tracheoesophageal speech. *The Annals of Otology, Rhinology, and Laryngology, 116*(4), 304–311.

Searl, J., & Evitts, P. M. (2004). Velopharyngeal aerodynamics of /m/ and /p/ in tracheoesophageal speech. *Journal of Voice, 18*(4), 557–566.

Searl, J., & Reeves, S. (2014). Nonsurgical voice restoration following total laryngectomy. In E. C. Ward & C. J. van As (Eds.), *Head and neck cancer: Treatment, rehabilitation, and outcomes* (2nd ed.). San Diego, CA: Plural Publishing.

Smith, B. E. (1986). Aerodynamic characteristics of Blom-Singer low-pressure voice prostheses. *Archives of Otolaryngology – Head & Neck Surgery, 112*(1), 50–52.

Snidecor, J. C. (1969). *Speech rehabilitation of the laryngectomized* (2nd ed.). Springfield, IL: Charles C. Thomas.

Snidecor, J. C., & Isshiki, N. (1965). Air volume and airflow relationships of six male esophageal speakers. *Journal of Speech and Hearing Disorders, 30*, 205–216.

Stepp, C. E., Heaton, J. T., & Hillman, R. E. (2008). Postlaryngectomy speech respiration patterns. *The Annals of Otology, Rhinology, and Laryngology, 117*(8), 557–563.

Stetson, R. H. (1937). Esophageal speech for any laryngectomized patient. *Archives of Otolaryngology, 26*, 132–142.

Stridsman, C., Mullerova, H., Skar, L., & Lindberg, A. (2013). Fatigue in COPD and the impact of respiratory symptoms and heart disease--a population-based study. *COPD, 10*(2), 125–132.

Struben, W., & van Gelder, L. (1958). Movements of the superior structures in the laryngectomized patient. *Archives of Otolaryngology, 67*, 655–659.

Swisher, W. E. (1980). Oral pressures, vowel durations, and acceptability ratings of esophageal speakers. *Journal of Communication Disorders, 13*(3), 171–181.

Tack, J. W., Qiu, Q., Schutte, H. K., Kooijman, P. G., Meeuwis, C. A., van der Houwen, E. B., … Verkerke, G. J. (2008). Clinical evaluation of a membrane-based voice-producing element for laryngectomized women. *Head & Neck, 30*(9), 1156–1166.

Tack, J. W., Rakhorst, G., van der Houwen, E. B., Mahieu, H. F., & Verkerke, G. J. (2007). In vitro evaluation of a double-membrane-based voice-producing element for laryngectomized patients. *Head & Neck, 29*(7), 665–674.

Tack, J. W., Verkerke, G. J., van der Houwen, E. B., Mahieu, H. F., & Schutte, H. K. (2006). Development of a double-membrane sound generator for application in a voice-producing element for laryngectomized patients. *Annals of Biomedical Engineering, 34*(12), 1896–1907.

Takeshita, T. K., Zozolotto, H. C., Ricz, H., Dantas, R. O., & Aguiar-Ricz, L. (2010). Correlation between tracheoesophageal voice and speech and intraluminal pharyngoesophageal transition pressure. *Pro Fono, 22*(4), 485–490.

Todisco, T., Maurizi, M., Paludetti, G., Dottorini, M., & Merante, F. (1984). Laryngeal cancer: Long-term follow-up of respiratory functions after laryngectomy. *Respiration, 45*(3), 303–315.

Togawa, K., Konno, A., & Hoshino, T. (1980). A physiologic study on respiratory handicap of the laryngectomized. *Archives of Oto-Rhino-Laryngology, 229*(1), 69–79.

van As, C. J., & Fuller, D. P. (2014). Prosthetic tracheoesophageal voice restoration following total laryngectomy. In E. C. Ward & C. J. van As (Eds.), *Head and neck cancer: Treatment, rehabilitation, and outcomes* (2nd ed., pp. 302–341). San Diego, CA: Plural Publishing.

Van den Berg, J., & Moolenaar-Bijl, A. J. (1959). Cricopharyngeal sphincter, pitch, intensity, and fluency in oesophageal speech. *Folia Phoniatrica, 10*, 65–84.

van den Boer, C., van Harten, M. C., Hilgers, F. J. M., van den Brekel, M. W. M., & Retèl, V. P. (2014). Incidence of severe tracheobronchitis and pneumonia in laryngectomized patients: A retrospective clinical study and a European-wide survey among head and neck surgeons. *European Archives of Oto-Rhino-Laryngology, 271*(12), 3297–3303.

van der Torn, M., de Vries, M. P., Festen, J. M., Verdonck-de Leeuw, I. M., & Mahieu, H. F. (2001). Alternative voice after laryngectomy using a sound-producing voice prosthesis. *Laryngoscope, 111*(2), 336–346.

van der Torn, M., van Gogh, C. D., Verdonck-de Leeuw, I. M., Festen, J. M., Verkerke, G. J., & Mahieu, H. F. (2006). Assessment of alaryngeal speech using a sound-producing voice prosthesis in relation to sex and pharyngoesophageal segment tonicity. *Head & Neck, 28*(5), 400–412.

Ward, E. C., Hartwig, P., Scott, J., Trickey, M., Cahill, L., & Hancock, K. (2007). Speech breathing patterns during tracheoesophageal speech. *Asia Pacific Journal of Speech Language Hearing, 10*, 33–42.

Weinberg, B., Horii, Y., Blom, E., & Singer, M. (1982). Airway resistance during esophageal phonation. *Journal of Speech and Hearing Disorders, 47*(2), 194–199.

Weinberg, B., & Moon, J. (1982). Airway resistance characteristics of Blom-Singer tracheoesophageal puncture prostheses. *Journal of Speech and Hearing Disorders, 47*(4), 441–442.

Weinberg, B., & Moon, J. (1984). Aerodynamic properties of four tracheoesophageal puncture prostheses. *Archives of Otolaryngology, 110*(10), 673–675.

Weinberg, B., & Moon, J. B. (1986). Airway resistances of Blom-Singer and Panje low pressure tracheoesophageal puncture prostheses. *Journal of Speech and Hearing Disorders, 51*(2), 169–172.

Woo, P., Colton, R. H., & Shangold, L. (1987). Phonatory airflow analysis in patients with laryngeal disease. *The Annals of Otology, Rhinology, and Laryngology, 96*(5), 549–555.

Wynder, E. L., Bross, I. J., & Day, E. (1956). Epidemiological approach to the etiology of cancer of the larynx. *Journal of the American Medical Association, 160*(16), 1384–1391.

Wynder, E. L., & Stellman, S. D. (1977). Comparative epidemiology of tobacco-related cancers. *Cancer Research, 37*(12), 4608–4622.

Xu, J. J., Chen, X., Lu, M. P., & Qiao, M. Z. (2009). Perceptual evaluation and acoustic analysis of pneumatic artificial larynx. *Otolaryngology and Head and Neck Surgery, 141*(6), 776–780.

Yohnnes, A. M., Chen, E., Moga, A. M., Leroi, I., & Connolly, M. J. (2017). Cognitive impairment in chronic obstructive pulmonary disease and chronic heart failure: A systematic review and meta-analysis of observational studies. *Journal of the American Medical Directors Association, 18*(5), 451.e1–451.e11.

Yuen, K. K., Sharma, A. K., Logan, W. C., Gillespie, M. B., Day, T. A., & Brooks, J. O. (2008). Radiation dose, driving performance, and cognitive function in patients with head and neck cancer. *Radiotherapy and Oncology, 87*, 304–307.

Zeleznik, J. (2003). Normative aging of the respiratory system. *Clinics in Geriatric Medicine, 19*(1), 1–18.

Zemlin, W. R. (1997). *Speech and hearing science: Anatomy and physiology* (4th ed.). Englewood Cliffs, NJ: Prentice Hall.

Zhang, X., Cai, X., Shi, X., Zheng, Z., Zhang, A., Guo, J., & Fang, Y. (2016). Chronic obstructive pulmonary disease as a risk factor for cognitive dysfunction: A meta-analysis of current studies. *Journal of Alzheimer's Disease, 52*(1), 101–111.

Zijlstra, R. J., Mahieu, H. F., van Lith-Bijl, J. T., & Schutte, H. K. (1991). Aerodynamic properties of the low-resistance Groningen button. *Archives of Otolaryngology – Head & Neck Surgery, 117*(6), 657–661.

Zraick, R. I., Smith-Olinde, L., & Shotts, L. L. (2012). Adult normative data for the KayPENTAX Phonatory Aerodynamic System Model 6600. *Journal of Voice, 26*(2), 164–176.

Zuur, J. K., Muller, S. H., de Jongh, F. H., van Zandwijik, N., & Hilgers, F. J. (2006). The physiological rationale of heat and moisture exchangers in postlaryngectomy pulmonary rehabilitation: A review. *European Archives of Oto-Rhino-Laryngology, 263*(1), 1–8.

Intelligibility in Postlaryngectomy Speech

14

Lindsay E. Sleeth and Philip C. Doyle

Introduction

A diagnosis of laryngeal cancer has far-reaching effects that will impact all areas of an individual's life including physical, emotional, psychological, economic, and social well-being (Bornbaum & Doyle, Chap. 5; Doyle, 1994, 2005; Doyle & MacDonald, Chap. 27; Eadie & Doyle, 2004, 2005; Meyer et al., 2004). Distinctive to a diagnosis of laryngeal cancer is the potential need to surgically remove the entire larynx leading to the loss of the individual's normal vocal mechanism and, subsequently, a loss of normal verbal communication. While cancer itself carries substantial disease burden, the loss of voice at the time of serious illness will create an added distress for the individual (Bornbaum et al., 2012; Doyle, 1994). Loss of verbal communication at the time of a health crisis is not typically experienced with other sites of cancer. For this reason, changes in verbal communication secondary to treatment for laryngeal cancer have long been of critical importance in postlaryngectomy rehabilitation.

Multiple studies have shown verbal communication to be one of the greatest predictors of quality of life (QOL) in individuals with laryngeal cancer (Eadie & Doyle, 2004; Karnell, Funk, & Hoffman, 2000; Meyer et al., 2004; Terrell et al., 2004; and others). The notion of QOL encompasses the areas of an individual's life within the physical, psychological, social, and spiritual domains of functioning. When expressed using the World Health Organization's (WHO, 2001) International Classification of Functioning, Disability and Health (ICF), issues secondary to the diagnosis and treatment of laryngeal cancer encompass all components of the ICF framework (body functions and structures, activities and participation, environmental factors, and personal factors). Eadie (2003) was the first to contextualize laryngeal cancer within the ICF framework, and she described the dramatic interactions that may emerge in one's postlaryngectomy functioning. Therefore, the ability to effectively restore an individual's verbal communication following removal of the larynx has the ability to positively impact a person's QOL. However, reacquisition of a new alaryngeal method of verbal communication does not in and of itself offer the sole index of postlaryngectomy rehabilitation success.

L. E. Sleeth (✉)
Voice Production and Perception Laboratory, Rehabilitation Sciences, Western University, London, ON, Canada

South West Local Health Integration Network, London, ON, Canada

P. C. Doyle
Voice Production and Perception Laboratory & Laboratory for Well-Being and Quality of Life, Department of Otolaryngology – Head and Neck Surgery and School of Communication Sciences and Disorders, Western University, Elborn College, London, ON, Canada

© Springer Nature Switzerland AG 2019
P. C. Doyle (ed.), *Clinical Care and Rehabilitation in Head and Neck Cancer*, https://doi.org/10.1007/978-3-030-04702-3_14

Understanding the loss of speech and its restoration through rehabilitative efforts raises numerous questions on the resultant effectiveness of postlaryngectomy communication. If social capacity is to be enhanced in the postlaryngectomy period, it cannot be achieved without at least a "good" level of SI – that is, good speech will not place excessive demands on the listener during communication (Evitts, Chap. 28). SI forms a core element underlying effective communication. For this reason, it is important that continued clinical efforts be directed at assessing and documenting postlaryngectomy speech rehabilitation outcomes. This includes that direct attention is paid to a variety of factors underlying its composite product, namely, intelligibility. Regardless of the method of alaryngeal speech acquired, whether it be the use of the artificial electrolarynx or esophageal or tracheoesophageal (TE) speech, a clinical focus on optimizing SI will form one of the foundational aspects of all head and neck cancer rehabilitation. Consequently, this chapter presents information related to SI with a specific focus on those are undergo total laryngectomy.

The concepts to be addressed herein have broad applications to all modes of postlaryngectomy voice and speech rehabilitation. In many respects today, information on TE speech is much more available in the literature, thus, TE speech has some prominence in the discussion to follow. This prominence is primarily based on the fact that TE speech is widely used; however, an additional factor also exists. That is, while considerable research on intelligibility related to TE speech was conducted in the first 25 years after its introduction (Singer & Blom, 1980), in recent years work in this area has been relatively sparse. It is also of value to note that while the historical literature on alaryngeal SI addressed comparative performance between methods (i.e., electrolaryngeal, esophageal, and TE), more recent comparative data are lacking. Thus, information on SI in postlaryngectomy speakers is the specific focus of subsequent sections of this chapter.

Postlaryngectomy Voice and Speech Rehabilitation

Alaryngeal Speech

When a total laryngectomy is required, an alternate method of postlaryngectomy "alaryngeal" voice and speech will need to be learned. Without doing so, the individual will be unable to communicate verbally and will be required to use writing or alternative or augmentative methods of communication (Childs, Palmer, & Fried-Oken, Chap. 15). At present, there are three primary methods of alaryngeal speech employed by laryngectomized individuals: (1) use of an artificial electrolarynx, (2) esophageal speech, and (3) tracheoesophageal (TE) speech. While multiple methods may be used by some speakers (e.g., use of esophageal speech and the electrolarynx), one method will almost certainly be identified by the individual as being their primary method of communication.

In 1980, the tracheoesophageal (TE) puncture voice restoration method and the first TE puncture voice prosthesis (Singer & Blom, 1980) was introduced as a new alaryngeal speech option. Briefly, the procedure involves creating a small, controlled midline puncture through the posterior wall of the trachea into the esophagus (Singer & Blom, 1980). A one-way, valved voice prosthesis is then inserted into the puncture to prevent closure of the site and to allow one-way flow of air from the trachea into the esophageal reservoir below the pharyngoesophageal (PE) segment (Blom, 1998). Upon exhalation, and when the tracheostoma is occluded by the individual's thumb or another "hands-free" device, pulmonary air is shunted into the esophagus, setting the PE segment into vibration and allowing for sound generation. Thus, while the alaryngeal tissue source is the same for both the esophageal and TE speech methods (the PE segment), it is the manner in which the system is placed into vibration and the amount of air available to continuously modulate that tissue prior to re-insufflation of the esophageal reservoir that distinguishes these two methods.

Since its introduction, TE voice restoration has become widely used as a postlaryngectomy speech rehabilitation method. In the early years following its introduction, the puncture was completed as a secondary procedure, that is, at some point following laryngectomy and full healing and postsurgical recovery. However, in the years to follow, use of the method as a primary procedure performed at the same time as the laryngectomy was increasingly pursued (Kao, Mohr, Kimmel, Getch, & Silverman, 1994; Singer, Blom, & Hamaker, 1983; Yoshida, Hamaker, Singer, Blom, & Charles, 1989). The larger influence, impact, and clinical implications of these approaches on postlaryngectomy voice and speech rehabilitation are addressed in greater detail elsewhere in this volume (see Graville, Palmer, & Bolognone, Chap. 11; Knott, Chap. 12). Consequently, in the section to follow, factors that may influence postlaryngectomy SI and the unique relationship of these factors to specific alaryngeal methods will be outlined.

Factors Influencing Speech Intelligibility: Preliminary Issues

SI is influenced by multiple factors. Normal SI is a result of a complex and highly coordinated interaction of physiologic systems under finely tuned neurological control. In the normal speech production system, intelligibility will be influenced by the power supply or driving source (the lungs), the vibratory element (the vocal folds), and a system of valves and filters (structures of the vocal tract including the oral cavity and its structures). The interaction of these systems provides for a maximal degree of flexibility that permits a wide range of acoustic changes which cross the frequency, intensity, and temporal domains. Postlaryngectomy voice and speech production will, therefore, present with alterations in the nature and interaction of all of these systems.

A breakdown in one component of the speech production system may create changes both upstream and downstream, with a net result on the final speech product. However, the loss of one's natural voice and decreases in the understandability of a new voicing source and the speech produced will result in substantial psychosocial changes. The impact of such changes in SI extend beyond the communication process itself to have a broader, negative influence on perceived QOL (Meyer et al., 2004). Yet each alaryngeal method needs to be considered independently in an effort to further understand the more refined aspects of why SI decreases.

Electrolaryngeal Speech For the electrolaryngeal speaker, the power supply and voicing source is now non-biologic (electronic) and external; this signal will be directed into the vocal tract (either via transcervical or intraoral application) where the sound source will be articulated into speech (see Nagle, Chap. 9). The electrolaryngeal voice source will be modified by the method of its transmission through neck tissues or through direct introduction into the oral cavity. The use of an electrolarynx voicing source also will be characterized by a relatively narrow range of frequencies (Nagle, Eadie, Wright, & Sumida, 2012), as well as a continuous "all voiced" signal source. Because of this continuous sound activation, perceptual challenges related to the listener's ability to make distinctions between voiced and voiceless cognate sounds (e.g., /p/ vs. /b/) will be observed (Weiss & Basili, 1985). Further, the unique nature of the electrolarynx with its robotic and monotone quality will influence the listener's perception of speech due to concerns related to its overall acceptability (Bennett & Weinberg, 1973). Thus, the interaction and impact of all three components of the physical analog system of speech production – the power supply, the voicing source, and the valves and filters – must be considered collectively in seeking to understand the intelligibility of the signal.

Esophageal speech For an esophageal speaker, the esophagus now becomes the driving source, but the capacity of this reservoir is limited, and it must be regularly replenished with air in order to continue producing speech (see Doyle & Finchem, Chap. 10). Additionally, esophageal speech will be generated by an anatomical voicing structure comprised of lower pharyngeal and upper esophageal tissues (the PE segment), one which does not have active adductory or abductory capabilities. Similar to the use of an electrolarynx, voiced-voiceless distinctions may be problematic because the PE segment cannot rapidly turn on and off; however, in esophageal speech, this also may be the result of limitations in both the power supply and the speaker's subsequent inability to generate adequate sound intensity, as well as the "all voiced" nature of the esophageal sound source (Christensen, Weinberg, & Alphonso, 1978; Connor, Hamlet, & Joyce, 1985). If the esophageal vibratory source is not fully powered by the air passing through it, a result of limited access to air within the esophagus that drives this tissue and then tissue oscillation for voicing will be incomplete and of reduced temporal duration. The reduced amplitude (intensity) of the esophageal voicing signal also has been shown to have a direct influence on phonetic quality (Blood, 1981). Again, interactions between the three analog systems of speech production cannot be underestimated in the context of understanding reductions in esophageal SI.

TE Speech Finally, the typical TE speaker has the capacity to exploit a very large volume of lung air to replenish the esophageal reservoir in a relatively continuous manner (see Bohnenkamp, Chap. 7; Searl, Chap. 13). Because the TE speaker has access to a pulmonary air supply, research data have most prominently documented increases in overall speech and syllable rates for TE speech when compared to esophageal speakers. In fact, word and syllable per minute measures for TE speakers have been shown to be at values approximating those of normal laryngeal speakers (Robbins, Fisher, Blom, & Singer, 1984). TE speakers typically are able to produce conversational speech without any unusual breaks in the flow of their speech.[1] This is in clear

contrast to even the most proficient esophageal speakers who will exhibit momentary stoppages in the flow of speech in order to re-insufflate the esophageal reservoir (Snidecor & Curry, 1960).

Further, because of the increased volume and pressure of air moving through the TE voice prosthesis into the esophageal reservoir, and the subsequent propagation of this signal into the vocal tract, the speaker may have the ability to produce voiceless sounds despite the continuous vibration of the PE voicing source (Doyle, Danhauer, & Reed, 1988). Doyle and colleagues hypothesized that this ability was secondary to the exploitation of air pressure within the upper vocal tract during TE speech production; that is, it was believed that some level of vocal tract turbulence[2] could be achieved during the TE speech process by manipulating the signal within the oral cavity during articulation. Results from studies by Doyle et al. (1988) and Searl and colleagues (Searl & Carpenter, 2002; Searl, Carpenter, & Banta, 2001) have shown that intelligibility issues commonly arise in the areas of voiced-voiceless distinctions of consonants (Gomyo & Doyle, 1989), as well as for the general consonant manner classes of stops, fricatives, and affricates.

The issue surrounding the voiced-voiceless distinction in alaryngeal speech in general (Jongmans, Hilgers, Pols, & van As-Brooks, 2006) involves confusing voiceless phonemes for voiced phonemes (e.g., perception of a /b/ when its voiceless cognate /p/ was intended). Doyle et al. (1988) hypothesized this to be a result of shortened voice onset time (VOT) in TE speakers, as well as a lag in the termination of voicing by the PE segment (Robbins, Christensen, & Kempster, 1986). As well, a study conducted by Doyle and Haaf (1989) found postvocalic consonants to be more intelligible than their prevocalic counterparts, suggesting that onset and offset phenomena must be considered. Doyle and Haaf (1989) also found voiced-voiceless confusions

---

[1] Electrolaryngeal speakers will also have the ability to generate a full phrase length that approximates that observed for the normal speaker. However, the signal itself may be monotone, and its mechanical quality may to some extent distract the listener.

[2] If air pressures and flows are of sufficient magnitude within the vocal tract, the speaker may be able to further compress that air during the act of articulation. If this does in fact occur, the compression of this air may be perceived by the listener as a voiceless sound despite the fact that the PE source has provided an energized, voiced signal.

and a manner of production intelligibility hierarchy similar to that found by Doyle et al. (1988). More recently, Searl et al. (2001) evaluated the intelligibility of stops and fricatives in TE speech; their findings were consistent with the two studies previously mentioned (Doyle et al., 1998; Doyle & Haaf, 1989) in that the most common errors emerged from the listeners' confusion of voiced for voiceless phonemes.

Speech Intelligibility

Kent, Weismer, Kent, and Rosenbek (1989) have defined SI as "the degree to which the speaker's intended message is recovered by the listener" (p. 483). Employing a more procedural definition, Hillman, Walsh, and Heaton (2005) have indicated that SI represents the percentage of speech items correctly identified by the listener. Regardless of the underlying etiology, reductions in SI have been a critical and longstanding concern in the area of speech disorders. When there is a breakdown in a speaker's ability to be easily understood by his or her communicative partner, many challenges will be experienced at multiple levels of communication functioning (Ackerstaff, Hilgers, Aaronson, & Balm, 1994). Reductions in SI will result in increased burden to both the speaker and the listener with a direct impact on social well-being. This concern is of particular importance to those who have undergone total laryngectomy and will be trained to use any alternative alaryngeal method of verbal communication (Doyle, 1994). However, numerous factors will influence any measure of SI.

Over the years, the intelligibility of alaryngeal speech has been studied by numerous researchers with varying populations of speakers, under a variety of conditions, and with a range of assessment of stimuli (Amster et al., 1972; Bridges, 1991; Clark & Stemple, 1982; Doyle et al., 1988; Filter & Hyman, 1975; Hillman, Walsh, Wolf, Fisher, & Hong, 1998; Hyman, 1955; Kalb & Carpenter, 1981; Miralles & Cervera, 1995; Tardy-Mitzell, Andrews, & Bowman, 1985; Weiss & Basili, 1985; and others). This includes multiple studies that have addressed individual methods of alaryn-

geal speech (esophageal, electrolaryngeal, and TE). A number of studies also have evaluated SI from a comparative perspective. The collective results of these studies have shown that SI has the potential to increase or decrease based on a range of factors such as the experience and training of speakers, the experience of the listeners, the type of stimuli, background noise and environmental conditions, speaker gender, type of postlaryngectomy speech mode, etc. (McColl, Fucci, Petrosino, Martin, & McCaffrey, 1998). Therefore, when considering the findings and implications of SI research in postlaryngectomy populations, it is important to consider the potential interaction of multiple factors (Yorkston & Beukelman, 1980). Doing so will allow one to contextualize the results of intelligibility testing in those who use alaryngeal speech. Interestingly, however, over the past 20 years, there has been an increasing paucity of information specific to SI issues that characterize postlaryngectomy speakers.

Interrelationships in Alaryngeal Speech Production

The previously outlined analog system and the inherent differences specific to each alaryngeal method will have a direct impact on SI. Perhaps the only level where intelligibility concerns do not exist in any substantial manner for postlaryngectomy speakers is related to vowel production.[3] The reason for this is that regardless of alaryngeal mode, the new voice source will always be voiced which is a fundamental requirement of vowels. However, changes in the amplitude and duration of vowels may impact the accuracy of their perception by the listener. For example, if the vowel signal is underpowered (e.g., during esophageal speech), it may carry insufficient information relative to its formant structure; similarly, if the temporal duration of the vowel is altered in either direction (reduced or extended),

---

[3]The exception here would be any laryngectomy procedure that includes the removal of any portion of the tongue or changes that occur secondary to resections at the base of the tongue.

intelligibility changes may occur (Sisty & Weinberg, 1972). Thus, the flow and continuity of TE speech that occurs due to access to pulmonary air has been shown to offer considerable perceptual advantages to listeners. When temporal components of alaryngeal speech production are optimized, durational aspects of sound production will also benefit (Doyle et al., 1988; Searl & Carpenter, 2002; Searl et al., 2001; and others).

While temporal speech advantages are well documented in the literature, TE speakers will also find some advantage in the frequency (pitch) and intensity (loudness) domains of the speech produced; however, these changes do in fact vary considerable from normal expectation. First, because of the TE speaker's access to a substantial volume of air from the lungs, the ability to "drive" pulmonary air through the PE segment at a greater pressure and rate of flow will result in the creation of an increased "duty cycle" specific to the vibratory source. As the duty cycle or rate of tissue vibration increases, the perceived pitch of TE voice will also be greater relative to esophageal speech despite use of the same vibratory (source tissues of the PE segment) for both methods. Even though the fundamental frequency of TE speech exceeds that of esophageal speakers, it will remain reduced from normal expectation. For this reason, gender considerations related to frequency for both esophageal and TE speakers must be considered (Bellandese, Lerman, & Gilbert, 2001; Eadie, Doyle, Hansen, & Beaudin, 2008). Secondly, the relative intensity of TE speech also will be increased because of greater short-term volumes of air that are available to the speaker.[4]

As a fundamental factor, the TE speaker's access to a large volume driving source (the lungs) to power the esophagus does have consid-

erable advantages across a variety of acoustic dimensions (Baggs & Pine, 1983; Qi & Weinberg, 1995; Robbins et al., 1984). The TE system is also able to be actively exploited by muscles of respiration which may then serve to fine-tune airflows through the vibratory source (Bohnenkamp, Chap. 7; Bohnenkamp, Forrest, Klaben, & Stager, 2012). Research has revealed that an esophageal speaker produces voice that is 10 dB-SPL lower for sustained vowels than that of a normal speaker (Weinberg, Horii, & Smith, 1980); this finding is a direct consequence of esophageal speakers not having access to vast volumes of air to drive the PE segment. Recall that an esophageal speaker will need to recharge the esophageal reservoir regularly as its volumetric capacity is only in the range of 60 cc (Diedrich, 1968).

Interestingly, Robbins et al. (1984) found that TE speakers produce voicing signals that are approximately 10 dB-SPL and 10 dB-A greater than normal speakers for vowels and conversational speech, respectively. From a simple acoustic perspective, this increase of "above normal" loudness may be interpreted as advantageous, yet it does carry with it limitations relative to real-life conversational interaction. More specifically, the increased vocal loudness associated with TE speech may limit a speaker's ability to maintain privacy when communicating with others. For that reason, a clinician's comprehensive knowledge related to the process of TE speech production, dynamic interactions between the new vibratory source and the vocal tract, and the resultant acoustic consequences (both negative and positive) are essential components underlying one's understanding of changes in SI. As stated by Weinberg, Horii, Blom, and Singer (1982, p. 1982) in relation to observed differences between esophageal and TE speakers, "*Since the voicing sources used to produce esophageal voices are regarded as surgical residue (Weinberg, 1980), we suggest that the operation of these residue sources has been maximized or optimized by alterations in respiratory drive state.*" Thus, clinicians must acknowledge that isolated components of the new alaryngeal speech process, regardless of mode, are likely to have unique consequences

---

[4]Although it is beyond the scope of the present chapter, increases in vocal loudness whether in a normal or esophageal-based alaryngeal system are directly correlated with one's ability to increase pressure below the point of vibration. Thus, the ability to modulate a relatively large volume of pulmonary air during TE voicing provides the speaker with an increase potential for achieving a wider range of vocal intensities.

that may directly influence SI. These changes may most often be detected in specific ways dependent upon the manner in which SI is evaluated (i.e., are stimuli comprised of words, sentences, etc.).

Does Alaryngeal Voice Quality Influence Intelligibility?

Despite the fact that the TE voicing process may mimic normal acoustic values for some dimensions (e.g., speech rate, increased pitch levels, etc.), it is critical to note that the "optimization" of voice/speech that Weinberg et al. (1980) identified *does not* result in a normal voice signal. All alaryngeal voices will be identified as being abnormal in regard to the overall perceived quality of the voice signal (Eadie & Doyle, 2002, 2005; Nagle & Eadie, 2012; McDonald, et al., 2010). And, data would suggest that the quality of the signal is the most significant factor relative to how a listener may judge the proficiency of a given speaker. Additionally, alaryngeal SI and the potential consequences that noise features which are simultaneously present in the signal may be quite variable both within and across alaryngeal methods. While clear distinctions in quality and performance will be observed between extrinsic (electrolaryngeal) and intrinsic (esophageal and TE) speech methods, it is important to note that each speech mode is highly variable. Even for individual speakers, ongoing signal variability will result in greater perceptual challenges for the listener who must work more to extract speech from noise (Doyle, 2017a). The importance of individual speaker variability across modes of speech was elegantly reported by Kalb and Carpenter (1981), and their work continues to hold merit today.

Even the most proficient esophageal or TE speaker will exhibit a voice quality that is almost certainly characterized by aperiodicity as part of the composite nature of the signal (Maryn, Dick, Vandenbruaene, Vauterin, & Jacobs, 2009; Smith, Weinberg, Feth, & Horii, 1978). This aperiodicity is a product of the variability of the tissue that comprises the PE segment (differences in location and mass) and its subsequent response to airflows

and pressures, factors that carry their own inherent degree(s) of variability (Doyle & Eadie, 2005; Moon & Weinberg, 1987). Thus, expectations of what any given alaryngeal speaker will sound like or how their intelligibility will manifest must be made with caution. Finally, the literature is rich with studies comparing a variety of features of the three alaryngeal methods, both to each other and to normal speech (Blom, Singer, & Hamaker, 1986; Clements, Rassekh, Seikaly, Hokanson, & Calhoun, 1997; Cullinan, Brown, & Blalock, 1986; Doyle et al., 1988; Robbins, 1984; Robbins et al., 1984; Tardy-Mitzell et al., 1985). When viewed together, the findings from these studies have often found TE speech to be judged as superior to the other alaryngeal modes in areas such as acceptability, overall intelligibility, pitch, intensity, and patient satisfaction, with ratings approaching those of normal speech in some instances. Nevertheless, it is also of importance to note that TE speech is not without substantial limitations.

As mentioned previously, esophageal and TE speakers will produce speech that is judged by listeners to be of lowered pitch. In fact, female esophageal and TE speakers tend to have pitch values similar to those of males, resulting in a voice that sounds more masculine (Bellandese et al., 2001; Trudeau, 1994). The loss of gender identity for a woman who undergoes total laryngectomy and uses alaryngeal speech may have a significantly negative impact on social performance and interaction and ultimately, one's judgment of their QOL. In addition, although TE speech often has shown to be highly acceptable when compared to other methods, it is clearly judged as less acceptable than laryngeal speech (Clark & Stemple, 1982; Finizia, Dotevall, Lundstrom, & Lindstrom, 1999; van As, Hilgers, Verdonck-de Leeuw, & Koopmans-van Beinam, 1998). Finally, even in the presence of several comparative advantages, TE speech has consistently been reported to be reduced in its intelligibility (Blom et al., 1986; Doyle et al., 1988; Pindzola & Cain, 1988; Robbins, 1984; Williams & Watson, 1985; and others). Thus, no one alaryngeal method is free of limitations; as a general rule, there will always be specific advantages and disadvantages to each method.

Clinical efforts that focus directly on increasing SI beyond basic "functional" levels are often disregarded in the contemporary rehabilitation setting. This is often a result of the cost associated with extra treatment sessions, limitations in the time available to skilled personnel, and sometimes, limitations related to general access to high quality and comprehensive alaryngeal speech rehabilitation services. SI is an area of inquiry that received generous attention when TE speech was first introduced, but unfortunately, it has been somewhat overlooked for the past 20 years. This in part may be a consequence of the fact that unless some unexpected complication occurs with TE voice restoration and its acquisition, most individuals will quickly acquire their new voice. Because voice and speech restoration in many instances is reacquired rather rapidly, efforts directed at refining speech may be pursued less often. It is, however, essential to reiterate that reduced SI has the potential to negatively impact a person's participation in society and it should remain an area of continued interest and exploration (Eadie et al., 2016). This problem is also applicable to those who use esophageal and electrolaryngeal methods.

Measuring Speech Intelligibility

As noted, a wide range of factors will potentially impact findings from SI assessments.[5] It is, therefore, important to understand and consider these factors before pursuing the clinical evaluation of alaryngeal speech, as well as when conducting research in this area. As stated by Subtelny (1977, p. 183) "Intelligibility is considered the most practical single index to apply in assessing competence in oral communication." Throughout history, intelligibility measurement has largely been obtained through two separate methods: scaling procedures and word identification (Schiavetti, 1992). Scaling procedures, such as the use of

equal-appearing interval (EAI) scales which allow the listener to make judgments about a speaker's intelligibility, were historically used more frequently due to their ease of application and scoring (Schiavetti, 1992).

Scaling Procedures Briefly, when intelligibility is assessed using the EAI scaling method, the listener judges intelligibility by selecting a discrete number that falls between two extreme anchors that represent the range of potential performance (e.g., "fully understandable" speech to "unable to understand"). Scales may range in numerical representation, for example, from 1 to 5 or from 1 to 7 or greater. The key to understanding the EAI method is that it ultimately asks the listener to assign a numeric rating that best represents their impression of where on the scale a speaker falls given the anchors provided. The simplicity of this type of rating task is beneficial, but it also allows for error on several fronts.

Recently, as intelligibility testing has continued to grow in many disordered speech populations, perceptual scaling procedures have received considerable attention and criticism. Although timely and efficient, scaling procedures often lack the ability to pinpoint specific areas of increased or decreased intelligibility. Intelligibility measures and the findings gathered from their application are, at times, also subject to misinterpretation and misrepresentation. As such, any approach to scaled assessments using the EAI method may have limited strength in accurately estimating an intelligibility score for each individual without also obtaining percentage values for the accurate retrieval of stimuli produced (Schiavetti, 1992). This suggests that in most instances, single approaches to evaluating SI must carry one or more caveats related to interpretation and use of the data.

A categorical judgment of intelligibility based on EAI scaling, regardless of the number that is selected from a given scale, may ultimately present a considerable range of performance. In considering any EAI scale, the question that often arises is that pertaining to, "what distinguishes or separates one number from the next?" Using an EAI scale, the question of what lies between any

---

[5] It should be noted that the factors which have been identified to influence measures of speech intelligibility apply to all communication disorders, not just in relationship to postlaryngectomy speakers.

two numbers on the scale in the context of the anchors provided is not easily discerned (see Stevens, 1975). Further, any scaled numeric assignment may not be consistent with measures obtained at the "word identification level." This potential problem in turn decreases the generalizability of findings gathered when using EAI scales to other studies conducted on intelligibility, as well as making it more difficult for both lay listeners and those who are experienced to rectify differences in their judgments. Thus, word identification testing procedures have increasingly become the method of choice when conducting intelligibility assessments and/or research, especially for alaryngeal speech. However, with only one exception (Weiss & Basili, 1985), there have not been specific measures developed for use with alaryngeal speakers. Given the types of factors identified herein that have the potential to influence speech production, it would seem that some consideration of developing specific types of evaluation instruments for alaryngeal speakers would be of value.

Direct Identification of Stimuli With application of the direct identification assessment method, listeners are required to transcribe each word, sentence, or phrase uttered by the speaker. Listener responses are then compared to the list of target stimuli produced by the speakers; these data are then subsequently converted into a percentage of incorrect and correct responses, resulting in an overall intelligibility score (Schiavetti, 1992. This measurement method has the clear advantage of being easily interpretable to not only clinicians but also naïve individuals and, perhaps more importantly, in conveying such information to those who use alaryngeal speech. If the stimuli and measurement procedure used are assessed in a consistent manner, changes over time or subsequent to therapy can be easily documented. Lastly, the measure is "objective" in nature which offers the potential for identification of what specific type(s) of intelligibility deficit(s) exist for each individual (Schiavetti, 1992). If, for example, an objective measure of intelligibility indicates that stop-plosive consonants are problematic (Gomyo & Doyle, 1989; Doyle & Haaf, 1989; Searl et al.,

2001), then efforts to remedy those deficits can be actively pursued. It is, however, important to acknowledge that despite the objective nature of such measures, the score obtained will always be contextually bound and may not easily be generalized to other types of stimuli or evaluation settings.

The determination of the loci or "where" intelligibility deficits exist (e.g., word-initial vs. word-final phonemes, relationships to vocalic elements, etc.) also must be considered with great care given the number of factors that can influence intelligibility judgments. Recent work by Doyle (2017b, unpublished data) has suggested that objective intelligibility scores can vary widely depending upon the construction of the test stimuli used, even if the word list is well-established and regularly used at the clinical level for intelligibility assessment. Nevertheless, the assumed sensitivity of word identification procedures and the ability to gain information solely from such measures has made this approach an obvious choice for many intelligibility investigations (Blom et al., 1986; Doyle et al., 1988; Pindzola & Cain, 1988; Smith & Calhoun, 1994; Tardy-Mitzell et al., 1985; and others).

Listener Experience Another area of intelligibility testing that may impact findings pertains to the influence of listener experience on the SI results obtained. Previous studies have employed the use of either naïve listeners (no prior educational experience with or formal exposure to the speaker population of interest) or experienced listeners typically, speech-language pathologists (SLPs) or physician/surgeons. Multiple studies with a variety of speaker populations have shown that intelligibility may be influenced by the sophistication of listeners (Beukelman & Yorkston, 1980; Doyle, Swift, & Haaf, 1989; Williams & Watson, 1985). These studies all suggest that assessment scores provided by SLPs reflect better speaker intelligibility than those made by inexperienced (naïve) listeners. Based on this observation, it has been suggested that the experienced listeners' prior exposure to the speaker population, and most likely the stimuli being evaluated as well, may potentially inflate their intelligibility scores. This makes the information less generalizable and possibly, less representative of the general listening population, a listener group that may have the most interaction with the speaker (Doyle et al., 1989). Yet the use of naïve listeners can influence findings as well.

First, since naïve listeners typically have had little exposure to alaryngeal speech (or other disorders for that matter), they may focus on the unnatural quality of the voice instead of the words or sounds being produced, a potentially confounding factor in the interpretation of the data. The quality of the vocal signal may in some way distract the listener from the stimuli they have been asked to assess. While all potential sources of distraction which may confound "pure" assessments of intelligibility cannot reasonably be excluded, recognition of the potential influence of this factor on listener judgments is of value. This issue has been raised in prior auditory-perceptual works associated with the dysarthrias (Darley, Aronson, & Brown, 1969, and others).

As well, naïve listeners may not be challenged by the task itself, and an internal desire to perform the task accurately, leading to "second guessing" confusions or errors, rather than lack of speaker intelligibility. Hence, the demands of the task that the listener is asked to perform must always be considered. This requires that efforts directed toward assessing intelligibility in alaryngeal speakers must weigh numerous factors and understand the potential strengths and weaknesses of any given approach to assessment. Within the dysarthria literature, the listener's familiarity with the stimuli has also been raised (Beukelman & Yorkston, 1980; Tjaden & Liss, 1995; Yorkston & Beukelman, 1978). There is not, however, a perfect method for intelligibility assessment in those who have undergone laryngectomy; similarly, and as noted there is no measure dedicated to the assessment of postlaryngectomy speech regardless of mode. Thus, when conducting intelligibility research or evaluating the validity of previous research on alaryngeal speakers, it is important to consider external factors that have the potential to influence results. In reference back to prior sections of this chapter, intelligibility assessments of alaryngeal speech must also carefully consider the nuances of each method and the potential impact that such alterations will have on measures obtained.

Findings from Alaryngeal Speech Intelligibility Research

Many studies have compared speaker performance across the three modes of alaryngeal speech, and results have indicated that TE speech is generally judged to be more intelligible than esophageal or electrolaryngeal speech (Blom et al., 1986; Doyle et al., 1988; Pindzola & Cain, 1988; Robbins, 1984; Robbins et al., 1984; Tardy-Mitzell et al., 1985; Williams & Watson, 1985). Blom et al. (1986) conducted a study assessing the intelligibility of individuals both before undergoing the TE puncture procedure and after. Prior to the procedure, these speakers were using either esophageal speech or an electrolarynx as their primary mode of communication. Following the TE voice restoration procedure, all individuals used TE speech to communicate. Intelligibility was determined by calculating the percentage of correct responses found using a multiple-choice response format test, the *Modified Rhyme Test* (House, Williams, Hecker, & Kryter, 1965).

Blom et al. (1986) reported a statistically significant improvement in the SI by the group following TE puncture, with preoperative mean intelligibility reported to be 78.15%, versus 91.51% mean intelligibility postoperatively (Blom et al., 1986). This not only illustrates the high intelligibility levels of those using TE speech but also the *potential advantages* of TE speech when compared to esophageal and artificial electrolaryngeal communication. In this context, it is important to note that the use of a forced-choice, closed set identification auditory-perceptual paradigm may influence results, thereby leading to higher intelligibility scores. That is, because the content of stimuli included in the test list was designed to assess particular types of perceptual errors, as well as the request for listeners to select a choice from a set of perceptual options, some "chance" occurrence of a correct response even when the signal has not been accurately detected may occur. This requires careful consideration of the data obtained (some margin of error must be acknowledged), and this will place greater importance on simultaneous assessments of within-listener agreement when they are asked to rate a subset of stimuli a second time.

Despite the early reports of Blom et al. (1986), TE speech is still less intelligible than speech produced by an individual with an intact larynx (Hillman et al., 2005). Studies have reported TE SI to range from 65% to 93% (Doyle et al., 1988; Pindzola & Cain, 1988; Tardy-Mitzell et al., 1985) dependent upon the procedures employed. Doyle et al. (1988) determined intelligibility through the assessment of consonant-vowel-consonant-vowel-consonant (CVCVC) nonsense syllables that were phonetically transcribed by naïve listeners using an open-response paradigm. This resulted in an average intelligibility of 65% (range 59–72%). The use of nonsense constructions as stimuli as well as the use of an open set response format clearly provided a more challenging task to the listeners, which in turn may have resulted in lower scores. However, while this more restrictive assessment process may reveal poorer intelligibility scores, it is in fact context stripped and may not accurately represent how a listener might perceive stimuli within a conversation or similar interaction with the speaker. In those circumstances, the listener can utilize context (grammatical) and employ what is equivalent to a Cloz procedure as part of a predictive process (Duffy & Giolas, 1974; Epstein, Giolas, & Owens, 1968; Giolas, Cooker, & Duffy, 1970). Thus, the choice of stimuli used to assess intelligibility is critical.

Pindzola and Cain (1988) used an entirely different method of intelligibility assessment by asking TE speakers to record monosyllabic English words from the *Multiple Choice Intelligibility Test* (Black & Haagen, 1963). Naïve listeners then identified their response a set of four options using a forced-choice paradigm. Their study reported an overall intelligibility of 93.20% across speakers. Tardy-Mitzell et al.

(1985) used a method similar to that of Pindzola and Cain (1988) with intelligibility judged from monosyllabic word lists (House et al., 1965). Once again, this study employed the forced-choice method with six possible response options for each stimulus word. Comparable intelligibility values were found with an average score of 93% (range 80.70–97.50%). As demonstrated in the above-cited studies, intelligibility has the potential to vary considerably based on internal and external factors and experimental design (stimuli, response format, listener familiarity, and context).

Continuing and Emerging Issues

Much of the research regarding TE SI was conducted in the mid- to late 1980s when the voice restoration procedure was emerging. As a new postlaryngectomy speech rehabilitation option, comparative data were necessary to assess the potential value and viability of this approach. Yet as TE puncture voice restoration became more popular, explorations of TE, as well as esophageal and electrolaryngeal SI, became less common. Since that time, however, very few new investigations have been conducted in relation to the intelligibility of alaryngeal speech. Over the past 20 years, many changes in the treatment of laryngeal cancer have occurred, improvements have been made to the design of TE puncture voice prostheses, esophageal speech may be more easily learned because of knowledge gained from TE speech failures (i.e., the identification of PE segment spasm), and refinements have been made to a several electrolaryngeal devices.

For the reasons noted, generalizing prior intelligibility research to the current generation of alaryngeal speakers is somewhat precarious. As well, a range of hands-free devices have been made available in recent years, removing the need for manual occlusion of the stoma when speaking (Lewis, Chap. 8; Graville, Palmer, & Bolognone, Chap. 11). These devices may differentially influence listener assessments of both SI and overall proficiency (Pauloski, Fisher, Kempster, & Blom, 1989) and are deserving of ongoing assessment. Thus, SI remains an important index of postlaryngectomy rehabilitation, and continuing its exploration is recommended.

Another factor that cannot be disregarded relative to intelligibility assessment is the fact that some who will undergo laryngectomy today may be performed following failed chemoradiation therapy. This, as well as other treatment-related factors such as the presence of postlaryngectomy complications (Damrose & Doyle, Chap. 3) and concomitant health comorbidities, may have a direct bearing on speech outcomes. In the current era of head and neck cancer surgery in general, and laryngectomy in specific, the use of more extensive reconstruction methods is increasingly common. As a result, the system that will be utilized for the production of any method of alaryngeal speech may be quite different than what has been reported in the past. It is our belief that continued explorations into SI provide not only a valuable area of clinical inquiry but one that will serve to better educate patients and provide the best opportunity for postlaryngectomy rehabilitation success.

At present, very little new research has been conducted with a focus on specific patterns of increased and decreased intelligibility that may exist across groups of alaryngeal speakers. Individual differences and the potential influence of very aperiodic or unusual quality signals can also serve to distract the listener's attention with a subsequent impact on intelligibility. The lack of current intelligibility research can be attributed, at least in part, to the wide use and relatively spontaneous acquisition of TE speech following puncture. As previously stated, by strict standards, TE speech has shown to be superior to the other alaryngeal methods in relation to the "fluent" nature of the speech produced, its increased overall acceptability, in addition to increased overall intelligibility, mean syllable length, pitch, intensity, and patient satisfaction (Blom et al., 1986; Clements et al., 1997; Cullinan et al., 1986; Doyle et al., 1988; Robbins, 1984; Robbins et al., 1984; Tardy-Mitzell et al., 1985). All of these factors contribute to a belief that intelligibility is relatively intact in all TE speakers. However, with the emerging potential that esophageal

speech is becoming much more viable as a non-prosthetic mode of alaryngeal speech, in addition to a number of refinements to electrolaryngeal devices (e.g., active frequency modulation), further research appears necessary.

In summary, it appears that the study of SI associated with alaryngeal speech has been overlooked to some extent in recent years. Accordingly, work specific to this important clinical area must be reignited. This inattention is unfortunate as the dissemination of information regarding intelligibility from the past may limit accurate representations at present. Of particular importance here is a concern that if faulty expectations of intelligibility are made, SLPs may limit their efforts to directly facilitate improvements in intelligibility. Regardless of which speech option any individual pursues, and despite the fact that no measurement "standard" currently exists, the formal assessment of intelligibility may provide the SLP with information that guides their ability to tailor individualized therapy (Christensen & Dwyer, 1990). This may involve tasks that center around targeting known error patterns (Doyle, Danhauer, & Lucks-Mendel, 1990) or contextual influences and the value of communication compensation and adaptations, with the result potentially creating more intelligible speech for each individual. The resultant increase in intelligibility has obvious clinical implications, as well as the potential to influence one's ability to fully participate in a variety of communication situations with benefit to perceived QOL.

Significance of Alaryngeal Speech Intelligibility Research

In past years, research has been conducted showing the potential impact speech and effective verbal communication can have on an individual with laryngeal cancer's QOL (Eadie & Doyle, 2004; Karnell et al., 2000; Meyer et al., 2004; Terrell et al., 2004).

The concept of QOL plays an important and prominent role in laryngeal cancer, particularly in relation to the loss of normal verbal communication. Past research has shown speech communication to be one of the most important predictors of perceived QOL in individuals with cancers of the head and neck (Terrell et al., 2004). A study conducted by Meyer et al. (2004) looked at the importance of effective communication in head and neck cancer survivors and found that decreased word intelligibility was statistically associated with decreases in survivors' enjoyment across many areas of functioning. This decreased ability to participate in normal daily activities increases the potential for disability among these individuals. Lower SI was also associated with a greater likelihood of altered QOL when compared to their more intelligible counterparts. Karnell et al. (2000) evaluated head and neck cancer survivors and found that speech and eating domains best predicted self-reported QOL scores, further reinforcing the importance of postlaryngectomy speech rehabilitation.

Finally, previous research has shown TE SI and acceptability to be positively correlated with one another, indicating that speech that is highly intelligible also tends to be perceived as highly acceptable to listeners (Pindzola & Cain, 1988). Therefore, highly intelligible speakers are not only more likely to be better understood but better accepted by the general public, in turn leading to a potentially increased QOL. The evidence presented in the studies above show that a relationship between highly intelligible speech and increased QoL exists among laryngeal cancer survivors. This, coupled with the fact that the fundamental objective of verbal communication is to be understood, creates a compelling argument as to why achieving effective and highly intelligible communication is so important for alaryngeal speakers and why continued research in this area is needed.

Conclusions

Loss of verbal communication presents a significant challenge in the presence of a potentially life-threatening disease such as laryngeal cancer. Thus, the ability to provide a functional means of verbal communication is an essential component of postlaryngectomy rehabilitation (Doyle,

1994). There has, however, been limited research conducted on alaryngeal SI over the past decade. This lack of more contemporary information is troublesome when one considers the significant changes that have occurred in the treatment of laryngeal cancer. Given research confirming the impact that communication effectiveness has on an individual's QOL, it is important that updated research on intelligibility be conducted. SLPs and physicians can benefit from more detailed information outlining the intelligibility patterns of those who use alaryngeal methods of speech. Alaryngeal speech continues to be characterized by multiple sound errors and that variability in sound intelligibility also exists specific to whether sounds appear within a word-initial or word-final position; these types of changes are further impacted by potential distractions secondary to the unusual quality of alaryngeal voice and speech, as well as how intelligibility is altered in conditions of competing noise. It is anticipated that clinical intervention can serve each individual to achieve the most intelligible speech possible. Information on various aspects of SI will allow healthcare professionals to better structure their treatment and therapy for each individual, providing them with the best opportunity to achieve the most intelligible speech possible, leading to more effective verbal communication, participation in society, and increased QOL.

References

Ackerstaff, A. H., Hilgers, F. J. M., Aaronson, N. K., & Balm, A. J. M. (1994). Communication, functional disorders and lifestyle changes after total laryngectomy. *Clinical Otolaryngology and Allied Sciences, 19*(4), 295–300.

Amster, W. W., Love, R. J., Menzel, O. J., Sandler, J., Sculthorpe, W. B., & Gross, F. M. (1972). Psychosocial factors and speech after laryngectomy. *Journal of Communication Disorders, 5*, 1–18.

Baggs, T. W., & Pine, S. J. (1983). Acoustic characteristics: Tracheoesophageal speech. *Journal of Communication Disorders, 16*(4), 299–307.

Bellandese, M. H., Lerman, J. W., & Gilbert, H. R. (2001). An acoustic analysis of excellent female esophageal, tracheoesophageal, and laryngeal speakers. *Journal of Speech, Language, and Hearing Research, 44*(6), 1315–1320.

Bennett, S., & Weinberg, B. (1973). Acceptability ratings of normal, esophageal, and artificial larynx speech. *Journal of Speech, Language, and Hearing Research, 16*(4), 608–615.

Beukelman, D. R., & Yorkston, K. M. (1980). Influence of passage familiarity on intelligibility estimates of dysarthric speech. *Journal of Communication Disorders, 13*, 33–41.

Black, J. W., & Haagen, C. H. (1963). Multiple choice intelligibility tests, forms A and B. *Journal of Speech and Hearing Disorders, 28*, 77–86.

Blom, E. D. (1998). Evolution of tracheoesophageal voice prostheses. In E. D. Blom, M. I. Singer, & R. C. Hamaker (Eds.), *Tracheoesophageal voice restoration following total laryngectomy* (pp. 1–8). San Diego, CA: Singular Publishing Group.

Blom, E. D., Singer, M. I., & Hamaker, R. C. (1986). A prospective study of tracheoesophageal speech. *Archives of Otolaryngology - Head and Neck Surgery, 112*, 440–447.

Blood, G. W. (1981). The interactions of amplitude and phonetic quality in esophageal speech. *Journal of Speech and Hearing Research, 24*, 308–312.

Bohnenkamp, T. A., Forrest, K., Klaben, B. K., & Stager, J. (2012). Chest wall kinematics during speech breathing in tracheoesophageal speakers. *Annals of Otology, Rhinology & Laryngology, 121*(1), 28–37.

Bornbaum, C. C., Fung, K., Franklin, J. H., Nichols, A., Yoo, J., & Doyle, P. C. (2012). A descriptive analysis of the relationship between quality of life and distress in individuals with head and neck cancer. *Supportive Care in Cancer, 20*(9), 2157–2165.

Bridges, A. (1991). Acceptability ratings and intelligibility scores of alaryngeal speakers by three listener groups. *British Journal of Disorders of Communication, 26*, 325–335.

Christensen, J. M., & Dwyer, P. E. (1990). Improving alaryngeal speech intelligibility. *Journal of Communication Disorders, 23*, 445–451.

Christensen, J. M., Weinberg, B., & Alfonso, P. J. (1978). Productive voice onset time characteristics of esophageal speech. *Journal of Speech and Hearing Research, 21*, 56–62.

Clark, J., & Stemple, J. (1982). Assessment of three modes of alaryngeal speech with a synthetic sentence identification task in varying message to competition ratios. *Journal of Speech and Hearing Research, 25*, 333–338.

Clements, K. S., Rassekh, C. H., Seikaly, H., Hokanson, J. A., & Calhoun, K. H. (1997). Communication after laryngectomy: An assessment of patient satisfaction. *Archives of Otolaryngology - Head and Neck Surgery, 123*, 493–496.

Connor, N. P., Hamlet, S. L., & Joyce, J. C. (1985). Acoustic and physiologic correlates of the voicing distinction in esophageal speech. *Journal of Speech and Hearing Disorders, 50*, 378–384.

Cullinan, W. L., Brown, C. S., & Blalock, P. D. (1986). Ratings of intelligibility of esophageal and tracheoesophageal speech. *Journal of Communication Disorders, 19*, 185–195.

Darley, F. L., Aronson, A. E., & Brown, J. R. (1969). Differential diagnostic patterns of dysarthria. *Journal of Speech, Language, and Hearing Research, 12*(2), 246–269.

Diedrich, W. M. (1968). The mechanism of esophageal speech. *Annals of the New York Academy of Sciences, 155*, 303–317.

Doyle, P. C. (1994). *Foundations of voice and speech rehabilitation following laryngeal cancer*. San Diego, CA: Singular.

Doyle, P. C. (1998). Postlaryngectomy rehabilitation: Clinical care following treatment for laryngeal cancer: The opening of doors. *Perspectives on Voice and Voice Disorders, 8*(3), 4–4.

Doyle, P. C. (2005). Rehabilitation in head and neck cancer: Overview. In P. C. Doyle & R. L. Keith (Eds.), *Contemporary considerations in the treatment and rehabilitation of head and neck cancer: Voice, speech and swallowing* (pp. 3–15). Austin, TX: PRO-ED, Incorporated.

Doyle, P. C. (2017a). Communication challenges in laryngeal cancer. In J. C. Friberg & L. A. Vinney (Eds.), *Laryngeal cancer: An interdisciplinary resource for practitioners* (pp. 73–89). Thorofare, NJ: Slack Inc.

Doyle, P. C. (2017b, unpublished data). The influence of formal test stimuli construction on assessments of tracheoesophageal speech intelligibility. Voice Production and Perception Laboratory, Western University, London, ON.

Doyle, P. C., Danhauer, J. L., & Lucks-Mendel, L. L. (1990). A SINDSCAL analysis of perceptual features for consonants produced by esophageal and tracheoesophageal talkers. *Journal of Speech and Hearing Disorders, 55*(4), 756–760.

Doyle, P. C., Danhauer, J. L., & Reed, C. G. (1988). Listeners' perceptions of consonants produced by esophageal and tracheoesophageal talkers. *Journal of Speech and Hearing Disorders, 53*, 400–407.

Doyle, P. C., & Eadie, T. L. (2005). Pharyngoesophageal segment function: A review and reconsideration. In P. C. Doyle & R. L. Keith (Eds.), *Contemporary considerations in the treatment and rehabilitation of head and neck cancer: Voice, speech and swallowing* (pp. 521–543). Austin, TX: PRO-ED, Incorporated.

Doyle, P. C., & Haaf, R. G. (1989). Perception of pre-vocalic and post-vocalic consonants produced by tracheoesophageal speakers. *The Journal of Otolaryngology, 18*(7), 350–353.

Doyle, P. C., Swift, E. R., & Haaf, R. G. (1989). Effects of listener sophistication on judgments of tracheoesophageal talker intelligibility. *Journal of Communication Disorders, 22*, 105–113.

Duffy, J. R., & Giolas, T. G. (1974). Sentence intelligibility as a function of key word selection. *Journal of Speech, Language, and Hearing Research, 17*(4), 631–637.

Eadie, T. L. (2003). The ICF: A proposed framework for comprehensive rehabilitation of individuals who use alaryngeal speech. *American Journal of Speech-Language Pathology, 12*(2), 189–197.

Eadie, T. L., & Doyle, P. C. (2002). Direct magnitude estimation and interval scaling of naturalness and severity in tracheoesophageal (TE) speakers. *Journal of Speech, Language, and Hearing Research, 45*(6), 1088–1096.

Eadie, T. L., & Doyle, P. C. (2004). Auditory-perceptual scaling and quality of life in tracheoesophageal speakers. *The Laryngoscope, 114*, 753–759.

Eadie, T. L., & Doyle, P. C. (2005). Quality of life in male tracheoesophageal (TE) speakers. *Journal of Rehabilitation Research and Development, 42*(1), 115–124.

Eadie, T. L., Doyle, P. C., Hansen, K., & Beaudin, P. G. (2008). Influence of speaker gender on listener judgments of tracheoesophageal speech. *Journal of Voice, 22*(1), 43–57.

Eadie, T. L., Otero, D., Cox, S., Johnson, J., Baylor, C. R., Yorkston, K. M., & Doyle, P. C. (2016). The relationship between communicative participation and postlaryngectomy speech outcomes. *Head & Neck, 38*(1), 1955–1961.

Epstein, R., Giolas, T. G., & Owens, E. (1968). Familiarity and intelligibility of monosyllabic word lists. *Journal of Speech and Hearing Research, 11*, 435–438.

Filter, M. D., & Hyman, M. (1975). Relationship of acoustic parameters and perceptual ratings of esophageal speech. *Perceptual and Motor Skills, 40*, 63–68.

Finizia, C., Dotevall, H., Lundstrom, E., & Lindstrom, J. (1999). Acoustic and perceptual evaluation of voice and speech quality. *Archives of Otolaryngology – Head and Neck Surgery, 125*, 157–163.

Giolas, T. G., Cooker, H. S., & Duffy, J. R. (1970). The predictability of words in sentences. *Journal of Auditory Research, 10*, 328–334.

Gomyo, Y., & Doyle, P. C. (1989). Perception of stop consonants produced by esophageal and tracheoesophageal speakers. *The Journal of Otolaryngology, 18*(4), 184–188.

Hillman, R. E., Walsh, M. J., & Heaton, J. T. (2005). Laryngectomy speech rehabilitation - A review of outcomes. In P. C. Doyle & R. L. Keith (Eds.), *Contemporary considerations in the treatment and rehabilitation of head and neck cancer: Voice, speech and swallowing* (pp. 75–90). Austin, TX: PRO-ED, Incorporated.

Hillman, R. E., Walsh, M. J., Wolf, G. T., Fisher, S. G., & Hong, W. K. (1998). Functional outcomes following treatment for advanced laryngeal cancer: Part I – voice preservation in advanced laryngeal cancer, part II – laryngectomy rehabilitation: The state of the art in the VA system. *The Annals of Otology, Rhinology & Laryngology, 107*(5), 2–21.

House, A. S., Williams, C. E., Hecker, M. H. L., & Kryter, K. D. (1965). Articulation testing methods: Consonantal differentiation with a closed response set. *Journal of the Acoustical Society of America, 37*(1), 158–166.

Hyman, M. (1955). An experimental study of artificial larynx and esophageal speech. *Journal of Speech and Hearing Disorders, 20*, 291–299.

Jongmans, P., Hilgers, F. J. M., Pols, L. C. W., & van As-Brooks, C. J. (2006). The intelligibility of tracheoesophageal speech, with an emphasis on voiced-voiceless distinction. *Logopedics Phoniatrics Vocology, 31*, 172–181.

Kalb, M. B., & Carpenter, M. A. (1981). Individual speaker influence on relative intelligibility of esophageal speech and artificial larynx speech. *Journal of Speech and Hearing Disorders, 46*, 77–80.

Kao, W. W., Mohr, R. M., Kimmel, C. A., Getch, C., & Silverman, C. (1994). The outcome and techniques of primary and secondary tracheoesophageal puncture. *Archives of Otolaryngology–Head & Neck Surgery, 120*(3), 301–307.

Karnell, L. H., Funk, G. F., & Hoffman, H. T. (2000). Assessing head and neck cancer patient outcome domains. *Head and Neck, 22*(1), 6–11.

Kent, R. D., Weismer, G., Kent, J. F., & Rosenbek, J. C. (1989). Toward phonetic intelligibility in dysarthria. *Journal of Speech and Hearing Disorders, 54*, 482–499.

Maryn, Y., Dick, C., Vandenbruaene, C., Vauterin, T., & Jacobs, T. (2009). Spectral, cepstral, and multivariate exploration of tracheoesophageal voice quality in continuous speech and sustained vowels. *The Laryngoscope, 119*(12), 2384–2394.

McColl, D., Fucci, D., Petrosino, L., Martin, D. E., & McCaffrey, P. (1998). Listener ratings of the intelligibility of tracheoesophageal speech in noise. *Journal of Communication Disorders, 31*(4), 279–289.

McDonald, R., Parsa, V., & Doyle, P. C. (2010). Objective estimation of tracheoesophageal speech ratings using an auditory model. *The Journal of the Acoustical Society of America, 127*(2), 1032–1041.

Meyer, T. K., Kuhn, J. C., Campbell, B. H., Marbella, A. M., Myers, K. B., & Layde, P. M. (2004). Speech intelligibility and quality of life in head and neck cancer survivors. *The Laryngoscope, 114*, 1977–1981.

Miralles, J. L., & Cervera, T. (1995). Voice intelligibility in patients who have undergone laryngectomies. *Journal of Speech and Hearing Research, 38*, 564–571.

Moon, J. B., & Weinberg, B. (1987). Aerodynamic and myoelastic contributions to tracheoesophageal voice production. *Journal of Speech, Language, and Hearing Research, 30*(3), 387–395.

Nagle, K. F., & Eadie, T. L. (2012). Listener effort for highly intelligible tracheoesophageal speech. *Journal of Communication Disorders, 45*(3), 235–245.

Nagle, K. F., Eadie, T. L., Wright, D. R., & Sumida, Y. A. (2012). Effect of fundamental frequency on judgments of electrolaryngeal speech. *American Journal of Speech-Language Pathology, 21*(2), 154–166.

Pauloski, B. R., Fisher, H. B., Kempster, G. B., & Blom, E. D. (1989). Statistical differentiation of tracheoesophageal speech produced under four prosthetic/occlusion speaking conditions. *Journal of Speech, Language, and Hearing Research, 32*(3), 591–599.

Pindzola, R. H., & Cain, B. H. (1988). Acceptability ratings of tracheoesophageal speech. *Laryngoscope, 98,* 394–397.

Qi, Y., & Weinberg, B. (1995). Characteristics of voicing source waveforms produced by esophageal and tracheoesophageal speakers. *Journal of Speech, Language, and Hearing Research, 38*(3), 536–548.

Robbins, J. (1984). Acoustic differentiation of laryngeal, esophageal, and tracheoesophageal speech. *Journal of Speech and Hearing Research, 27,* 577–585.

Robbins, J., Christensen, J. M., & Kempster, G. (1986). Characteristics of speech production after tracheoesophageal puncture: Voice onset time and vowel duration. *Journal of Speech and Hearing Research, 20,* 499–504.

Robbins, J., Fisher, H. B., Blom, E. C., & Singer, M. I. (1984). A comparative acoustic study of normal, esophageal, and tracheoesophageal speech production. *Journal of Speech and Hearing Disorders, 49,* 202–210.

Schiavetti, N. (1992). Scaling procedures for the measurement of speech intelligibility. In R. D. Kent (Ed.), *Intelligibility in speech disorders* (pp. 11–34). Philadelphia, PA: John Benjamins Publishing Co.

Searl, J. P., & Carpenter, M. A. (2002). Acoustic cues to the voicing feature in tracheoesophageal speech. *Journal of Speech, Language, and Hearing Research, 45,* 282–294.

Searl, J. P., Carpenter, M. A., & Banta, C. L. (2001). Intelligibility of stops and fricatives in tracheoesophageal speech. *Journal of Communication Disorders, 34,* 305–321.

Singer, M. I., & Blom, E. D. (1980). An endoscopic technique for restoration of voice after laryngectomy. *Annals of Otology, Rhinology, and Laryngology, 89,* 529–533.

Singer, M. I., Blom, E. D., & Hamaker, R. C. (1983). Voice rehabilitation after total laryngectomy. *The Journal of Otolaryngology, 12*(5), 329–334.

Sisty, N. L., & Weinberg, B. (1972). Formant frequency characteristics of esophageal speech. *Journal of Speech, Language, and Hearing Research, 15*(2), 439–448.

Smith, B. E., Weinberg, B., Feth, L. L., & Horii, Y. (1978). Vocal roughness and jitter characteristics of vowels produced by esophageal speakers. *Journal of Speech, Language, and Hearing Research, 21*(2), 240–249.

Smith, L. F., & Calhoun, K. H. (1994). Intelligibility of tracheoesophageal speech among naïve listeners. *Southern Medical Journal, 87*(3), 333–341.

Snidecor, J. C., & Curry, E. T. (1960). How effectively can the laryngectomee expect to speak? *The Laryngoscope, 70*(1), 62–67.

Stevens, S. S. (1975). *Psychophysics: Introduction to its perceptual.* New York, NY: Neural and Social Prospects Wiley.

Subtelny, J. (1977). Assessment of speech with implications for training. In F. Bess (Ed.), *Childhood deafness* (pp. 183–194). New York, NY: Grune & Stratton.

Tardy-Mitzell, S., Andrews, M. L., & Bowman, S. A. (1985). Acceptability and intelligibility of tracheoesophageal speech. *Archives of Otolaryngology, 111*(4), 213–215.

Terrell, J. E., Ronis, D. L., Fowler, K. E., Bradford, C. R., Chepeha, D. B., Prince, M. E., … Duffy, S. A. (2004). Clinical predictors of quality of life in patients with head and neck cancer. *Archives of Otolaryngology – Head and Neck Surgery, 130,* 401–408.

Tjaden, K. K., & Liss, J. M. (1995). The role of listener familiarity in the perception of dysarthric speech. *Clinical Linguistics & Phonetics, 9*(2), 139–154.

Trudeau, M. D. (1994). The acoustical variability of tracheoesophageal speech. In R. L. Keith & F. L. Darley (Eds.), *Laryngectomy rehabilitation* (pp. 383–394). Austin, TX: Pro-Ed, Incorporated.

van As, C. J., Hilgers, F. J. M., Verdonck-de Leeuw, I. M., & Koopmans-van Beinam, F. J. (1998). Acoustical analysis and perceptual evaluation of tracheoesophageal prosthetic voice. *Journal of Voice, 12,* 239–248.

Weinberg, B. (1980). *Readings in speech following total laryngectomy.* University Park Press.

Weinberg, B., Horii, Y., Blom, E., & Singer, M. (1982). Airway resistance during esophageal phonation. *Journal of Speech and Hearing Disorders, 47*(2), 194–199.

Weinberg, B., Horii, Y., & Smith, B. E. (1980). Long-time spectral and intensity characteristics of esophageal speech. *The Journal of the Acoustical Society of America, 67*(5), 1781–1784.

Weiss, M. S., & Basili, A. G. (1985). Electrolaryngeal speech produced by laryngectomized subjects: Perceptual characteristics. *Journal of Speech and Hearing Research, 28,* 294–300.

Williams, S., & Watson, J. B. (1985). Differences in speaking proficiencies in three laryngectomy groups. *Archives of Otolaryngology, 111,* 216–219.

World Health Organization. (2001). *ICF: International Classification of Functioning, Disability and Health.* Geneva, Switzerland: Author.

Yorkston, K. M., & Beukelman, D. R. (1978). A comparison of techniques for measuring intelligibility of dysarthric speech. *Journal of Communication Disorders, 11,* 499–512.

Yorkston, K. M., & Beukelman, D. R. (1980). A clinician-judged technique for quantifying dysarthric speech based on single-word intelligibility. *Journal of Communication Disorders, 13,* 15–31.

Yoshida, G. Y., Hamaker, R. C., Singer, M. I., Blom, E. D., & Charles, G. A. (1989). Primary voice restoration at laryngectomy: 1989 update. *The Laryngoscope, 99*(10), 1093–1095.

Communication Support Before, During, and After Treatment for Head and Neck Cancer

15

15

Jana M. Childes, Andrew D. Palmer,
and Melanie B. Fried-Oken

Introduction

Many individuals who undergo treatment for head and neck cancer (HNC) experience alterations in their communication, either as a result of the cancer itself or the treatment that they receive (Kreeft, Van Der Molen, Hilgers, & Balm, 2009). For some individuals, these changes may be mild and persist only temporarily, while for others there may be significant changes that will impact verbal communication for the rest of their lives. It is now widely recognized that effective communication is an essential component of patient safety and quality care (The Joint Commission, 2010). In addition to communication impairments that affect health outcomes, patient engagement, and perceived satisfaction with one's care, those with communication vulnerabilities in the healthcare system also may present with limited English literacy, limited health literacy, cultural differences, and contextual or situational challenges (Blackstone, Beukelman, & Yorkston, 2015). In prospective studies of speech outcomes after HNC sur-

gery, there is often a dramatic decrease in speech intelligibility and communication for months after surgery (Borggreven et al., 2005; Eadie, Chap. 29; Hillman, Walsh, Wolf, Fisher, & Hong, 1998; List et al., 1996; Pauloski et al., 1994). During radiation and chemoradiation, there often is a progressive worsening of voice and speech during treatment followed by a gradual improvement, but function typically does not return to pretreatment levels (Jacobi, van der Molen, Huiskens, Van Rossum, & Hilgers, 2010). Many long-term survivors of HNC continue to have persistent problems with communication more than 5 years after treatment (Meyer et al., 2004). During hospitalization, many individuals with communication challenges experience feelings of anger, fear, frustration, and loss of control (Carroll, 2004; Doyle & MacDonald, Chap. 27). Those who are unable to resume the ability to speak after HNC treatment tend to have the lowest levels of satisfaction, not only with their ability to communicate but also with their overall quality of life (Clements, Rassekh, Seikaly, Hokanson, & Calhoun, 1997; Doyle, 1994; Evitts, Chap. 28; Hillman et al., 1998; Palmer & Graham, 2004). Difficulties communicating in the inpatient medical setting may place an individual at significant risk. According to one study of multiple medical facilities, patients with communication impairments were three times more likely to experience a preventable adverse medical event than patients without a communication impairment (Bartlett, Blais, Tamblyn, Clermont, & MacGibbon, 2008). Consequently, clinicians must work to facili-

J. M. Childes · A. D. Palmer (✉)
Northwest Center for Voice and Swallowing, Department of Otolaryngology – Head & Neck Surgery, Oregon Health and Science University, Portland, OR, USA
e-mail: palmeran@ohsu.edu

M. B. Fried-Oken
Departments of Neurology, Pediatrics, Biomedical Engineering & Otolaryngology & Institute on Development and Disability, Oregon Health & Science University, Portland, OR, USA

tate communication across a variety of settings and respond to changes in their patients' communication needs over time.

Many patients who experience speechlessness in the acute-care setting during a hospitalization prefer to use writing, mouthing, and gestures for expression, as these strategies are familiar and require the least amount of effort and new learning (Happ, Roesch, & Kagan, 2005). Since medical providers often underestimate the degree of communication difficulty experienced by their patients, providing guidance to medical staff and communication partners regarding how to promote simple, effective communication is often beneficial (Rodriguez & Blischak, 2010). The risk of being unable to effectively communicate wants, needs, and wishes or to summon help in an emergency is greater in this context for those who have cognitive impairments, low levels of literacy, impaired vision, and poor strength or coordination of the upper extremities. The use of a range of communication options can be very effective for patients who will have a prolonged course of rehabilitation or ultimately will not be able to regain a verbal method of communication (Fox & Rau, 2001). A combination of communication options might include simple low-tech and no-tech strategies often supplemented by text-to-speech applications or software, dedicated speech-generating devices, and telephone communication devices. Increasing numbers of HNC survivors and their families have computers and internet access and are using these technologies to access health information and to communicate with their healthcare providers (Kagan, Clarke, & Happ, 2005; Lea, Lockwood, & Ringash, 2005). With the advent of widespread, affordable technology for text-to-speech applications, instant messaging, and videoconferencing, nonverbal communication options are also more readily accessible than ever before (Light & McNaughton, 2014). Evidence suggests that HNC survivors are increasingly turning to these technologies to meet their communication needs (Childes, Palmer, Fried-Oken, & Graville, 2017).

The speech-language pathologist (SLP) is uniquely positioned to address the needs of the HNC survivor and his or her family. Although many of the techniques and strategies that SLPs use are the same as those used for other clinical populations (e.g., those with dysarthria), the rehabilitation of the HNC survivor is qualitatively different. Knowledge about the impact of HNC and its treatment are essential in designing an effective treatment program (Graville, Palmer, & Andersen, 2016). In order to be successful, therapy goals should shift over time from more immediate priorities, such as the communication of wants and needs during the acute phase of cancer treatment, to more comprehensive rehabilitation once acute side effects have diminished (Kearney & Cavanagh, Chap. 20). HNC treatment is usually multidisciplinary, involving a large number of medical specialties and a process that must be coordinated for optimal outcomes (Light et al., 2017). Previous research has shown that a multidisciplinary treatment approach is often beneficial (Fox & Rau, 2001). In doing so, clinicians must take into consideration the individual's psychosocial and communication needs and his or her professional and personal priorities and be responsive to that particular individual's changing needs over the course of recovery.

To date, there is little information about individuals who may use technology for communication, either in addition to or in place of speech, outside the hospital or clinic setting (Happ, Roesch, & Kagan, 2004). In a recent investigation, individuals who had undergone total laryngectomy and used technology to supplement verbal communication (either in person or over the telephone) were surveyed about their reasons for doing so (Childes et al., 2017). Although it had been assumed that the majority of these individuals would not have a viable method of spoken communication, this proved not to be the case. The majority of respondents (65%) listed an alaryngeal speech method as their primary method of communication, whereas a minority (35%) relied on a nonverbal method as their primary communication method (e.g., an SGD, writing, or mouthing words). It had been assumed that most people would have initiated communication device use during the first 6 months after surgery and this proved to be the case (53%). Nonetheless, it was notable that many individuals began using adopted devices at a later date, 6–12 months after surgery (24%) or even later (24%), often to meet a specific communication need such as telephone use, returning to work, or as a backup method for emergencies. In addition, they described use of communication devices in an impressive range of contexts, including when outdoors and in the car, for volunteer and professional work, during medical appointments and hospitalizations, and at support group meetings, sporting events, family gatherings, and holiday parties. Although imperfect, the use of a communication device was associated with a range of positive psychological emotions, such as an increased sense of security, independence, and control. Compared to a matched reference group, individuals who used technology to support verbal communication had undergone more aggressive cancer treatment and tended to use more communication methods. Encouragingly, however, the two groups did not differ significantly in the frequency or success of their communication. Although most of the respondents reported that an SLP had been involved in selecting or obtaining a device (47%), a minority received training by an SLP (24%), and over a third of the respondents reported that they had received no training in the use of the device (39%). It appears that currently many HNC patients are adopting these technologies with minimal support and training, perhaps due to a lack of awareness on the part of clinicians who work with this population.

Communication Supports: General Overview and Terminology

According to the American Speech-Language-Hearing Association (n.d.):

Augmentative and alternative communication (AAC) is an area of clinical practice that addresses the needs of individuals with significant and complex communication disorders characterized by impairments in speech-language production and/or comprehension, including spoken and written modes of communication. AAC is composed of a variety of techniques and tools, including picture communication boards, line drawings, speech-generating devices (SGDs), tangible objects, manual signs, gestures, and finger spelling, to help the individual express thoughts, wants and needs, feelings, and ideas. AAC is augmentative when used to supplement existing speech and alternative when used in place of speech that is absent or not functional. AAC may be temporary, as when used by patients postoperatively in intensive care, or permanent, as when used by an individual who will require the use of some form of AAC throughout his or her lifetime.

Understanding the nature and purpose of the different types of communication supports is critical in selecting the most appropriate strategies, methods, and devices for each individual. First, it is helpful to understand the distinction between *aided* and *unaided supports*. Unaided supports are those communication strategies that can be completed without an external tool, such as gestures, head nods, attention-getting signals, and facial expressions. In contrast, aided supports are those that are completed with the use of a communication tool that is external to the body. These tools may include no-technology, low-technology, or high-technology methods. *No-technology* methods are those nonelectronic communication supports that do not produce speech but provide the communication partner with visual information, such as writing, drawing, communication books, topic cards, and alphabet boards. *Low-technology* and *high-technology* methods employ speech-generating devices, which are electronic and produce voice output. Low-technology supports include speech-generating devices with a limited number of communication topics or mes-

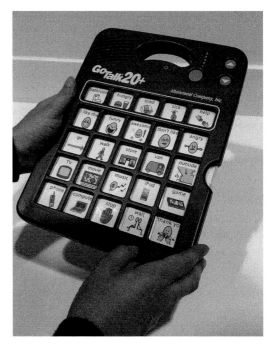

Fig. 15.1 An example of a dedicated speech-generating device with digitized speech. (GoTalk 20+, Attainment Company, Verona, WI)

sages, often utilizing *digitized* speech, where whole messages are recorded for subsequent playback without the ability to combine words or phrases to create novel messages (Fig. 15.1). High-technology SGDs integrate numerous topics and messages for *synthesized* speech output, where the device employs a text-to-speech strategy to provide voice output for each message using a rule-based algorithm (Beukleman, Garrett, & Yorkston, 2007). High-technology SGDs are often more flexible and beneficial to persons with unlimited topic and vocabulary needs, requiring a platform that allows for novel message creation through free spelling and/or the combination of whole words and phrases. These devices also may facilitate other written communication functions such as word processing, text messaging, and email. Additionally, high-technology SGDs include both *dedicated devices*, which are designed for the primary purpose of operating as a communication device (Fig. 15.2), and *integrated devices*, where a commercially available mobile technique (e.g., tablet, laptop, etc.) is able to operate as an SGD through the addition of a speech-generating software program or application (Fig. 15.3).

Traditionally, a number of other types of prosthetic devices have been used to facilitate spoken communication after HNC (Sullivan, Gaebler, & Ball, 2007). These include the artificial larynx/electrolarynx and tracheoesophageal voice pros-

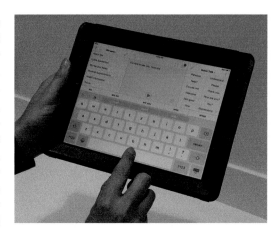

Fig. 15.3 An example of an integrated device serving as a speech-generating device. (An iPad with the text-to-speech application, Proloquo4text © 2013–2018, AssistiveWare)

thesis for individuals who have undergone laryngectomy (see Nagle, Chap. 9, and Graville, Palmer & Bolognone, Chap. 11, respectively), intraoral prosthetics for the tongue or soft palate (Leeper, Gratton, Lapointe, & Armstrong, 2005), as well as amplification devices. These would fall under the categories of no-technology or low-technology augmentative devices. As these topics are dealt with elsewhere, they will not be covered in this chapter.

Intervention

As verbal communicators, most people naturally employ multiple aided and unaided communication methods to meet their daily communication needs, often without conscious thought or effort. When faced with the prospect of a short-term or chronic loss of verbal communication secondary to HNC treatment, many individuals feel that they are losing their only communication modality. It is important that SLPs help their HNC patients to identify the range of communication methods that are already at their disposal, such as writing, gesture, facial expression, email, and text messaging. Identification of these familiar methods may demonstrate to an individual that, even though voice or speech may be comprised, he or she already has multiple methods in place and will be able to continue to utilize them. Upon making this realization,

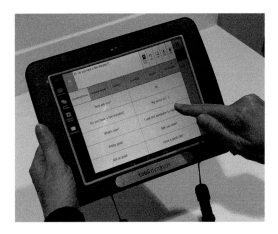

Fig. 15.2 An example of a dedicated speech-generating device with synthesized speech. (Tobii Dynavox T-10, Tobii Dynavox, Pittsburgh, PA)

some individuals become more receptive to the use of other novel communication methods.

The timeline for communication intervention for individuals can vary widely, based upon the nature of their HNC treatment and individual needs. Some individuals may be seen prior to the initiation of HNC treatment, while others may be seen at a later time. Based upon when the patient is referred, the SLP might provide AAC intervention at one or more of the following timepoints: (a) preparation for altered communication before HNC treatment is initiated, (b) during HNC treatment as communication needs change, (c) after HNC treatment is completed, either during rehabilitation or in response to long-term changes in communication needs or abilities over time. Each of these areas will be addressed more fully in subsequent sections.

Communication support prior to HNC treatment Pretreatment counseling by the SLP has been established as an important part of the protocol in preparation for HNC treatment whether medical (i.e., radiation and/or chemotherapy) or surgical (Doyle, 1994; Glaze, 2005). The SLP will typically provide education about the anticipated physiologic and functional changes to speech, voice, resonance, breathing, and swallowing. Through communication with the medical team, the SLP should understand the patient's medical history, diagnosis, and anticipated treatment plan, including the proposed treatment modalities and anticipated timeline for recovery. Taken together, this will allow the SLP to more fully anticipate the nature and duration of that individual's temporary or permanent loss of verbal communication. Through education about these anticipated communication changes, SLPs have an opportunity to introduce the concept of communication supports and discuss how they might be beneficial within the patient's specific treatment program.

The pretreatment counseling session provides an opportunity to evaluate the patient's baseline communication, including areas such as language and literacy skills, pretreatment speech intelligibility, and current use of all modes of communication (Doyle, 1994). It is also beneficial to gain a general understanding of the patient's computer

literacy and access to computers or other forms of technology. A full environmental assessment should be completed (Beukelman & Mirenda, 2013) to identify current communication partners and the contexts in which communication occurs, current and future employment status, social activities, hobbies, and interests in order to ascertain the range of their communication activities. For persons who already have access to a tablet device, smartphone, or laptop computer, these mobile technologies could function as an integrated speech-generating device with the addition of a speech-generating software program or application (see Case One). The patient and any accompanying caregivers may begin to identify strategies to facilitate communication during treatment and begin to acquire any necessary items (such as a wipe-off board, favorite pens and

Case One

Barbara is a 64-year-old woman who was seen for preoperative counseling before undergoing total laryngectomy. She was pleased to learn that her iPad could be used as a communication tool after her surgery, either with a speech-generating app or with a drawing app to use like a whiteboard for writing messages. Despite feeling overwhelmed about the upcoming surgery, Barbara selected and downloaded *Proloquo4text*, a speech-generating app. Familiarizing herself with the speech-generating app operations and messages before surgery helped her to use these strategies while in the hospital and upon her return home. She also reported that researching apps and programming messages before surgery allowed her to be proactive in a situation where she felt powerless. She eventually resumed verbal communication with the use of an electrolarynx but reported that "I now use the electrolarynx or the iPad, depending on where I am. If we are in a place with a lot of background noise or where I can't be understood, I then use my iPad."

paper, or a Boogie Board™) which are readily available commercially in most locales. This is of particular importance when an individual is about to undergo surgery, and it is anticipated that verbal communication will be lost for some period of time due to anatomic changes from surgery or the placement of a tracheostomy tube. Whenever possible, a communication board should be provided for the patient to take home and learn how to use prior to their hospitalization. Previous research in neurologic populations has shown that learning any new method is not easy when an individual is unwell and unfamiliar with it (Fried-Oken, Howard, & Stewart, 1991). Guidelines for pretreatment assessment and intervention are summarized in Table 15.1.

It is not uncommon for care partners who are eager to support their loved one to offer to purchase a mobile technology, such as a tablet or smartphone, for the patient to use during this time. While well-intentioned, this may become a source of additional stress if the patient is expected to learn to use a novel technology during the acute stages of HNC treatment. Further, this may also be a source of frustration for caregivers if the provided technology is not utilized effectively. Consequently, it is often preferable to rely on lower-technology strategies until their long-term communication needs have been identified and the patient is able to participate in the process of selecting the most appropriate device.

Table 15.1 Guidelines and considerations for communication support prior to HNC intervention

Consider short-term as well as long-term needs and prognosis for recovery
Assess functional reading/writing skills briefly, and consider barriers to communication (both short- and long-term) including cognition, vision, hearing, and manual dexterity for writing
Ask about technology ownership including home computers, laptops, mobile, and/or smartphones that could be used as a communication device
Ask about landline phone ownership, and begin TTY application, if appropriate
Provide an example of a communication board used during hospitalization if expected to be nonvocal (note: If a non-native English speaker, provide one with space for native words to be written in next to English to facilitate the use of the communication board without a translator present)

If the family wishes to trial other options, the SLP should encourage consideration of technology that is already familiar to the patient or to borrow mobile technology if available (e.g., a smartphone or tablet that is not currently being used) rather than buying a device that might not be suitable. For those patients for whom severe, long-term alterations in communication are anticipated, the role and nature of SGDs should be introduced in greater detail, guided by the patient's readiness to discuss their future needs. Most importantly, the patient and their caregivers should be reassured that they will be supported by the SLP across the course of treatment with the primary goal of maintaining functional communication, whether verbally or through an alternative means.

Individuals who know in advance that they may lose their ability to communicate verbally can record phrases in their own voices for eventual use on an SGD, a procedure known as *message banking*. A similar process, known as *voice banking*, refers to a process in which customized synthetic speech is generated based on the user's own voice. To date, most of the literature regarding the use of these technologies has been conducted in patients with progressive neurological disease (Fried-Oken, Mooney, & Peters, 2015). Khan and colleagues (2011) reported a case study in which voice banking prior to surgery was used to subsequently reconstruct the voice of a woman ("BC") after total laryngectomy. In this case, a 7-min audio recording of BC reading aloud from a novel was used as the basis for the synthesized voice. Despite the low quality of the original recording, naïve and familiar listeners rated the synthesized voice as moderately acceptable. Further, BC herself reported that it was a distinct improvement over the voice quality of her electrolarynx which she found "embarrassing to use because it did not fit with her personality and affected her social relationships" (p. 65). The speech technology to pre-store messages and to create synthetic voices has improved substantially since BC's report. This is now a viable, inexpensive, and accessible option that should be examined by SLPs and patients before surgery, though most patients are not familiar with options (Oosthuizen, Dada, Bornman, & Koul, 2017).

Costello and Dimery (2014) have outlined the specific equipment and procedures needed to preserve a patient's pre-surgical voice and messages.

Communication support during HNC treatment The stress and anxiety related to a cancer diagnosis and its treatment are significant and pervasive (Hammerlid et al., 1999). Anxiety levels of individuals about to undergo HNC surgery have been shown to be comparable to those of persons admitted to a psychiatric facility for acute anxiety reactions (Dropkin, 2001). The early postoperative period is one of the crises for many individuals as they adjust to the physical changes after surgery, and levels of distress may be substantial for both patients and their caregivers (Bornbaum, 2013; Bornbaum et al., 2012; Verdonck-de Leeuw et al., 2007). In addition to dealing with postoperative side effects such as pain, these individuals and their families also must learn various degrees of self-care and prepare for the transition home (Hughes, Hodgson, Muller, Robinson, & McCorkle, 2000; Ziegler, Newell, Stafford, & Lewin, 2004). At the same time, they must begin adapting to new methods of communication and learning new ways to interact with others, a previously simple task that can now be effortful, time-consuming, and burdensome (Evitts, Chap. 28; Fletcher, Cohen, Schumacher, & Lydiatt, 2012). The early introduction of new methods of speech communication during this time may be perceived as an additional stressor by patients and an additional burden by hospital staff (de Maddalena, 2002; Happ et al., 2005). In the acute-care setting, problems communicating about pain management can often be ineffective, resulting in increased levels of frustration and dissatisfaction with care (Rodriguez, 2003). Some SLPs recommend providing topic-specific message boards, such as "questions about pain management," so that patients have a way to get information without needing to learn new communication methods (Hurtig, Nilsen, Happ, & Blackstone, 2015). Since prospective studies have shown that progress toward developing functional speech or alternative communication occurs over at least the first 6 months postoperatively, most of the "work" of rehabilitation occurs after this initial period of time, typically on an outpatient basis (Armstrong et al., 2001). For those who undergo nonsurgical treatment, the course is usually different, typically with a gradual increase in voice- and speech-related changes, often to the point where communication is difficult for a variety of reasons including pain, edema, dry mouth, and thick secretions and sometimes the need for tracheostomy or intubation (Fletcher et al., 2012; Kreeft et al., 2009).

During and after HNC treatment, whether surgical or medical (i.e., radiation and/or chemotherapy treatment), many patients will experience changes in their communication ranging from minor disruption to a complete loss of functional voice and speech. Aided and unaided communication supports may be particularly beneficial during this period (see Case Two). Patients may be encouraged to use gestures, head nods, and facial expressions along with vocalizations or

Case Two
Debbie, a 66-year-old woman who underwent a total glossectomy, initially refused to consider an SGD as she was "not tech savvy at all." She used writing as her primary communication method immediately after her surgery and benefited from creation of a small communication book with high-frequency words and messages. However, once she returned home she realized that she did not have a way to communicate by telephone. This was important to her as she frequently called her elderly mother who lived in another state. She requested a trial with an SGD at her next appointment. She appreciated the word and phrase prediction features to increase her typing efficiency as she was "not a fast typist." She selected a dedicated SGD, the Tobii Dynavox T-15, and obtained funding through insurance. She used visual scene displays with a selected number of messages in a grid-based layout. Debbie found the visual display and a limited number of messages increased her comfort using the device initially. She increased the number of message choices per page as she felt more confident operating a computerized device.

limited speech (Happ, 2001). Writing and drawing are the most commonly used aided strategies during this period, as they are familiar and readily available. However, paper and pencil communication methods may be challenging for a number of reasons, including low baseline literacy, visual impairment, and difficulty holding or manipulating a pen or pencil due to positioning issues, arthritis, or reductions in arm mobility after a neck dissection (see Boulougouris & Doyle, Chap. 23). Further, factors such as pain, location of IV site, and wound dressings after radial forearm free flap tissue transfer may create additional challenges. Thus, exploring a variety of functional options is required. Guidelines and considerations for communication support during hospitalization or admission to a rehabilitation setting are summarized in Table 15.2.

As many communicative interactions in the hospital setting are quite predictable, they may lend themselves to the use of a communication board or book. In an effort to ease the burden of creating such a tool, it is helpful to provide a communication board or book that includes phrases that are likely to be used in this setting, such as those related to pain management, breathing, positioning, environmental control, etc. This allows for quick and efficient communication of these topics without the added burden of handwriting. The SLP should orient the patient and family to this tool and provide practice opportunities. In addition to messages related to the patient's care and environment, there should also be blank spaces for patients and families to add personalized messages. For non-English speakers a communication board can be customized by asking a translator or family member to add translations of English words underneath each item in the patient's own language. HNC patients have been shown to prioritize messages that facilitate communication related to psychosocial needs and participation in social exchanges during postoperative hospitalization (Rodriguez & Blischak, 2010). In addition to practical communication needs such as pain, breathing problems/suctioning, toileting, and requesting clarification, many individuals also want to be able to exchange social information. Many individuals want to be able to express greetings and thanks and also to be able to request information, such as a person's name or the reason for their visit. Resources that permit patients to communicate about their emotional experiences and share feelings are often of great importance in the recovery and rehabilitation process and have been shown to be associated with higher levels of patient satisfaction (Stovsky, Rudy, & Dragonette, 1988).

The use of a SGD in the acute phase, while undergoing and recovering from HNC treatment, should be considered carefully. Factors affecting the decision to intervene at this point include the patient's medical status, communication needs, and readiness to adopt this type of communication method. Many patients may own or have access to some form of mobile technology, such as a smartphone, tablet, or laptop, and may plan to use these as an integrated SGD during this time.

Communication support following HNC treatment: Initial rehabilitation and beyond Once HNC treatment is completed and some of the acute side effects of treatment have begun to subside, the focus of communication rehabilitation increasingly turns from short- to long-term needs.

Table 15.2 Guidelines and considerations for communication support during hospitalization or admission to rehabilitative setting

Begin or continue all of the above in Table 15.1
Ensure access to writing materials, communication boards, call light, and/or other low-tech options, and ensure that staff members know that individual is nonspeaking. Provide counseling about optimal use of communication materials/strategies in order to get message across quickly/efficiently in order to reduce anxiety and frustration
Consider post-discharge communication needs. If individual has technology that will be useful as a communication device, recommend downloading apps/software suited to immediate needs, and begin orientation to basic functions
If appropriate for speech rehabilitation, begin when medically appropriate
If not a candidate for speech rehabilitation, or anticipated to have a prolonged course of recovery, or not willing/able to participate in speech rehabilitation, consider formal AAC evaluation and investigation of funding options whenever feasible

Many individuals will resume functional verbal communication, and speech rehabilitation has been shown to be effective even in those with extensive oral cavity resections (Furia et al., 2001; Kreeft et al., 2009). Those with extensive surgical resections and multiple treatment modalities (i.e., surgery radiation and chemotherapy), however, may exhibit significant limitations in verbal communication despite significant efforts (Pauloski et al., 1994) and, therefore, may benefit from additional communication options (see Case Three). Guidelines and considerations for communication support during initial posttreatment intervention are summarized in Table 15.3.

In addition to missing dentition and altered anatomy after surgery, communication can be negatively impacted by long-term side effects of treatment, such as chronic pain, xerostomia, soft tissue fibrosis following radiation therapy, and lymphedema (see Kearney & Cavanagh, Chap.

Table 15.3 Guidelines and considerations for communication support during initial speech rehabilitation

Begin or continue all of the above in Tables 15.1 and 15.2
Even if there is a good prognosis for recovery of spoken communication, consider the full range of their short-term needs, including familial, social, and vocational communication with familiar and unfamiliar adults, particularly over the telephone, and ensure that these needs are addressed
Address environmental barriers to communication wherever possible (e.g., hearing loss, background noise), counsel good communication practices in frequent communication partners (e.g., face-to-face communication, establish topic of conversation, "three-strikes rule" – Allow a maximum of two repetitions before writing the message and then continuing with speech), and consider amplification needs
For those using communication devices, initiate teaching/training, and ensure knowledge of useful features (e.g., storing messages, word prediction, etc.) that may improve speed and accuracy
Prioritize AAC evaluation and funding requests for those who do not have a functional method of speech, have a poor prognosis for speech recovery, and/or have significant barriers to therapy participation (e.g., delayed healing, multiple comorbidities, as well as financial, transportation, or other barriers to therapy participation)

Case Three

Ted is a 71-year-old man with a history of surgical resection and radiation therapy for tonsil cancer. He worked extensively in speech rehabilitation, but, due to difficulty with both dysarthria and dysphonia, his verbal communication was limited to short utterances. He frequently used writing to communicate in group situations due to difficulty being understood, but the time required to compose a handwritten message meant that the conversation frequently moved on before he could take his turn. He benefited from the use of a Tobii Dynavox T-10, a dedicated SGD with a text-based communication layout, which allowed for quick selection of programmed messages to access from a grid-based display as well as free spelling novel messages via an onscreen keyboard. Ted found that this significantly increased his participation in large group and family gatherings because "now I can sit and take part in the conversation without holding it up." Most meaningful was the ability to program, save, and then play jokes and messages about his life experiences that he could share with his grandchildren, especially the youngest members of the family who were not yet able to read.

20; Smith, Chap. 22). The posttreatment period can be one of stress and anxiety as individuals struggle to return to previous personal and professional roles, which increases communication demands for interactions with both familiar and unfamiliar communication partners in a variety of settings (Fletcher et al., 2012; Fox & Rau, 2001). Initially following treatment, friends and family members may be strongly motivated to help the individual, a phenomenon known as "support mobilization" (Dunkel-Schetter & Skokan, 1990; Eckenrode, 1983), resulting in an increase in social support from friends, family, and healthcare providers (Fletcher et al., 2012). Once the acute period of treatment has concluded, however, patients may have less frequent contact and support from their clinicians and also experience decreased support from family and friends, a phenomenon known as the "erosion of support" (Bolger, Foster, Vinokur, & Ng, 1996), which may result in greater feelings of distress (Sanchez-Salazar & Stark, 1972). Consistent with this phenomenon, caregiver strain and burden have been shown to increase steadily and reach its peak 1 year after laryngeal cancer treatment (Blood, Simpson, Dineen, Kauffman, & Raimondi, 1994). Distress does not necessarily decrease over time and may, in fact, increase particularly for patients with communication impairments and their partners (Bornbaum, 2013; Bornbaum et al., 2012; Krouse, Krouse, & Fabian, 1990; Rapoport, Kreitler, Chaitchik, Algor, & Weissler, 1993; Verdonck-de Leeuw et al., 2007). Some individuals may require additional communication support, long after their HNC treatment has been completed, due to changes in health status, the impact of comorbidities, or changes in communication ability due to the long-term side effects of HNC treatment (Childes et al., 2017). In such a situation, communication needs and abilities should be reassessed and intervention provided (Table 15.4).

Table 15.4 Guidelines and considerations for communication support for long-term/late speech rehabilitation and/or re-evaluation

Begin or continue all of the above in Tables 15.1, 15.2 and 15.3
Consider changes in the individual's needs as they interact with more people in a greater variety of settings. Evaluate the efficacy of communication methods across these contexts, and intervene if there are situations that the individual cannot manage or avoid (e.g., telephone communication, noisy backgrounds, unfamiliar partners)
Also consider changes in communication ability over time. Previously functional methods may become less so, due to changes in health status, vision, hearing, cognition, manual dexterity, etc.
The attitudes of communication partners may also change over time. Options that were previously rejected or favored may not remain so, and other alternatives may become more acceptable
Reevaluate as needed

For many HNC survivors, a variety of communication contexts pose particular challenges, such as being understood over the telephone, in background noise, in the car, and while outdoors (Childes et al., 2017). As patients become more medically stable, they tend to visit the HNC clinic and their SLP less often. Ideally, the SLP should continue to follow the individual through this period and evaluate their current communication methods to ensure that they meet these increasing communication demands. The HNC survivor should continue to be encouraged to use multiple communication methods and select the most appropriate method for any given communicative environment. The SLP should emphasize that everyone is now using communication technology for verbal interchanges, so the use of apps or SGDs has become commonplace. Even those who resume functional verbal communication in quiet environments with familiar communication partners, or for short durations, may benefit from use of an SGD app on their smartphone as a secondary method for clarification and conversational repair. Others may benefit from an SGD in place of verbal communication in specific situations such as over the telephone or for private interchanges. The choice to use SGDs or communication supports for different communication environments and a range of partners is a critical and fluid treatment decision that must be made by the patient, family, and medical team. The person-centered approach is different for each patient. As general societal communication continues to include more personal technology, SGDs, apps, and tools for information transfer have become increasingly ubiquitous and may be more acceptable to the HNC patient as a result.

In summary, the communication needs of HNC patients are complex, regardless of treatment modality. Some individuals experience a period of speechlessness during the acute period that may exacerbate the feelings of anxiety and distress resulting from the other physical, emotional, and physiologic side effects of treatment. It is critical to maintain functional communication during this time, and this is often achieved through the use of multiple communication methods. For some individuals, the introduction of any new communication method may be an additional stressor and may be rebuffed in favor of more familiar methods (de Maddalena, 2002). For others, using simple unaided methods or written text may reduce stress and isolation. The SLP should provide education regarding these communication options and then support the patient in their preferred method(s). However, it is also important that the SLP revisits the need for aided and/or speech-generating communication supports to address long-term communication needs as the patient's medical status stabilizes. During treatment, the use of a SGD may provide successful communicative interactions that reduce frustration, increase independence, and promote increased engagement in speech rehabilitation.

Communication Device and Application Selection

While it is difficult for most SLPs (even those who routinely provide AAC services) to remain abreast of all of the different apps and devices available, clinicians should understand the characteristics of different types of communication apps in order to match that person's communication needs to the most suitable software program. The SLP should consider the anticipated duration of use, cost, and programming requirements. There are many well-designed apps that are available free or at low cost which allow the patient to try an app without significant investment; this is especially true in the text-to-speech category. Text-to-speech apps are often simple in design and fairly easy to learn to use. Consequently, these apps may be used "out of the box" and can provide an introduction to speech-generating technology without significant demands for operational learning or programming. In contrast, the cost of more comprehensive apps will vary widely and can be significant. More advanced apps also carry the potential for increased demands related to the amount of programming and associated operational learning required for use. In many instances, the features and use of apps may be accessed through online videos pro-vided by the company's website or posted on YouTube. Before buying, therefore, it is often advisable to begin with the use of free or "lite" versions of the app that are available for a short-term trial period. It is important to be aware of the fact that the free version of some apps may not include all the features of the full version or may use a synthesized voice of lower quality. Nonetheless, a short-term trial may allow the patient, their caregivers, and the clinician time to explore the app before investing additional time and money. At the time of writing, in the United States, Medicare or private insurance funding is not available for the purchase of mobile technology that will be used as an integrated SGD, but some private insurance plans provide reimbursement for the purchase of a comprehensive communication app.

According to Ball, Kent-Walsh, and Harrington (2016), there are a number of characteristics of the HNC population that differentiate them from other populations that may be good candidates for AAC devices. As a result, they recommend eight key features of communication devices that should be prioritized during the process of device selection as they are likely to be associated with higher rates of success (Table 15.5).

AAC and the Changing Role of the SLP

With the widespread availability of commercially available technology (e.g., a laptop computer, tablet, or smartphone), it will be increasingly common for a patient to present the SLP with a device that they have already acquired and wish to use as a SGD. This may occur at any point within the course of rehabilitation. Dedicated SGDs are no longer the only option. Consequently, these technologies are more accessible than ever before for communication (Light & McNaughton, 2014). Even though the SLP may not have helped with device selection, the clinician is still critical for device training and implementation. The widespread availability and ease of acquisition of integrated SGD devices may cause the need for

Table 15.5 Characteristics of AAC devices recommended for HNC patients

Characteristic	Rationale
1. Portability	For individuals who are physically active and living independently in the community, lightweight portability is an essential feature. This is less of a concern for those who are wheelchair dependent or who will use the device in a single setting
2. Direct access	Most individuals will have sufficient manual dexterity to type or directly tap and select onscreen images from a visual array. The display or keyboard should be large enough to minimize the number of errors
3. High-quality display	The display screen should be legible for those with visual impairment and in a variety of lighting contexts (e.g., allow for changing font settings or tilting the screen to minimize glare)
4. High-quality voice output	For those who will be using the device in challenging communication contexts (e.g., while traveling in a car, over background noise, etc.), high-quality voice output with adjustable volume or options for external amplification are essential features
5. Traditional orthography	Individuals with adequate literacy will likely prefer standard orthography for message generation due to its familiarity. Those with typing skills may prefer a QWERTY layout, while others may prefer the letters to be arranged alphabetically
6. Novel message generation	Due to the wide variety of messages that may need to be conveyed, the ability to generate novel messages is likely essential. Message banking may be useful in addition to store high-frequency messages
7. Rate acceleration	Generating novel messages on an AAC device is typically much slower than natural speech, and any features that can increase the speed of message generation (e.g., word and phrase prediction) are often highly valued by patients
8. Ease of use	Most individuals do not wish to spend significant amounts of time learning to use and program the new device. Simplicity and the ability to use the device "out of the box" are highly desirable

Adapted from Ball et al. (2016)

device training to be overlooked (Atticks, 2012). As people who rely on AAC have reported: "Assistive technology without training is not assistive" (R. Creech, personal communication). Light's (1989) framework of user competence provides a helpful guide for the identification of treatment targets. It is not uncommon for patients or family members to purchase a mobile technology that is completely unfamiliar to the user. Consequently, significant time and effort may be required to master the operating system, download and configure the speech-generating program, and determine how to best utilize the device to meet a patient's specific communication needs. For some individuals, an SGD will be used to augment verbal communication. For others, the SGD might be an alternative to speech. Regardless of the SGD, it is the SLP's role to match the most appropriate communication method with a variety of settings and partners in order to demonstrate competence, as discussed below (Table 15.6).

Communication Competence

Extending the seminal work of Hymes (1972) which highlighted the importance of context to communication, Janice Light (1989) proposed a definition of communication competence for people who rely on AAC that has four domains: (1) linguistic competence, (2) operational competence, (3) social competence, and (4) strategic competence. Collectively, the consideration of these domains underlies fundamental components of successful rehabilitation and functional communication. Each of these domains will be addressed briefly in the sections to follow.

Linguistic competence Linguistic competence implies mastery of the linguistic code of both the individual's native language and the language in the communication system. In the HNC population, most patients have mastered their native language and retain an intact linguistic system posttreatment. Therefore, clinical emphasis

Table 15.6 Different types of apps and their use for communication

Application type	Description	Application for HNC patients	Sample apps
Symbol-based communication apps			
Symbol-based grid systems Communication narratives	1. Topics and messages may be organized in a traditional grid layout or accessible through communication narratives or visual scenes 2. Vocabulary is supported by picture icons. 3. Voice output may utilize digitized or synthesized speech 4. The ability to create new messages through combination of whole words or free spelling may or may not be included	When considering HNC patients, apps of this type are frequently beneficial for persons with limited baseline literacy skills for reading or writing or those with a co-occurring language or cognitive impairment	*GoTalk now* *Scene & Heard* *SoundingBoard* *Talking tiles* *TouchChat*
Text-based communication apps			
Simple text-to-speech apps	1. Onscreen keyboard allows the user to type a message and speak it aloud. 2. May include word prediction or a limited number of frequently used messages	Beneficial for use during immediately following surgery due to simplicity of use and low cost. These apps may be useful as a supplement to verbal communication for clarification or conversational repair, or may be used in place of verbal communication in challenging environments, such as when outdoors, communicating over noise, etc.	*Speak it* iSpeech *TTS* *Talk app*
Comprehensive text-based apps	1. Communication is achieved through a combination of typing novel messages as well as accessing frequently used messages for a variety of topics 2. Word and/or phrase prediction likely included to include speed and accuracy of novel message production. 3. Phrases and topics may be personalized 4. May include conversational interjections or "quick chat" phrases to facilitate conversational participation	Beneficial as a primary communication method for persons who are unable to regain functional verbal communication after HNC treatment. Persons who frequently use a text-based app in addition to speech may benefit from quick access to frequently used messages. In addition, word/phrase prediction and whole messages are beneficial for persons with poor spelling or typing abilities.	*Verbally* *Predictable* *Compass* (from Tobii Dynavox) *Proloquo4Text*

should be placed on the mastery of the vocabulary related to the patient's specific SGD and where messages, words, or symbols are placed in the device. For people who are "generative" spellers, linguistic competence is based on their literacy skills. For people who rely on dynamic screens that store messages by topic or grammatical category, they must learn how to recall the words or symbols based on their semantic or syntactic correspondences. For non-native English speakers, digital recordings of languages are always available, and most speech-generating devices now have synthetic voice in multiple languages. One responsibility of the SLP is to determine that the people who rely on the SGD have the receptive and expressive language skills to generate speech output with the device.

Operational competence Operational competence refers to the technical skills required to operate a specific SGD. This includes the basic operations of turning a device on and off, launching the communication software, checking the battery level, and the adjusting volume, as well as more advanced operations such as programming personalized messages, creating or editing message pages, problem-solving, and device maintenance. For those who use high-tech SGDs, operational competence includes knowledge about the features that maximize the speed of message generation (e.g., word and phrase prediction and easy access to whole messages) to facilitate the natural "flow" of a conversation. An SLP who introduces an SGD to a patient must either be operationally competent or rely on the expertise of a manufacturer representative, colleague, or the patient's family/support.

Social competence Social competence relates to the skills required to successfully navigate social exchanges, including the use of etiquette and polite social utterances, information sharing, and exchanges that promote social closeness. Social competence includes the use of discourse strategies (e.g., initiating, maintaining, and ending interactions, turn taking, continuing conversation) and specific pragmatic functions (e.g., requesting information, denying, negating, or agreeing). Sociorelational skills, such as the ability to join a conversation and the desire or will to communicate, are included in this domain, as well.

Strategic competence Strategic competence refers to the appropriate use of strategies that promote successful communication. This includes the selection of a communication method to meet the needs of a specific interaction, as well as the use of strategies to manage that interaction effectively. The strategy chosen depends on the partners, situation, and the nature of the message that is being shared. For example, writing a private message might be a great strategy in a noisy bar with your friend but would not be appropriate in a group setting to tell a joke. Many HNC patients utilize multiple communication methods, both during and after treatment, possibly choosing between writing, verbal communication, and the use of SGDs (Childes et al., 2017). It has been shown that the majority of alaryngeal speakers use more than one method of communication on a daily basis, with some routinely using three methods or more (Palmer & Graham, 2004).

Similarly, Sullivan and colleagues (1993) reported that many alaryngeal speakers use a variety of speaking methods, typically relying on more than one method of communication as the difficulty of the communication situation increased. Some HNC patients, therefore, may already demonstrate strategic competence, as demonstrated by their ability to switch between different communication methods depending on the situation. In addition to the decision-making process of selecting the most appropriate communication method for the interaction, strategic competence also refers to the use of appropriate strategies for managing the interaction (e.g., requesting time to compose a message, clarification, and the use of conversational repair). With the introduction of new modalities, it is the SLP's responsibility to teach strategic competence to promote optimal communication across settings.

Addressing Multiple Rehabilitative Needs

Many HNC patients experience debilitating side effects from treatment that make participation in rehabilitation difficult. In one qualitative study, HNC survivors reported that there was a time when the "storm of symptoms" that they experienced "trumped" attempts to communicate, because these attempts were often effortful, painful, or unsuccessful (Fletcher et al., 2012). In the words of one participant: "You get through the storm. I just did the best I could and tried not to talk" (p. 128). Blood, Luther, and Stemple (1992) reported that those who were overwhelmed by the experience of dealing with cancer were least likely to be able to participate effectively in alaryngeal speech therapy. Despite this fact, the authors emphasized the importance of continued participation since therapy "serves as a necessary anchor for the patients at a time when they need some way to gain control over their lives" (p. 68). Even though the ability of an individual to participate may be limited and the gains in therapy may be small, the importance of therapy during this time is not diminished. Bryant (1991) described the entire course of therapy of a single client, a 40-year-old woman with severe speech and swallowing deficits as a result of surgery and radiation for HNC. Week by week over the course of several months, the therapeutic voice, speech, and swallowing goals were adjusted to enable her to manage her secretions, resume an oral diet, and regain the ability to communicate verbally. Bryant's description is an accurate depiction of the potentially long and frustrating course of rehabilitation that many individuals must undertake following treatment for HNC.

Frequently, the SLP must balance competing goals and determine an appropriate therapeutic regimen that balances the client's needs with the impact of side effects such as pain and fatigue which may interfere with progress. Over the course of treatment, the client's needs will typically change as they return to a wider range of daily activities. This may include the need for increased contact with strangers, use of the telephone, and communication in less supportive environments. Fox and Rau (2001) describe a case study in which John, a 45-year-old architect, went through a prolonged "grieving process" after losing the ability to speak following total laryngectomy with total glossectomy. A multidisciplinary treatment approach was designed to address his psychosocial and communication needs and enable him to continue working in his professional field. In this example, the rehabilitation team "did not always agree with John on the priorities for his communication system" but realized the importance of allowing him to direct the course of his recovery and elected to "adjust the pace and practices of their intervention" accordingly (p. 165). As mentioned previously, in a recent investigation, individuals who had undergone total laryngectomy and used technology to supplement verbal communication (either in person or over the telephone) were surveyed about their reasons for doing so (Childes et al., 2017). Many described initiating the use of a communication device outside the initial postoperative period to meet a specific need such as telephone use and returning to work or as a backup method for use in emergencies. Although communication devices were used by a minority of individuals surveyed, device use was not limited to individuals who were unable to communicate verbally, nor was it restricted to the immediate postoperative period. Consequently, it appears that there is a subset of individuals employing technology to support verbal communication very successfully after HNC treatment for various purposes and in combination with other methods of communication.

In the past, there has been a general stereotypical view that HNC patients are poor candidates for AAC intervention or that devices are likely to be acceptable only to those who are nonverbal. In the past 25 years, however, there has been a dramatic increase in the range of communication options and technologies that can be adapted to the needs of individuals with communication disorders (Ball et al., 2016; Light & McNaughton, 2014). Technology access and usage among this population are increasing, and HNC survivors, like other groups, are using computers for a wide variety of purposes (Kagan et al., 2005; Lea et al., 2005). There is an increasing trend to use multimedia and mobile devices in this capacity which may be more acceptable in general because of their widespread use and cultural cachet (Atticks, 2012) and also because they can be used "off the shelf" (Frankoff & Hatfield, 2011). Previous research has shown that HNC survivors often do not agree with SLPs about which devices are most suited to their needs (Fox & Rau, 2001; Happ et al., 2005). Consequently, a better understanding of the priorities of HNC survivors, the changes in their communication needs over time, and what types of intervention may be most beneficial at different times in the rehabilitative process is long overdue.

Summary

This chapter has addressed the issue of how communication support can be used effectively for a wide variety of HNC patients across the course of treatment. To date, this remains an area that is under-researched, and consequently there is a paucity of information about optimal practice patterns. In the past 25 years, however, there has been a dramatic increase in the range of communication options and technologies that can be adapted to the needs of individuals with a variety of communication disorders. Recent research has shown that there are a small group of individuals adopting these technologies to meet their communication needs after HNC treatment but it appears that these types of communication intervention remain underutilized and it is likely that a number of barriers to usage continue to exist. These barriers include the stereotype of the HNC population as "technology averse," the consideration of AAC interventions only for those who are not expected to regain verbal communication, and the lack of AAC training and awareness of many SLPs who work with the HNC population. In the future, a better understanding of the priorities of HNC survivors, the changes in their communication needs over time, and the types of intervention that are most beneficial at different times in the rehabilitative process should guide the development of evidence-based protocols to enable better and more comprehensive care.

References

American Speech-Language Hearing Association. (n.d.). ASHA practice portal: augmentative and alternative communication. Retrieved from: https://www.asha.org/Practice-Portal/Professional-Issues/Augmentative-and-Alternative-Communication/

Armstrong, E., Isman, K., Dooley, P., Brine, D., Riley, N., Dentice, R., … Khanbhai, F. (2001). An investigation into the quality of life of individuals after laryngectomy. *Head & Neck, 23,* 16–24.

Atticks, A. H. (2012). Therapy session 2.0: From static to dynamic with the iPad. *Perspectives on Gerontology, 17,* 84–93. Rockville, MD: American Speech Language Hearing Association.

Ball, L. J., Kent-Walsh, J., & Harrington, N. A. (2016). Consideration of communication options in head and neck cancer: Augmentative and alternative. In B. H. Ruddy, H. Ho, C. Sapienza, & J. J. Lehman (Eds.), *Cases in head and neck cancer: A multidisciplinary approach* (pp. 207–217). San Diego, CA: Plural Publishing.

Bartlett, G., Blais, R., Tamblyn, R., Clermont, R. J., & MacGibbon, B. (2008). Impact of patient communication problems on the risk of preventable adverse events in acute care settings. *Canadian Medical Association Journal, 178*(12), 1555–1562.

Beukleman, D. R., Garrett, K. L., & Yorkston, K. M. (2007). *Augmentative communication strategies for adults with acute or chronic medical conditions.* Baltimore, MD: Paul H. Brookes Publishing Co.

Beukelman, D. R., & Mirenda, P. (2013). *Augmentative and alternative communication: Supporting children and adults with complex communication needs* (3rd ed.). Baltimore, MD: Paul H. Brookes Publishing Co.

Blackstone, S. W., Beukelman, D. R., & Yorkston, K. M. (2015). *Patient-provider communication: Roles for speech-language pathologists and other health care professionals.* San Diego, CA: Plural Publishing.

Blood, G. W., Luther, A. R., & Stemple, J. C. (1992). Coping and adjustment in alaryngeal speakers. *American Journal of Speech-Language Pathology, 1,* 63–69.

Blood, G. W., Simpson, K. C., Dineen, M., Kauffman, S. M., & Raimondi, S. C. (1994). Spouses of individuals with laryngeal cancer: Caregiver strain and burden. *Journal of Communication Disorders, 27*(1), 19–35.

Bolger, N., Foster, M., Vinokur, A. D., & Ng, R. (1996). Close relationships and adjustment to a life crisis: The case of breast cancer. *Journal of Personality and Social Psychology, 70,* 283–294.

Borggreven, P. A., Verdonck-de Leeuw, I., Langendijk, J. A., Doornaert, P., Koster, M. N., de Bree, R., & Leemans, C. R. (2005). Speech outcome after surgical treatment for oral and oropharyngeal cancer: A longitudinal assessment of patients reconstructed by a microvascular flap. *Head & Neck, 27*(9), 785–793.

Bornbaum, C.C. (2013). *Measuring the sixth vital sign: A descriptive analysis of distress in individuals with head and neck cancer and their caregivers.* Unpublished master's thesis. University of Western Ontario, London, Ontario, Canada.

Bornbaum, C. C., Fung, K., Franklin, J. H., Nichols, A., Yoo, J., & Doyle, P. C. (2012). A descriptive analysis of the relationship between quality of life and distress in individuals with head and neck cancer. *Support Care Cancer, 20*(9), 2157–2165.

Bryant, M. (1991). Biofeedback in the treatment of a selected dysphagic patient. *Dysphagia, 6*(3), 140–144.

Carroll, S. M. (2004). Nonvocal ventilated patients' perceptions of being understood. *Western Journal of Nursing Research, 26*(1), 85–103.

Clements, K. S., Rassekh, C. H., Seikaly, H., Hokanson, J. A., & Calhoun, K. H. (1997). Communication after laryngectomy: An assessment of patient satisfaction. *Archives of Otolaryngology–Head & Neck Surgery, 123*(5), 493–496.

Childes, J. M., Palmer, A. D., Fried-Oken, M., & Graville, D. J. (2017). The use of technology for phone and face-to-face communication after total laryngectomy. *American Journal of Speech-Language Pathology, 26*(1), 99–112.

Costello, J., & Dimery, K. (2014). Preserving legacy: A guide to message banking in a patient's voice. *International Society for Augmentative and Alternative Communication.*

de Maddalena, H. (2002). The influence of early speech rehabilitation with voice prostheses on the psychological state of laryngectomized patients. *European Archives of Oto-Rhino-Laryngology, 259*, 48–52.

Doyle, P. C. (1994). *Foundations of voice and speech rehabilitation following laryngeal cancer.* San Diego, CA: Singular Publishing Group.

Dropkin, M. J. (2001). Anxiety, coping strategies, and coping behaviors in patients undergoing head and neck cancer surgery. *Cancer Nursing, 24*(2), 143–148.

Dunkel-Schetter, C., & Skokan, L. A. (1990). Determinants of social support provision in personal relationships. *Journal of Social and Personal Relationships, 7*(4), 437–450.

Eckenrode, J. (1983). The mobilization of social supports: Some individual constraints. *American Journal of Community Psychology, 11*, 509–528.

Fletcher, B. S., Cohen, M. Z., Schumacher, K., & Lydiatt, W. (2012). A blessing and a curse: Head and neck cancer survivors' experiences. *Cancer Nursing, 35*, 126–132.

Fox, L. E., & Rau, M. T. (2001). Augmentative and alternative communication for adults following glossectomy and laryngectomy surgery. *AAC Augmentative and Alternative Communication, 17*, 161–166.

Frankoff, D. J., & Hatfield, B. (2011). Augmentative and alternative communication in daily clinical practice: Strategies and tools for management of severe communication disorders. *Topics in Stroke Rehabilitation, 18*, 112–119.

Fried-Oken, M., Howard, J., & Stewart, S. R. (1991). Feedback on AAC intervention from adults who are temporarily unable to speak. *Augmentative and Alternative Communication, 7*(1), 43–50.

Fried-Oken, M., Mooney, A., & Peters, B. (2015). Supporting communication for patients with neurodegenerative disease. *NeuroRehabilitation, 37*(1), 69–87.

Furia, C. L., Kowalski, L. P., Latorre, M. R., Angelis, E. C., Martins, N. M., Barros, A. P., & Ribeiro, K. C. (2001). Speech intelligibility after glossectomy and speech rehabilitation. *Archives of Otolaryngology–Head & Neck Surgery, 127*(7), 877–883.

Glaze, L. E. (2005). Counseling the laryngectomized patient and family: Considerations before, during, and after treatment. In P. C. Doyle & R. L. Keith (Eds.), *Contemporary considerations in the treatment and rehabilitation of head and neck cancer: Voice, speech, and swallowing* (pp. 353–378). Austin, TX: Pro-Ed.

Graville, D. J., Palmer, A. D., & Andersen, P. E. (2016). Rehabilitation of the head and neck cancer patient. In A. F. Johnson & B. H. Jacobson (Eds.), *Medical speech-language pathology: A practitioner's guide* (3rd ed., pp. 180–205). New York, NY: Thieme.

Hammerlid, E., Ahlner-Elmqvist, M., Bjordal, K., Biörklund, A., Evensen, J., Boysen, M., … Westin, T. (1999). A prospective multicentre study in Sweden and Norway of mental distress and psychiatric morbidity in head and neck cancer patients. *British Journal of Cancer, 80*(5–6), 766–774.

Happ, M. B. (2001). Communicating with mechanically ventilated patients: State of the science. *AACN Advanced Critical Care, 12*(2), 247–258.

Happ, M. B., Roesch, T. K., & Kagan, S. H. (2004). Communication needs, methods, and perceived voice quality following head and neck surgery. *Cancer Nursing, 27*, 1–9.

Happ, M. B., Roesch, T. K., & Kagan, S. H. (2005). Patient communication following head and neck cancer surgery: A pilot study using electronic speech-generating devices. *Oncology Nursing Forum, 32*(6), 1179–1187.

Hillman, R. E., Walsh, M. J., Wolf, G. T., Fisher, S. G., & Hong, W. K. (1998). Functional outcomes following treatment for advanced laryngeal cancer. *The Annals of Otology, Rhinology & Laryngology. Supplement, 172*, 1–27.

Hughes, L. C., Hodgson, N. A., Muller, P., Robinson, L. A., & McCorkle, R. (2000). Information needs of elderly postsurgical cancer patients during the transition from hospital to home. *Journal of Nursing Scholarship, 32*(1), 25–30.

Hurtig, R. R., Nilsen, M. L., Happ, M. B., & Blackstone, S. W. (2015). Adult acute care and intensive care in hospitals. In S. W. Blackstone, D. R. Beukelman, & K. M. Yorkston (Eds.), *Patient-provider communication: Roles for speech-language pathologists and other health care professionals.* San Diego, CA: Plural Publishing.

Hymes, D. H. (1972). On communicative competence. In J. B. Pride & J. Holmes (Eds.), *Sociolinguistics* (pp. 269–293). Harmondsworth, UK: Penguin Books.

Jacobi, I., van der Molen, L., Huiskens, H., Van Rossum, M. A., & Hilgers, F. J. (2010). Voice and speech outcomes of chemoradiation for advanced head and neck cancer: A systematic review. *European Archives of Oto-Rhino-Laryngology, 267*(10), 1495–1505.

Joint Commission, The. (2010). *Advancing effective communication, cultural competence, and patient- and family-centered care: A roadmap for hospitals.* Oakbrook Terrace, IL: The Joint Commission.

Kagan, S. H., Clarke, S. P., & Happ, M. B. (2005). Head and neck cancer patient and family member interest in and use of E-mail to communicate with clinicians. *Head & Neck, 27*, 976–981.

Khan, Z. A., Green, P., Creer, S., & Cunningham, S. (2011). Reconstructing the voice of an individual following laryngectomy. *Augmentative and Alternative Communication, 27*(1), 61–66.

Kreeft, A. M., Van Der Molen, L., Hilgers, F. J., & Balm, A. J. (2009). Speech and swallowing after surgical treatment of advanced oral and oropharyngeal carcinoma: A systematic review of the literature. *European Archives of Oto-Rhino-Laryngology, 266*(11), 1687–1698.

Krouse, J., Krouse, H., & Fabian, R. (1990). Adaptation to surgery for head and neck cancer. *Laryngoscope, 99*, 789–794.

Lea, J. L., Lockwood, G., & Ringash, J. (2005). Survey of computer use for health topics by patients with head and neck cancer. *Head & Neck, 27*, 8–14.

Leeper, H. A., Gratton, D. G., Lapointe, H. J., & Armstrong, J. E. (2005). Maxillofacial rehabilitation for oral cancer. In P. C. Doyle & R. L. Keith (Eds.), *Contemporary considerations in the treatment and rehabilitation of head and neck cancer* (pp. 261–313). Austin, TX: Pro-Ed.

Light, J. (1989). Toward a definition of communicative competence for individuals using augmentative and alternative communication systems. *Augmentative and Alternative Communication, 5*(2), 137–144.

Light, J., & McNaughton, D. (2014). Communicative competence for individuals who require augmentative and alternative communication: A new definition for a new era of communication? *Augmentative and Alternative Communication, 30*, 1–18.

Light, T., Rassi, E. E., Maggiore, R. J., Holland, J., Reed, J., Suriano, K., … Clayburgh, D. (2017). Improving outcomes in veterans with oropharyngeal squamous cell carcinoma through implementation of a multidisciplinary clinic. *Head & Neck, 39*(6), 1106–1112.

List, M. A., Ritter-Sterr, C. A., Baker, T. M., Colangelo, L. A., Matz, G., Pauloski, B. R., & Logemann, J. A. (1996). Longitudinal assessment of quality of life in laryngeal cancer patients. *Head & Neck, 18*, 1–10.

Meyer, T. K., Kuhn, J. C., Campbell, B. H., Marbella, A. M., Myers, K. B., & Layde, P. M. (2004). Speech intelligibility and quality of life in head and neck cancer survivors. *Laryngoscope, 114*(11), 1977–1981.

Oosthuizen, I., Dada, S., Bornman, J., & Koul, R. (2017). Message banking: Perceptions of persons with motor neuron disease, significant others and clinicians. *International Journal of Speech-Language Pathology*, 1–10. https://www.tandfonline.com/doi/full/10.1080/17549507.2017.1356377.

Palmer, A. D., & Graham, M. S. (2004). The relationship between communication and quality of life in alaryngeal speakers. *Journal of Speech-Language Pathology and Audiology, 28*, 6–24.

Pauloski, B. R., Logemann, J. A., Rademaker, A. W., McConnel, F., Stein, D., Beery, Q., … Graner, D. (1994). Speech and swallowing function after oral and oropharyngeal resections: One-year follow-up. *Head & Neck, 16*(4), 313–322.

Rapoport, Y., Kreitler, S., Chaitchik, S., Algor, R., & Weissler, K. (1993). Psychosocial problems in head-and-neck cancer patients and their change with time since diagnosis. *Annals of Oncology, 4*(1), 69–73.

Rodriguez, C. S. (2003). Pain measurement in elderly head and neck cancer patients with communication impairments. (Doctoral dissertation, University of South Florida, 2003). USF Special Collections-Tampa USF Thesis and Dissertation Collection LD1801.F6p 2003 R64.

Rodriguez, C. S., & Blischak, D. M. (2010). Communication needs of nonspeaking hospitalized postoperative patients with head and neck cancer. *Applied Nursing Research, 23*, 110–115.

Sanchez-Salazar, V., & Stark, A. (1972). The use of crisis intervention in the rehabilitation of laryngectomees. *The Journal of Speech and Hearing Disorders, 37*, 323–328.

Stovsky, B., Rudy, E., & Dragonette, P. (1988). Comparison of two types of communication methods used after cardiac surgery with patients with endotracheal tubes. *Heart & Lung, 17*(3), 281–289.

Sullivan, M. D., Beukelman, D. R., & Mathy-Laikko, P. (1993). Situational communicative effectiveness of rehabilitated individuals with total laryngectomies. *Journal of Medical Speech-Language Pathology, 1*, 73–80.

Sullivan, M. D., Gaebler, C., & Ball, L. J. (2007). AAC for people with head and neck cancer. In D. R. Beukleman, K. L. Garrett, & K. M. Yorkston (Eds.), *Augmentative communication strategies for adults with acute or chronic medical conditions* (pp. 347–367). Baltimore, MD: Paul H. Brookes Publishing Co.

Verdonck-de Leeuw, I. M., Eerenstein, S. E., Van der Linden, M. H., Kuik, D. J., de Bree, R., & Leemans, C. R. (2007). Distress in spouses and patients after treatment for head and neck cancer. *Laryngoscope, 117*(2), 238–241.

Ziegler, L., Newell, R., Stafford, N., & Lewin, R. (2004). A literature review of head and neck cancer patients' information needs, experiences and views regarding decision-making. *European Journal of Cancer Care, 13*(2), 119–126.

Speech Deficits Associated with Oral and Oropharyngeal Carcinomas

Gabriela Constantinescu and Jana M. Rieger

Introduction

Head and neck cancer (HNCa) treatment and rehabilitation require some of the most complex care in patient survivorship (WHO, 2014). Despite this, current rehabilitation services continue to lack coordination and integration and are inconsistently offered (McEwen et al., 2015). Recommendations in caring for HNCa patients stem, for the most part, from systematic reviews (Cohen et al., 2016); however, quality, standardized assessments with longer follow-ups are necessary to drive strong guidelines. Since HNCa treatment involves structures critical to speech production, an understanding of the speech problems faced by patients is key to improving post-cancer quality of life (Dwivedi et al., 2009). This chapter summarizes the expected speech difficulties associated with HNCa treatment, assessment methods, and outcomes for speech in oral and oropharyngeal cancers.

G. Constantinescu · J. M. Rieger (✉)
Institute for Reconstructive Sciences in Medicine (iRSM), Misericordia Community Hospital and Department of Communication Sciences and Disorders, Faculty of Rehabilitation Medicine, University of Alberta, Edmonton, AL, Canada

Department of Communication Sciences and Disorders, Faculty of Rehabilitation Medicine University of Alberta, and Institute for Reconstructive Sciences in Medicine (iRSM), Misericordia Community Hospital, Edmonton, AB, Canada
e-mail: constant@ualberta.ca; jana.rieger@ualberta.ca

Reporting on cancers of the oral cavity and oropharynx separately has been challenging, as the anatomical definitions are not always clearly or consistently delineated in the literature (Chi, Day, & Neville, 2015). For the purposes of this chapter, the oral cavity includes the lips, buccal mucosa, floor of mouth, alveolar ridge, gingiva, anterior two thirds of the tongue, maxilla, and retromolar trigone. Oropharyngeal tumors include those originating or invading the soft palate, base of tongue (or posterior one third), palatine tonsils, palatoglossal folds, valleculae, and posterior pharyngeal wall (Chi et al., 2015). As in the case of any cancer, the primary concern is disease-free survival, which involves an aggressive multidisciplinary approach.

Cancer Treatment and Speech

Treatments for oral and oropharyngeal cancers vary depending on different factors including the etiology of the tumor, the size and location of the lesion, the philosophy of the treating center, the patient's age, and their treatment preference. Intervention can involve surgical resection, radiation therapy, chemotherapy, or a combination of these treatment modalities. Most oral cancers are treated with surgery, with advanced cancers requiring adjuvant radiation or chemoradiation therapy. Early-stage oropharyngeal cancers may be treated either with radiation therapy or surgery

© Springer Nature Switzerland AG 2019
P. C. Doyle (ed.), *Clinical Care and Rehabilitation in Head and Neck Cancer*,
https://doi.org/10.1007/978-3-030-04702-3_16

alone. In early-stage tumors of the tonsils, these two treatment modalities have been shown to provide comparable survival after 5 years (Cohan et al., 2009). Late-stage oropharyngeal tumors may be treated with surgery as the primary modality, followed by a combination of adjuvant therapies (Chi et al., 2015). This multimodal approach is used as surgery alone provides superior local control when compared to radiation alone; however, the rate of local recurrence remains high in the absence of adjuvant therapy (Cohan et al., 2009).

Regardless of treatment modality, speech function is often negatively impacted. The production of speech requires the rapid, precise, and coordinated movement of more than 100 muscles within the respiratory, laryngeal, velopharyngeal, and oral mechanisms (Levelt, 1989). Primary inspiratory and expiratory muscles ensure a constant supply of airstream from the lungs required for speech. The movement of this airstream past the vocal folds generates a sound wave, which is then propagated along the vocal tract. This wave is modulated by the natural resonating characteristics of anatomical structures in the pharynx and oral cavity (Redford, 2015).

Surgical treatment involves the resection and removal of the tumor along with affected anatomies, such as the tongue, mandible, or soft palate. Larger tumors requiring more extensive resections, especially of the mobile tongue, result in poorer speech outcomes than smaller tumors (Borggreven et al., 2005; Colangelo, Logemann, & Rademaker, 2000; Perry, Shaw, & Cotton, 2003; Su, Hsia, Chang, Chen, & Sheng, 2003). Larger defects can be reconstructed with tissue flap from another part of the body, such as radial forearm or fibular free flaps. When the reconstructive flap replaces a muscle, speech may be negatively impacted because of the loss of motor control associated with that muscle and an immobile flap that relies on residual muscles for passive movement (Markkanen-Leppanen et al., 2006). In addition to the surgical removal of muscle, nerves innervating these structures may be resected or transected during surgery or as part of the defect (Hiiemae & Palmer, 2003; Loewen, Boliek, Harris, Seikaly, & Rieger, 2010; Piagkou,

Demesticha, Skandalakis, & Johnson, 2011). This can have deleterious effects on the sensorimotor integration that is vital to articulatory precision.

For many years, surgery was the treatment of choice for HNCa until organ preservation protocols, using chemoradiation, were introduced as a primary treatment modality. It was hypothesized that preservation of function would follow the preservation of anatomical structures since they were not surgically altered. Over time, as more data were collected, it was apparent that this was not always the case (Hutcheson et al., 2012; Tschiesner, 2012). Radiation therapy can result in fibrosis, soreness, and peripheral neuropathy (Elghouche et al., 2016; Epstein, Wilkie, Fischer, Kim, & Villines, 2009; Krisciunas et al., 2016; Lin, Jen, & Lin, 2002), side effects that may directly affect speech function. Finally, surgery and radiation therapy are associated with scarring, xerostomia, and mucositis (Chi et al., 2015). It is apparent then that speech will be more impaired following a combination of these treatments than subsequent to surgery alone or radiation therapy alone (Morton, 2003; Perry et al., 2003). Multiple factors weigh into the speech impairment experienced by patients, such as the extent and degree of different treatment modalities, as well as how these treatments are combined with one another.

Impacts on speech can originate from a number of insults to the respiratory, laryngeal, velopharyngeal, and/or oral mechanisms. For example, comorbidities associated with HNCa that affect the respiratory system, such as chronic obstructive pulmonary disease (COPD) and lung infections, can negatively impact subglottal pressure and, thus, also influence speech (Hoit, Lansing, Dean, Yarkosky, & Lederle, 2011). The acoustic response of the oral and oropharyngeal cavities also may change as a result of surgical modifications to the vocal tract shape, length, and cross-sectional area and could lead to atypical resonances. Misarticulations can result from the resection, reconstruction, and irradiation of several muscles. For example, precise articulation of /f/, a voiceless fricative, requires the action of the inferior orbicularis oris (for labiodental contact);

superior longitudinal muscles, genioglossus, and geniohyoid (for oral tongue positioning); as well as the levator veli palatini and pharyngeal constrictors (for adequate velopharyngeal closure). Any type of phoneme error can be observed in HNCa patients: substitutions (e.g., patient has a tethered anterior tongue reconstruction and now substitutes "ah" for /r/), distortions (e.g., patient had a hemiglossectomy and now lateralizes all sibilants), additions (e.g., patient overemphasizes parts of a word, such as /bʌlu/ for /blu/), and omissions (e.g., patient had a glossectomy and can only produce bilabial consonant phonemes: /paɪ/ for /plaɪ/). The heterogeneity of this patient population, the variety of treatment approaches, and the relatively small numbers of patients – 4300 new cases in Canada in 2015 (Canadian Cancer Society's Advisory Committee on Cancer Statistics, 2015) – make studying this population particularly difficult. For this reason, a comprehensive and standardized approach to speech evaluation is important.

Standardized speech evaluations provide baseline measures of pretreatment or pre-therapy function. They help clinicians recognize changes in function resulting from cancer treatment or rehabilitation, identify goals for therapy, and carry out cross-study comparisons. Standardized evaluations also help identify patients requiring additional or immediate supports (Perry & Frowen, 2006). A good clinical speech assessment is thorough, valid, and reliable and uses a variety of modalities (i.e., questionnaires, perceptual evaluation, acoustic evaluation) (Shipley & McAfee, 2004).

Assessment Tools

Although deglutition following oncological treatment for HNCa has been extensively studied, research on speech function is less comprehensive. A PubMed search for the phrase "speech head and neck cancer" resulted in 2898 articles, almost half the number following a search for "swallowing head and neck cancer" (Fig. 16.1). This bias makes intuitive sense; that is, a swallowing impairment can result in medical complications, such as malnutrition, dehydration, aspiration pneumonia, and choking. On the other hand, impairments in the speech domain have no such explicit physical health consequences. However, when asked, HNCa survivors placed speech as one of their top five priorities (Tschiesner et al., 2013). This finding was confirmed to be especially true for those with late-stage oral cancer (Metcalfe, Lowe, & Rogers, 2014). In other studies, oral and oropharyngeal cancer patients rated speech as the top third important issue (above swallowing) 1 year following treatment and beyond 18 months (Zuydam, Lowe, Brown, Vaughan, & Rogers, 2005). Radford et al. also noted that issues with speech ranked higher than those with swallowing at 6 months posttreatment (Radford, Woods, Lowe, & Rogers, 2004). Speech following treatment for HNCa has been a high priority for patients and speech-language pathologists for the past four to five decades, and management of this function has evolved to represent increasingly more precise and comprehensive evaluations.

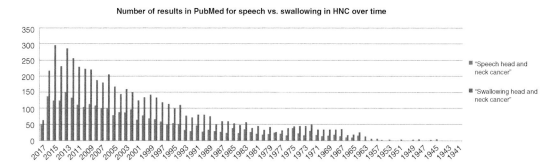

Fig. 16.1 Comparison of publications in speech vs. swallowing relative to head and neck cancer

Historical Viewpoint

To understand current speech evaluation practice for this population, it is important to appreciate the progression in the field over time. During the 1970s, when speech-language pathologists first began practicing in medical settings (Miller & Groher, 1993), the first reports of speech outcomes following HNCa were documented (Massengill, Maxwell, & Pickrell, 1970; Skelly, 1973). Over time, the focus shifted from informal speech assessments to more objective ones. For example, clinicians' overall impressions of a patient's speech were replaced with standardized assessments including intelligibility and associated inquiry specific to phoneme production, resonance, and acoustics. These approaches, however, focus on clinician-derived outcomes, areas that experts consider important and that they expect will be altered by cancer treatment. To add depth to an evaluation, patient-derived outcomes also should be considered alongside the clinician-derived ones (see Eadie, Chap. 29; Radford et al., 2004). Clinical practice has revealed that patient perceptions might differ from clinician impressions of severity. As such, assessments have shifted to capture patient perceptions of speech alongside objective clinical measures (Govender, Breeson, Tuomainen, & Smith, 2013). Efforts that seek to address both types of concerns can serve to provide a more comprehensive understanding of speech deficits that exist posttreatment (see Doyle, Chap. 17).

Dwivedi et al. (2009) organized evaluation of speech in HNCa patients into three main modalities: perceptual clinical evaluation, acoustic evaluation, and questionnaire evaluation. Ideally, assessment tools from two or more of these categories should be administered; however, most articles in the literature include only one modality, such as questionnaires or perceptual evaluations (Dwivedi et al., 2009). Furthermore, a majority of studies reporting speech outcomes in HNCa are retrospective in nature (Dwivedi et al., 2009). While a limitation to some degree, retrospective reports have provided important starting points for prospective work. The next sections describe various types of speech assessment modalities including subjective rating scales (which are considered to be general impressions of the attending clinician), clinician-driven assessments, patient-driven evaluations, and, finally, population perceptions.

Subjective Rating Scales

Subjective ratings and impressions of speech are usually provided by clinicians, either informally in the medical chart (e.g., "speech was easy to understand") or by recording the patient's speech and having one or more naïve raters score how easy it was to understand the patient's speech on an ordinal scale (Dios, Feijoo, Ferreiro, & Alvarez, 1994). Evaluating speech in this manner is fast and simple; however, it lacks objectivity and precision. What is "somewhat unintelligible" to one clinician may be rated as "normal speech" by another. In their review of functional outcomes in HNCa patients, Lam Tang and colleagues found that the majority of researchers assessed speech outcomes using study-specific, nonstandardized, subjective rating scales (Lam Tang, Rieger, & Wolfaardt, 2008). This limitation is problematic because it makes comparison across studies and between clinicians difficult, thus, reducing the external validity of such findings. Furthermore, subjective ratings do not provide insight into which aspects of speech (e.g., articulation, resonance, acoustics, or voice) were altered by treatment and where treatment can have the greatest impact. For example, a patient's assessment may reveal high intelligibility scores, but poor resonance outcomes, meaning that a naïve listener can understand this individual but will still find his/her speech quality atypical. In this situation, speech assessment that focuses on overall intelligibility alone will fail to capture what is really causing the disturbance for the listener.

One widely used scale that is both valid and reliable is the Frenchay Dysarthria Assessment (FDA), which was originally developed for patients with neurological impairments (McKinstry & Perry, 2003). A second scale, the London Speech Evaluation (LSE), is the first speech-specific perceptual evaluation tool developed and validated for HNCa patients (Dwivedi, Rose, et al., 2012). Tools such as these are quick to administer and require little to no post-appointment analysis, making them an attractive approach for busy clinicians. Some researchers and clinicians, however, prefer to carry out more objective and in-depth evaluations of speech. Within this chapter, these will be referred to as clinician-driven assessments and detailed in the following section.

Clinician-Driven Assessments

Oral Mechanism Examination No speech evaluation would be complete without a comprehensive oral mechanism examination to understand the current limitations and potential influence of altered anatomy and physiology on speech production. The main structures of interest are the tongue, mandible, soft and hard palates, teeth, and lips. The oral mechanism examination can complement auditory-perceptual evaluation and assess kinematic events (e.g., the displacement, direction, and speed of movement of oral structures). Clinicians should pay particular attention to missing tissues, scar tissue or reconstruction that potentially limits mobility, and fistulas that affect resonance. Clinicians also should check for neurological weakness and fasciculation, which can sometimes be a result of chemotherapy or radiation-induced neuropathy (Lin et al., 2002). In addition, xerostomia, missing or damaged dentition, ill-fitting dentures, and obvious lesions also should be carefully evaluated, as any of these factors may affect intelligibility or result in maladaptive articulation. Following the oral mechanism evaluation, the clinician may use a battery of standardized methods to assess various aspects of speech such as intelligibility, articulation, acoustics, and resonance (Dwivedi et al., 2009).

Intelligibility Intelligibility, or how easy it is to understand a person, is the most commonly evaluated perceptual domain. The reason for this may be because intelligibility is the result of the efficient integration and coordination of motor

speech processes and also the primary aim of most speech therapy (Robertson & Thomson, 1986). Intelligibility has been assessed in HNCa patients using a variety of tools, such as the *Computerized Assessment of Intelligibility of Dysarthric Speech* (CAIDS) (Yorkston, Beukelman, & Traynor, 1984), component VI of the Robertson Dysarthria Profile (Robertson & Thomson, 1986), and the Munich Intelligibility Profile from Ziegler and Hartmann (as cited in Mády, Sader, Hoole, Zimmermann, & Horch, 2009).

The CAIDS includes single word level (i.e., words without context) and sentence level (i.e., words provided in context) stimuli. The patient is asked to read a series of words and sentences. The words are randomly generated from a closed set of 12 other similar sounding words. Sentences vary in length from 5 to 15 words each; two sentences of each length are provided as a stimulus. The patient's speech is recorded and later transcribed by a naïve listener. Percent intelligibility is determined by calculating the number of correctly identified words divided by the total number of words in the stimuli presented. One advantage of CAIDS and other tools like it is that they provide a ratio level of measurement. That is, measures obtained reflect a continuous scale, allowing for the use of parametric statistics in a research context. On the other hand, the Robertson Dysarthria Profile (Revised) uses seven tasks to measure intelligibility. The first three ask the patient to read five words of increasing phoneme length, three phrases, and then read a passage. The remaining four tasks are used to gather ratings for rate, intonation, rhythm, and stress; these ratings are made by three judges: the clinician, someone familiar to the patient, and a stranger (Robertson & Thomson, 1986).

Some difficulties posed by these assessments include the need for an unfamiliar listener for analysis or rating, as well as the requirement that patients are able to read. Furthermore, speech that is read is different from conversational speech and, therefore, has been criticized as having poor external validity (Connoly, 1986). Nevertheless, intelligibly measures mentioned above have several advantages: they are relatively easy to administer and analyze; they allow us to compare outcomes across cancer treatment modalities with greater sensitivity than subjective ratings scales; and they allow us to compare current function to baseline (Yorkston et al., 1984). One important consideration is that assessment of intelligibility does not capture atypical but intelligible speech. For example, a patient may obtain a high sentence intelligibility score on the CAIDS, but still have high nasalance scores, indicating hypernasality or atypical speech quality (Seikaly et al., 2003). In other cases, "sounding different" could be related to articulation. Therefore, the clinician should focus on assessments that also capture these features of speech, the topics of our next three sections: articulation, acoustics, and resonance.

Articulation Speech sound errors can be evaluated using a more standard articulation assessment, such as the *Fisher-Logemann Test of Articulation* (FLTA) *Competence* (Fisher & Logemann, 1971). Different measures can be obtained by using this tool, such as the percent correct for consonants and vowels, the type of articulation errors, and common contexts for these misarticulations. The FLTA includes testing of consonants in all phonetic positions (initial, medial, and final). The FLTA also can provide clinicians with an in-depth understanding of which phonemes the patient is able to produce with ease, with effort and/or distortion, or not at all. It also offers a good starting point for structuring a program for speech intervention. One disadvantage of administering the FLTA is that it can be time-consuming; for this reason, it may be more feasible to administer FLTA or other tests of articulation in situations that warrant a more extensive evaluation of this speech domain. For example, the clinician may encounter patients who are easy to understand, but who may be lecturers at a university, sales personnel, or radio announcers. These patients may request speech therapy even if highly intelligible. The clinician may wish to administer the FLTA to understand which phonemes should be targeted in therapy and how to order contexts into a hierarchy. Tests

of articulation often focus on consonant phonemes; however, vowel space and vowel production also contribute to intelligibility. Acoustic evaluations provide a means to understand these parameters.

Acoustics This type of assessment includes measurement of spectral characteristics of formant frequencies. The first three formant frequencies are of greatest interest in clinical speech evaluation. These three formants are identified acoustically as F1, F2, and F3. These formant values and their ranges are related to tongue height and advancement as well as subsequent changes in the size of the oral and oropharyngeal cavities. Treatment for HNCa can limit the range of movement of the tongue and consequently alter acoustics. Therefore, because formants can be affected by cancer and its treatment and because they are an indirect way to evaluate articulatory aspects of speech, acoustic evaluation in HNCa patients is an important modality to consider (Dwivedi et al., 2016).

Acoustic assessment, however, is the most uncommon clinical evaluation modality in HNCa patients (Dwivedi et al., 2009).

In their review, Dwivedi et al. found that only 4 of 70 studies evaluated acoustics, all of which were for oral cancer patients and were conducted retrospectively. In these four studies, the parameters reported included fundamental frequencies (F0), formant frequencies, the range of F2, and noise-to-harmonic ratio (Dwivedi et al., 2009). Laaksonen and colleagues used acoustic analysis to evaluate vowels, diphthongs, and sibilants (Laaksonen et al., 2009; Laaksonen, Rieger, Happonen, Harris, & Seikaly, 2010). In one study, the group evaluated a patient with a history of anterior tongue resection that was reconstructed with a radial forearm free flap and treated with a palatal augmentation prosthesis (this type of prosthesis is described later in this chapter). The authors analyzed the first and second formants (F1, F2) of three vowels (/i/, /ʌ/, /u/) and phrases, in contexts where these vowels were preceded by /h/ and final /d/ (e.g., "Say heed again," where the vowel of interest is /i/) (Peterson & Barney, 1952).

This /h/-vowel-/d/ structure was purposively selected to facilitate identification of the vowel in analysis. /h/ is a voiceless consonant, making the onset vowel visually clear; however, production of /h/ in a word-final position was deemed too difficult, and as a result, /d/, a voiced stop, was selected as another obvious marker on a spectrograph. The authors also calculated the acoustic vowel space areas or vowel quadrilaterals in Hz^2. The details of this approach go beyond the scope of this chapter, but the reader is directed to the original article for this methodology as well as additional rationale for selecting these specific vowel targets (Laaksonen et al., 2009).

In a second study, the same group evaluated oral cancer patients longitudinally. In this case, in addition to F1 and F2, the authors also reported on the fundamental frequency (F0) and duration of vowels and diphthongs (Laaksonen et al., 2010). Although time-consuming, acoustic measures may provide important information about changes in the resonating tract following cancer treatment. Furthermore, acoustic analysis may be used in treatment. For example, a clinician may wish to understand what a sound error looks like acoustically and use that information to provide feedback to the patient on what the target phoneme should look like, so that the patient can try to approach that target. Another parameter that may impact speech quality, and sometimes intelligibility, is resonance.

Resonance Resonance in patients with HNCa can be affected by changes to either the palatal structures or the tongue. Defects of the soft palate (velum) that have been reconstructed with a bulky flap may result in hyponasality. On the other hand, hypernasality may result at any point where either the maxilla or the structures of the soft palate prevent inappropriate transmission of sound through the nasal cavity (e.g., due to the soft palate insufficiency or incompetence). Cul-de-sac resonance can occur with changes to the base of tongue that result in a bulky flap being carried posteriorly into the pharynx. This type of resonance also can arise from surgery resulting in a widening of the pharynx where the acoustic transmission of sound is resonated within that chamber before passing through the lips.

Velopharyngeal insufficiency (VPI) typically describes a palate where tissue is insufficient to achieve adequate closure with the pharyngeal walls, thus, providing inadequate separation between the oral and nasal cavities during speech. VPI may be the result of surgical treatment, radiation therapy, or of surgery and/or adjuvant radiation therapy. On the other hand, velopharyngeal incompetence is a label used for inadequate closure in the absence of structural limitations. It is often associated with neurogenic disorders and tends to be more rare in patients with HNCa but could be seen in patients receiving radiation therapy, where the nerve innervation has been compromised by that treatment.

In order to prevent a resonance disorder, the soft palate may be reconstructed with a flap, or the velopharyngeal insufficiency may be rehabilitated using a pharyngeal obturator (Rieger et al., 2009). Cancer of the maxilla is often treated with surgical resection and either reconstruction with a bone-containing flap (osseous flap) or rehabilitation with a maxillary obturator. If the separation between the oral and nasal cavities is at all compromised by either a fistula (in the case of surgical reconstruction) or ill-fitting prostheses (in the case of a maxillary obturators), hypernasality will result.

Ongoing evaluation of resonance in conjunction with imaging techniques (e.g., nasoendoscopy, videofluoroscopy) should be carried out to ensure that these approaches were successful in addressing hypernasality. Evaluation of resonance and velopharyngeal closure may include nasal endoscopy and measures of nasalance using a nasometer (KayPENTAX, Lincoln Park, NJ) (Fig. 16.2). Clinician-driven evaluations, such as the ones mentioned above, are an excellent approach to assessing and monitoring speech function over time. However, as mentioned earlier, clinicians also need to consider patient-reported outcomes in the event a discrepancy exists between a clinician's judgment of function and the patient's perception of that impairment.

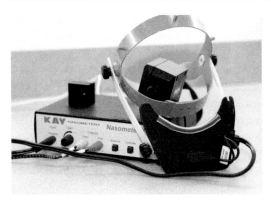

Fig. 16.2 KayPENTAX Nasometer™ assessment system

Patient-Driven Assessments

Previous research and clinical experience have shown that some patient perceptions of speech function are discordant with auditory-perceptual evaluations generated by clinicians. This disagreement may depend on patient personality, background, self-efficacy, and expectations of treatment outcome (Bandura, 1997). A function-specific questionnaire is the Speech Handicap Index (SHI), a 30-item tool that has been shown to be valid and reliable with HNCa patients (Dwivedi, St Rose, et al., 2012). The SHI yields an overall score, as well as two sub-scales scores for the speech and psychosocial domains. An additional question on the SHI (not related to the overall, composite score) asks patients to describe the quality of their own speech from the following choices: excellent, good, average, and bad.

In addition to function-specific patient-reported measures, quality of life questionnaires specific to HNCa exist (e.g., European Organization for Research and Treatment of Cancer Head and Neck-specific module – QLQ-H&N35); however, these tools have few speech-specific questions (Bjordal et al., 1999). Another commonly used, HNCa-specific questionnaire is the UW-QOL (Rogers, Laher, Overend, & Lowe, 2002), which contains one question on speech among 12 other domains including pain, recreation, and swallowing (see Arrese & Schieve, Chap. 19). An interesting aspect of the UW-QOL is that it asks patients to select the three areas

that were most important to them in the past week.

In a further effort to ensure comprehensive and valid evaluation of function, a recently developed International Classification of Functioning, Disability and Health (ICF) core set specific to HNCa patients was created through the consensus of an international multidisciplinary consortium of professionals (Tschiesner, Rogers, Dietz, Yueh, & Cieza, 2010). Core sets such as this one are created by selecting categories from an otherwise extensive and comprehensive list of more than 1400 categories that pertain to the needs of a particular patient group; this allows ICF-based tools to be tailored and thus more easily applicable (Tschiesner et al., 2010). For example, body functions such as sensation of pain (code b280) and body structures such as the mouth (code s320) and pharynx (code s330) can impact speech (code d330), family relationships (code d760), and economic self-sufficiency (code d870) (Tschiesner et al., 2010). This ICF core set can be used to rate the content validity of existing assessment tools, as well as to guide the development of new ones (Tschiesner et al., 2013). This approach provides a common framework and language between clinicians, researchers, and patients in describing speech function and the restrictions in quality of life associated with dysfunction (see Doyle & MacDonald, Chap. 27 and Eadie, Chap. 29).

Population-Based Perception of Speech

Another important aspect of speech evaluation is population-based perception of speech. This aspect can include ratings on the acceptability of speech, social perception of speech (e.g., annoying, intimidating) (Bressman, Jacobs, Quintero, & Irish, 2009; Rieger et al., 2006), and other behaviors that the patient actively initiates to make herself/himself understood (e.g., slowing down, facial expressions, gestures, self-advocacy). For example, a patient may indicate that he/she sounds "like a cartoon character," while another patient may openly share that he/she has a history of HNCa resulting in difficulties with speaking. A clinician should be sensitive to comments made by patients in relation to how their speech is perceived by others and, when appropriate, work with a psychologist to build confidence and self-advocacy.

Clinicians should also comment on the patient's social awareness with respect to whether or not listeners understand. Furthermore, it is important to assess the patient's ability to compensate for a breakdown in communication by providing clues, slowing down, or pairing speech with written communication or gestures. Functional goals, such as those that enhance the flow of conversation and social participation for patients, may be combined with more targeted, phoneme-specific therapy.

Future Directions for Assessment

The need for multimodal, structured, and standardized evaluation of speech that includes a baseline and long-term follow-up has been well documented in the literature (Dwivedi et al., 2009; Jacobi, van der Molen, Huiskens, van Rossum, & Hilgers, 2010; Schuster & Stelzle, 2012). Ideally, assessment should include an oral mechanism examination, auditory-perceptual and acoustic evaluations, speech-specific questionnaires, and patient-reported outcomes, as well as impressions from a population-based perception of speech. It has been recommended that, at a minimum, speech evaluation should include an oral mechanism examination and assessments of articulation, resonance, and intelligibility (Hutcheson & Lewin, 2013). These assessments are ideally conducted pretreatment and at 1, 6, 12, 18, and 24 months posttreatment (Dwivedi et al., 2009). Now that the reader is familiar with speech assessment, the following section will cover outcomes that clinicians can expect to find.

Speech Outcomes

Few prospective studies with follow-up longer than 5 years have been conducted on speech outcomes in patients with HNCa. One example is the longitudinal study carried out by Kraaijenga and colleagues with patients receiving chemoradiation for advanced-stage cancer of the oral cavity, oropharynx, or hypopharynx (Kraaijenga et al., 2016). The paucity (i.e., low number) and heterogeneity (i.e., combining oral and oropharyngeal patient groups and/or using a variety of outcome measures) in the literature are problematic as information on functional outcomes is often used when selecting cancer treatment modalities to optimize speech (Schuster & Stelzle, 2012). Furthermore, tumors originating in the oral cavity and the oropharynx differ in their cause, treatment, and prognosis (Chi et al., 2015). The next sections provide a summary of speech outcomes following surgery and chemoradiation.

Surgery

Surgical treatment is more common in association with cancers of the oral cavity (Chi et al., 2015). As these resections often involve the oral tongue, speech production is most impaired. Although intelligibility has been shown to remain high when linguistic context is presented (i.e., sentences), even for patients with advanced-stage oral cancer, speech is still said to be atypical (Hutcheson & Lewin, 2013). When affected, intelligibility is influenced by the type of reconstruction, the bulk and mobility of the reconstruction, as well as whether or not the flap is sensate (Nicoletti et al., 2004; Pauloski et al., 1998; Perry & Frowen, 2006). For example, as a general rule, free flap reconstructions result in less tethering of the residual tongue to the floor of the mouth or gingiva and, thus, better speech outcomes (Urken, Moscoso, Lawson, & Biller, 1994). However, it is important to note that variability does exist in postsurgical outcomes.

Zuydam and colleagues sought to identify predictors of speech and swallowing function following primary surgery for oral and oropharyngeal cancer (Zuydam et al., 2005). These authors used the UW-QOL as their outcome measure, although they recognized its limitations. Univariate statistics identified that tumor size (but not tumor site), radiation therapy, primary closure/laser surgery, and extent of neck dissection were predictive of speech outcomes at 1-year posttreatment. Multivariate stepwise logistic regression in the same study found that primary closure/laser surgery was the only predictor of good speech (Zuydam et al., 2005). Collectively, these data indicate that primary closures result in good speech-related quality of life; however, this reconstruction approach is not always feasible (e.g., large resection). Furthermore, clinicians should be aware of variability in outcomes despite general trends.

Articulatory precision has been linked to the extent of tongue resection; resections that preserve half or more of the native tongue have been associated with good intelligibility (Hutcheson & Lewin, 2013). Bressman and colleagues identified the critical point for the size of tongue defect that would result in poor speech acceptability as being more than 20.4% (Bressman et al., 2009). Specific articulation errors have not been extensively explored, and the few case studies reporting on compensatory substitutions are not recent (Georgian, Logemann, & Fisher, 1982; Morrish, 1988). As cancer therapies have changed substantially since the 1980s, it is important to report on current articulatory adaptations made by those treated for HNCa.

Although most studies have found that reconstruction using sensate flaps result in better speech outcomes (e.g., word intelligibility), a lack of consensus exists in the literature on whether innervated free flaps offer an advantage in preservation of intelligibility (Namin & Varvares, 2016). Elfring and colleagues studied patients with base of tongue cancers whose defects were reconstructed with radial forearm free flaps and the impact that nerve status had on quality of life. They found that although transected lingual and hypoglossal nerves can impact quality of life in domains such as swallowing and social contact, no differences were found in the speech domain between patients with transected, repaired, or intact nerves (Elfring et al., 2014). These findings support previous research: sensate flaps do not necessarily provide an advantage in speech tasks (Markkanen-Leppanen et al., 2006).

In their review of speech literature, Dwivedi et al. found that unless the larynx is in the field of radiation, there is little change in voice fundamental frequency (F_0). When F_0 is impacted, it may be due to surgery or radiation therapy affecting the suprahyoid muscles and leading to altered forces acting on the laryngeal muscles (Dwivedi et al., 2009). In a study conducted by the same team on acoustic parameters in oral and oropharyngeal cancer patients, a difference by gender was found. Males had higher F1 and F2 values, whereas females had lower values for the same formants when compared to healthy adults. Furthermore, acoustic evaluations were not found to correlate with auditory-perceptual or questionnaire evaluations, once again highlighting the importance of multimodal assessment of speech (Dwivedi et al., 2016).

With respect to tumor involvement of the palatopharyngeal sphincter, intelligibility may be restored to preoperative levels in some patients (Seikaly et al., 2003); however, acoustic and aeromechanical measures remain altered, particularly when resections include over half of the soft palate (Rieger et al., 2008). These types of findings, once again, support the expansion of speech evaluation beyond measures of intelligibility alone (see Searl, Chap. 13).

Using the SHI questionnaire, researchers have found that intelligibility was the primary concern for both oral and oropharyngeal cancer patients treated with surgery as the primary modality, while poor articulation was an issue for oral cavity patients (Dwivedi, St Rose, et al., 2012). Oral cavity cancer patients also experienced more severe speech-related psychosocial impairment. The predominant psychosocial issues in both oral and oropharyngeal patients were feelings of incompetence and feeling upset because of impaired speech. Understanding the patient's perception of his/her own speech impairment and additional concerns such as the unpredictable fluctuations in intelligibility throughout the day (Dwivedi, St Rose, et al., 2012) is crucial to rehabilitation. Due to the obvious impacts that surgical treatment has on the structures so intimately involved in speech, chemoradiation protocols were turned to as a potential way to preserve anatomy and, with it, function.

Chemoradiation

Treatment with chemoradiation alone, referred to as organ preservation, also results in detriments in speech function. Patient-reported speech problems on the SHI have been found in 55% (Rinkel et al., 2016) to 77% (Kraaijenga et al., 2016) of patients who have undergone this treatment modality. Impact on speech appears to be contingent on radiation technique, as intensity-modulated radiation therapy (IMRT) was associated with significantly better speech outcomes than that found using conventional radiation therapy (Kraaijenga et al., 2016; Rinkel et al., 2016). In addition to the type of radiation, mean doses to the tongue and velopharynx also were found to be related to speech function. For example, mean radiation doses to the base of tongue, oral cavity, and velopharynx related to changes in tongue grooving and strength, laryngeal height, palatalization, and degree of pharyngeal constriction (Jacobi et al., 2016). Regarding articulation, stridents and velars were the consonant phonemes identified as being the most difficult for patients with advanced HNCa (Mittal et al., 2001).

With respect to the continuum of follow-up, it is difficult to piece together how speech function changes, as some studies use patient-reported outcomes and others use objective measures. For example, researchers found that SHI ratings were poorest at 3 months posttreatment but improved at 6 months posttreatment. Dry mouth was reported by patients to have a negative impact on speech (Lazarus et al., 2014). Studies using SHI and other patient-perceived outcomes, however, should be interpreted with caution as these reports may not be a true reflection of improvement and may suggest an adaptation to posttreatment speech that has in fact not changed or worsened. When using acoustic evaluations, researchers found that 1 year after treatment, there was no recovery in the deviations noted in vowel space; consonant articulation had deterio-

rated (Jacobi, van Rossum, van der Molen, Hilgers, & van den Brekel, 2013). When followed for 10 years or longer, auditory-perceptual assessment, speech intelligibility, and articulation were impaired in 86% of patients (Kraaijenga et al., 2016). Finally, anecdotal evidence revealed that patients treated with high-dose radiation therapy return for speech evaluation after several years, exposing resonance issues.

Speech Rehabilitation

Provision of speech therapy to this patient population is crucial; data have shown that naïve listeners use speech quality to form negative impressions of patients who have been treated for HNCa (Rieger et al., 2006). Although speech therapy can be effective at improving intelligibility (Furia et al., 2001), very few studies have been conducted to date on the ideal timing, approach, and patient candidacy. It has been suggested that rehabilitation should begin as soon as suture lines have healed (Perry & Frowen, 2006). Therapy may focus on maximizing residual function or achieving alternative manner of articulation using electropalatography and/or audio recordings for visual and auditory biofeedback.

In some circumstances, speech therapy may be paired with intraoral prosthetic rehabilitation. This includes palatal lifts (used to lift the soft palate for patients with velopharyngeal incompetence), pharyngeal obturators (used to seal the velopharyngeal port in patients with velopharyngeal insufficiency), and palatal augmentation prostheses (PAPs). Whereas lifts and obturators address issues with resonance, they also may indirectly impact articulation by removing the need for compensatory misarticulations (Markkanen-Leppanen et al., 2006). PAPs lower the palatal vault and are especially useful for patients with large tongue defects (Laaksonen et al., 2009). All of the aforementioned prostheses can be fabricated to clip on the patient's natural dentition or, in some cases, can be created as part of a full upper denture. In many cases of dentures, dental implant retention will be necessary to support the biomechanical requirements of a lift or obturator. Prosthetic rehabilitation requires interdisciplinary collaboration between speech-language pathologists and prosthodontists (see Cardosa & Chambers, Chap. 21). Candidacy and dental status must be assessed beforehand, and appropriate expectations should be communicated with patients for the impact of prosthetic rehabilitation on speech, as well as swallowing.

Conclusions

Speech evaluations that are standardized and comprehensive provide baseline measures, assist clinicians in monitoring changes in function over time, and allow for a deeper understanding of how speech function is impacted by different cancer treatment modalities. Parameters such as articulation, acoustics, and resonance should be evaluated alongside intelligibility. Assessments should address both clinician and patient concerns, adding a deeper understanding to the issues faced by patients and identifying those requiring additional or immediate supports. Finally, long-term follow-ups are necessary to understand how speech changes as a result of cancer treatment in the patient's survivorship.

References

Bandura, A. (1997). *Self-efficacy the exercise of control*. New York, NY: W. H. Freeman and Company.

Bjordal, K., Hammerlid, E., Ahlner-Elmqvist, M., de Graeff, A., Boysen, M., & Evensen, J. F. (1999). Quality of life in head and neck cancer patients: Validation of the European Organization for Research and Treatment of cancer quality of life questionnaire-H&N35. *Journal of Clinical Oncology, 17*(3), 1008–1019.

Borggreven, P. A., Verdonck-de Leeuw, I., Langendijk, J. A., Doornaert, P., Koster, M. N., de Bree, R., & Leemans, C. R. (2005). Speech outcome after surgical treatment for oral and oropharyngeal cancer: A longitudinal assessment of patients reconstructed by a microvascular flap. *Head & Neck, 27*(9), 785–793. https://doi.org/10.1002/hed.20236

Bressman, T., Jacobs, H., Quintero, J., & Irish, J. C. (2009). Speech outcomes for partial Glossectomy surgery: Measures of speech articulation and listener perception. *Canadian Journal of Speech-Language Pathology and Audiology, 33*(4), 204–210.

Canadian Cancer Society's Advisory Committee on Cancer Statistics. (2015). *Canadian cancer statistics 2015*. Toronto, ON: Canadian Cancer Society. Retrieved from http://www.cancer.ca/en/cancer-information/cancer-type/

Chi, A. C., Day, T. A., & Neville, B. W. (2015). Oral cavity and oropharyngeal squamous cell carcinoma–an update. *CA: A Cancer Journal for Clinicians, 65*(5), 401–421. https://doi.org/10.3322/caac.21293

Cohan, D. M., Popat, S., Kaplan, S. E., Rigual, N., Loree, T., & Hicks, W. L. (2009). Oropharyngeal cancer: Current understanding and management. *Current Opinion in Otolaryngology & Head and Neck Surgery, 17*(2), 88–94. https://doi.org/10.1097/MOO.0b013e32832984c0

Cohen, E. E., LaMonte, S. J., Erb, N. L., Beckman, K. L., Sadeghi, N., Hutcheson, K. A., … Pratt-Chapman, M. L. (2016). American Cancer Society head and neck cancer survivorship care guideline. *CA: A Cancer Journal for Clinicians, 66*(3), 203–239. https://doi.org/10.3322/caac.21343

Colangelo, L. A., Logemann, J. A., & Rademaker, A. W. (2000). Tumor size and pretreatment speech and swallowing in patients with resectable tumors. *Otolaryngology-Head and Neck Surgery, 122*(5), 653–661. https://doi.org/10.1067/mhn.2000.104014

Connoly, J. H. (1986). 1986 Connolly intelligibility: A linguistic review.pdf. *British Journal of Disorders of Communication, 21*, 371–376.

Dios, P. D., Feijoo, J. F., Ferreiro, M. C., & Alvarez, J. A. (1994). Functional consequences of partial Glossectomy. *Journal of Oral and Maxillofacial Surgery, 52*, 12–14.

Dwivedi, R. C., Kazi, R. A., Agrawal, N., Nutting, C. M., Clarke, P. M., Kerawala, C. J., … Harrington, K. J. (2009). Evaluation of speech outcomes following treatment of oral and oropharyngeal cancers. *Cancer Treatment Reviews, 35*(5), 417–424. https://doi.org/10.1016/j.ctrv.2009.04.013

Dwivedi, R. C., Rose, S. S., Chisholm, E. J., Kerawala, C. J., Clarke, P. M., Nutting, C. M., … Kazi, R. (2012). Development and validation of first-ever speech-specific perceptual speech evaluation tool for patients with head and neck cancer: The London speech evaluation (LSE) scale. *Head & Neck, 34*(1), 94–103. https://doi.org/10.1002/hed.21683

Dwivedi, R. C., St Rose, S., Chisholm, E. J., Bisase, B., Amen, F., Nutting, C. M., … Kazi, R. (2012). Evaluation of speech outcomes using English version of the Speech Handicap Index in a cohort of head and neck cancer patients. *Oral Oncology, 48*(6), 547–553. https://doi.org/10.1016/j.oraloncology.2012.01.001

Dwivedi, R. C., St Rose, S., Chisholm, E. J., Clarke, P. M., Kerawala, C. J., Nutting, C. M., … Harrington, K. J. (2016). Acoustic parameters of speech: Lack of correlation with perceptual and questionnaire-based speech evaluation in patients with oral and oropharyngeal cancer treated with primary surgery. *Head & Neck, 38*(5), 670 676. https://doi.org/10.1002/hed.23956

Elfring, T., Boliek, C. A., Winget, M., Paulsen, C., Seikaly, H., & Rieger, J. M. (2014). The relationship between lingual and hypoglossal nerve function and quality of life in head and neck cancer. *Journal of Oral Rehabilitation, 41*(2), 133–140. https://doi.org/10.1111/joor.12116

Elghouche, A., Shokri, T., Qin, Y., Wargo, S., Citrin, D., & Van Waes, C. (2016). Unilateral cervical polyneuropathies following concurrent Bortezomib, Cetuximab, and radiotherapy for head and neck cancer. *Case Reports in Otolaryngology, 2016*, 2313714. https://doi.org/10.1155/2016/2313714

Epstein, J. B., Wilkie, D. J., Fischer, D. J., Kim, Y. O., & Villines, D. (2009). Neuropathic and nociceptive pain in head and neck cancer patients receiving radiation therapy. *Head & Neck Oncology, 1*, 26. https://doi.org/10.1186/1758-3284-1-26

Fisher, H. B., & Logemann, J. A. (1971). *The fisher-Logemann test of articulation competence.* Boston, MA: Houghton Mifflin.

Furia, C. L. B., Kowalski, L. P., Latorre, M. R. D. O., Angelis, E. C., Martins, N. M. S., Barros, A. P. B., & Ribeiro, K. C. B. (2001). Speech intelligibility after Glossectomy and speech rehabilitation. *Archives of Otolaryngology – Head & Neck Surgery, 127*, 877–883.

Georgian, D. A., Logemann, J. A., & Fisher, H. B. (1982). Compensatory articulation patterns of a surgically treated oral cancer patient. *Journal of Speech and Hearing Disorders, 47*(2), 154–159.

Govender, R., Breeson, L., Tuomainen, J., & Smith, C. H. (2013). Speech and swallowing rehabilitation following head and neck cancer: Are we hearing the patient's voice? Our experience with ten patients. *Clinical Otolaryngology, 38*, 381–442.

Hiiemae, K. M., & Palmer, J. B. (2003). Tongue movements in feeding and speech. *Critical Reviews in Oral Biology & Medicine, 14*(6), 413–429.

Hoit, J. D., Lansing, R. W., Dean, K., Yarkosky, M., & Lederle, A. (2011). Nature and evaluation of dyspnea in speaking and swallowing. *Seminars in Speech and Language, 32*(1), 5–20. https://doi.org/10.1055/s-0031-1271971

Hutcheson, K. A., & Lewin, J. S. (2013). Functional assessment and rehabilitation: How to maximize outcomes. *Otolaryngologic Clinics of North America, 46*(4), 657–670. https://doi.org/10.1016/j.otc.2013.04.006

Hutcheson, K. A., Lewin, J. S., Barringer, D. A., Lisec, A., Gunn, G. B., Moore, M. W., & Holsinger, F. C. (2012). Late dysphagia after radiotherapy-based treatment of head and neck cancer. *Cancer, 118*(23), 5793–5799. https://doi.org/10.1002/cncr.27631

Jacobi, I., Navran, A., van der Molen, L., Heemsbergen, W. D., Hilgers, F. J., & van den Brekel, M. W. (2016). Radiation dose to the tongue and velopharynx predicts acoustic-articulatory changes after chemo-IMRT treatment for advanced head and neck cancer. *European Archives of Oto-Rhino-Laryngology, 273*(2), 487–494. https://doi.org/10.1007/s00405-015-3526-8

Jacobi, I., van der Molen, L., Huiskens, H., van Rossum, M. A., & Hilgers, F. J. (2010). Voice and speech outcomes of chemoradiation for advanced head and neck cancer: A systematic review. *European Archives of Oto-Rhino-Laryngology, 267*(10), 1495–1505. https://doi.org/10.1007/s00405-010-1316-x

Jacobi, I., van Rossum, M. A., van der Molen, L., Hilgers, F. J., & van den Brekel, M. W. (2013). Acoustic analysis of changes in articulation proficiency in patients with advanced head and neck cancer treated with Chemoradiotherapy. *Annals of Otology, Rhinology & Laryngology, 122*(12), 754–762.

Kraaijenga, S. A., Oskam, I. M., van Son, R. J., Hamming-Vrieze, O., Hilgers, F. J., van den Brekel, M. W., & van der Molen, L. (2016). Assessment of voice, speech, and related quality of life in advanced head and neck cancer patients 10-years+ after chemoradiotherapy. *Oral Oncology, 55*, 24–30. https://doi.org/10.1016/j.oraloncology.2016.02.001

Krisciunas, G. P., Platt, M., Trojanowska, M., Grillone, G. A., Haines, P. C., & Langmore, S. E. (2016). A novel in vivo protocol for molecular study of radiation-induced fibrosis in head and neck cancer patients. *Annals of Otology, Rhinology & Laryngology, 125*(3), 228–234. https://doi.org/10.1177/0003489415607527

Laaksonen, J. P., Loewen, I. J., Wolfaardt, J., Rieger, J., Seikaly, H., & Harris, J. (2009). Speech after tongue reconstruction and use of a palatal augmentation prosthesis: An acoustic case study. *Canadian Journal of Speech-Language Pathology and Audiology, 33*(4), 196–203.

Laaksonen, J. P., Rieger, J., Happonen, R. P., Harris, J., & Seikaly, H. (2010). Speech after radial forearm free flap reconstruction of the tongue: A longitudinal acoustic study of vowel and diphthong sounds. *Clinical Linguistics & Phonetics, 24*(1), 41–54. https://doi.org/10.3109/02699200903340758

Lam Tang, J., Rieger, J., & Wolfaardt, J. (2008). A review of functional outcomes related to prosthetic treatment after maxillary and mandibular reconstruction in patients with head and neck cancer. *International Journal of Prosthodontics, 21*, 337–354.

Lazarus, C. L., Husaini, H., Hu, K., Culliney, B., Li, Z., Urken, M., … Harrison, L. (2014). Functional outcomes and quality of life after chemoradiotherapy: Baseline and 3 and 6 months post-treatment. *Dysphagia, 29*(3), 365–375. https://doi.org/10.1007/s00455-014-9519-8

Levelt, W. J. M. (1989). *Speaking: From intention to articulation.* Cambridge, MA: The MIT Press.

Lin, Y. S., Jen, Y. M., & Lin, J. C. (2002). Radiation-related cranial nerve palsy in patients with nasopharyngeal carcinoma. *Cancer, 95*(2), 404–409. https://doi.org/10.1002/cncr.10668

Loewen, I. J., Boliek, C. A., Harris, J., Seikaly, H., & Rieger, J. M. (2010). Oral sensation and function: A comparison of patients with innervated radial forearm free flap reconstruction to healthy matched controls. *Head & Neck, 32*(1), 85–95. https://doi.org/10.1002/hed.21155

Mády, K., Sader, R., Hoole, P. H., Zimmermann, A., & Horch, H. H. (2009). Speech evaluation and swallowing ability after intra-oral cancer. *Clinical Linguistics & Phonetics, 17*(4–5), 411–420. https://doi.org/10.1080/0269920031000079921

Markkanen-Leppanen, M., Isotalo, E., Makitie, A. A., Asko-Seljavaara, S., Pessi, T., Suominen, E., & Haapanen, M. L. (2006). Changes in articulatory proficiency following microvascular reconstruction in oral or oropharyngeal cancer. *Oral Oncology, 42*(6), 646–652. https://doi.org/10.1016/j.oraloncology.2005.11.004

Massengill, R., Maxwell, S., & Pickrell, K. (1970). An analysis of articulation following partial and total glossectomy. *Journal of Speech and Hearing Disorders, 35*, 170–173.

McEwen, S. E., Davis, A. M., Jones, J. M., Martino, R., Poon, I., Rodriguez, A. M., & Ringash, J. (2015). Development and preliminary evaluation of a rehabilitation consult for survivors of head and neck cancer: An intervention mapping protocol. *Implementation Science, 10*, 6. https://doi.org/10.1186/s13012-014-0191-z

McKinstry, A., & Perry, A. (2003). Evaluation of speech in people with head and neck cancer: A pilot study. *International Journal of Language & Communication Disorders, 38*(1), 31–46. https://doi.org/10.1080/1368282021000014877

Metcalfe, C. W., Lowe, D., & Rogers, S. N. (2014). What patients consider important: Temporal variations by early and late stage oral, oropharyngeal and laryngeal subsites. *Journal of Cranio-Maxillofacial Surgery, 42*(5), 641–647. https://doi.org/10.1016/j.jcms.2013.09.008

Miller, R. M., & Groher, M. E. (1993). Speech-language pathology and dysphagia: A brief historical perspective. *Dysphagia, 8*, 180–184.

Mittal, B. B., Kepka, A., Mahadevan, A., Kies, M., Pelzer, H., List, M. A., ... Logemann, J. (2001). Tissue/dose compensation to reduce toxicity from combined radiation and chemotherapy for advanced head and neck cancers. *International Journal of Cancer, 96*(Suppl), 61–70. https://doi.org/10.1002/ijc.10360

Morrish, E. C. E. (1988). Compensatory articulation in a subject with total glossectomy. *British Journal of Disorders of Communication, 23*, 13–22.

Morton, R. (2003). Studies in the quality of life of head and neck cancer patients: Results of a two-year longitudinal study and a comparative cross-sectional cross-cultural survey. *Laryngoscope, 113*, 1091–1103.

Namin, A. W., & Varvares, M. A. (2016). Functional outcomes of sensate versus insensate free flap reconstruction in oral and oropharyngeal reconstruction: A systematic review. *Head & Neck, 38*(11), 1717–1721. https://doi.org/10.1002/hed.24494

Nicoletti, G., Soutar, D. S., Jackson, M. S., Wrench, A. A., Robertson, G., & Robertson, C. (2004). Objective assessment of speech after surgical treatment for oral cancer: Experience from 196 selected cases. *Plastic and Reconstructive Surgery, 113*(1), 114–125. https://doi.org/10.1097/01.PRS.0000095937.45812.84

Pauloski, B. R., Logemann, J. A., Colangelo, L. A., Rademaker, A. W., McConnel, F. M. S., Heise, M. A., ... Esclamado, R. (1998). Surgical variables affecting speech in treated patients with Oral and oropharyngeal cancer. *Laryngoscope, 108*, 908–916.

Perry, A., & Frowen, J. (2006). Speech and swallowing function in head and neck cancer patients: What do we know? *Cancer Forum, 30*(3), 178–183.

Perry, A. R., Shaw, M. A., & Cotton, S. (2003). An evaluation of functional outcomes (speech, swallowing) in patients attending speech pathology after head and neck cancer treatment(s): Results and analysis at 12 months post-intervention. *Journal of Laryngology & Otology, 117*(5), 368–381. https://doi.org/10.1258/002221503321626410

Peterson, G. E., & Barney, H. L. (1952). Control methods used in a study of the vowels. *The Journal of the Acoustical Society of America, 24*(2), 175–184.

Piagkou, M., Demesticha, T., Skandalakis, P., & Johnson, E. O. (2011). Functional anatomy of the mandibular nerve: Consequences of nerve injury and entrapment. *Clinical Anatomy, 24*(2), 143–150. https://doi.org/10.1002/ca.21089

Radford, K., Woods, H., Lowe, D., & Rogers, S. N. (2004). A UK multi-Centre pilot study of speech and swallowing outcomes following head and neck cancer. *Clinical Otolaryngology, 29*, 376–381.

Redford, M. A. (2015). *The handbook of speech production*. West Sussex, UK: Wiley Blackwell.

Rieger, J., Bohle, G., Huryn, J., Lam Tang, J., Harris, J., & Seikaly, H. (2009). Surgical reconstruction versus prosthetic Obturation of extensive soft palate defects: A comparison of speech outcomes. *International Journal of Prosthodontics, 22*, 566–572.

Rieger, J., Dickson, N., Lemire, R., Bloom, K., Wolfaardt, J., Wolfaardt, U., & Seikaly, H. (2006). Social perception of speech in individuals with oropharyngeal reconstruction. *Journal of Psychosocial Oncology, 24*(4), 33–51. https://doi.org/10.1300/J077v24n04_03

Rieger, J. M., Zalmanowitz, J. G., Li, S. Y., Tang, J. L., Williams, D., Harris, J., & Seikaly, H. (2008). Speech outcomes after soft palate reconstruction with the soft palate insufficiency repair procedure. *Head & Neck, 30*(11), 1439–1444. https://doi.org/10.1002/hed.20884

Rinkel, R. N., Verdonck-de Leeuw, I. M., Doornaert, P., Buter, J., de Bree, R., Langendijk, J. A., ... Leemans, C. R. (2016). Prevalence of swallowing and speech problems in daily life after chemoradiation for head and neck cancer based on cut-off scores of the patient-reported outcome measures SWAL-QOL and SHI. *European Archives of Oto-Rhino-Laryngology, 273*(7), 1849–1855. https://doi.org/10.1007/s00405-015-3680-z

Robertson, S. J., & Thomson, F. (1986). *Working with dysarthrics: A practical guide to therapy for dysarthria*. Bicester: Winslow Press.

Rogers, S. N., Laher, S. H., Overend, L., & Lowe, D. (2002). Importance-rating using the University of Washington quality of life questionnaire in patients treated by primary surgery for oral and oropharyngeal cancer. *Journal of Cranio-Maxillofacial Surgery, 30*(2), 125–132. https://doi.org/10.1054/jcms.2001.0273

Schuster, M., & Stelzle, F. (2012). Outcome measurements after oral cancer treatment: Speech and speech-related aspects–an overview. *Oral and Maxillofacial Surgery, 16*(3), 291–298. https://doi.org/10.1007/s10006-012-0340-y

Seikaly, H., Rieger, J., Wolfaardt, J., Moysa, G., Harris, J., & Jha, N. (2003). Functional outcomes after primary oropharyngeal cancer resection and reconstruction with the radial forearm free flap. *Laryngoscope, 113*, 897–904.

Shipley, K. G., & McAfee, J. G. (2004). *Assessment in speech-language pathology*. Clifton Park, NY: Delmar Learning.

Skelly, M. (1973). *Glossectomee speech rehabilitation*. Springfield, IL: Charles Thomas.

Su, W. F., Hsia, Y. J., Chang, Y. C., Chen, S. G., & Sheng, H. (2003). Functional comparison after reconstruction with a radial forearm free flap or a pectoralis major flap for cancer of the tongue. *Otolaryngology-Head and Neck Surgery, 128*(3), 412–418. https://doi.org/10.1067/mhn.2003.38

Tschiesner, U. (2012). Preservation of organ function in head and neck cancer. *GMS Current Topics in Otorhinolaryngology – Head and Neck Surgery, 11*, 1–18.

Tschiesner, U., Rogers, S., Dietz, A., Yueh, B., & Cieza, A. (2010). Development of ICF core sets for head and neck cancer. *Head & Neck, 32*(2), 210–220. https://doi.org/10.1002/hed.21172

Tschiesner, U., Sabariego, C., Linseisen, E., Becker, S., Stier-Jarmer, M., Cieza, A., & Harreus, U. (2013). Priorities of head and neck cancer patients: A patient survey based on the brief ICF core set for HNC. *European Archives of Oto-Rhino-Laryngology, 270*(12), 3133–3142. https://doi.org/10.1007/s00405-013-2446-8

Urken, M. L., Moscoso, J. F., Lawson, W., & Biller, H. F. (1994). A systematic approach to functional reconstruction of the Oral cavity following partial and Total Glossectomy. *Archives of Otolaryngology – Head & Neck Surgery, 120*, 589–601.

WHO. (2014). Head and Neck Cancer: Union for International Cancer Control 2014 Review of Cancer Medicines of the WHO List of Essential Medicines. *2014 Review of Cancer Medicines of the WHO List of Essential Medicines*. Retrieved from http://www.who.int/selection_medicines/committees/expert/20/applications/cancer/en/

Yorkston, K., Beukelman, D., & Traynor, C. (1984). *Assessment of intelligibility of dysarthric speech*. Portland, OR: CC Publications.

Zuydam, A. C., Lowe, D., Brown, J. S., Vaughan, E. D., & Rogers, S. N. (2005). Predictors of speech and swallowing function following primary surgery for oral and oropharyngeal cancer. *Clinical Otolaryngology, 30*, 428–437.

Documenting Voice and Speech Outcomes in Alaryngeal Speakers

17

Philip C. Doyle

Introduction

The Oxford English Dictionary succinctly defines the term *"outcome"* as "The way a thing turns out; a consequence" (2018). Communication loss following total laryngectomy is one of the most significant consequences of laryngeal cancer; it is an outcome that will persist for the remainder of one's life. Fortunately, multiple postlaryngectomy speech rehabilitation options exist, namely, esophageal speech, tracheoesophageal (TE) speech, or the use of artificial electrolarynx. Regardless of which method(s) of alaryngeal voice and speech rehabilitation is acquired, even the most proficient and "superior" alaryngeal speaker will exhibit reductions in their overall communication proficiency and effectiveness.

Communication, broadly defined, provides the fundamental concern underlying the information to follow. Verbal communication will always involve a speaker and a listener, and ideally, there will be no disruption in how the signal is generated (voice) and modulated (speech) or how it is received (hearing and comprehension). The con-

tent of this chapter directly acknowledges that the measurement of parameters that physically characterize alaryngeal voice and speech signal is necessary and meaningful; however, such measures may not represent the full range of one's ability or represent the ideal index of postlaryngectomy communication outcomes. In the sections to follow, specific recommendations on the need for four areas of measurement are outlined. This includes a discussion of acoustic measures, the auditory-perceptual (A-P) evaluation, the need for assessments of speech intelligibility, and the value of self-reported instruments in documenting voice-related outcomes. Consequently, the goal of this chapter seeks to provide support for the continuing need to gather data on voice, speech, and communication functioning in those who use alaryngeal speech regardless of the method used.

A Brief History of the Development of Medical Outcomes

Since the late 1980s, there has been a substantial and continued interest in the measurement of patient "status" secondary to medical intervention (Kotronoulas et al., 2014). Research conducted over a period of almost four decades on medical outcomes has in large part been statistically oriented (Ryan et al., 2012; Tarlov et al., 1989; Ware Jr et al., 1995). As with any statistical undertaking, the analysis of larger datasets

P. C. Doyle (✉)
Voice Production and Perception Laboratory & Laboratory for Well-Being and Quality of Life, Department of Otolaryngology – Head and Neck Surgery and School of Communication Sciences and Disorders, Western University, Elborn College, London, ON, Canada
e-mail: pdoyle@uwo.ca

© Springer Nature Switzerland AG 2019
P. C. Doyle (ed.), *Clinical Care and Rehabilitation in Head and Neck Cancer*,
https://doi.org/10.1007/978-3-030-04702-3_17

offers the potential for subsequent determinations from those data to be made with greater confidence. That is, prediction of outcomes may be enhanced.

Outcomes research is most often associated with and frequently serves to monitor or track the "success or failure" of any given treatment approach, but these data are also used to inform other areas of health care (e.g., funding decisions for personnel, service access, etc.). In speech-language pathology, clinical outcomes specific to voice and speech rehabilitation in those treated for laryngeal cancer form a key index of treatment success. However, regardless of the method(s) of treatment, changes in voice and speech will always occur following total laryngectomy (Angel, Doyle, & Fung, 2011).

Efforts directed at developing measurement instruments that quantify the consequences of treatment have been observed with increasingly prominence across all aspects of health care. This has included interest in the conceptual underpinnings of outcomes and interest in the clinical data gathered. In the present context, documenting the consequences of a treatment through a variety of "lenses" and the subsequent attempt to logically seek coherence in what otherwise may be seen as disparate bits of information may offer the best index of one's true outcome.

The collective body of clinical explorations related to laryngeal cancer crosses an incredibly wide and multidisciplinary literature. This includes topics ranging from the physical and biological value of a particular medical treatment procedure to those related to patient satisfaction and to those that might be more broadly considered as "quality of life" considerations (Doyle & MacDonald, Chap. 27). In this regard, comprehensive clinical outcomes in those treated for laryngeal cancer must address physical, psychological, social, and spiritual domains of functioning (deBoer, McCormick, Pruyn, Ryckman, & van den Borne, 1999). However, a fundamental issue in those who are treated for laryngeal cancer will center around the individual's capacity for verbal communication and the intersection of this factor with social performance and participation (Eadie, Chap. 29).

Communication: Beyond Voice and Speech Production

Reed (1983) has suggested that the primary objective of postlaryngectomy rehabilitation should seek to assist the individual in leading as normal a life as possible. Yet when the larynx is lost, normal communication will never again occur. Voice and speech deficits secondary to laryngectomy will in some instances have devastating consequences, some directly relating to how others will respond to one's new method of verbal communication. Alterations in voice and speech have the direct potential to negatively influence personal, social, emotional, and psychosocial health. With that in mind, the value of gathering outcomes that more fully represent the constructs of the "biopsychosocial" model of health becomes clear. The biopsychosocial model provides clinicians with the opportunity to consider the impact of a larger and interrelated set of factors in order to more fully and accurately define posttreatment outcomes (Engel, 1977).[1] Given the complex relationships between all domains of functioning associated with laryngeal cancer and the consequences of its treatment, the willingness to extend the assessment of outcomes beyond solely objective acoustic measures of voice and speech outcome is essential (Doyle, 1999).

Communication is a social act that occurs between at least two people (a dyad). Thus, the relationship between the speaker and the listener involves more than verbal signals exchanged between individuals. If the verbal signal is without disruption, information can be conveyed in an efficient and effective manner. At the most basic level of interaction, speech intelligibility is required (see Sleeth & Doyle, Chap. 14). Beyond the linguistic content of the information communicated between one or more people, acoustic features of the speech signal as well as the

---

[1] In order to appreciate the complexities of the biopsychosocial model in relationship to laryngeal cancer, the reader is encouraged to read the excellent review by Eadie (2003) concerning the application of the International Classification of Functioning (ICF, World Health Organization, 2001) in this population.

collective "quality" of the voice are readily detected during a communication exchange. When a deviation from normal exists in either the voice or speech signal (or both), communication will be influenced.

When a voice or speech disorder exists, it will also carry with it reciprocal changes that will challenge the listener. As stated by Charles Van Riper (1978, p. 43) "…speech is abnormal when it deviates so far from the speech of other people that it calls attention to itself, interferes with communication, or causes the speaker or his listeners to be distressed." Using Van Riper's definition, the concept of "speech" can be expanded to include one's "voice." Thus, while the inherent acoustic properties of speech (frequency, intensity, and temporal characteristics) and the dynamic A-P composite it creates (voice quality) can be measured, the more dramatic personal impact that such deviations have on the act of communication may not be fully realized. Further, the changes that may occur in the listener are also likely to increase in response to increases in the overall severity or unusual presentation of the disorder.

When considering alaryngeal speech, there is a plethora of clinical and research data that consistently indicates that the signal is grossly abnormal in one or more parameters of measurement (Doyle, 1994). Although variation across alaryngeal speakers does exist (some speakers are in fact better than others), all methods of alaryngeal speech will be identified as abnormal by the listener. When a grossly abnormal signal is detected by the listener, additional changes in the communication process will occur (see Evitts, Chap. 28). Furthermore, Doyle (1994) raised the issue of differential societal penalty when one considers gender (i.e., men may be less penalized than women for abnormal vocal quality), and this suspicion has been confirmed experimentally in alaryngeal speakers (Eadie & Doyle, 2004, 2005a). In the current era of treatment, as surgical resections for laryngeal cancers are extended, particularly in relation to the use of free-flap procedures, the nature of voice and speech may be even more varied across a variety of traditional acoustic measures. This is one of the reasons why a continuing need remains for the acquisition of a range of new data on voice and speech outcomes secondary to the treatment for laryngeal cancer.

Rehabilitation as a Process

It is increasingly well recognized that recovery and rehabilitation following the treatment for laryngeal cancer is a continuous process. The consequences of treatment will always result in some level of disability, and these changes will remain for the duration of the individual's life. That is, simply stated, laryngeal cancer and the consequences of its treatment will result in a chronic health condition. For this reason, efforts directed toward documenting one's more comprehensive rehabilitation status are essential. This documentation must involve active consideration of a variety of dimensions including those that may positively or negatively influence either short- or long-term outcomes.

As a simple example, as one learns any alaryngeal method, there will be a learning curve. But, it may also be safely assumed that each speaker will exhibit a "ceiling" in the proficiency of their voice, speech, and overall communication effectiveness. Again, all of this must be considered with the recognition that both the speaker and listener will influence outcomes. Similar to the evaluation of quality of life (Doyle & MacDonald, Chap. 27), any documentation of alaryngeal voice and speech rehabilitation success must consider multiple aspects of the speaker's overall communication functioning and its potential impact on social participation (Eadie, Chap. 29). The attributes that ultimately form a traditional rehabilitation outcome for individuals treated for laryngeal malignancies will most often involve assessments of specific tasks and activities at given points in time. But a more contemporary view is that such assessments also should be employed with comprehensive targets, most specifically at the level of social participation (Baylor, Burns, Eadie, Britton, & Yorkston, 2011; Eadie et al., 2016; Eadie, Day, Sawin, Lamvik, & Doyle, 2013).

Despite an extensive and longstanding clinical literature on postlaryngectomy voice and speech rehabilitation, the need to acquire, analyze, and document new data on treatment outcomes persists. This need is made more urgent due to changes in laryngeal cancer treatment protocols, advances in microsurgical reconstruction, the limits of applying historical objective data to contemporary voice and speech capabilities, and the value of providing extended data on communication performance when using postlaryngectomy methods of speech. The acquisition of any method of alaryngeal voice and speech is not a static event; rather, skills, proficiency, and compensation will continue to develop over time; this too will require additional research.

One of the most significant changes in the surgical treatment of laryngeal cancer over the past two decades has been observed in the application of extended surgical procedures along with the use of various microvascular, free-tissue transfer reconstruction procedures. Clinical research has demonstrated the range of voice and speech changes that will occur secondary to these types of procedures (Alam, Vivek, & Kmiecik, 2008; Deschler, Doherty, Reed, & Singer, 1998; Deschler, Herr, Kmiecik, Sethi, & Bunting, 2015; Divi, Lin, Emerick, Rocco, & Deschler, 2011; Emerick, Herr, & Deschler, 2014; Fung et al., 2007; Sethi, Kozin, Lam, Emerick, & Deschler, 2014; and others). As treatment methods become more extensive, most notably in the area of surgical intervention, the A-P characteristics of post-treatment voice and speech may be impacted more dramatically.

Additionally, this need also extends to broader considerations of communication and social capacity, as well as to placing vocal outcomes within the larger context of rehabilitation and one's long-term well-being. Effective communication may hold the most significant factor influencing positive psychosocial functioning for those who are laryngectomized. Changes in voice will carry with it a greater risk of psychosocial changes and associated changes in coping, adjustment, and adaptation following laryngectomy (Blanchard, Albrecht, Rucksdeschel, Grant, & Hammick, 1995; Blood, Luther, & Stemple,

1992; Doyle, 1994; Langius et al., 1994; Mathieson, Stam, & Scott, 1990; Plumb & Holland, 1977; Rohe, 1994; Salmon, 1986; Shanks, 1995; Shapiro & Kornfeld, 1987).

Excluding these types of concerns and/or failing to address them in relation to "how" the alaryngeal voice influences the speaker and disrupts the communication dyad is a significant omission. Recalling Van Riper's (1978) definition, if one's postlaryngectomy communication creates distress for the listener, then it is not unreasonable to assume that the speaker will be at increased risk of psychological and psychiatric problems. In fact, research has documented that social withdrawal is a strong predictive factor for depression and the significant consequences that may occur (D'Antonio et al., 1998; Henderson & Ord, 1997; Lydiatt, Moran, & Burke, 2009; Vokes, Weichselbaum, Lippman, & Hong, 1993; Zeller, 2006). Further, this risk is not only associated with the early period following cancer diagnosis and treatment, but may exist for the remainder of the individual's life (Bjordal & Kaasa, 1995; Gritz et al., 1999).

Gathering Outcome Measures

In the early periods post-diagnosis and during treatment, as well as following the completion of treatment, more generalized outcome measures (i.e., symptom screens, quality of life assessments) may be of substantial value. While the direct focus of these types of measures does not always center on specific aspects of one's voice or speech, some measurement instruments do in fact address areas that have overlay to communication issues. For example, many quality of life measures seek information related to whether the respondent is avoiding interactions with others or whether they are doing less socially. In cases where the individual indicates that such changes have occurred, the string of events that have potentially led to it must be identified. Sometimes these reductions in social activity or social participation may be due to factors such as fatigue or physical pain or similar issues. However, in other instances, concerns about communication may drive the individual's choice of withdrawing from activities. Of particular importance here is when this observation exists in the situation of an alaryngeal speaker who has been "professionally" judged to be a very good or excellent speaker, one whose communication is not significantly impacted by reduced intelligibility. Withdrawal in such circumstances goes beyond communication.

Under the above-cited circumstances, the question of "why" one is withdrawing must be explored. Questions should seek to determine if the individual speaker is finding the response of listeners to be problematic or if other observations during communication interactions have been altered (e.g., people avoiding conversations, terminating verbal interactions quickly, etc.). Similarly and directly in line with Van Riper (1978) is the possibility that the listener has withdrawn because of their discomfort with the speaker's new voice or that they become distressed when interacting with an alaryngeal speaker. All of these types of concerns can be drawn back to disruptions in how the communication dyad functions or breaks down (Doyle & Baker, 2018).

One of the most frequently raised concerns about the gathering of any clinical measure relates to time demands. This concern is understandable given the increasing demands placed on clinicians. However, the collection of data specific to voice, speech, and communication outcomes can often be effectively structured to coincide with regular follow-up and oncologic monitoring.[2] In some instances, assessment can be done during the course of ongoing treatment (e.g., radiotherapy, postsurgery, etc.). Assessment can also take place without great burden to either the patient or the clinician at those intervals where regular, posttreatment outpatient surveillance will occur. In seeking to document postlaryngectomy rehabilitation status and/or the extent of progress secondary to the completion of treatment for laryngeal can-

cer, verbal communication always will be a primary objective.

Those who wish to document voice and speech rehabilitation outcomes and associated functioning must also carefully consider aspects of other areas of functioning and assess levels of disability. This will include a careful exploration related to the resumption, or lack thereof, in one's social functioning, including inquiry regarding one's vocational and avocational activities. If such logical relationships between communication and social functioning are not made, the interpretation of isolated voice and speech rehabilitation outcomes may be subject to substantial error. At the very least, inattention to broad communication issues with a focus solely on voice and speech measures alone may be narrow in scope and potentially context-stripped.

Communication Outcomes and Quality of Life

Comprehensive care for those treated for laryngeal cancer and the ability to monitor their rehabilitation progress cannot focus solely on objective, parametric measures (e.g., assessments of fundamental frequency, intensity, speech rate, etc.). Rather, when data from parametric assessments are paired with assessments of how others judge one's voice/speech or how vocal changes influence personal functioning, an enhanced understanding of outcomes may be possible. Additionally, the use of additional measures that assess the intersection of "voice-related" functioning and quality of life may offer valuable information on potential deficits that may exist. Collectively, this information may offer insights into why the problem exists (e.g., the listener may have some degree of hearing impairment), may serve to identify strategies to reduce or eliminate reported problems (e.g., encouraging the speaker to talk more slowly), or suggest potential accommodations to improve communication in specific environments (e.g., the presence of background noise); these types of recommendations can be very helpful to the speaker and may improve overall rehabilitation outcomes.

[2]Computer based online technology also provides an excellent vehicle for regular data collection and monitoring, however, privacy concerns must be considered.

Outcomes as Clinical Targets

Several observations suggest that continuing attempts to document outcomes in this clinical population should be actively pursued. The first pertains to the fact that no clear data exist on what describes and defines the upper performance limits of postlaryngectomy voice and speech for any given alaryngeal method – electrolaryngeal speech, esophageal speech, or TE speech. The second emerges directly from changes in how laryngeal cancer is treated medically today. With the acceptance of chemoradiation treatment protocols comes the potential that voice and speech may be differentially influenced should there be a recurrence of cancer and a total laryngectomy is required. Third, should complications occur as a result of treatment, there may be additional voice and speech implications.

It must also be recognized that those who undergo conservative treatment methods (radiation therapy alone, endoscopic resection of tumors, or CRT) may also experience changes in voice quality (Finizia, Dotevall, Lundström, & Lindström, 1999). In those who have undergone conservation treatment, voice quality may be substantially disrupted; however, speech will likely be unchanged. Thus, efforts that seek to document these types of changes secondary to treatment can provide substantial information to both the individual who is treated and for the clinician. At the very least, baseline (pretreatment) measures should always be obtained; assessments at regular intervals (during posttreatment medical surveillance visits) can also serve to document changes that may require medical follow-up (e.g., unusual changes in specific parameters of voice, or alterations in voice quality may represent a recurrence of disease). But, regular basic voice (and speech) assessments may identify changes in the individual's voice that could be the result of purposeful compensations. In circumstances where compensatory vocal behaviors result in negative changes in voice quality, more traditional, direct voice therapy approaches can be offered by the SLP (Doyle, 1997).

Because of the breadth of concerns related to "how one does" following treatment for cancer of the larynx, there is continued debate on what constitutes the best index of success. Clearly, the ability to reacquire one or more methods of alaryngeal speech production is essential. But it is equally important to acknowledge that the reacquisition of verbal communication, even if by all technical measurement standards is excellent, does not insure that a successful patient outcome has been achieved. Consequently, the ability to monitor the bigger picture of communication outcomes, or those that seek to identify specific changes in one's social use of voice, can be of substantial benefit.

Finally, the relationship of voice and speech, its uniqueness relative to obvious changes in postlaryngectomy voice quality, and how these changes affect the listener and potentially how that interacts with the communication process remain important when considering treatment outcomes. Because of this, component parts must be partitioned at times in order to document the change (either negative or positive) in one or more factors or features while at the same time indexing any functional limitations related to one's ability to return to as normal a life as possible. The potential points of importance across this continuum may in fact be numerous, with a likelihood of substantial interaction.[3]

Reducing Vulnerability as an Outcome

With loss of the normal spoken voice, individuals treated for laryngeal cancer are increasingly vulnerable to stigma and isolation (Ablon, 1981). This may evolve from a number of factors, but it may be most directly related to the individual's self-perception of their non-normal method of verbal communication and obvious physical changes as a consequence of the laryngectomy. These issues and associated concerns of how the listener may react to them are of great importance

---

[3]The author acknowledges that eating and swallowing changes in this population are common, and intervention in this area is also within the professional purview of the SLP.

to the success of rehabilitation. Stigmatizing conditions cannot be overlooked because they threaten the individual's judgment of self, which might then pose a risk to relationships in the individual's own social milieu (Goffman, 1963). Laryngectomy is disfiguring, which further threatens the person's identity. Although the treatment of other sites of cancer may be hidden, the sequelae of treatment for laryngeal are easily observed both visually and auditorily.

Fear, anxiety, and emotional burden can only be addressed directly through verbal communication. Thus, one can appreciate the emotional challenges that will be experienced following laryngectomy. The ability to "talk things out" with another, whether that be a family member, friend, SLP, or other health-care professional, is often of significant importance over the course of the cancer journey; thus, a reduction in one's ability to communicate effectively or more critically the total inability to communicate may have devastating consequences.

Alaryngeal Voice and Speech Outcomes

While it is beyond the scope of the present chapter, there is a large historical literature on acoustic measures obtained from speakers using the artificial electrolarynx (a variety of commercially available devices), esophageal speech, and TE speech. Doyle (1994) provided a comprehensive summary of findings that addressed comparative measures of performance by artificial laryngeal, esophageal, and TE speakers, including information on A-P evaluation (acceptability, preference, and prosodic features) and speech intelligibility. Despite the fact that Doyle's (1994) summary is more than 20 years old, with exception of the additional information on the acoustic characteristics of TE puncture voice restoration, particularly in relation to multiple types of flap reconstruction, there have been limited acoustic data reported in the intervening period of time. This observation provides support for the recommendation that acquisition of a new body of data from all who undergo total laryngectomy and use

alaryngeal methods of verbal communication is mandatory.

If such data can be obtained and if careful subgroupings of speakers can be generated based on specified factors (treatment modality, the presence of specific complications, etc.), the goal of defining the upper limits of vocal performance may be possible, and expectations can be more accurately determined. Consequently, the discussion to follow outlines a summary of the types of measures to be obtained. Initially, the acquisition of a standard speech sample is presented along with the information on the recording process and tasks involved. In regard to the information on acoustic measures that can be generated from the sample, basic procedural details of collection and analysis are provided. Relative to the other measures discussed herein, namely, A-P methods and the evaluation of speech intelligibility, a more general discussion describing their use and interpretation is offered.

Gathering the Alaryngeal Voice and Speech Sample

Recording process and tasks Acoustic evaluation of alaryngeal speech provides the most basic index of postlaryngectomy voice/speech outcomes. This includes the evaluation of fundamental frequency (f_0), measures of vocal intensity, and a variety of temporal measures. Efforts must always be made to obtain the sample in a quiet environment and, ideally, obtain repeated recordings in the same environment whenever possible. All efforts should be made to maintain a constant mouth-to-microphone distance during recordings. This may be achieved using a small, fixed microphone stand, by positioning a small electret microphone on a light, neck-mounted holder, or by simply holding the microphone at a fixed distance just off of one corner of the speaker's mouth.

Recording environment While the speaker sample of interest to the present discussion is unique, the acquisition and recording of stimuli and the analysis procedures employed are essentially consistent with most clinically based efforts to gather voice samples for acoustic assessment. Gathering the voice and speech sample under consistent procedural conditions in a sound-treated environment is certainly recommended; however, in a busy clinical setting, it is acknowledged that the environment may be less of a confound. But all efforts to maintain a consistent yet not always experimentally controlled process are acceptable in an effort to gather descriptive data.

Recording and analysis software At present, a variety of free web-based programs may be used to record directly to a personal computer or tablet; some very good and easy to use programs are also available as applications for cell phones. The selection of program is a personal choice, but the clinician should confirm that any recording software or application that is selected does not compress the digital signal, and digitization rates should be sufficient (minimally exceeding 20 kHz). Please keep in mind that a recording could be made on any device and then transferred over to another software program for analysis. While several options for signal processing and analysis do exist, one common program that is available online without charge is Praat[4]; this program provides numerous analysis options that range from simple to much more advanced measures.

Microphone placement As noted, all efforts should be made to maintain a consistent mouth-to-microphone distance of 6 inches (15 cm) during the entire recording. All recordings, regardless of the task, should be completed by asking the speaker to produce each stimulus without any unusual alteration in their voice. That is, the speaker should provide the sample in a manner that is representative of their regular, typical (habitual) speech pattern. A demonstration of all tasks should be provided by the clinician. If problems are encountered, reinstruction should be provided by the clinician if it is determined that some type of change or variation in the speaker's voice is detected in comparison with other conversational interactions with the individual.

---

[4]http://www.fon.hum.uva.nl/praat/download_win.html

Stimuli The basic recording protocol should include three specific types of samples: vowels, an oral reading, and a short monologue. Begin the recording by asking the speaker to produce three vowels (/a/, /i/, /u/) three times each. The speaker should be asked to produce each vowel for approximately 6 s, with a short pause in between. TE speakers should be instructed to take a "normal" inspiration rather than taking a large breath prior to any given task. Each vowel should be produced in sequence (i.e., /a/–/a/–/a/, etc.). There is no need to record each sample as a separate digital file as the entire sample can be edited at some point following the recording.

Next, a standard reading passage, either the *Rainbow Passage* (Fairbanks, 1960) or the *Grandfather Passage* (Darley, Aronson, & Brown, 1975), should be obtained. It is advised that you allow the speaker to read the passage aloud one time to ensure that they understand the content and do not mispronounce any of the words contained in the passage. Following the oral reading, the clinician should request the speaker to produce a short monologue sample; this may involve asking the speaker to talk about family, a hobby, the work that they do, a trip to a special place, etc. The topic covered in the monologue itself is not critical, but rather, it is desired that speaker produce a running speech sample of approximately 1 min without lengthy pauses. An experienced clinician who is familiar with the stimuli and protocol described can gather the sample in approximately 5 min.

Analyzing the Voice and Speech Sample: Acoustic Measures

Frequency measures Once all samples have been obtained, they can be transferred in order to edit samples and conduct analyses. For each vowel, the middle 2 s of the sample should be extracted; doing so will avoid any unusual variations in the sample due to the initiation of voice or its termination. These extracted nine samples (three vowels x three samples) should then be analyzed for f_0. Dependent upon the analysis program used, minimum and maximum frequency measures for the sample may also be provided. Similarly, perturbation measures in the frequency (jitter) and amplitude (shimmer) domains may be gathered (Globlek, Stajner-Katusic, Musura, Horga, & Liker, 2004; Horii & Weinberg, 1975; Ng, Liu, Zhao, & Lam, 2009; Robbins, 1984). It should be noted, however, that for very "noisy" alaryngeal samples, perturbation measures may be difficult to obtain because the cycle-to-cycle tracking capacity of some programs may not be able to deal with the extreme signal aperiodicity. Finally, and if it is an option on the analysis program used, a signal-to-noise ratio (SNR) or harmonics-to-noise ratio (HNR) should be obtained.

For the reading passage, one can determine an average frequency level, as well as identify the range of frequency variation in the sample obtained. While this can be conducted on the entire reading passage, it is recommended that one sentence of either reading be extracted and analyzed. For the *Rainbow Passage*, this has typically been the second sentence ("The rainbow is a division of white light into many beautiful colors.").

Lastly, the same analysis procedure used with the reading passage can be employed with the monologue. However, if significant silent pauses occur during the monologue sample, it is recommended that those silent periods be edited out prior to analysis as at times, and dependent upon the analysis program used, acoustic measures gathered may be influenced.

Spectral measures The use of more comprehensive spectral analyses, those that consider the interactions between the voicing source and the influence of the vocal tract, has been conducted with postlaryngectomy speakers. These types of measures provide the opportunity to document changes that occur in multiple acoustic domains (frequency, amplitude, and duration) through simultaneous signal processing. Assessments of acoustic properties of speech samples using an analysis method termed *long-term average spectrum* (LTAS) measures have formed the most prominent area of exploration in the literature. However, as a general rule, these types of analyses are typically more elaborate and tend to have been conducted as part of empirical investiga-

tions related to alaryngeal speech (Imaizumi, Boku, Koike, & Ohta, 1983; Qi & Weinberg, 1991, 1995; Qi, Weinberg, & Bi, 1995; van Gogh, Festen, Verdonck-de Leeuw, Parker, Traissac, Cheesman, Mahieu, 2005; Weinberg, Horii, & Smith, 1980).

Because of the use of an intrinsic, biological voicing source for esophageal and TE speech, most of the published work in the area of acoustics has been done with those two populations (Van der Torn, De Vries, Festen, Verdonck-de Leeuw, & Mahieu, 2001). Nevertheless, the capacity to evaluate signals using analyses of the composite spectrum holds the potential of providing further information on alaryngeal speech in that such measures may be correlated to A-P judgments by listeners (van As, Hilgers, Verdonck-de Leeuw, & Koopmans-van Beinum, 1998). Research focused on identifying potential relationships between LTAS and similar spectral measures with listener judgments has been conducted with a variety of other, non-alaryngeal populations who exhibit voice disorders (Cannito, Buder, & Chorna, 2005; Tjaden, Sussman, Liu, & Wilding, 2010). When the collective findings from studies in this area are examined, it would appear that similar applications to alaryngeal speakers may provide further insights into the degree of variation that characterizes any given alaryngeal method.

In reconsidering the pressing need to define and perhaps redefine what constitutes a superior speaker for any given alaryngeal speech method, these types of measures may be of particular value. While LTAS measures form a specific type of voice and speech analysis, other types of signal evaluation methods have emerged and been employed by those with interest in alaryngeal speech signals (Huang, Falk, Chan, Parsa, & Doyle, 2009; Maryn, Dick, Vandenbruaene, Vauterin, & Jacobs, 2009; McDonald, Parsa, & Doyle, 2010). These modifications and expansions are based on the desire to more fully analyze and document a variety of independent acoustic parameters and their possible interactions, particularly in those with very aperiodic and noisy speech signals (Ali, Parsa, Doyle, & Berkane, 2017).

Intensity While intensity measures can be extracted from all of the above-referenced samples, the measures obtained from any sample will be a relative index. That is, loudness obtained during these clinically based tasks will not be referenced to a known intensity level in sound pressure level (SPL). If there is a desire to gather explicit SPL measures of intensity in alaryngeal speakers, experimental requirements and all the technical needs to do so will be required. However, if general information on one's habitual speaking level is desired or if a given speaker's dynamic range is needed (determining the speaker's ability to vary intensity), assessment tasks that mirror those of many clinical measures will suffice. As a caveat here, it is rare that intensity samples are obtained clinically for those who use an electrolarynx; the reason for this is that intensity control is done manually on the device.

Briefly, with the speaker seated at a fixed distance in front of a portable sound level meter, she/he is asked to provide several bursts or trials of the vowel /a/. While directly observing the sound level meter during productions, the clinician will note the value indicated on the meter. Dependent on the type of sound level meter used, either a sweep-needle type of measure or more commonly a discrete digital, numeric readout will be provided. In regard to speaker's dynamic range, first they will be requested to produce their softest production of a vowel (again, typically an /a/) and then their loudest production. The loudest sample will be short in duration because it will quickly deplete air when using esophageal or TE speech. Several practice trials may be of benefit prior to taking the formal measures. Once each value is determined, they should be noted; the absolute difference between the two samples (the value of the loudest sample minus the softest value) will represent the speaker's dynamic intensity range.

Temporal measures The assessment of alaryngeal speech within the temporal domain can range from those that are quite simple (absolute reading time for a passage of known length) to more refined measures that identify the number of syllables produced per minute (the # of syllables in a given utterance divided by total time from start to finish) or other increasingly more refined timing measures. However, it is important to note that in samples of running speech, pauses will exist. Thus, speech rates can be calculated at a true syllabic level (pause time removed) or as a combined timing measure (pauses included). An added measure that can be gleaned from the above is the calculation of the simple ratio of speaking time to pause time. This type of measure may be very beneficial in identifying the need for clinical training and monitoring and, in the case of TE speakers, can often be referenced to normal values available in the literature.

As a simple example of the utility of these types of timing measures, consider an esophageal speaker who is in the early phases of acquiring speech (Doyle & Finchem, Chap. 10). Silent periods in the speech signal may not only be numerous in occurrence, but the length of such pauses can be long at times. This is the result of the speaker learning the process of insufflating the esophagus and then moving that air back through the pharyngoesophageal segment in order to generate "esophageal" voice. Documenting changes in these temporal relationships provides direct guidance on how to adjust training tasks, with the ability to further document changes over time. Finally, temporal measures may be employed for very specific types of assessment or evaluation. This would include measures of voice onset time (VOT) or vowel duration, as well as timing relationships associated with other consonants (Christensen & Weinberg, 1976; Christensen, Weinberg, & Alphonso, 1978; Robbins, Christensen, & Kempster, 1986; Scarpino & Weinberg, 1981; and others). However, as a rule, these types of measures are more descriptive in nature rather than being of direct value as a clinical outcome.

Auditory-Perceptual Measures

There is an extensive literature on A-P evaluation of alaryngeal speech that extends back almost 50 years. Prior to the 1980s when TE puncture voice restoration was introduced, the majority of published data pertained to esophageal speech and speech produced using the electronic artificial larynx. After the 1980s, A-P work on TE speech prevailed, although several studies were designed as comparative explorations with TE and other methods of alaryngeal speech. A review of those studies is not appropriate in the present context, but A-P measures may provide the most significant single index of alaryngeal voice and speech outcomes. Ultimately, listener judgments of a range of perceptual features can assess the composite voice and speech signal, such as "acceptability" (Bennett & Weinberg, 1973). In doing so, and with very few exceptions (e.g., more parametric assessments of features such as vocal pitch, speech rate, etc.), A-P evaluation is focused on "quality" considerations. Measures of this type which seek to quantify collective aspects of the alaryngeal signal may have the greatest value because they are likely to best represent how members of the lay public may perceive postlaryngectomy voice and speech (Eadie & Doyle, 2002, 2004).

Increasing interest in the A-P characteristics of all methods of alaryngeal voice and speech has grown considerably over the past 20 years, including comparative work that also has addressed conservation laryngectomy procedures from a perceptual perspective (Doyle, Leeper, Houghton-Jones, Heeneman, & Martin, 1995; Keith, Leeper, & Doyle, 1995). In most instances, the stimuli used for a majority of these studies come from listener evaluations of a standard reading passage (either in whole or part); over the past 15 years, this has most often involved the second sentence of the *Rainbow Passage.* Therefore, in regard to a need for postlaryngectomy voice and speech outcome measures, a clinician's careful planning in designing their recording protocol to document outcomes can offer substantial efficiencies.

In the present case, the reading passage stimuli can be used for both acoustic analyses and A-P evaluation. While such evaluation does not need to be conducted in a extensively controlled, research-like manner, the ability to ask others (most often coworkers) to make assessments of one or more well-defined A-P feature(s) can reduce some clinician bias from the assessment process. But assessments by professionals, or those who have increased levels of experience with an exposure to alaryngeal speakers, can introduce bias into the data obtained (Doyle, Swift, & Haaf, 1989; and others). However, finding the balance between eliminating potential sources of listener bias and the practicality of clinically based measures must always be considered.

Currently, there is no clearly identified, ideal A-P feature described in the literature for use with alaryngeal speakers. The feature of "acceptability" has been used in alaryngeal speech and likely remains a viable and useful metric today (Bennett & Weinberg, 1973; Eadie & Doyle, 2002, 2005b; Shipp, 1967). Yet the use of other features that might help to distinguish or better characterize variation within specific speaker groups is also needed. For example, the A-P feature of "effort" has been employed in recent years and does appear to have clinical value (Nagle & Eadie, 2012). That is, if an A-P assessment indicates that in the listener's judgment the speaker is using too much effort (e.g., a TE speaker who has access to pulmonary air), it may explicitly reflect that the speaker is in fact working too hard to produce voice. Clinical intervention that seeks to reduce the speaker's effort in generating voice may then track in a positive manner with other perceptual features (e.g., acceptability, pleasantness, etc.). Listener comfort has also been explored in relation to severity judgments of TE speakers by Doyle and colleagues (Doyle et al., 2011). Clinical assessments of A-P features that can find utility as a meaningful outcome measure, as well as serve to identify clinical remediation tasks, are of greatest benefit.

Finally, what currently emerges as the most important concern related to A-P evaluation relates to the measurement procedure itself. Historically, many studies have involved the use of scaled procedures as a manner of documenting speaker performance. This has most frequently been done using equal-appearing interval (EAI) scaling procedures. Although EAI scales may be appropriate in some instances, its use for many A-P features may be inappropriate. The issue that emerges relative to scaling methods is dictated primarily by the feature being assessed and whether it is an additive psychophysical dimension or one that is substitutive, dimensions that are identified as *prothetic* and *metathetic*, respectively. For this reason, EAI scaling may not be the ideal choice for the documentation of some A-P features of alaryngeal voice and speech (Metz, Schiavetti, & Sacco, 1990).

Based on existing information in the literature, it appears that the best procedural approach for gathering A-P outcomes for alaryngeal speakers would be based on the application of visual analogue scale (VAS) methodology; empirical evidence indicates the advantage of VAS scaling methods for A-P evaluation of all categories of disordered voice. This would include postlaryngectomy voice and speech in that VAS methods are valid for both prothetic and metathetic dimensions. For further details regarding the importance of this issue and related scaling concerns, the reader is referred to the foundational work of Stevens (1975) pertaining to psychophysical methods and relative to voice and speech considerations, the work of Kent (1992, 1996) and others (Schiavetti, 1992; Schiavetti, Sacco, Metz, & Sitler, 1983; Toner & Emanuel, 1989; Whitehill, Lee, & Chun, 2002).[5]

Speech Intelligibility Measures

It is widely agreed that speech intelligibility (SI) forms an essential metric of postlaryngectomy voice and speech; hence, measuring it forms one of the most important approaches to documenting outcomes. Despite a large and well-established literature addressing SI, there is no consensus on the best method of gathering these data for alaryngeal speakers. What is understood about the assessment of SI is that it almost certainly does not lend itself to assessment via the use of scaling methods. This includes methods that involve partitioning a judgment according to an interval scale regardless of its length or in relation to making global judgments of intelligibility that would be represented along a continuum of arbitrarily assessed percentage values ranging from 0% to 100%. Schiavetti (1992, p. 27) has explicitly noted that "...neither interval scaling or percentage estimation judgment of speech intelligibility is a viable technique for the clinical or research measurement of speech intelligibility." This indicates that other forms of evaluating SI will provide the most valid means of generating outcome data regardless of underlying etiology of the disorder (McLeod, Harrison, & McCormack, 2012).

A review of the literature on alaryngeal SI shows that a variety of stimuli (words and sentences and nonsense syllables), whether or not the stimuli are produced using a carrier phrase, whether they are present in noise, the manner of listener response (scaling vs. direct transcription, etc.), and the sophistication of the listener (naïve vs. experienced), as well as other strategies have been used to document SI performance (Doyle et al., 1989; Doyle, Danhauer, & Reed, 1988; Horii & Weinberg, 1975; Schiavetti, Sitler, Metz, & Houde, 1984). But as noted in another chapter that addresses issues of SI in greater detail (Sleeth & Doyle, Chap. 14), there is no agreement on the "best" method of documenting SI outcomes.

At the very least, future explorations of SI should minimally consider the following issues. First, there is ample experimental and clinical evidence from the past five decades that clearly define the types of issues that characterize alaryngeal voice and speech. Much of this work is foundational in nature and represents parameters outlined previously in this chapter (i.e., frequency, intensity, temporal measures, etc.). These data provide information that should guide the development of a more specific type of intelligibility measure or set of measures that are designed to address the factors that make alaryngeal voice and speech unique. Additionally, relationships between SI and functional voice-related concern should be explored more fully (Eadie, Otero, Bolt, Kapsner-Smith, & Sullivan, 2016).

To date, the only existing English word list that was designed specifically for use with a group of alaryngeal speakers is that reported by Weiss and Basili (1985). Their list was used with electrolaryngeal speakers with a focus on the intelligibility of word-initial and word-final con-

---

[5]The conceptual concerns relating to auditory-perceptual scaling of voice and speech quality or inherent features that culminate in the listener's characterization of quality also apply to measures of speech intelligibility.

sonants. The list is comprised of 66 monosyllabic English words with all consonants except "zh" represented in both word-initial and word-final positions, with exception of those that cannot appear in both positions due to linguistic rules (e.g., "ng" and "h" cannot be used in word-initial or word-final phonetic contexts, respectively). But application of this word list as an SI measure has not gained large acceptance. If this list or others can be used in a consistent manner, information on SI may provide a more sensitive metric that will allow for comparative measures to be obtained with greater interpretive accuracy. Based on the above information, there continues to be a need for standardization of approaches to gathering and documenting outcomes related to SI in alaryngeal speakers. From a development perspective, the content of any specialized tests of alaryngeal SI should be designed based on existing acoustic knowledge on esophageal, TE, and artificial laryngeal speech.

Self-Assessed Voice-Related Outcomes

Documenting postlaryngectomy voice and speech outcomes can always be enhanced through the use of self-reported measures or those which are often termed "patient-reported outcomes" (see Eadie, Chap. 29). These types of measures offer important insights into individualized concerns or challenges faced by the alaryngeal speaker. Similar to other areas of outcome measurement discussed previously, there does not appear to be any consensus-based approach or protocol for gathering such information.

The primary criticism of self-reported measures has usually been directed to the fact that they represent a "subjective" impression by the individual of their own capabilities or performance. However, if the measure being used has been assessed carefully relative to its psychometric properties, there is no reason to discount the validity of such assessments. In fact, it may be argued that self-reports may provide the best and most accurate manner of documenting alaryngeal speech and communication outcomes. As an

example, what a professional deems as representative of "excellent" alaryngeal voice and speech or outstanding postlaryngectomy communication skills may not always transfer across to the individual's perception of their communicative capacity. Hence, the ability to document outcomes through convergent information that is derived from objective and subjective indices may provide a more representative picture of one's true postlaryngectomy status.

One self-reported measure that has gained increasing use with postlaryngectomy speakers is the *Voice-Related Quality of Life* (V-RQOL) instrument originally developed and reported by Hogikyan and Sethuraman (1999). Although originally developed to assess laryngeal-based voice disorders (e.g., vocal fold paralyses, benign mass lesions, etc.), Doyle and his colleagues have argued that the structure of the measure can be extended to postlaryngectomy populations. The reasoning behind this recommendation was derived from a belief that the questions posed in this simple ten-item measure essentially reflect self-judgments to questions that address voice and communication-based disability (Bornbaum, Day, & Doyle, 2014; Cox & Doyle, 2014; Day & Doyle, 2010; Moukarbel et al., 2011).

One of the advantages of the V-RQOL is that the measure is constructed to provide both "physical" (six questions) and "social-emotional" (four questions) subscores, as well as a total score. Through a proprietary scoring algorithm for the V-RQOL, an assessment of one's voice-related deficits can be determined for all three scores. However, research conducted by Bornbaum et al. (2014) has provided empirical data which suggest that a slight modification in the application of the scoring algorithm be employed when the measure is applied to alaryngeal speakers. At the very least, this measure can provide an ongoing index of one's function specific to their use of alaryngeal voice and speech. And, given its brevity, it can be easily gathered as part of any regular follow-up visit with ease.

Moukarbel et al. (2011) assessed a group of 75 alaryngeal speakers using the V-RQOL. Speaker groups representing all three postlaryngectomy speech modes were included in the study. Data obtained indicated that speakers who used intrinsic methods (esophageal and TE) had better scores (less disability) than did those who used the electrolarynx. However, substantial variability in scores was observed regardless of speech mode. The V-RQOL has also been used in a descriptive manner for other populations who have undergone laryngectomy. Similarly, V-RQOL scores have also been employed in relation to combined assessments of coping in those who have been laryngectomized (Eadie & Bowker, 2012). Thus, these types of comparative and descriptive data may provide a point of reference when the V-RQOL is used clinically as an individual outcome measure. As with any other type of outcome measures, continued exploration of self-reported instruments in the context of postlaryngectomy voice and speech performance and general communication is recommended.

Summary

This chapter has addressed the topic of documenting alaryngeal voice and speech outcomes. However, as part of this stated need, further understanding and research pertaining to the broader concern of postlaryngectomy communication is necessary. Speech-language pathology has traditionally centered its focus on those areas that underlie verbal communication. Given the numerous changes in current treatment protocols and extended surgical reconstructions, as well as other considerations, there exists a continuing need to gather contemporary data on voice, speech, and communication outcomes. This will include acoustic evaluation, A-P assessment, measures of speech intelligibility, and self-reported instruments that may serve to index voice-related disability secondary to the treatment for laryngeal cancer. Despite the obvious relevance of gathering objective, parametric measures of voice and speech, these measures alone may be inadequate in documenting rehabilitation success. Documenting postlaryngectomy voice and speech outcomes must be viewed in a more comprehensive manner relative to communicative functioning with considerations of both the speaker and the listener. Finally, there remains a critical need for the collection and analysis of a new body of voice and speech outcome measures in those who use alaryngeal speech. Efforts directed toward this objective will be of substantial benefit to the process of postlaryngectomy rehabilitation.

References

Ablon, J. (1981). Stigmatized health conditions. *Social Science and Medicine, 15B*, 5–9.

Alam, D. S., Vivek, P. P., & Kmiecik, J. (2008). Comparison of voice outcomes after radial forearm free flap reconstruction versus primary closure after laryngectomy. *Otolaryngology—Head and Neck Surgery, 139*(2), 240–244.

Ali, Y. S. E., Parsa, V., Doyle, P. C., & Berkane, S. (2017, April). Disordered speech quality estimation using the matching pursuit algorithm. In: *Electrical and computer engineering (CCECE), 2017 IEEE 30th Canadian conference*, (pp. 1–5). IEEE.

Angel, D., Doyle, P. C., & Fung, K. (2011). Measuring voice outcomes following treatment for laryngeal cancer. *Expert Review of Pharmacoeconomics & Outcomes Research, 11*(4), 415–420.

Baylor, C., Burns, M., Eadie, T., Britton, D., & Yorkston, K. (2011). A qualitative study of interference with communicative participation across communication disorders in adults. *American Journal of Speech-Language Pathology, 20*(4), 269–287.

Bennett, S., & Weinberg, B. (1973). Acceptability ratings of normal, esophageal, and artificial larynx speech. *Journal of Speech and Hearing Research, 16*, 608–615.

Bjordal, K., & Kaasa, S. (1995). Psychological distress in head and neck cancer patients 7–11 years after curative treatment. *British Journal of Cancer, 71*(3), 592.

Blanchard, C. G., Albrecht, T., Ruckdeschel, J., Grant, D., & Hammick, R. (1995). The role of social support in adaptation to cancer and to survival. *Journal of Psychosocial Oncology, 13*, 75–95.

Blood, G. W., Luther, A. R., & Stemple, J. C. (1992). Coping and adjustment in alaryngeal speakers. *American Journal of Speech–Language Pathology, 1*, 63–69.

Bornbaum, C. C., Day, A. M., & Doyle, P. C. (2014). Examining the construct validity of the V-RQOL in speakers who use alaryngeal voice. *American Journal of Speech-Language Pathology, 23*(2), 196–202.

Bornbaum, C. C., Doyle, P. C., Skarakis-Doyle, E., & Theurer, J. A. (2013). A critical exploration of the International Classification of Functioning, Disability, and Health (ICF) framework from the perspective of oncology: Recommendations for revision. *Journal of Multidisciplinary Healthcare, 6*, 75–86.

Bornbaum, C. C., Fung, K., Franklin, J. H., Nichols, A., Yoo, J., & Doyle, P. C. (2012). A descriptive analysis of the relationship between quality of life and distress in individuals with head and neck cancer. *Supportive Care in Cancer, 20*(9), 2157–2165.

Cannito, M., Buder, E., & Chorna, L. (2005). Spectral amplitude measures of adductor spasmodic dysphonic speech. *Journal of Voice, 19*, 391–410.

Christensen, J. M., & Weinberg, B. (1976). Vowel duration characteristics of esophageal speech. *Journal of Speech, Language, and Hearing Research, 19*(4), 678–689.

Christensen, J. M., Weinberg, B., & Alphonso, P. J. (1978). Productive voice onset time characteristics of esophageal speech. *Journal of Speech and Hearing Research, 21*, 52–62.

Cox, S. R., & Doyle, P. C. (2014). The influence of electrolarynx use on postlaryngectomy voice-related quality of life. *Otolaryngology–Head and Neck Surgery, 150*(6), 1005–1009.

D'Antonio, L. L., Long, S. A., Zimmerman, G. J., Peterman, A. H., Petti, G. H., & Chonkich, G. D. (1998). Relationship between quality of life and depression in patients with head and neck cancer. *Laryngoscope, 108*, 806–811.

Darley, F. L., Aronson, A. E., & Brown, J. E. (1975). *Motor speech disorders*. Philadelphia, PA: W.B. Saunders.

Day, A. M., & Doyle, P. C. (2010). Assessing self-reported measures of voice disability in tracheoesophageal speakers. *Journal of Otolaryngology-Head & Neck Surgery, 39*(6), 762–768.

deBoer, M. F., McCormick, L. K., Pruyn, J. F. A., Ryckman, R. N., & van den Borne, B. W. (1999). Physical and psychosocial correlates of head and neck cancer: A review of the literature. *Otolaryngology – Head and Neck Surgery, 120*, 427–436.

Deschler, D. G., Doherty, E. T., Reed, C. G., & Singer, M. I. (1998). Quantitative and qualitative analysis of tracheoesophageal voice after pectoralis major flap reconstruction of the neopharynx. *Otolaryngology—Head and Neck Surgery, 118*(6), 771–776.

Deschler, D. G., Herr, M. W., Kmiecik, J. R., Sethi, R., & Bunting, G. (2015). Tracheoesophageal voice after total laryngopharyngectomy reconstruction: Jejunum versus radial forearm free flap. *Laryngoscope, 125*(12), 2715–2721.

Divi, V., Lin, D. T., Emerick, K., Rocco, J., & Deschler, D. G. (2011). Primary TEP placement in patients with laryngopharyngeal free tissue reconstruction and salivary bypass tube placement. *Otolaryngology–Head and Neck Surgery, 144*(3), 474–476.

Doyle, P. C. (1994). *Foundations of voice and speech rehabilitation following laryngeal cancer*. San Diego, CA: Singular.

Doyle, P. C. (1997). Voice refinement following conservation surgery for cancer of the larynx: A conceptual framework for treatment intervention. *American Journal of Speech-Language Pathology, 6*(3), 27–35.

Doyle, P. C. (1999). Postlaryngectomy speech rehabilitation: Contemporary considerations in clinical care. *Journal of Speech–Language Pathology and Audiology, 23*, 109–116.

Doyle, P. C., & Baker, A. M. H. (2018, November). *Postlaryngectomy communication competence and disability secondary to tracheoesophageal puncture voice restoration*. Paper presented at the annual convention of the American Speech-Language-Hearing Association, Boston, MA.

Doyle, P. C., Danhauer, J. L., & Reed, C. G. (1988). Listeners' perceptions of consonants produced by esophageal and tracheoesophageal talkers. *Journal of Speech and Hearing Disorders, 53*(4), 400–407.

Doyle, P. C., Leeper, H. A., Houghton-Jones, C., Heeneman, H., & Martin, G. F. (1995). Perceptual characteristics of hemilaryngectomized and near-total laryngectomized male speakers. *Journal of Medical Speech-Language Pathology, 3*(2), 131–143.

Doyle, P. C., Skidmore, E., Elliott, H., Senchuk, C., Day, A. M. B., Bornbaum, C., Dzioba, A., & Sleeth, L. (2011, November). *Relationships between listener comfort and voice severity in tracheoesophageal speech*. Presented at the annual convention of the American Speech-Language-Hearing Association, San Diego, CA.

Doyle, P. C., Swift, E. R., & Haaf, R. G. (1989). Effects of listener sophistication on judgments of tracheoesophageal talker intelligibility. *Journal of Communication Disorders, 22*(2), 105–113.

Eadie, T. L. (2003). The ICF: A proposed framework for comprehensive rehabilitation of individuals who use alaryngeal speech. *American Journal of Speech-Language Pathology, 12*(2), 189–197.

Eadie, T. L., & Bowker, B. C. (2012). Coping and quality of life after total laryngectomy. *Otolaryngology–Head and Neck Surgery, 146*(6), 959–965.

Eadie, T. L., Day, A. M., Sawin, D. E., Lamvik, K., & Doyle, P. C. (2013). Auditory-perceptual speech outcomes and quality of life after total laryngectomy. *Otolaryngology–Head and Neck Surgery, 148*(1), 82–88.

Eadie, T. L., & Doyle, P. C. (2002). Direct magnitude estimation and interval scaling of pleasantness and severity in dysphonic and normal speakers. *Journal of the Acoustical Society of America, 112*(6), 3014–3021.

Eadie, T. L., & Doyle, P. C. (2004). Auditory–perceptual scaling and quality of life in tracheoesophageal speakers. *Laryngoscope, 114*, 753–759.

Eadie, T. L., & Doyle, P. C. (2005a). Quality of life in male tracheoesophageal (TE) speakers. *Journal of Rehabilitation Research and Development, 42*(1), 115.

Eadie, T. L., & Doyle, P. C. (2005b). Scaling of voice pleasantness and acceptability in tracheoesophageal speakers. *Journal of Voice, 19*(3), 373–383.

Eadie, T. L., Otero, D., Cox, S., Johnson, J., Baylor, C. R., Yorkston, K. M., & Doyle, P. C. (2016). The relationship between communicative participation and postlaryngectomy speech outcomes. *Head & Neck, 38*(S1), E1955–E1961.

Eadie, T. L., Otero, D. S., Bolt, S., Kapsner-Smith, M., & Sullivan, J. R. (2016). The effect of noise on relationships between speech intelligibility and self-reported communication measures in tracheoesophageal speakers. *American Journal of Speech-Language Pathology, 25*(3), 393–407.

Emerick, K. S., Herr, M. A., & Deschler, D. G. (2014). Supraclavicular flap reconstruction following total laryngectomy. *Laryngoscope, 124*(8), 1777–1782.

Engel, G. L. (1977). The need for a new medical model: A challenge for biomedicine. *Science, 196*(4286), 129–136.

Fairbanks, G. (1960). *Voice and articulation handbook.* New York, NY: Harper & Row.

Finizia, C., Dotevall, H., Lundström, E., & Lindström, J. (1999). Acoustic and perceptual evaluation of voice and speech quality: A study of patients with laryngeal cancer treated with laryngectomy vs irradiation. *Archives of Otolaryngology–Head & Neck Surgery, 125*(2), 157–163.

Fung, K., Teknos, T. N., Vandenberg, C. D., Lyden, T. H., Bradford, C. R., Hogikyan, N. D., … Chepeha, D. B. (2007). Prevention of wound complications following salvage laryngectomy using free vascularized tissue. *Head & Neck, 29*(5), 425–430.

Globlek, D., Stajner-Katusic, S., Musura, M., Horga, D., & Liker, M. (2004). Comparison of alaryngeal voice and speech. *Logopedics Phoniatrics Vocology, 29*(2), 87–91.

Goffman, E. (1963). *Stigma: Notes on the management of a spoiled identity.* Englewood Cliffs, NJ: Prentice Hall.

Gritz, E. R., Carmack, C. L., de Moor, C., Coscarelli, A., Schacherer, C. W., Meyers, E. G., & Abemayor, E. (1999). First year after head and neck cancer: Quality of life. *Journal of Clinical Oncology, 17*, 352–360.

Henderson, J. M., & Ord, R. A. (1997). Suicide in head and neck cancer patients. *Journal of Oral and Maxillofacial Surgery, 55*(11), 1217–1221.

Hogikyan, N. D., & Sethuraman, G. (1999). Validation of an instrument to measure voice-related quality of life (V-RQOL). *Journal of Voice, 13*(4), 557–569.

Horii, Y., & Weinberg, B. (1975). Intelligibility characteristics of superior esophageal speech presented under various levels of masking noise. *Journal of Speech and Hearing Research, 18*, 413–419.

Huang, A., Falk, T. H., Chan, W. Y., Parsa, V., & Doyle, P. C. (2009, September). Reference-free automatic quality assessment of tracheoesophageal speech. In: *Engineering in Medicine and Biology Society, 2009. EMBC 2009. Annual international conference of the IEEE,* (pp. 6210–6213). IEEE.

Imaizumi, S., Boku, S., Koike, Y., & Ohta, F. (1983). Multidimensional analysis of alaryngeal voice quality. *Journal of the Acoustical Society of Japan (E), 4*(3), 139–148.

Keith, R. L., Leeper, H. A., & Doyle, P. C. (1995). Microanalytic acoustical voice characteristics of near-total laryngectomy. *Otolaryngology–Head and Neck Surgery, 113*(6), 689–694.

Kent, R. D. (Ed.). (1992). *Intelligibility in speech disorders: Theory, measurement and management* (Vol. 1). Amsterdam: John Benjamins Publishing.

Kent, R. D. (1996). Hearing and believing: Some limits to the auditory-perceptual assessment of speech

and voice disorders. *American Journal of Speech-Language Pathology, 5*(3), 7–23.

Kotronoulas, G., Kearney, N., Maguire, R., Harrow, A., Di Domenico, D., Croy, S., & MacGillivray, S. (2014). What is the value of the routine use of patient-reported outcome measures toward improvement of patient outcomes, processes of care, and health service outcomes in cancer care? A systematic review of controlled trials. *Journal of Clinical Oncology, 32*(14), 1480–1501.

Lydiatt, W. M., Moran, J., & Burke, W. J. (2009). A review of depression in the head and neck cancer patient. *Clinical Advances in Hematology and Oncology, 7*(6), 397–403.

Maryn, Y., Dick, C., Vandenbruaene, C., Vauterin, T., & Jacobs, T. (2009). Spectral, cepstral, and multivariate exploration of tracheoesophageal voice quality in continuous speech and sustained vowels. *Laryngoscope, 119*(12), 2384–2394.

Mathieson, C. M., Stam, H. J., & Scott, J. P. (1990). Psychosocial adjustment after laryngectomy: A review of the literature. *Journal of Otolaryngology, 19*, 331–336.

McDonald, R., Parsa, V., & Doyle, P. C. (2010). Objective estimation of tracheoesophageal speech ratings using an auditory model. *Journal of the Acoustical Society of America, 127*(2), 1032–1041.

McLeod, S., Harrison, L. J., & McCormack, J. (2012). The intelligibility in context scale: Validity and reliability of a subjective rating measure. *Journal of Speech, Language, and Hearing Research, 55*(2), 648–656.

Metz, D. E., Schiavetti, N., & Sacco, P. R. (1990). Acoustic and psychophysical dimensions of the perceived speech naturalness of nonstutterers and post-treatment stutterers. *Journal of Speech and Hearing Disorders, 55*(3), 516–525.

Moukarbel, R. V., Doyle, P. C., Yoo, J. H., Franklin, J. H., Day, A. M. B., & Fung, K. (2011). Voice-related quality of life (V-RQOL) outcomes in laryngectomees. *Head & Neck, 33*(1), 31–36.

Nagle, K. F., & Eadie, T. L. (2012). Listener effort for highly intelligible tracheoesophageal speech. *Journal of Communication Disorders, 45*(3), 235–245.

Ng, M. L., Liu, H., Zhao, Q., & Lam, P. K. (2009). Long-term average spectral characteristics of Cantonese alaryngeal speech. *Auris Nasus Larynx, 36*(5), 571–577.

Plumb, M. M., & Holland, J. C. (1977). Comparative studies of psychological function in patients with advanced cancer. 1. Self-reported depressive symptoms. *Psychosomatic Medicine, 39*, 264–276.

Qi, Y., & Weinberg, B. (1991). Spectral slope of vowels produced by tracheoesophageal speakers. *Journal of Speech, Language, and Hearing Research, 34*(2), 243–247.

Qi, Y., & Weinberg, B. (1995). Characteristics of voicing source waveforms produced by esophageal and tracheoesophageal speakers. *Journal of Speech, Language, and Hearing Research, 38*(3), 536–548.

Qi, Y., Weinberg, B., & Bi, N. (1995). Enhancement of female esophageal and tracheoesophageal speech. *Journal of the Acoustical Society of America, 98*(5), 2461–2465.

Reed, C. G. (1983). Surgical-prosthetic techniques for alaryngeal speech. *Communicative Disorders, 8,* 109–124.

Robbins, J. (1984). Acoustic differentiation of laryngeal, esophageal, and tracheoesophageal speech. *Journal of Speech and Hearing Research, 27,* 577–585.

Robbins, J., Christensen, J. M., & Kempster, G. (1986). Characteristics of speech production after tracheoesophageal puncture: Voice onset time and vowel duration. *Journal of Speech and Hearing Research, 20,* 499–504.

Rohe, D. E. (1994). Loss, grief, and depression after laryngectomy. In R. L. Keith & F. L. Darley (Eds.), *Laryngectomy rehabilitation* (3rd ed., pp. 487–514). Austin, TX: PRO-ED.

Ryan, P. B., Madigan, D., Stang, P. E., Marc Overhage, J., Racoosin, J. A., & Hartzema, A. G. (2012). Empirical assessment of methods for risk identification in healthcare data: Results from the experiments of the observational medical outcomes partnership. *Statistics in Medicine, 31*(30), 4401–4415.

Salmon, S. J. (1986). Adjusting to laryngectomy. *Seminars in Speech and Language, 7,* 67–94.

Scarpino, J., & Weinberg, B. (1981). Junctural contrasts in esophageal and normal speech. *Journal of Speech, Language, and Hearing Research, 24*(1), 120–126.

Schiavetti, N. (1992). Scaling procedures for the measurement of speech intelligibility. In R. Kent (Ed.), *Intelligibility in speech disorders: Theory, measurement and management* (pp. 11–34). Amsterdam: John Benjamins Publishing.

Schiavetti, N., Sacco, P. R., Metz, D. E., & Sitler, R. W. (1983). Direct magnitude estimation and interval scaling of stuttering severity. *Journal of Speech, Language, and Hearing Research, 26*(4), 568–573.

Schiavetti, N., Sitler, R. W., Metz, D. E., & Houde, R. A. (1984). Prediction of contextual speech intelligibility from isolated word intelligibility measures. *Journal of Speech, Language, and Hearing Research, 27*(4), 623–626.

Sethi, R. K., Kozin, E. D., Lam, A. C., Emerick, K. S., & Deschler, D. G. (2014). Primary tracheoesophageal puncture with supraclavicular artery island flap after total laryngectomy or laryngopharyngectomy. *Otolaryngology–Head and Neck Surgery, 151*(3), 421–423.

Shanks, J. C. (1995). Coping with laryngeal cancer. *Seminars in Speech and Language, 16*(3), 180–190.

Shapiro, P. A., & Kornfeld, D. S. (1987). Psychiatric aspects of head and neck cancer surgery. *Psychiatric Clinics of North America, 10,* 87–100.

Shipp, T. (1967). Frequency, duration, and perceptual measures in relation to judgments of alaryngeal speech acceptability. *Journal of Speech and Hearing Research, 10,* 417–427.

Stevens, S. S. (1975). *Psychophysics: Introduction to its perceptual, neural and social prospects.* New York, NY: Riley.

Tarlov, A. R., Ware, J. E., Greenfield, S., Nelson, E. C., Perrin, E., & Zubkoff, M. (1989). The medical outcomes study. *JAMA, 262*(7), 925–930.

The Oxford English Dictionary. (2018). Retrieved June 8, 2018. https://en.oxforddictionaries.com/definition/outcome

Tjaden, K., Sussman, J. E., Liu, G., & Wilding, G. (2010). Long-term average spectral (LTAS) measures of dysarthria and their relationship to perceived severity. *Journal of Medical Speech-Language Pathology, 18*(4), 125–134.

Toner, M. A., & Emanuel, F. W. (1989). Direct magnitude estimation and equal appearing interval scaling of vowel roughness. *Journal of Speech, Language, and Hearing Research, 32*(1), 78–82.

van As, C. J., Hilgers, F. J., Verdonck-de Leeuw, I. M., & Koopmans-van Beinum, F. J. (1998). Acoustical analysis and perceptual evaluation of tracheoesophageal prosthetic voice. *Journal of Voice, 12*(2), 239–248.

Van der Torn, M., De Vries, M. P., Festen, J. M., Verdonck-de Leeuw, I. M., & Mahieu, H. F. (2001). Alternative voice after laryngectomy using a sound-producing voice prosthesis. *Laryngoscope, 111*(2), 336–346.

Van Gogh, C. D., Festen, J. M., Verdonck-de Leeuw, I. M., Parker, A. J., Traissac, L., Cheesman, A. D., & Mahieu, H. F. (2005). Acoustical analysis of tracheoesophageal voice. *Speech Communication, 47*(1–2), 160–168.

Van Riper, C. (1978). *Speech correction: Principles and methods.* Englewood Cliffs, NJ: Prentice-Hall.

Vokes, E. E., Weichselbaum, R. R., Lippman, S. M., & Hong, W. K. (1993). Head and neck cancer. *New England Journal of Medicine, 328*(3), 184–194.

Ware, J. E., Jr., Kosinski, M., Bayliss, M. S., McHorney, C. A., Rogers, W. H., & Raczek, A. (1995). Comparison of methods for the scoring and statistical analysis of SF-36 health profile and summary measures: Summary of results from the Medical Outcomes Study. *Medical Care, 33,* AS264–AS279.

Weinberg, B., Horii, Y., & Smith, B. E. (1980). Long-time spectral and intensity characteristics of esophageal speech. *Journal of the Acoustical Society of America, 67*(5), 1781–1784.

Weiss, M. S., & Basili, A. C. (1985). Electrolaryngeal speech produced by laryngectomized subjects: Perceptual characteristics. *Journal of Speech, Language, and Hearing Research, 28*(2), 294–300.

Whitehill, T. L., Lee, A. S., & Chun, J. C. (2002). Direct magnitude estimation and interval scaling of hypernasality. *Journal of Speech, Language, and Hearing Research, 45*(1), 80–88.

World Health Organization. (2001). *The international classification of functioning, disability and health: ICF.* Geneva: World Health Organization.

Zeller, J. L. (2006). High suicide risk found for patients with head and neck cancer. *JAMA, 296*(14), 1716–1717.

Swallowing Disorders and Rehabilitation in Patients with Laryngeal Cancer

18

Heather M. Starmer

Introduction

Dysphagia is common sequelae of laryngeal cancer as well as the treatments employed to eradicate it. Treatment for laryngeal cancer may include single- or multimodality treatments including surgery, radiation, and chemotherapy. In general, the greater the number of treatments implemented, the greater the potential for negative consequences such as dysphagia (Burnip, Owen, Barker, & Patterson, 2013). As a result, efforts have been ongoing to identify less toxic treatment regimens while maintaining comparable cure rates. Unfortunately, larynx cancer survival rates have remained relatively stable over the past 40 years despite treatment advances (Fig. 18.1) (Howlader, 2016). As a result, efforts to de-intensify treatment in order to minimize toxicity must be balanced with the primary goal of cure/survival. Treatment-related dysphagia remains a major concern for individuals with larynx cancer, with significant possible impacts on nutrition, pulmonary health, and quality of life. In the chapter to follow, several specific issues will be discussed including the incidence of dysphagia in those treated for laryngeal cancer and how dysphagia varies and is treated depending upon treatment modality.

Baseline Swallowing Characteristics

Swallowing function prior to treatment for laryngeal cancer is heavily influenced by stage of disease. While patients with small volume disease (T1-2) often have limited pre-treatment dysphagia, those with locally advanced disease (T3-4) have a significant risk of pre-treatment dysphagia (Starmer, Gourin, Lua, & Burkhead, 2011) (Fig. 18.2). Pre-treatment swallowing issues may involve pharyngeal impairment and poor airway closure leading to aspiration with its inherent pulmonary risks (Starmer et al., 2011; Stenson et al., 2000). Because changes in swallowing function including aspiration are often silent, it is imperative that instrumental assessment of baseline swallowing precede oncologic therapy, particularly in patients with advanced-stage laryngeal cancer. In particular, in the case of patients being considered for "larynx preservation" treatments such as radiation or partial laryngectomy, it is crucial to ensure the larynx is functioning and worth preserving. Patients with significant baseline swallowing issues and aspiration may be poor candidates for partial surgeries or radiation-based treatment as those swallowing difficulties are likely to be amplified

H. M. Starmer (✉)
Department of Otolaryngology – Head and Neck Surgery, Head and Neck Speech and Swallowing Rehabilitation, Stanford Cancer Center, Stanford, CA, USA
e-mail: hstarmer@stanford.edu

© Springer Nature Switzerland AG 2019
P. C. Doyle (ed.), *Clinical Care and Rehabilitation in Head and Neck Cancer*,
https://doi.org/10.1007/978-3-030-04702-3_18

Fig. 18.1 Laryngeal cancer survival rates between 1975 and 2013. (From Howlader et al. (2016))

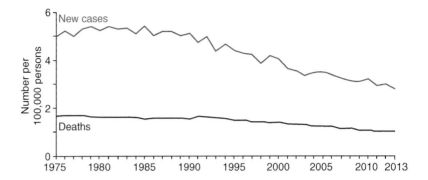

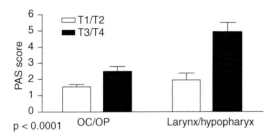

Fig. 18.2 Pre-treatment swallowing penetration-aspiration scale scores by site and stage of disease (OC, oral cavity; OP, oropharynx). (From Starmer et al. (2011), Figure 1, with permission of John Wiley and Sons)

following treatment (Frowen, Cotton, Corry, & Perry, 2010). As a result, the speech-language pathologist (SLP) plays an important role on the multidisciplinary team in assessing pre-treatment function in order to prognosticate post-treatment function (see Box 18.1).

Because of the risk of silent aspiration in this population, instrumental assessment is critical in the pre-treatment setting. This may involve either videofluoroscopic swallowing study (VFSS) or fiberoptic endoscopic evaluation of swallowing (FEES). VFSS utilizes radiographic imaging to provide real-time video assessment of the coordinated oral, pharyngeal, and cervicoesophageal phases of swallowing. In contrast, FEES utilizes endoscopic imaging of the pharynx and larynx during swallowing. Both assessment procedures have been shown to have comparable ability in detecting laryngeal penetration/aspiration (Langmore, Schatz, & Olsen, 1991). Laryngeal penetration occurs when bolus material enters the laryngeal vestibule but remains above the true vocal folds, while aspiration refers to any bolus

Box 18.1 SLP Assessment Influences Oncologic Treatment Decisions
RG is a 76-year-old male diagnosed with a T3N2b squamous cell carcinoma of the supraglottic larynx. He was referred to a multidisciplinary head and neck cancer center for discussion of treatment options. Prior to meeting with the SLP, three options appeared feasible from an oncologic perspective: open supraglottic laryngectomy, total laryngectomy, and concurrent chemoradiation. During his MBS study, the patient was found to have a delayed swallow onset, poor closure of the laryngeal vestibule, and poor pharyngeal clearance leading to aspiration both during and after the swallow. Considering these findings, his history of COPD, and difficulty following directions for compensatory strategies during the MBS, it was deemed that he was not a good candidate for organ preservation. Total laryngectomy was chosen as the safest option for functional reasons.

material dropping below the level of the vocal folds. While VFSS offers the advantage of visualization of the interrelated oral, pharyngeal, and cervical esophageal stages of swallowing, FEES offers direct visualization of the larynx and associated structures. Both of these instrumental options may play an important role in evaluating the baseline swallowing function of patients with laryngeal cancer. Choices regarding which tool to utilize should depend on the availability of the tool, clinician experience/training with the tool, and goals of the swallowing study (see Tables 18.1 and 18.2).

Prior to onset of cancer treatment, the SLP will play an important role not just in evaluating baseline function but also in educating the patient regarding expectations during/after treatment. While data are currently not available, in the case of patients undergoing surgical procedures, teaching compensatory strategies prior to surgery may facilitate their use postoperatively. For example, FEES can be used as visual feedback to demonstrate the treatment target (e.g., tight closure of the glottis using a supraglottic swallow) in order to facilitate good approximation of the target postoperatively. Additionally, the SLP can provide estimated timelines for anticipated recovery and should outline the rehabilitation process both during hospitalization and following discharge. It is critical for the patient to have a basic understanding of timelines for recovery to ensure realistic expectations of when they will resume

Table 18.1 Advantages and disadvantages of FEES

Pros	Cons
No radiation exposure	*No visualization of oral phase*
Portable/can be taken to bedside	*No visualization of the esophagus*
Provides valuable anatomic information	*Missed visualization during the swallow due to whiteout*
Clear visualization of residue patterns	*Difficult to perform in infants, young children, or noncooperative adults*
Foods not limited	*Difficult to directly visualize physiology such as hyoid excursion*

Table 18.2 Advantages and disadvantages of VFSS

Pros	Cons
Visualization of oral, pharyngeal, and esophageal phases	*Radiation exposure*
Can be done from infancy through adults	*Difficulties with transportation of some patients*
Visualization of hyolaryngeal excursion	*May miss events when fluoroscopy is off*
Visualization of cricopharyngeus	*Requires the use of barium*

different levels of oral intake and how intensive their rehabilitation may be. Setting realistic expectations may lead to greater patient satisfaction with outcomes.

In the case of patients undergoing nonsurgical intervention (i.e., radiation or chemoradiation), pre-treatment education and counseling is critical for adoption of a preventative dysphagia treatment regime. That is, the patient must be informed regarding acute treatment toxicities, the potential for long-term changes in swallowing, and the benefit of exercises to mitigate this risk. Information dissemination prior to treatment will help the patient to adopt realistic expectations, thus, reducing potential frustration and anxiety during and after treatment. In order for the SLP to educate the patient regarding expectations and recovery, the SLP must possess a comprehensive understanding of how different treatments may impact swallowing. Therefore, in the following sections, we will discuss specific treatments of larynx cancer, their likely impact on swallowing, and strategies the SLP can use to rehabilitate dysphagia.

Management of Laryngeal Cancer

Larynx cancer can be managed through both surgical and nonsurgical treatments. For patients undergoing primary surgery, swallowing outcomes vary significantly based upon the extent and location of resection. Surgical procedures may include limited laryngeal resection, supraglottic laryngectomy, and total laryngectomy, among others. Each procedure brings its own unique impact on swallowing. The larynx can be anatomically divided into three regions: the supraglottis, the glottis, and the subglottis. Cancers arising from the supraglottic larynx (structures superior to the vocal folds) are surgically managed through either the supraglottic or supracricoid laryngectomy (Ferlito et al., 2000; Spriano et al., 1997) or alternatively may be treated with radiation ± chemotherapy (Meyers & Alvi, 1996). Surgery to the supraglottic larynx may include resection of parts of the hyoid bone, epiglottis, aryepiglottic folds, and false (ventricular) vocal folds. The supraglottic region is critical for closure of the laryngeal vestibule, which provides the initial point of entry to the airway. Therefore surgery in this region commonly may impact airway protection, leading to aspiration and its associated risks.

In contrast to tumors of the supraglottic region, cancers arising from the glottis (true vocal folds) may require minimally invasive surgery, vertical hemilaryngectomy, total laryngectomy (TL), or radiation-based treatment (Hartl, 2012). It should be noted at this point that approximately 75% of all laryngeal cancers arise from the glottis. Because glottal closure is the last gate of defense against aspiration, surgery to this region may lead to direct issues with aspiration, as well as changes in voice production and quality.

Finally, cancers extending to, or arising from, the subglottic larynx (those areas inferior to the vocal fold and the conus elasticus) will often require total laryngectomy or radiation-based treatment, and these may exhibit reduced survival. TL will be discussed at length later in this chapter; however, it is typically associated with reduced swallowing efficiency, rather than safety, due to surgical separation of the airway and swallowing passage. For patients undergoing any surgical resection, the SLP should refer to the operative note to glean information about exactly what was resected and how the patient was reconstructed; such information may provide valuable insights into the types of deficits that may be reported and observed.

Minimally Invasive Resection

Minimally invasive resections typically involve endoscopic visualization and transoral resection in order to avoid entry to the larynx through an open incision in the neck. Resection is increasingly accomplished with laser technology. Transoral laser microsurgery (TLM) is one treatment option employed for early-stage glottic cancer. It is frequently used as a substitute for radiation therapy due to its lower potential morbidity, treatment time, and cost (Mendenhall,

Werning, Hinerman, Amdur, & Villaret, 2004). The impact of endoscopic laser surgery on swallowing is generally agreed to be minimal, as this approach allows for relative preservation of laryngeal and pharyngeal movement and sensation in contrast to other treatment options. However, it is important to note that size and location of the tumor are associated with swallowing outcomes with more advanced (larger) tumors associated with poorer swallowing function (Bernal-Sprekelsen, Vilaseca-Gonzalez, & Blanch-Alejandro, 2004; Hoffman & Buatti, 2004). In these instances, temporary use of a nasogastric (NG) feeding tube is generally limited to less than 3 weeks, with the duration of use related to extent of surgery (Jepsen et al., 2003).

Despite attempts to minimize the risk of dysphagia using minimally invasive approaches, postoperative dysphagia may occur. Postoperative dysphagia may include aspiration from reduced airway closure, reduced pharyngeal constrictor function, and impaired sensation due to scarring and edema (Brehmer & Laubert, 1999). SLP treatment in the early postoperative stage may include efforts to improve airway closure during the swallow. The use of a volitional breath hold procedure and supraglottic swallow strategies may be helpful in the early period following surgery to enhance airway protection. Endoscopy can then be used for biofeedback to assist the patient in knowing when adequate airway closure is achieved. In addition, glottal closure exercises can be performed; this includes approaches such as the modified Valsalva and adduction exercises (McCulloch, Perlman, Palmer, & Van Daele, 1996). If SLP intervention is unable to accomplish glottic closure, medialization procedures such as vocal fold injections and medialization thyroplasty may be offered by the otolaryngologist (Siu, Tam, & Fung, 2016).

Partial Laryngectomy

More advanced laryngeal tumors often require more aggressive surgical management such as vertical hemilaryngectomy, supraglottic laryngectomy, or supracricoid laryngectomy (Harris,

Bhuskute, Rao, Farwell, & Bewley, 2016). Details regarding these three conservation approaches can be found below. Based on existing information, a predictable pattern of deficits exists depending upon the procedure chosen. Additionally, the size of resection and the need for postoperative radiation therapy may influence outcomes. Rehabilitative treatments employed by the SLP will also differ depending on the nature and extent of resection. In the following section, each of these procedures will be discussed in greater detail.

Vertical Hemilaryngectomy

Vertical hemilaryngectomy is a procedure that was used frequently as a primary treatment for advanced laryngeal cancer prior to the advent of chemoradiation protocols. In recent years, however, this procedure has largely fallen out of fashion due to comparatively poor voice outcomes in contrast to the use of radiation. However, this conservative approach is still a viable surgical option for some patients and necessarily warrants brief discussion. Vertical hemilaryngectomy essentially involves the removal of one half of the larynx in the vertical plane. For example, this may include removal of the one side of the epiglottis, aryepiglottic fold, false vocal fold, and true vocal fold. Following this type of resection, airway closure during swallowing is the primary concern. Despite this limitation, functional swallowing results after hemilaryngectomy are generally favorable relative to other partial laryngectomy procedures. For example, 1 year following hemilaryngectomy, Rademaker et al. (1993) reported that 75% of patients demonstrated normal swallowing function and 92% returned to their preoperative diet level with feeding tube removal. In contrast, only 57% of those patients undergoing extended supraglottic resection achieved baseline diet or normal swallow.

Because of the removal of one half of the larynx, the goal in rehabilitation directed at safe swallowing seeks to accomplish apposition between the intact side and the operated side. Compensatory strategies are typically necessary

in the early postoperative phase and may include a head turn to the operated side and/or a chin tuck to narrow the laryngeal inlet (Logemann, 1997). Effortful, volitional airway closure is another therapeutic target to minimize aspiration risk. Because adaptation is likely, the use of compensatory strategies is often temporary following hemilaryngectomy. However, the need for additional and/or refined swallowing intervention should be applied based on physiologic findings during instrumental swallowing assessment.

Supraglottic Laryngectomy

Supraglottic laryngectomy involves removal of structures above the level of the glottis; therefore, the true vocal folds, arytenoids, and tongue base are the only remaining structures that can be used to achieve airway closure. Supraglottic laryngectomy can be accomplished through traditional, open surgical approaches through the neck or via endoscopic/laser resections through the oral cavity. Following traditional open supraglottic laryngectomy, patients may initiate oral intake within 1 month of surgery but often require up to 3 months to return to a full oral diet (Lazarus, 2000; Logemann et al., 1994). Inferior or superior extension of surgical resection is associated with prolonged recovery and increased dysphagia severity, sometimes lasting up to 2 years for some patients (Lazarus, 2000; Wasserman, Murry, Johnson, & Myers, 2001). Higher T-stage supraglottic tumors (i.e., those >T3) are typically associated with longer duration of feeding tube use (Bernal-Sprekelsen et al., 2004). Fortunately, advances in surgical technology (such as endoscopic resection) have led to improved functional outcomes and more rapid recovery for selected patients.

In contrast to traditional open surgical approaches, endoscopic laser resection of supraglottic tumors is associated with more rapid return to oral intake and better overall swallowing outcomes in the long term (Jepsen et al., 2003; Sasaki, Leder, Acton, & Maune, 2006). One explanation for improved outcomes in patients undergoing endoscopic resection is related to the preservation of the superior laryngeal nerve and, thus, maintenance of laryngeal sensation, which may impact the glottic closure reflex. In patients undergoing endoscopic supraglottic laryngectomy, the glottic closure reflex was observed in most patients within 72 h of surgery, while the majority of patients undergoing open surgery never recovered full function, even up to 12 years postsurgery (Sasaki et al., 2006). Minimally invasive supraglottic laryngectomies (see Table 18.3) have been categorized to better describe the extent of resection (Remacle et al., 2009), and these categories are associated with different swallowing outcomes. Aspiration is infrequent in patients undergoing Type I–II surgeries, but it is seen in 7% of those with Type III resection and nearly one-half of those patients undergoing Type IV supraglottic resection (Piazza et al., 2016).

Aspiration due to lack of supraglottic airway closure is the primary swallowing deficit associated with supraglottic laryngectomy. If surgery is extended to include part or all of the hyoid bone, laryngeal elevation may be reduced, compounding issues with airway closure. If resection includes the tongue base, oropharyngeal transit and/or bolus control may be impacted resulting in the presence of residue after the swallow and/or risk of penetration and aspiration before and after the swallow. Damage to the superior laryngeal nerve may lead to reduced sensation. Based on the pattern of the dysphagia observed, the SLP will need to tailor swallowing intervention to include compensatory strategies, therapeutic exercises, and dietary modifications as deemed necessary (Box 18.2).

Clinical training of the supraglottic and super-supraglottic swallowing maneuvers is critical for airway closure rehabilitation following supraglottic laryngectomy. These techniques aim to facilitate glottal airway closure prior to, as well as during the swallow; this is followed by a throat clear to expel any residual material on the superior aspect of the vocal folds prior to inhalation (Ohmae, Logemann, Kaiser, Hanson, & Kahrilas, 1996). The super-supraglottic swallow adds an increase in effort in order to further narrow the laryngeal inlet through apposition of the tongue base to the arytenoids.

In addition to swallowing maneuvers, the SLP should utilize therapeutic exercises to address physiologic deficits noted from the instrumental swallowing study. Commonly, exercises may include effortful swallow, Masako, and the Mendelsohn maneuver. Additionally, cricopharyngeal myotomy at the time of partial

Table 18.3 European Laryngological Society classification of transoral supraglottic laryngectomies (Remacle et al., 2009)

Type	Description
I	Limited excision of one supraglottic subsite (suprahyoid epiglottis, aryepiglottic fold, arytenoid, ventricular fold)
IIa	Suprahyoid epiglottectomy without resection of the pre-epiglottic space
IIb	Total epiglottectomy without resection of the pre-epiglottic space
IIIa	Complete supraglottic laryngectomy with resection of the pre-epiglottic space without extension to the ventricular fold
IIIb	Complete supraglottic laryngectomy with resection of the pre-epiglottic space and extension to the ventricular fold
IVa	Lateral supraglottic laryngectomy without arytenoid resection
IVb	Lateral supraglottic laryngectomy including resection of the arytenoid cartilage

Box 18.2 Postoperative Management Following Supraglottic Laryngectomy

FL is a 64-year-old male diagnosed with a T2 N1 squamous cell carcinoma of the supraglottic larynx. Baseline swallowing function was good, and he proceeded to a transoral, laser supraglottic laryngectomy. Patient consulted with SLP on postoperative day (POD) 1, and the supraglottic swallow strategy was reviewed. On POD 2, he completed a FEES examination, and laryngeal penetration was observed prior to/during the swallow. Using a supraglottic swallow technique, he was able to prevent aspiration. He initiated a soft diet with thin liquids and advanced to regular solids 1 week following surgery.

laryngectomy has been associated with reduced incidence of cricopharyngeal spasm and, therefore, better bolus clearance into the esophagus in this population (Ceylan, Koybasioglu, Asal, Kizil, & Inal, 2003).

Supracricoid Laryngectomy

The supracricoid laryngectomy is based on the philosophy that the cricoarytenoid unit (arytenoid cartilage, cricoarytenoid joint, posterior and lateral cricoarytenoid muscles, and recurrent and superior laryngeal nerves) is the functional anatomic unit of the larynx (Tufano, 2002). This surgical procedure includes the removal of the true and false vocal folds bilaterally, the entire thyroid cartilage, and at times the epiglottis and one arytenoid (cricohyoidepiglottopexy). This procedure, when used with stringent patient selection criteria, can lead to high local cancer control while avoiding the need for a permanent tracheostoma (Zacharek et al., 2001). Based on existing reports in the literature, this can result in improvement in overall quality of life in contrast to those undergoing total laryngectomy (Weinstein et al., 2001).

Following supracricoid laryngectomy, there is loss of airway closure at all levels due to resection of the supraglottic and glottic regions of the larynx. As a result, therapeutic intervention focuses on establishing a new pattern of airway protection. Accomplishing airway closure will rely on training contact between the remaining arytenoid and the base of the tongue (or epiglottis if not resected). Training this new mechanism of airway closure is often slow and stepwise, starting with managing secretions and subsequently advancing slowly from thicker items like purees to thinner liquids. The use of endoscopic biofeedback also can be quite beneficial as it allows the patient to visualize and improve airway closure. Despite poor airway protection after supracricoid laryngectomy, with prudent patient selection, return to functional oral intake is possible for the majority of patients (Farrag et al., 2007; Zacharek et al., 2001).

Total Laryngectomy and Swallowing

As the airway and the swallowing passages are surgically separated during total laryngectomy (TL), airway safety is not typically a concern; however, swallowing efficiency can be markedly diminished (Fig. 18.3) (InHealth Technologies). A study of 110 laryngectomees in Australia revealed 71% self-reported some degree of dysphagia following TL (Maclean, Cotton, & Perry, 2009). Further, these authors demonstrated that those patients reporting dysphagia were more likely to have depression, anxiety, and stress in contrast to those who did not report dysphagia after TL. Patients with dysphagia following TL may report an increased sense of social isolation due to the combined impact of their communication and swallowing difficulties (Doyle, 1994). As such, it is important for the SLP working with laryngectomees to remain mindful about possible swallowing difficulties and its impact on those who undergo TL. It is particularly important for the SLP to note that swallowing difficulties associated with surgery may be further compounded by side effects of radiation (see Kearney & Cavanagh, Chap. 20).

The videofluoroscopic swallowing study (VFSS) is one common, effective method for evaluating swallowing following TL. VFSS is preferred over FEES in this population as it allows for greater visualization of the upper esophageal sphincter (UES) and cervical esophagus. It should be emphasized that the intent of VFSS with laryngectomees is not to evaluate for aspiration but rather to assess for other factors such as the presence of postoperative fistulas, strictures, aspects of bolus flow efficiency, and pseudovallecula. VFSS can also be used to assess the cervical esophagus in relation to tracheoesophageal voice prosthesis issues. With the rising incidence of salvage laryngectomy following radiation-based treatment, VFSS is increasingly utilized postoperatively to assess for healing issues and potential complications such as pharyngocutaneous fistula. Historically, pharyngocutaneous fistula was uncommon and impacted less than 20% of patients; however, in the era of

Fig. 18.3 Anatomic changes following total laryngectomy (note lack of connection between the trachea and esophagus). (Image courtesy of InHealth Technologies©)

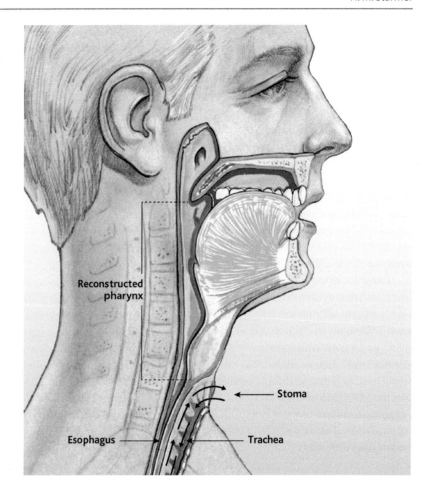

salvage surgery, rates have risen to close to 30% (Hasan et al., 2017; Paydarfar & Birkmeyer, 2006). The presence of a postoperative fistula will delay initiation of oral intake. A prolonged nothing by mouth (NPO) status may result in swallowing issues such as atrophy, fibrosis, and stricture leading to further delays in diet advancement.

While pharyngocutaneous fistula has a marked impact on oral intake, it is typically a transient condition which resolves over time. Disruption of typical pharyngeal physiologic function is anticipated following laryngectomy, but it is a greater long-term concern. Removal of the hyolaryngeal complex reduces traction forces to open the UES resulting in poorer bolus clearance into the esophagus. Additionally, reduced pharyngeal pressures due to disruption of the

pharyngeal constrictors will result in lower bolus driving pressures. These factors may lead to impaired UES relaxation and, therefore, creation of an increased volume of pharyngeal residue. Typically, however, a myotomy procedure will be completed during TL to reduce resistance at the level of the UES in a preventative manner (Horowitz & Sasaki, 1993).

Manometric assessment has recently contributed to our understanding of pressure changes following TL. Most notably, manometry has demonstrated that intrabolus pressures are consistently high following laryngectomy, a finding that suggests an obstruction of bolus flow at the level of the UES (Zhang et al., 2016). In addition to the alteration of muscular influences leading to reduced traction of and pressure against the UES, stricture may further restrict bolus flow into the esophagus. A stricture is a narrow region in the pharynx or upper esophagus that limits bolus passage, particularly with solid foods in contrast to liquids. Stricture is a common challenge after TL. Strictures are particularly common in patients undergoing salvage surgery, with hypopharyngeal primary tumors, closed primarily rather than with free tissue transfer, in females, and in those requiring extended laryngectomy (Nyquist, Hier, Dionisopoulos, & Black, 2006; Vu et al., 2008; Wulff et al., 2015). Dilation or stretching of the region of stricture has been the primary treatment approach; however, in order to adequately manage stricture, dilation may need to be repeated multiple times (Zhang et al., 2016).

Another possible contributor to post-laryngectomy dysphagia is the formation of a pseudoepiglottis/pseudovallecula. This is a structural byproduct of vertical closure and appears much like a normal epiglottis/vallecula on videofluoroscopy (Fig. 18.4) (Davis, Vincent, Shapshay, & Strong, 1982). As the pseudoepiglottis is an immobile structure, foods and liquids may build up in the pseudovallecular space. When this buildup is severe enough, it may result in backflow of contents into the oral or nasal

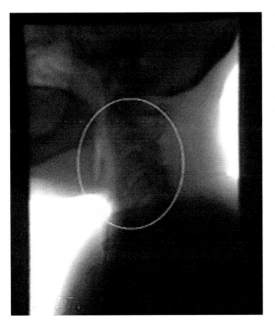

Fig. 18.4 MBS image of pseudoepiglottis and pseudovallecula

> **Box 18.3 Dysphagia Following Total Laryngectomy**
> HR is a 67-year-old female who underwent primary laryngectomy for T4 N0 squamous cell carcinoma of the glottic larynx followed by postoperative radiation. She had primary closure of the surgical defect. Swallowing was difficult during radiation due to pain and dry mouth, and she relied on a feeding tube for ~50% of her nutritional needs. Approximately 2 months following radiation, she had her feeding tube removed and started to advance to a regular diet. She presented to the speech pathologist with complaints of a sense of dry solids and pills sticking in her throat. A MBS was completed and revealed a pseudoepiglottis with collection of residual material in the pseudovallecula (see Fig. 18.4). She was referred back to her surgeon who performed a laser resection of the scar band leading to greater ease of swallowing.

cavities. If warranted, laser resection may be offered to eliminate this problem (Box 18.3).

While structural changes following TL are typically not impacted by behavioral intervention, the SLP working with laryngectomees should consider therapeutic intervention and compensatory strategies that may help improve bolus flow. Swallowing exercises targeting tongue strength and base of tongue retraction may improve bolus clearance and reduce the severity of dysphagia. Compensations are commonly recommended by the SLP and may include alternating liquids and solids and the avoidance of problematic food items.

Radiation-Associated Dysphagia

Prior to the 1990s, patients with advanced laryngeal cancer were typically treated with total laryngectomy as primary treatment. With publication of the VA Larynx Trial and RTOG

91-11, chemoradiation as a primary treatment option rose in popularity given comparable cure rates between those receiving nonoperative treatment and those undergoing TL (Forastiere et al., 2003; Wolf et al., 1991). Since this major shift in oncologic management of advance laryngeal cancer, it has become increasingly clear that preservation of structures through the use of nonoperative treatments does not necessarily equate to preservation of function. Dysphagia has increasingly been identified as a common toxicity of radiation-based treatment including acute swallowing-related toxicities, chronic dysphagia, and late-onset dysphagia (Hutcheson et al., 2012; Logemann et al., 2006). These issues may contribute to long-term health and nutrition problems and diminished quality of life (Eisbruch et al., 2011; Gillespie et al., 2005).

There are three primary ways in which radiation can impact swallowing function. Initially, during treatment, patients may swallow less frequently due to treatment-related side effects such as pain and dry mouth (xerostomia). As a result of reduced use, the muscles involved with deglutition may weaken and atrophy. Further, tissues exposed to radiation may develop fibrosis over time, which may reduce the pliability of soft tissue and the range of motion of musculature. Fibrosis is essentially a maladaptive healing process during which excessive collagen deposits form in a region of inflammation, leading to scar formation. Fibrosis is generally quite resistant to typical therapeutic exercise and, therefore, must be prevented whenever possible. Finally, in a smaller subset of patients, progressive cranial neuropathy may develop, further impacting muscle strength and function. Progressive neuropathy is typically observed many years after the completion of radiation therapy. Each of these pathophysiologic causes of radiation-associated dysphagia should be treated differently, with strengthening techniques being the target intervention for atrophy, maintenance of mobility being the target for prevention of fibrosis, and compensation being the mainstay treatment when cranial neuropathies emerge.

Physiologic changes to the swallowing apparatus after radiation-based treatment for larynx cancer have been well-documented in the literature (Starmer, Tippett, & Webster, 2008). Issues such as reductions in base of tongue retraction, anterior-posterior tongue movement, laryngeal elevation, and cricopharyngeal opening as well as delayed pharyngeal swallow have been found to be more common in patients treated for laryngeal cancer, leading to higher rates of percutaneous endoscopic gastrostomy (PEG) tube dependence (Logemann et al., 2006). Reduced airway protection and deficits in pharyngeal clearance also contribute to elevated levels of laryngeal penetration and aspiration. Aspiration pneumonia as a consequence of radiation-associated dysphagia has been reported to occur in up to 25% of patients who have undergone chemoradiation and is associated with a 42% increase in the risk of death (Xu et al., 2015). Ten-year follow-up data from the RTOG 91-11 trial discussed previously demonstrated a higher death rate from noncancer causes in patients receiving concurrent chemoradiation (Forastiere et al., 2013). The addition of chemotherapy to radiation treatment protocols has been associated with higher dysphagia rates (Jiang, Zhang, Li, Zhao, & Eisele, 2016), and it has been postulated that aspiration events may account for this higher long-term death rate in chemoradiation patients.

The importance of prophylactic swallowing therapy during radiation-based treatment for laryngeal cancer is increasingly better understood. A retrospective case control study by Carroll et al. (2008) demonstrated that individuals performing exercises prior to and during chemoradiation demonstrated a more normal tongue base apposition to the posterior pharyngeal wall during swallowing, as well as more normal epiglottic inversion. A randomized controlled trial by Kotz et al. (2012) further demonstrated that those patients receiving prophylactic swallowing therapy had more favorable diet levels 3–6 months following completion of treatment in comparison with those who received exercises after completion of treatment. When viewed together, these two reports demonstrated that both physiology (Carroll et al., 2008) and function (Kotz et al., 2012) are optimized with application of preventative dysphagia exercises.

Additional evidence on the benefit of prophylactic swallowing exercises came from Carnaby-Mann, Crary, Schmalfus, & Amdur (2012) "pharyngocise" study. In the active treatment arm of this randomized control trial, patients performed swallowing exercises twice daily over the duration of treatment. Results indicated that there was less structural change in the genioglossus, hyoglossus, and mylohyoid muscles than in patients who received either a sham treatment or no active treatment. Further, individuals in the active treatment group were more likely to continue with an oral diet during treatment. In addition to measuring differences in posttreatment anatomy/physiology, a composite measure was designed to designate a favorable swallowing-related outcome. This measure included <10% weight loss, the maintenance of oral diet, and a change of <10 points on the Mann Assessment of Swallowing Ability (MASA). In the active treatment arm of the study, 86% of patients achieved this desirable outcome, while only 47% of those who were not actively engaged in swallowing treatment achieved the same outcome. Carnaby-Mann et al.'s data revealed a 36% absolute risk reduction for loss of swallowing ability for those who participated in preventative exercise. These studies serve as compelling evidence that patients receiving radiation-based treatment should be actively engaged in swallowing therapy prior to the start of treatment.

Speech-language pathologists working with patients with laryngeal cancer need to have a firm and comprehensive understanding of swallowing physiology and the structures impacted by treatment in order to devise an appropriate treatment plan. In the absence of clinical trials demonstrating superiority of particular exercises, the SLP must enlist their knowledge and expertise to select the most appropriate exercises. However, adherence to treatment recommendations is often limited (Shinn et al., 2013); therefore, the SLP should be mindful to devise an efficient, feasible therapy plan (see Messing, Ward, & Lazarus, Chap. 6, and Starmer, Chap. 24). The swallowing exercises that are most frequently used in laryngeal cancer patients who are undergoing radiation include the Masako maneuver, effortful swallow, effortful pitch glide, Mendelsohn maneuver, and Shaker exercises. Although evidence of a direct link between lymphedema and swallow function does not currently exist, it is possible that submental lymphedema seen following radiation for larynx cancer may inhibit laryngeal elevation (see Smith, Chap. 22). As there is evidence of benefit from decongestive therapies on lymphedema (Smith et al., 2015), application of lymphedema therapy by trained personnel may offer another treatment that is worthy of consideration.

In addition to the performance of swallowing exercises for proactive prevention of radiation-associated dysphagia, there is evidence that continuing oral intake during treatment has a positive impact on swallowing outcomes. Posttreatment diet level has been associated with maintenance of oral intake during treatment in that those who maintained at least some oral intake had significantly more advanced diet levels following treatment (Langmore, Krisciunas, Miloro, Evans, & Cheng, 2012). Additional evidence supporting the relationship between oral intake and posttreatment diet level was provided by Hutcheson et al. (2013). This study demonstrated that eating and performing swallowing exercises during radiation-based treatments provided protective benefit for maintenance of diet following treatment. For individuals who were not eating and not exercising, only 65% reported a return to normal diet following radiation. In contrast, for those who both ate and exercised during treatment, 92% returned to a normal oral diet. Thus, it is clear that the SLP should be involved in the care of patients with laryngeal cancer prior to the start of radiation with the goal of providing swallowing exercises and to encourage continued oral intake.

Unfortunately, despite the clear importance of the SLP in assessing pre-treatment and posttreatment swallowing function, administering prehabilitative and rehabilitative exercises, and prescribing compensatory strategies and dietary modifications, patients with laryngeal cancer may have limited interaction with SLP over the course of their care. In a study using Medicare Surveillance, Epidemiology, and End Result

(SEER) data to evaluate the use and impact of SLP care on patients with laryngeal cancer over the age of 65 in the United States, only 6% were seen by SLP between diagnosis and 6 months following completion of primary therapy (Starmer et al., 2015). Further, less than a quarter of patients were seen by an SLP at some point between cancer diagnosis and 5 years later. However, patients were most likely to consult with SLP during the initial treatment phase if undergoing TL or if presenting with dysphagic symptoms. Long-term SLP care was seen most in individuals with dysphagia, TL, tracheostomy, or salvage surgery. Yet, when SLP care was provided, it significantly reduced the risk of stricture, weight loss, dysphagia, and aspiration pneumonia. Finally, SLP care was associated with reduced risk of death. These data not only collectively support the value of the SLP in caring for the patient with laryngeal cancer but also highlight the underutilization of SLPs in older patients with laryngeal cancer. It serves as a reminder that SLPs must continue to advocate for their patients to ensure timely referral for services that can increase the likelihood of an improved posttreatment outcome.

Conclusion

Patients with laryngeal cancer are at substantial risk for developing swallowing difficulties both prior to and following treatment. Patients at highest risk for dysphagia include those with advanced-stage disease and those requiring extensive and multimodal treatment. While patient care should be individualized, standard protocols are recommended; this includes pretreatment instrumental evaluation, pre-treatment education and counseling, posttreatment instrumental evaluation, and the implementation of evidence-based treatment plans including rehabilitative exercise and training of compensatory strategies. Aspiration risk is elevated in patients with laryngeal cancer, but it can often be well managed when compensatory strategies are employed. Finally, the SLP plays a vital role on the head and neck care team and, therefore,

should advocate for their early involvement and long-term rehabilitation services in order to optimize functional swallowing recovery.

References

Bernal-Sprekelsen, M., Vilaseca-Gonzalez, I., & Blanch-Alejandro, J. L. (2004). Predictive values for aspiration after endoscopic laser resections of malignant tumors of the hypopharynx and larynx. *Head & Neck, 26*, 103–110.

Brehmer, D., & Laubert, A. (1999). Diagnosis of postoperative dysphagia and aspiration. Fiberoptic endoscopic controlled methylene blue drinking. *HNO, 47*, 479–484.

Burnip, E., Owen, S. J., Barker, S., & Patterson, J. M. (2013). Swallowing outcomes following surgical and non-surgical treatment for advanced laryngeal cancer. *The Journal of Laryngology and Otology, 127*, 1116–1121.

Carnaby-Mann, G., Crary, M. A., Schmalfus, I., & Amdur, R. (2012). "Pharyngocise": Randomized control trial of preventative exercises to maintain muscle structure and swallowing function during head and neck chemoradiotherapy. *International Journal of Radiation Oncology, Biology, Physics, 83*, 210–219.

Carroll, W. R., Locher, J. L., Canon, C. L., Bohannon, I. A., McColloch, N. L., & Magnuson, J. S. (2008). Pretreatment swallowing exercises improve swallow function after chemoradiation. *Laryngoscope, 118*, 39–43.

Ceylan, A., Koybasioglu, A., Asal, K., Kizil, Y., & Inal, E. (2003). The effects of pharyngeal neurectomy and cricopharyngeal myotomy on postoperative deglutition in patients undergoing horizontal supraglottic laryngectomy. *Kulak Burun Boğaz Ihtisas Dergisi, 11*, 170–174.

Davis, R., Vincent, M., Shapshay, S., & Strong, M. (1982). The anatomy and complications of "T" closure versus vertical closure of the hypopharynx after laryngectomy. *Laryngoscope, 92*, 16–22.

Doyle P.C. (1994) Foundations of voice and speech rehabilitation following laryngeal cancer. San Diego, CA: Singular.

Eisbruch, A., Kim, H. M., Feng, F. Y., Lyden, T. H., Haxer, M. J., … TenHaken, R. K. (2011). Chemo-IMRT of oropharyngeal cancer aiming to reduce dysphagia: Swallowing organs, late complication probabilities, and dosimetric correlates. *International Journal of Radiation Oncology, Biology, Physics, 81*, e93–e99.

Farrag, T. Y., Koch, W. M., Cummings, C. W., Goldenberg, D., Abou-Jaoude, P. M., Califano, J. A., … Tufano, R. P. (2007). Supracricoid laryngectomy outcomes: The Johns Hopkins experience. *Laryngoscope, 117*, 129–132.

Ferlito, A., Silver, C. E., Howard, D. J., Laccourreye, O., Rinaldo, A., & Owen, R. (2000). The role of partial laryngeal resection in current management of laryngeal cancer: A collective review. *Acta Oto-Laryngologica, 120*, 456–465.

Forastiere, A. A., Goepfert, H., Maor, M., Pajak, T. F., Weber, R., Morrison, W., … Cooper, J. (2003). Concurrent chemotherapy and radiotherapy for organ preservation in advanced laryngeal cancer. *The New England Journal of Medicine, 349*, 2091–2098.

Forastiere, A. A., Zhang, Q., Weber, R. S., Maor, M. H., Goepfert, H., Pajak, T. F., … Cooper, J. S. (2013). Long-term results of RTOG 91-11: A comparison of three nonsurgical treatment strategies to preserve the larynx in patients with locally advanced larynx cancer. *Journal of Clinical Oncology, 31*, 845–852.

Frowen, J., Cotton, S., Corry, J., & Perry, A. (2010). Impact of demographics, tumor characteristics, and treatment factors on swallowing after (chemo) radiotherapy for head and neck cancer. *Head & Neck, 32*, 513–528.

Gillespie, M., Brodsky, M. B., Day, T. A., Sharma, A. K., Lee, F., & Martin-Harris, B. (2005). Laryngeal penetration and aspiration during swallowing after the treatment of advanced oropharyngeal cancer. *Archives of Otorhinolaryngology Head and Neck Surgery, 131*, 615–619.

Harris, B. N., Bhuskute, A. A., Rao, S., Farwell, D. G., & Bewley, A. F. (2016). Primary surgery for advanced-stage laryngeal cancer: A stage and sub-site specific survival analysis. *Head & Neck, 38*, 1380–1386.

Hartl, D. M. (2012). Evidence-based practice: Management of glottic cancer. *Otolaryngologic Clinics of North America, 45*, 1143–1161.

Hasan, Z., Dwivedi, R. C., Gunaratne, D. A., Virk, S. K., Palme, C. E., & Riffat, F. (2017). Systematic review and meta-analysis of the complications of salvage total laryngectomy. *European Journal of Surgical Oncology, 43*, 42–51.

Hoffman, H. T., & Buatti, J. (2004). Update on the management of laryngeal cancer. *Current Opinion in Otolaryngology & Head and Neck Surgery, 12*, 525–531.

Horowitz, J. B., & Sasaki, C. T. (1993). Effect of cricopharyngeus myotomy on postlaryngectomy pharyngeal contraction pressures. *Laryngoscope, 103*, 138–140.

Howlader, N., Noone, A. M., Krapcho, M., Miller, D., Bishop, K., Altekruse, S. F., … Cronin, K. A. (2016). *SEER cancer statistics review, 1975–2013*. Bethesda, MD: National Cancer Institute. Retrieved from http://seer.cancer.gov/csr/1975_2013/.

Hutcheson, K. A., Bhayani, M. K., Beadle, B. M., Gold, K. A., Shinn, E. H., Lai, S. Y., & Lewin, J. (2013). Eat and exercise during radiotherapy or chemoradiotherapy for pharyngeal cancers. Use it or lose it. *JAMA Otolaryngology. Head & Neck Surgery, 139*, 1127–1134.

Hutcheson, K. A., Lewin, J. S., Barringer, D. A., Lisec, A., Gunn, G. B., Moore, M. W., & Holsinger, F. C. (2012). Late dysphagia after radiotherapy-based treatment of head and neck cancer. *Cancer, 118*, 5793–5799.

Jepsen, M. C., Gurushanthaiah, D., Roy, N., Smith, M. E., Gray, S. D., & Davis, R. K. (2003). Voice, speech, and swallowing outcomes in laser-treated laryngeal cancer. *Laryngoscope, 113*, 923–928.

Jiang, N., Zhang, L. J., Li, L. Y., Zhao, Y., & Eisele, D. W. (2016). Risk factors for late dysphagia after (chemo) radiotherapy for head and neck cancer: A systematic methodological review. *Head & Neck, 38*, 792–800.

Kotz, T., Federman, A. D., Kao, J., Milman, L., Packer, S., Lopez-Prieto, C., … Genden, E. M. (2012). Prophylactic swallowing exercises in patients with head and neck cancer undergoing chemoradiation: A randomized trial. *Archives of Otolaryngology – Head & Neck Surgery, 138*, 376–382.

Langmore, S., Krisciunas, G. P., Miloro, K. V., Evans, S. R., & Cheng, D. M. (2012). Does PEG cause dysphagia in head and neck cancer patients? *Dysphagia, 27*, 251–259.

Langmore, S. E., Schatz, K., & Olsen, N. (1991). Endoscopic and videofluoroscopic evaluations of swallowing and aspiration. *The Annals of Otology, Rhinology, and Laryngology, 100*, 678–681.

Lazarus, C. L. (2000). Management of swallowing disorders in head and neck cancer patients: Optimal patterns of care. *Seminars in Speech and Language, 21*, 293–309.

Logemann, J. A. (1997). *Evaluation and treatment of swallowing disorders*. Austin, TX: Pro Ed.

Logemann, J. A., Gibbons, P., Rademaker, A. W., Pauloski, B. R., Kahrilas, P. J., Bacon, M., … McCracken, E. (1994). Mechanisms of recovery of swallow after supraglottic laryngectomy. *Journal of Speech and Hearing Research, 37*, 965–974.

Logemann, J. A., Rademaker, A. W., Pauloski, B. R., Lazarus, C. L., Mittal, B. B., Brockstein, B., … Liu, D. (2006). Site of disease and treatment protocol as correlates of swallowing function in patients with head and neck cancer treated with chemoradiation. *Head & Neck, 28*, 64–73.

Maclean, J., Cotton, S., & Perry, A. (2009). Dysphagia following a total laryngectomy: The effect on quality of life, functioning, and psychological well-being. *Dysphagia, 24*, 314–321.

McCulloch, T. M., Perlman, A. L., Palmer, P. M., & Van Daele, D. J. (1996). Laryngeal activity during swallow, phonation, and the Valsalva maneuver: And electromyographic analysis. *Laryngoscope, 106*, 1351–1358.

Mendenhall, W. M., Werning, J. W., Hinerman, R. W., Amdur, R. J., & Villaret, D. B. (2004). Management of T1-T2 glottic carcinomas. *Cancer, 100*, 1786–1792.

Meyers, E. N., & Alvi, A. (1996). Management of carcinoma of the supraglottic larynx: Evolution, current concepts, and future trends. *Laryngoscope, 106*, 559–567.

Nyquist, G. G., Hier, M. P., Dionisopoulos, T., & Black, M. J. (2006). Stricture associated with primary tracheoesophageal puncture after pharyngolaryngectomy and free jejunal interposition. *Head & Neck, 28*, 205–209.

Ohmae, Y., Logemann, J. A., Kaiser, P., Hanson, D. G., & Kahrilas, P. J. (1996). Effects of two breath-holding maneuvers on oropharyngeal swallow. *The Annals of Otology, Rhinology, and Laryngology, 105*, 123–131.

Paydarfar, J. A., & Birkmeyer, N. J. (2006). Complications in head and neck surgery: A meta-analysis of postlaryngectomy pharyngocutaneous fistula. *Archives of Otolaryngology – Head & Neck Surgery, 132*, 67–72.

Piazza, C., Barbieri, D., Del Bon, F., Grazioli, P., Perotti, P., Paderno, A., ... Peretti, G. (2016). Functional outcomes after different types of transoral supraglottic laryngectomy. *Laryngoscope, 126*, 1131–1135.

Rademaker, A. W., Logemann, J. A., Pauloski, B. R., Bowman, J. B., Lazarus, C. L., Sisson, G. A., ... Collins, S. L. (1993). Recovery of postoperative swallowing in patients undergoing partial laryngectomy. *Head & Neck, 15*, 325–334.

Remacle, M., Hantzakos, A., Eckel, H., Evrard, A. S., Bradley, P. J., Chevalier, D., ... Werner, J. (2009). Endoscopic supraglottic laryngectomy: A proposal for a classification by the working committee on nomenclature, European Laryngological Society. *European Archives of Ororhinolaryngology, 266*, 993–998.

Sasaki, C. T., Leder, S. B., Acton, L. M., & Maune, S. (2006). Comparison of the glottic closure reflex in traditional "open" versus endoscopic laser supraglottic laryngectomy. *The Annals of Otology, Rhinology, and Laryngology, 115*, 93–96.

Shinn, E. H., Basen-Engquist, K., Baum, G., Steen, S., Bauman, R. F., Morrison, W., ... Lewin, J. S. (2013). Adherence to preventative exercises and self-reported swallowing outcomes in post-radiation head and neck cancer patients. *Head & Neck, 35*, 1707–1712.

Siu, J., Tam, S., & Fung, K. (2016). A comparison of outcomes in interventions for unilateral vocal fold paralysis: A systematic review. *Laryngoscope, 126*, 1616–1624.

Smith, B. G., Hutcheson, K. A., Little, L. G., Skoracki, R. J., Rosenthal, D. I., Lai, S. Y., & Lewin, J. S. (2015). Lymphedema outcomes in patients with head and neck cancer. *Otolaryngology and Head and Neck Surgery, 152*, 284–291.

Spriano, G., Antognoni, P., Piantanida, R., Varinelli, D., Luraghi, R., Cerizza, L., & Tordiglione, M. (1997). Conservative management of T1-T2N0 supraglottic cancer: A retrospective study. *American Journal of Otolaryngology, 18*, 229–305.

Starmer, H. M., Gourin, C. G., Lua, L. L., & Burkhead, L. (2011). Pretreatment swallowing assessment in head and neck cancer patients. *Head & Neck, 121*, 1208–1211.

Starmer, H. M., Quon, H., Simpson, M., Webster, K., Tippett, D., Herbert, R. J., ... Gourin, C. G. (2015). Speech-language pathology care and short- and long-term outcomes of laryngeal cancer treatment in the elderly. *Laryngoscope, 125*, 2756–2763.

Starmer, H. M., Tippett, D. C., & Webster, K. T. (2008). Effects of laryngeal cancer on voice and swallowing. *Otolaryngologic Clinics of North America, 41*, 793–818.

Stenson, K. M., MacCracken, E., List, M., Haraf, D. J., Brockstein, B., Weichselbaum, R., & Vokes, E. E. (2000). Swallowing function in patients with head and neck cancer prior to treatment. *Archives of Otolaryngology – Head & Neck Surgery, 126*, 371–377.

Tufano, R. (2002). Organ preservation for laryngeal cancer. *Otolaryngologic Clinics of North America, 35*, 1067–1080.

Vu, K. N., Day, T. A., Gillespie, M. B., Martin-Harris, B., Sinha, D., Stuart, R. K., & Sharma, A. K. (2008). Proximal esophageal stenosis in head and neck cancer patients after total laryngectomy and radiation. *ORL Journal Otorhinolaryngol Specialty, 70*, 229–235.

Wasserman, T., Murry, T., Johnson, J. T., & Myers, E. N. (2001). Management of swallowing in supraglottic and extended supraglottic laryngectomy patients. *Head & Neck, 23*, 1043–1048.

Weinstein, G. S., El-Sawy, M. M., Ruiz, C., Dooley, P., Chalian, A., El-Sayed, M. M., & Goldberg, A. (2001). Laryngeal preservation with supracricoid partial laryngectomy results in improved quality of life when compared with total laryngectomy. *Laryngoscope, 111*, 191–199.

Wolf, G., Hong, K., Fisher, S., Hong, W. K., Hillman, R., Spaulding, M., ... Henderson, W. G. (1991). Induction chemotherapy plus radiation compared with surgery plus radiation in patients with advanced laryngeal cancer: The Department of Veterans Affairs Laryngeal Cancer Study Group. *The New England Journal of Medicine, 324*, 1685–1690.

Wulff, N. B., Kristensen, C. A., Andersen, E., Charabi, B., Sorensen, C. H., & Homoe, P. (2015). Risk factors for postoperative complications after total laryngectomy following radiotherapy or chemoradiation; a 10-year retrospective longitudinal study in Eastern Denmark. *Clinical Otolaryngology, 40*, 662–671.

Xu, B., Boero, I. J., Hwang, L., Le, Q. T., Moiseenko, V., Sanghvi, P. R., ... Murphy, J. D. (2015). Aspiration pneumonia after concurrent chemoradiotherapy for head and neck cancer. *Cancer, 121*, 1303–1311.

Zacharek, M. A., Pasha, R., Meleca, R. J., Dworkin, J. P., Stachler, R. J., Jacobs, J. R., ... Garfield, I. (2001). Functional outcomes after supracricoid laryngectomy. *Laryngoscope, 111*, 1558–1564.

Zhang, T., Szczeniak, M., Maclean, J., Bertrand, P., Wu, P. I., Omari, T., & Cook, I. J. (2016). Biomechanics of pharyngeal deglutitive function following total laryngectomy. *Otolaryngology and Head and Neck Surgery, 155*, 295–302.

Dysphagia Management of Head and Neck Cancer Patients: Oral Cavity and Oropharynx

19

Loni C. Arrese and Heidi Schieve

Dysphagia is a prevalent and serious sequela of head and neck cancer (HNC) and its treatments. The presence of head and neck malignancy often disrupts normal anatomy, yielding oropharyngeal dysphagia resulting from mass effect, nerve involvement, and/or tumor-related pain. The treatment modalities for HNC, which include surgery, radiotherapy, and/or chemoradiation, also often result in dysphagia or exacerbate a pre-existing dysphagia. However, these life-saving treatment modalities often have adverse effects that negatively influence one's overall functional status, which includes swallowing and quality of life (QOL). This chapter will focus on anticipated swallowing impairments and dysphagia treatment as it relates to oral and oropharyngeal cancers. In doing so, we will maintain the assumption that oral cavity cancers are primarily treated surgically followed by adjuvant radiotherapy or chemoradiation for advanced stage disease, while oropharynx tumors are most often treated with nonsurgical multimodality intervention (e.g., chemoradiation).

The incidence of dysphagia within the HNC population is high, with symptoms first appearing at the time of HNC diagnosis in up to 40% of patients with advanced stage tumors (Stenson et al., 2000). This baseline dysphagia is directly related to tumor size and location (Stenson et al., 2000). Tumor invasion into the pharynx and/or larynx may lead to impaired bolus clearance and impaired airway closure by way of mass effect or obstruction, while oropharynx tumors more often yield disruptions with bolus propulsion and transport. Dysphagia symptoms are then typically intensified or caused by oncologic treatment.

Following oncologic intervention, it is reported that a wide range of as many as 39–64% of all HNC patients are left with some degree of permanent swallowing problems (Caudell et al., 2009; Francis, Weymuller, Parvathaneni, Merati, & Yueh, 2010; Hutcheson et al., 2014). However, it has been suggested that the reported incidence is underestimated due to discrepancies between patient perception and objective findings of swallow pathophysiology via instrumental assessment (Arrese, Carrau, & Plowman, 2017; Rogus-Pulia, Pierce, Mittal, Zecker, & Logemann, 2014). This discrepancy appears to be related to the neurosensory deficits (e.g., silent aspiration) resulting from either direct tumor invasion or neuromuscular posttreatment toxicities. Regardless of cause, disruptions in motor and sensory pathways often result in silent

L. C. Arrese (✉)
Department of Medicine at the University of Wisconsin School of Medicine and Public Health, Madison, WI, USA

H. Schieve
Otolaryngology, The Ohio State University, Columbus, OH, USA
e-mail: Heidi.schieve@osumc.edu

© Springer Nature Switzerland AG 2019
P. C. Doyle (ed.), *Clinical Care and Rehabilitation in Head and Neck Cancer*,
https://doi.org/10.1007/978-3-030-04702-3_19

aspiration, which has been reported to be as high as 18.5% at the time of HNC diagnosis and may range from 22% to 60% after specific cancer treatment (Denaro, Merlano, & Russi, 2013). Thus, the occurrence of dysphagia within the HNC population is highly variable and represents a growing clinical problem (see Starmer, Chap. 18).

Dysphagia management for HNC patients begins with a comprehensive pretreatment evaluation of swallowing safety and efficiency. This includes an instrumental swallow evaluation via videofluoroscopy, a method known as a modified barium swallow study, or via fiber-optic endoscopic evaluation of swallowing (FEES) coupled with standardized ratings for oral intake and patient-reported outcomes (PROs). The baseline objective swallow assessment serves to guide the medical plan of care, to establish dysphagia-related needs, and to counsel the patient effectively for anticipated posttreatment challenges and functional outcomes. In the event of subclinical findings (i.e., not overt or those without medical consequence), the baseline assessment assists the clinician in determining if alternative methods of nutrition are required and/or anticipated during or following treatment. Further, if an individual presents with swallowing deficits unrelated to tumor invasion (e.g., presbyphagia), they might have an increased likelihood of swallow dysfunction following oncologic intervention due to reduced ability for compensation (Pauloski, 2008). In the sections to follow, a framework for dysphagia management of (1) surgically treated and (2) nonsurgically treated HNC patients will be provided.

Surgical Treatment for Head and Neck Cancer

Surgery for HNC may alter an individual's cosmetic appearance, as well as their QOL and functional ability to speak, smell, chew, and/or swallow. In general, changes due to surgery can be predicted based on tumor location and size (Colangelo, Logemann, Pauloski, Pelzer, & Rademaker, 1996; Pauloski, 2008). Functional

deficits resulting from surgical intervention are typically limited to specific anatomic and related neurophysiologic changes caused by the surgery itself. The predictable nature of postsurgical deficits allows individualized counseling and education regarding postoperative expectations to be provided to patients. This is important in regard to the comprehensiveness of patient care, as effective preoperative education positively influences long-term QOL outcomes for this patient population (Llewellyn, McGurk, & Weinman, 2006).

The primary goal of surgical intervention for treatment of HNC is to cure the patient of his/her malignancy while minimizing functional loss. Surgical intervention is an option for treatment of HNC when a negative surgical resection margin can be achieved (Schoppy et al., 2017). A negative resection margin refers to the complete removal of the tumor and the surrounding normal tissue, thus decreasing the risk for leaving microscopic or macroscopic cancer tissue behind. In contrast, positive surgical resection margins are associated with higher mortality rates (Byers, Bland, Borlase, & Luna, 1978; Haque, Contreras, McNicoll, Eckberg, & Petitti, 2006; Jesse & Sugarbaker, 1976; Luryi et al., 2015). Should the extent of the surgical intervention require removal of vital anatomic structures important for function and QOL, surgical intervention may be suboptimal. However, it is important to note that removal of tumor and surrounding tissue in the situation of HNC may necessitate the sacrifice of critical anatomical structures responsible for efficient bolus preparation and transfer as well as airway protection required when swallowing (see Shavolar, Yeh, & Fung, Chap. 1).

While oral cavity cancers are typically treated with surgical resection as the primary intervention, oropharynx cancers are largely treated nonsurgically due to anticipated beneficial oncological response with organ preservation via definitive radiation or chemoradiation (Argiris, Karamouzis, Raben, & Ferris, 2008). One important difference in the functional outcomes of these treatment modalities is that an individual's swallow function typically improves after surgery, while it tends to worsen after radiotherapy

(Pauloski et al., 1994; Pauloski, Rademaker, Logemann, & Colangelo, 1998). However, at this time, compensatory (Table 19.1) and rehabilitative techniques (Table 19.2) for dysphagia remain the same regardless of chosen treatment modality. Of note, a combined modality approach that employs adjuvant therapy (i.e., surgery followed by additional treatment via radiation with or

Table 19.1 Compensatory strategies and the intended response

Compensatory strategy	Intended response
Head tilt to non-affected or stronger side	Gravity keeps bolus to non-affected or stronger portion of oral cavity for improved containment and anterior-posterior (AP) oral pressure drive; reduces oral residue
Posterior head tilt	Gravity assists AP transport and oral pressure drive to reduce oral residue
Bolus delivery modifications	Placement to non-affected side or posterior oral placement improves bolus manipulation and AP oral pressure drive directed at bolus; reduces oral residue Ease of placement can be assisted with utensil modification (see below)
Utensil modifications: type and/or smaller size	Modified utensils typically consist of tongue blades, smaller silverware, syringes, or straws Helps to improve oral bolus acceptance Assists with directing bolus to dentition, gums, or native structures for manipulation or mastication
Effortful swallow	May increase pharyngeal pressure drive by assisting contact of base of tongue with posterior pharyngeal wall and improving pharyngeal contraction; may increase upper esophageal sphincter (UES) duration of opening (Hind, Nicosia, Roecker, Carnes, & Robbins, 2001)
Liquid wash and/or liquid assist	Helps to clear residue in oral cavity and/or pharynx Aids bolus formation in the presence of hyposalivation
Manual lip closure	Improves labial seal, which, in turn, can improve bolus containment, increase intraoral pressure drive, and reduce oral residue
Palatal drop/ augmentation prosthesis	Improves tongue (or neo-tongue) to palate contact for increased AP oral pressure drive
Palatal obturator device/ palatal lift device	Creates complete or improved closure of hard palate to nasal cavity and/or velopharyngeal port for increased oropharyngeal pressure drive
Reduced bolus volume	Improves ease of mastication and oral bolus formation Improves oral bolus acceptance with trismus and/or microstomia
Manual nares occlusion	Helps to generate increased pharyngeal pressure drive for patients with impaired or absent velopharyngeal closure
Head turn (to affected/ weaker side)	Aids in blocking/closing off affected or weaker side of the pharynx while redirecting bolus to stronger side Improves true vocal fold approximation during glottic adduction Increases cricopharyngeus (CP) distension by reducing resting pressure directed on this muscle (Ohmae, Ogura, Kitahara, Karaho, & Inouye, 1998) May improve pharyngeal bolus efficiency overall, thereby reducing airway events (i.e., penetration/aspiration) with residuals after the swallow
Chin tuck	Keeps bolus anterior in oral cavity slightly longer Moves the epiglottis and base of tongue posteriorly to narrow laryngeal vestibule while widening the vallecular space May improve airway protection and reduce airway events before the swallow (Pauloski, 2008)
Volitional oral hold	Alters swallow initiation in both the timing and location of the food bolus relative to the airway (Palmer, Hiiemae, Matsuo, & Haishima, 2007) Can aid in reducing guarding of pharyngeal swallow due to pain response
Supraglottic swallow maneuver	Improves true vocal fold adduction to prevent aspiration during the swallow (Pauloski, 2008) Variation of super-supraglottic swallow maneuver helps to prevent aspiration before and during the swallow (Ohmae, Logemann, Kaiser, Hanson, & Kahrilas, 1996), as effortful breath hold increases arytenoid approximation to epiglottic petiole with improved laryngeal vestibule closure before and during the swallow
Multiple swallows	Improves oropharyngeal bolus clearance, thereby reducing likelihood of airway events with residual

Table 19.2 Rehabilitative considerations and the intended response

Rehabilitative option	Intended response
Labial range of motion	Protrusion posture improves labial seal for improved swallow efficiency (Logemann, Pauloski, Rademaker, & Colangelo, 1997) Retraction likely to increase oral aperture for improved bolus acceptance
Labial strengthening	Targets strength/tightness of labial seal for generation of intraoral bolus pressure Resistance can be achieved via tongue blade as indicated Can monitor via Iowa Oral Performance Instrument (IOPI®) (IOPI® Medical, LLC, Redmond, WA) (Solomon, Clark, Makashay, & Newman, 2008)
Lingual range of motion	Aids oral bolus control and formation; increases anterior-posterior (AP) oral bolus propulsion Can help prevent scar band formation or tethering at surgical site Lingual pullback targets base of tongue mobility for improved contact with posterior pharyngeal wall; recommend assessment of most effective cue with direct visualization (e.g., fluoroscopy or nasoendoscopy)
Lingual strengthening	Improves lingual pressure generated during the swallow (Robbins et al., 2005, 2007), which is suspected to improve AP oral bolus propulsion Increases endurance to avoid fatigue during meals Can use tongue blades as manual resistance in different planes depending on therapy targets IOPI® or Swallow STRengthening OropharyNGeal (SwallowSTRONG) (Swallow Solutions, LLC, Madison, WI) devices can be used for objective monitoring of lingual strength over time as well as tool for patient biofeedback
Mendelsohn maneuver	Improves hyolaryngeal elevation and excursion Aids in opening and increasing duration time of CP muscle (Kahrilas, Logemann, Krugler, & Flanagan, 1991)
Shaker technique: isometric and isokinetic	Increases CP distension with indirect (non-swallow) task to target musculature involved in hyolaryngeal elevation/excursion (Shaker et al., 1997)
Effortful pitch glides	Indirect (non-swallow) task to increase engagement of musculature involved in hyolaryngeal elevation and pharyngeal contraction (Miloro, Pearson, & Langmore, 2014)
Jaw range of motion, including sustained mandibular extension	Enhances ease of oral bolus acceptance and mastication of solids Sustained mandibular extension can be assisted with use of stacked tongue blades or devices such as TheraBite® Jaw Motion Rehabilitation System™ (Atos Medical, New Berlin, WI) Can objectively monitor via jaw ROM scales
Effortful swallow exercise	Targets base of tongue contact with posterior pharyngeal wall Increases pharyngeal contraction (Hind et al., 2001)
Masako maneuver	Enhances superior posterior pharyngeal wall engagement to improve contact with base of tongue (Pauloski, 2008)

without chemotherapy) is indicated for curative intent of advanced stage tumors.

The site and size of the resection considered in combination with an individual's baseline swallow function help to predict postoperative swallow function. The location and degree of surgical resection will define the structures and cranial nerve pathways impacted and subsequently provide the dysphagia clinician with important information regarding the resultant impact of surgery on swallow function (Arrese & Lazarus, 2013). For example, in general, patients with oropharyngeal cancers and/or advanced stage tumors (T3– T4) have increased swallow deficits following surgical intervention when compared to oral cavity cancers and early-stage tumors (T2) (Borggreven et al., 2007). Postoperatively, collaboration with the surgical team prior to initiating a per oris (PO) diet, or liquid/food intake by mouth, is essential, as liquids and foods can cause unwanted irritation/damage to the surgical site. The early goals of dysphagia management in the postoperative phase focus primarily on nutritional intake and airway protection. Priority is placed on nutritional goals to promote healing and achieve homeostasis for the patient. In addition, in order to minimize risk of respiratory complications (e.g., aspiration pneumonia), attention to airway protection is essential. This is typically achieved via compensatory interventions while the patient is in the acute postoperative phase. Compensatory interventions primarily consist of diet modifications and postural strategies used to alter bolus flow (Logemann, 1999). Additionally, rehabilitative goals are established in order to target deficits noted on examination.

Depending on surgical site and anticipated dysphagia, a patient may rely on short- or long-term alternative methods of nutrition such as a nasogastric (NG) tube or percutaneous endoscopic gastrostomy (PEG) tube. Should a long-term alternative method of nutrition be indicated via PEG, intraoperative placement following tumor extirpation is preferred to avoid potential complications and decrease the likelihood of patient discomfort (Raynor, Williams, Martindale, & Porubsky, 1999). In addition to the previous discussion of acute postoperative outcomes, further implications and considerations in long-term functional outcomes from surgical reconstruction will be discussed in the section to follow.

Impact of Surgical Reconstruction

If surgical resection is minimal, primary wound closure can be achieved. However, if tumor burden is large, skin grafts and/or microvascular flap reconstruction is required in order to obtain wound closure and preserve function. Reconstruction can lead to an adynamic segment of tissue in resected areas as well as reduced sensation postoperatively. Flap reconstruction can, therefore, result in sensory deficits that will influence bolus formation and the timing of swallow initiation. In addition, scarring at the surgical site may further alter the integrity and dynamic movement of the impacted structures. Whether a consequence of tumor involvement, surgical excision, or nerve manipulation intraoperatively, interruptions in nerve pathways can result in reduced or absent motor and/or sensory function of related areas. That is, disruptions to afferent and efferent neurological pathways will directly impact func-

tional capacity. Thus, anatomical changes, scar formation, and alterations to nerve pathways often result in significant bolus flow changes with the potential for impaired swallow efficiency and reduced airway protection.

The following section will provide a framework for anatomical changes and related functional expectations, compensatory strategies, and dysphagia rehabilitation options in regard to tumor site. Of note, tumors may extend to multiple sites simultaneously, resulting in varied effects. Further, multimodality treatments add an additional layer of tissue and neuromuscular changes that may impact swallowing function. Therefore, the compensatory strategies and rehabilitative options listed are offered as suggestions for consideration rather than as definitive and comprehensive modifications and therapy targets.

Dysphagia Based on Surgical Site

Please see Table 19.1 for further descriptions of recommended compensatory strategies and Table 19.2 for associated rehabilitative options.

Oral Cavity

Lip

Anatomical Changes/Functional Expectations

The lips create a sphincter-like seal important for oral bolus containment and anterior-posterior (AP) oral pressure drive. The orbicularis oris muscle aids in constriction of the lips to create the labial seal. Poor or incomplete re-approximation of this muscle during reconstruction following tumor resection increases the risk of anterior bolus escape and may limit the bolus from remaining at the anterior oral cavity. The same scenario can also occur with damage to the marginal mandibular nerve, impacting movement of the lower lip, or similarly, injury to the mental nerve influencing lower lip sensation. In such instances, manage-

Table 19.3 Compensatory strategies and rehabilitative considerations for lip resection

Compensatory strategies	Rehabilitative considerations
Manual lip closure	Labial range of motion exercises (Logemann et al., 1997)
Head tilt to non-affected side	Labial strengthening exercises (Solomon et al., 2008)
Utensil modifications	
Bolus delivery modifications	

Table 19.4 Compensatory strategies and rehabilitative considerations for floor of mouth resection

Compensatory strategies	Rehabilitative considerations
Head tilt to non-affected side	Lingual range of motion exercises
Effortful swallow	Lingual strengthening exercises (Robbins et al., 2005, 2007)
Liquid assist and/or liquid wash	With sacrifice of hyolaryngeal elevator musculature:
Utensil modifications	Mendelsohn maneuver (Kahrilas et al., 1991)
Bolus delivery modifications	Effortful pitch glides (Miloro et al., 2014)
	Shaker technique (isometric and isokinetic) (Shaker et al., 1997)

ment of secretions may become problematic with the possibility of anterior oral pooling and eventual labial escape of secretions. The surgical complication of reduced oral aperture, that is, microstomia, can also occur, a deficit that can lead to reduced oral bolus acceptance, difficulty with denture placement, and poor oral hygiene. See Table 19.3 for compensatory and rehabilitative considerations.

Floor of the Mouth

Anatomical Changes/Functional Expectations

Floor of mouth (FOM) surgery can influence bolus formation, AP bolus propulsion, and airway protection. The floor of mouth sulcus aids in oral bolus retention and formation. The elimination or a reduction in size of this sulcus can lead to impairments in oral bolus containment and preparation. In addition, reconstruction may involve suturing the tongue to the neo-FOM, leading to reduced lingual range of motion and loss of stabilization of the hyolaryngeal complex. The floor of mouth musculature, specifically the mylohyoid and geniohyoid muscles, aids in elevation and excursion of the hyoid bone. With dissection or elimination of these muscles, reduced hyolaryngeal elevation/excursion is anticipated, leading to potential for incomplete laryngeal vestibule closure, reduced airway protection, and impaired upper esophageal opening. Additionally, there is potential for hyposalivation, and its resultant impacts on

bolus formation, as sublingual glands are located in the floor of the mouth and contribute to saliva production. See Table 19.4 for compensatory and rehabilitative considerations.

Oral Tongue

Anatomical Changes/Functional Expectations

The oral tongue contributes to both anterior and posterior oral bolus containment and significantly affects AP oral bolus propulsion. Without adequate lingual range of motion and strength, oral bolus control can be impaired with anterior escape of bolus and reduced propulsion into the pharynx. The amount and location of the surgical resection impacts functional outcomes. The extent of the oral tongue resection is directly associated with oropharyngeal swallow efficiency (McConnel et al., 1994). Minimal impact on pharyngeal swallow function is observed when resection is limited to the anterior tongue (Pauloski et al., 1993). Should tumor size and therefore resultant defect warrant free flap reconstruction, flap size can also affect oral manipulation; adequate flap size is essential to allow for oral bolus acceptance while maintaining flap-to-palate contact for pressure drive on the bolus. See Table 19.5 for compensatory and rehabilitative considerations.

Table 19.5 Compensatory strategies and rehabilitative considerations for oral tongue resection

Compensatory strategies	Rehabilitative considerations
Head tilt to non-affected side	Lingual range of motion exercises of remnant tongue to prevent scarring/tethering of the surgical site
Posterior head tilt	Lingual strengthening exercises of remnant tongue (Robbins et al., 2005, 2007)
Palatal drop/augmentation prosthesis	
Utensil modifications	
Bolus delivery modifications	

Mandible

Anatomical Changes/Functional Expectations

Mandibular resection will necessitate removal of dentition in affected areas, leading to impairments for mastication of solid foods. Alterations to the normal mandibular structure may result in impaired occlusion, which further impacts mastication as well as overall jaw stability required for efficient swallowing, oral containment, and laryngeal elevation (Arrese & Lazarus, 2013). Jaw range of motion, a function that is necessary for mandibular extension for oral bolus acceptance and mastication, is particularly impaired when surgical resection includes the region involving the temporomandibular joint. Surgical reconstruction can include a free flap containing bone to replace the resected native mandible. Mandibular reconstruction with a microvascular osteocutaneous flap can improve outcomes in terms of chewing, swallowing, and cosmesis (Buchbinder et al., 1989). However, mastication efficiency of the neomandible due to lack of dentition, possible reduction in jaw range of motion, and impaired occlusion or unavoidable size mismatch between the native mandible and flap used for reconstruction may be impaired. Mastication of any solids can prove to be difficult following mandibular resection, with patients requiring alterations to pattern of mastication or relying on

Table 19.6 Compensatory strategies and rehabilitative considerations for mandible resection

Compensatory strategies	Rehabilitative considerations
Utensil modifications	Jaw range of motion exercises
Reduced bolus amount	
Soft solids	

diet modifications. See Table 19.6 for compensatory and rehabilitative considerations.

Maxilla/Hard Palate

Anatomical Changes/Functional Expectations

Tumors that involve the maxilla typically require bony resection for removal. When this occurs, the division between the oral cavity and nasal cavity is interrupted. Nasal regurgitation can occur through the aperture created. The use of obturators (Fig. 19.1) or, in some cases, surgical flaps can help to reduce or prevent nasal regurgitation. It should be noted that the extent of resection, including dentition and soft/hard tissue involved, can impact anticipated functional outcomes with palatal obturator use (Goiato, Pesqueira, Ramos da Silva, Gennari Filho, & Micheline Dos Santos, 2009). These factors, therefore, impact an individual's candidacy for palatal obturator placement. See Table 19.7 for compensatory and rehabilitative considerations.

Parotid Gland and Retromolar Trigone

Anatomical Changes/Functional Expectations

The parotid gland is an important source of serous or watery saliva, and this region houses the pathway of the facial nerve. With removal of the parotid, hyposalivation and an increase in viscosity of saliva can occur. If the facial nerve is dissected, reduced or absent motor movement on the ipsilateral lower face will also occur. The retromolar trigone is housed in an area close to the parotid gland. Excision and reconstruction of the retromolar trigone can lead to scar formation with reduced structural flexibility and associated range of motion of the

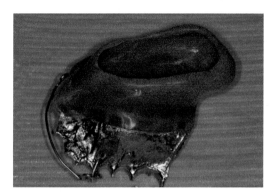

Fig. 19.1 Obturator. (Courtesy of L. Arrese)

Table 19.7 Compensatory strategies and rehabilitative considerations for maxilla resection

Compensatory strategies	Rehabilitative considerations
Use of obturator device	Not applicable
Head tilt to non-affected side and/or posterior head tilt	

Table 19.8 Compensatory strategies and rehabilitative considerations for parotid gland and retromolar trigone resection

Compensatory strategies	Rehabilitative considerations
Head tilt to non-affected side	Jaw range of motion exercises
Utensil modifications	
Reduced bolus amount	
Liquid assist and/or liquid wash	

impacted area. Trismus, or restricted mandibular opening, with reduced oral bolus acceptance is a consideration for this population due to the proximity with key musculature (i.e., masseter, lateral pterygoid, medial pterygoid) involved in mandibular extension within the surgical site. Furthermore, mastication can become difficult due to movement deficits in jaw mobility. See Table 19.8 for compensatory and rehabilitative considerations.

Oropharynx

Velum

Anatomical Changes/Functional Expectations

Movement of the velum during the act of swallowing serves to close the passage between the nasal cavity and the pharynx. Therefore, any resection of the velum can lead to impaired closure of the velopharyngeal port. This then leads to reduced pharyngeal pressure drive with anticipated increased pharyngeal bolus residue. Depending on the extent of resection, retrograde flow through the velopharyngeal port can occur due to these pressure changes, resulting in nasal regurgitation, particularly with thin liquids. A palatal lift prosthesis can aid in improved velopharyngeal closure to reduce or eliminate nasal regurgitation. This prosthesis is most effective when lateral and pharyngeal walls are preserved in surgical resection (Lazarus, 2000), as the movement of this musculature also aids in velopharyngeal closure. See Table 19.9 for compensatory and rehabilitative considerations.

Tonsil

Anatomical Changes/Functional Expectations

In the acute period following surgery, pain response with tonsillar resection is the most significant barrier to rehabilitation (Toma, Blanshard, Eynon-Lewis, & Bridger, 1995). Due to guarding, or delayed initiation of pharyngeal swallow due to anticipated pain with this action,

Table 19.9 Compensatory strategies and rehabilitative considerations for velum resection

Compensatory strategies	Rehabilitative considerations
Manual nares occlusion	Not applicable
Use of obturator device	
Use of palatal lift device	

Table 19.10 Compensatory strategies and rehabilitative considerations for tonsil resection

Compensatory strategies	Rehabilitative considerations
Head turn to affected side	Effortful swallow (should formation of scarring postoperatively be anticipated)
Chin tuck	
Volitional oral hold	

Table 19.11 Compensatory strategies and rehabilitative considerations for base of tongue resection

Compensatory strategies	Rehabilitative considerations
Head turn to affected side	Masako maneuver
Chin tuck	Effortful swallow
Chin tuck in combination with head turn to affected side	Lingual range of motion exercises
Effortful swallow	Oral tongue strengthening exercises
Volitional oral hold	
Supraglottic swallow maneuver	

premature spillage is common immediately postoperatively, particularly with thin liquids. This subsequently leads to impaired airway protection with increased likelihood of airway events (i.e., penetration or aspiration). Furthermore, surgical resection of this area can result in scarring of the adjacent pharyngeal wall, leading to decreased lateral pharyngeal wall contraction. See Table 19.10 for compensatory and rehabilitative considerations.

Base of Tongue

Anatomical Changes/Functional Expectations

Base of tongue (BOT) resections can lead to significant changes in oropharyngeal swallow function in relation to both bolus efficiency and airway protection. Surgery can result in reduced bulk of and/or scar formation to the BOT, which leads to decreased oropharyngeal bolus pressure due to incomplete contact between the BOT and posterior pharyngeal wall. Reduced driving force typically results in incomplete pharyngeal bolus clearance. Furthermore, aspiration risk increases in this patient population, particularly if the size of BOT resection is >50% (Smith et al., 2008). Of note, the size and type of this resection classically warrants reconstruction with a free flap to provide adequate manipulability and volume of the reconstructed area (Haughey, Taylor, & Fuller, 2002). While required for reconstruction, flap placement typically results in an adynamic segment with reduced sensation, particularly in the acute postoperative period. However, it is important to note

that the bulk of the flap can be essential in improving pharyngeal swallow function by creating consistent contact to the posterior pharyngeal wall during swallowing. This contact leads to reduced pharyngeal residue and directing the bolus away from the airway (O'Connell et al., 2008). In conclusion, resection of the BOT can lead to devastating effects, but the extent of resection and reconstruction should be taken into consideration when counseling patients on anticipated swallow outcomes. See Table 19.11 for compensatory and rehabilitative considerations.

Pharynx

Pharyngeal Wall

Anatomical Changes/Functional Expectations

Surgical changes to the pharyngeal wall typically result in impaired muscle contraction directed at the bolus, leading to reduced pharyngeal pressure drive and impaired bolus efficiency. Unilateral deficits, including unilateral bulging of the posterior pharyngeal wall, are common if involvement is limited to one side. Scar bands forming postoperatively lead to a reduction in the pharyngeal stripping wave or the sequential contraction of the superior, medial,

Table 19.12 Compensatory strategies and rehabilitative considerations for pharyngeal wall resection

Compensatory strategies	Rehabilitative considerations
Head turn to affected side	Masako maneuver
Effortful swallow	Effortful swallow
Multiple swallows	Mendelsohn maneuver
Supraglottic swallow maneuver	Effortful pitch glides
	Shaker technique (isometric and isokinetic)

and inferior pharyngeal constrictor musculature to squeeze the bolus down. This further contributes to incomplete pharyngeal bolus clearance. Surgery also can require sacrifice of the palatopharyngeus and stylopharyngeus muscles, which contributes to impairment of airway protection, as these muscles contribute to hyolaryngeal elevation. This surgical intervention can therefore have significant impact on the pharyngeal phase of the swallow overall as well as increase aspiration risk postoperatively. See Table 19.12 for compensatory and rehabilitative considerations.

Nonsurgical Treatment for Head and Neck Cancer

Treatment of HNC has shifted over the past decades to focus on "organ sparing" or conservation therapies, specifically radiotherapy with or without chemotherapy. Great efforts have been directed toward the development of these "less invasive" oncologic treatments to (1) minimize radiation dose to critical structures of the swallowing mechanism via the use of intensity-modulated radiotherapy (IMRT) and (2) reduce regimen-related toxicities through the use of targeted chemotherapy agents (Bonner et al., 2006; Eisbruch et al., 2011; Villa & Sonis, 2016). However, despite these efforts, it is estimated that 39–64% of patients are left with chronic swallowing deficits due to the adverse effects of treatment (Caudell et al., 2009; Francis et al., 2010; Hutcheson et al., 2014). Furthermore, dysphagia

may present at various time points across the continuum of care and survivorship. For purposes of the subsequent section, we will provide a framework for speech pathology services across three distinct timeframes: (1) proactive dysphagia management, (2) persistent radiation-associated dysphagia (RAD), and (3) surveillance dysphagia management.

Proactive Dysphagia Management

The importance of early treatment and even proactive swallowing therapy is increasingly recognized by oncology service providers. This concept is supported in the literature, including several observational studies and randomized control trials (Carnaby-Mann, Crary, Schmalfuss, & Amdur, 2012; Carroll et al., 2008; Duarte, Chhetri, Liu, Erman, & Wang, 2013; Hutcheson et al., 2013; Kotz et al., 2012; Kulbersh et al., 2006; van der Molen et al., 2011; Virani, Kunduk, Fink, & McWhorter, 2015), which have demonstrated that early dysphagia therapy and management is a means to maintaining oropharyngeal function (see Fig. 19.2). Dysphagia clinicians have adopted the phrase "Use it or Lose it" (Hutcheson et al., 2013), a principle of neuroplasticity that refers to remodeling and local wiring of the brain that occur as one acquires a new skill. Persistent practice or repetitive challenge is required to prevent degeneration of a given capacity. Disuse of the swallowing musculature, as often seen during chemoradiation primarily due to odynophagia resulting from oral mucositis, can result in loss of skill and endurance by way of muscular wasting. Additionally, immobilization of the aerodigestive track may exacerbate the onset of muscle fibrosis and is related to reduced QOL (Gillespie, Brodsky, Day, Lee, & Martin-Harris, 2004; Hutcheson et al., 2013).

Acute toxicities of chemoradiation include mucositis, salivary dysfunction, and dysgeusia, which make eating unpleasant and often painful (odynophagia). Commonly, patients stop eating or limit their intake to liquid supplements during

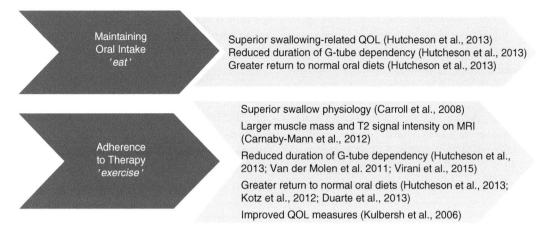

Fig. 19.2   Evidence to support proactive swallowing therapy

treatment. This results in reducing the load and muscular force generation required for swallowing. Further, it is estimated that at least half of the patients require a feeding tube during treatment secondary to the acute toxicities of chemoradiation (Bhayani, Hutcheson, Barringer, Lisec, et al., 2013; Bhayani, Hutcheson, Barringer, Roberts, et al., 2013). Therefore, in addition to patient education and symptom management, dysphagia therapy during the course of chemoradiation has two primary facilitation goals: (1) *eating* and (2) *exercise* (Hutcheson et al., 2013). Hutcheson et al. (2013) also suggest that eating and exercising during chemoradiation both independently and significantly predict better short- and long-term functional outcomes. Specifically, their work demonstrated that individuals who either maintained PO intake or performed swallowing exercises during chemoradiation had more favorable function outcomes when compared to those who did neither. Further, individuals who both *ate* and *exercised* had better outcomes than those who did only one or the other. It is, however, of importance to mention that in an effort to promote a patient's ability to eat and exercise throughout treatment, adequate pain management is essential. Though outside the scope of this chapter, a multidisciplinary approach to pain management is essential for optimal performance (De Sanctis et al., 2016).

Management of Persistent Radiation-Associated Dysphagia (RAD)

Acute and persistent RAD in the first several months posttreatment can vary significantly in its severity and presentation; however, traditionally this appears to reflect varying degrees of muscle edema, fibrosis, and disuse atrophy (Rosenthal, Lewin, & Eisbruch, 2006). Rehabilitation needs are driven by patient goals and expectations, the functional profile of the patient, and findings of the posttreatment instrumental swallowing study. Unfortunately, due to aberrant physiology of the swallowing musculature within the previously radiated field (sclerosis, fibrosis, and/or atrophy), our traditional therapy tools alone are largely ineffective to address persistent RAD (Langmore & Pisegna, 2015). In addition, our traditional swallowing regimens often lack the required principles of (1) motor learning and (2) exercise physiology. Exercise efforts must challenge the neuromuscular system beyond the level of usual or normal activity in order to elicit adaptations. Specifically, exercise paradigms must progressively overload the swallowing musculature in order to improve muscle strength and force generation for swallowing. Unfortunately, there is no reliable way to measure and continually challenge the swallowing musculature using traditional and often home-based, swallowing protocols. Thus, a standard program consisting solely of traditional swallowing exercises is often insufficient in managing these persistent swallow deficits. Fortunately, in investigational settings with selected heterogeneous patient populations, intensive device-driven and/or bolus-driven swallowing therapies have shown promise toward improving functional swallowing status and QOL of patients with persistent posttreatment RAD (Table 19.13). These intensive therapy protocols require mass practice of functional tasks under conditions that require a progressive workload over time. Thus, such treatment approaches may represent an effective *exercise-based* training protocol in the presence of posttreatment atrophy, myopathy, potential neuropathies, and sensory deficits. Many of these studies represent preliminary outcomes (Hutcheson et al., 2017; Thompson et al., 2016; Van Nuffelen et al., 2015); thus, further research and replication of results is required in order to generalize outcomes to clinical practice. Incorporating such treatment approaches into daily practice should be aligned with goal-directed therapies targeting specific pathophysiology detected on instrumental assessment.

Table 19.13 Bolus- and device-driven regimens

Author	Intervention	Conclusion
Bolus-driven intervention studies with HNC patients		
Crary, Carnaby, LaGorio and Carvajal (2012)	McNeill Dysphagia Therapy Program	Improved swallowing performance posttreatment
Carnaby-Mann and Crary (2010)	McNeill Dysphagia Therapy Program and sEMG	Superior outcomes compared with traditional dysphagia therapy supplemented with sEMG biofeedback
Device-driven intervention studies with HNC patients		
Hutcheson et al. (2017)	Expiratory muscle strength training (EMST)	Improved swallow safety as indexed by the DIGEST
Thompson, Divyak, Zielinski and Rogus-Pulia (2016) *ASHA presentation*	Lingual strengthening via the SwallowSTRONG device	Improved swallow safety as indexed by the penetration-aspiration scale
Martin-Harris et al. (2015)	Respiratory training via visually guided feedback	Improved airway protection and bolus clearance
Van Nuffelen et al. (2015)	Lingual strengthening via the IOPI®	Ongoing randomized control trial assessing lingual strength training at 60, 80, or 100% of a patient's maximal tongue strength

Surveillance Dysphagia Management

The need for dysphagia surveillance throughout survivorship has increased given the epidemiological shift of the HNC population attributed to the human papillomavirus (HPV). Due to increased survival rates and decreased age of diagnosis, this epidemic has the potential to result in a population of young, otherwise healthy cancer survivors, challenged by long-term swallowing deficits (see Theurer, this volume). While most patients will attenuate their expectations and establish a "new normal" baseline level of functioning in the presence of xerostomia, the progressive development or late-onset dysphagia is yet not well understood. A case series by Hutcheson et al. (2014) reported a median latency for the development of late radiation-associated dysphagia (late-RAD) after oropharyngeal radiotherapy to be 5.8 years; others have reported a latency of lower cranial neuropathies to range from 1 to 34 years for HNC patients who had received treatment with definitive radiotherapy (Jaruchinda, Jindavijak, & Singhavarach, 2012; Kong et al., 2011). It has, therefore, been suggested that the development of late-RAD follows a long interval (often >5 years) of adequate functioning per patient report (Hutcheson, Yuk, Holsinger, Gunn, & Lewin, 2015).

However, given the known discrepancy between patient-perceived impairment and physiological findings via instrumental assessment (Arrese et al., 2017), surveillance monitoring of swallowing function is warranted in contemporary practice with this growing population in an effort to provide early intervention as deficits arise. Objective assessments for surveillance would therefore determine if there are subclinical findings indicative of late-RAD, allowing for early intervention in an effort to maintain swallow function and prevent further decline.

Conclusion

This chapter has provided a framework for evidence-based dysphagia management of surgically treated oral cavity and oropharynx cancers and nonsurgically treated oropharynx cancers. Swallowing deficits are known adverse effects of oral and oropharyngeal cancer management. Therefore, early establishment of expectations, symptom management, and mobilization of the swallowing musculature aid to optimize rehabilitation and improve survivorship for HNC patients in the settings of both surgical and nonsurgical treatments. While treatment planning requires an individualized approach specific to each patient, this chapter has provided knowledge to guide assessment and rehabilitation of this specialized population based on tumor location and treatment modality. Anticipated outcomes are reviewed to aid in patient counseling and expectations. Compensatory and rehabilitative techniques are described in depth to enable the clinician to intervene appropriately postoperatively, during chemoradiotherapy, and following completion of chemoradiotherapy. In conclusion, an evidence-based approach to evaluation and treatment of dysphagia with this patient population can result in improved functional swallowing outcomes as the patient is undergoing and has completed life-saving treatment for oral and oropharynx cancers.

References

Argiris, A., Karamouzis, M. V., Raben, D., & Ferris, R. L. (2008). Head and neck cancer. *The Lancet, 371*(9625), 1695–1709. https://doi.org/10.1016/S0140-6736(08)60728-X

Arrese, L. C., Carrau, R., & Plowman, E. K. (2017). Relationship between the eating assessment Tool-10 and objective clinical ratings of swallowing function in individuals with head and neck cancer. *Dysphagia, 32*(1), 83–89. https://doi.org/10.1007/s00455-016-9741-7

Arrese, L. C., & Lazarus, C. L. (2013). Special groups: Head and neck cancer. *Otolaryngologic Clinics of North America, 46*(6), 1123–1136. https://doi.org/10.1016/j.otc.2013.08.009

Bhayani, M. K., Hutcheson, K. A., Barringer, D. A., Lisec, A., Alvarez, C. P., Roberts, D. B., … Lewin, J. S. (2013). Gastrostomy tube placement in patients with oropharyngeal carcinoma treated with radiotherapy or chemoradiotherapy: Factors affecting placement and dependence. Head & Neck, 35(11), 1634–1640. https://doi.org/10.1002/hed.23200

Bhayani, M. K., Hutcheson, K. A., Barringer, D. A., Roberts, D. B., Lewin, J. S., & Lai, S. Y. (2013). Gastrostomy tube placement in patients with hypopharyngeal cancer treated with radiotherapy or chemoradiotherapy: Factors affecting placement and dependence. *Head & Neck, 35*(11), 1641–1646. https://doi.org/10.1002/hed.23199

Bonner, J. A., Harari, P. M., Giralt, J., Azarnia, N., Shin, D. M., Cohen, R. B., … Ang, K. K. (2006). Radiotherapy plus cetuximab for squamous-cell carcinoma of the head and neck. *New England Journal of Medicine, 354*(6), 567–578. https://doi.org/10.1056/NEJMoa053422

Borggreven, P. A., Verdonck-de Leeuw, I., Rinkel, R. N., Langendijk, J. A., Roos, J. C., David, E. F., … Leemans, C. R. (2007). Swallowing after major surgery of the oral cavity or oropharynx: A prospective and longitudinal assessment of patients treated by microvascular soft tissue reconstruction. *Head & Neck, 29*(7), 638–647. https://doi.org/10.1002/hed.20582

Buchbinder, D., Urken, M. L., Vickery, C., Weinberg, H., Sheiner, A., & Biller, H. (1989). Functional mandibular reconstruction of patients with oral cancer. *Oral Surgery, Oral Medicine and Oral Pathology, 68*(4 Pt 2), 499–503; discussion 503–494.

Byers, R. M., Bland, K. I., Borlase, B., & Luna, M. (1978). The prognostic and therapeutic value of frozen section determinations in the surgical treatment of squamous carcinoma of the head and neck. *American Journal of Surgery, 136*(4), 525–528.

Carnaby-Mann, G., Crary, M. A., Schmalfuss, I., & Amdur, R. (2012). "Pharyngocise": Randomized controlled trial of preventative exercises to maintain muscle structure and swallowing function during head-

and-neck chemoradiotherapy. *International Journal of Radiation Oncology, Biology, Physics, 83*(1), 210–219. https://doi.org/10.1016/j.ijrobp.2011.06.1954

Carnaby-Mann, G. D., & Crary, M. A. (2010). McNeill dysphagia therapy program: A case-control study. *Archives of Physical Medicine and Rehabilitation, 91*(5), 743–749. https://doi.org/10.1016/j.apmr.2010.01.013

Carroll, W. R., Locher, J. L., Canon, C. L., Bohannon, I. A., McColloch, N. L., & Magnuson, J. S. (2008). Pretreatment swallowing exercises improve swallow function after chemoradiation. *The Laryngoscope, 118*(1), 39–43. https://doi.org/10.1097/MLG.0b013e31815659b0

Caudell, J. J., Schaner, P. E., Meredith, R. F., Locher, J. L., Nabell, L. M., Carroll, W. R., ... Bonner, J. A. (2009). Factors associated with long-term dysphagia after definitive radiotherapy for locally advanced head-and-neck cancer. *International Journal of Radiation Oncology, Biology, Physics, 73*(2), 410–415. https://doi.org/10.1016/j.ijrobp.2008.04.048

Colangelo, L. A., Logemann, J. A., Pauloski, B. R., Pelzer, J. R., & Rademaker, A. W. (1996). T stage and functional outcome in oral and oropharyngeal cancer patients. *Head & Neck, 18*(3), 259–268.

Crary, M. A., Carnaby, G. D., LaGorio, L. A., & Carvajal, P. J. (2012). Functional and physiological outcomes from an exercise-based dysphagia therapy: A pilot investigation of the McNeill Dysphagia Therapy Program. *Archives of Physical Medicine and Rehabilitation, 93*(7), 1173–1178. https://doi.org/10.1016/j.apmr.2011.11.008

De Sanctis, V., Bossi, P., Sanguineti, G., Trippa, F., Ferrari, D., Bacigalupo, A., ... Lalla, R. V. (2016). Mucositis in head and neck cancer patients treated with radiotherapy and systemic therapies: Literature review and consensus statements. *Critical Reviews in Oncology/Hematology, 100*, 147–166. https://doi.org/10.1016/j.critrevonc.2016.01.010

Denaro, N., Merlano, M. C., & Russi, E. G. (2013). Dysphagia in head and neck cancer patients: Pretreatment evaluation, predictive factors, and assessment during radio-chemotherapy, recommendations. *Clinical and Experimental Otorhinolaryngology, 6*(3), 117–126. https://doi.org/10.3342/ceo.2013.6.3.117

Duarte, V. M., Chhetri, D. K., Liu, Y. F., Erman, A. A., & Wang, M. B. (2013). Swallow preservation exercises during chemoradiation therapy maintains swallow function. *Otolaryngology- Head and Neck Surgery, 149*(6), 878–884. https://doi.org/10.1177/0194599813502310

Eisbruch, A., Kim, H. M., Feng, F. Y., Lyden, T. H., Haxer, M. J., Feng, M., ... Ten Haken, R. K. (2011). Chemo-IMRT of oropharyngeal cancer aiming to reduce dysphagia: Swallowing organs late complication probabilities and dosimetric correlates. *International Journal of Radiation Oncology, Biology, Physics, 81*(3), e93–e99. https://doi.org/10.1016/j.ijrobp.2010.12.067

Francis, D. O., Weymuller, E. A., Parvathaneni, U., Merati, A. L., & Yueh, B. (2010). Dysphagia, stricture, and pneumonia in head and neck cancer patients: Does treatment modality matter? *Annals of Otology, Rhinology & Laryngology, 119*(6), 391–397.

Gillespie, M. B., Brodsky, M. B., Day, T. A., Lee, F. S., & Martin-Harris, B. (2004). Swallowing-related quality of life after head and neck cancer treatment. *The Laryngoscope, 114*(8), 1362–1367. https://doi.org/10.1097/00005537-200408000-00008

Goiato, M. C., Pesqueira, A. A., Ramos da Silva, C., Gennari Filho, H., & Micheline Dos Santos, D. (2009). Patient satisfaction with maxillofacial prosthesis. Literature review. *Journal of Plastic, Reconstructive & Aesthetic Surgery, 62*(2), 175–180. https://doi.org/10.1016/j.bjps.2008.06.084

Haque, R., Contreras, R., McNicoll, M. P., Eckberg, E. C., & Petitti, D. B. (2006). Surgical margins and survival after head and neck cancer surgery. *BMC Ear, Nose and Throat Disorders, 6*, 2. https://doi.org/10.1186/1472-6815-6-2

Haughey, B. H., Taylor, S. M., & Fuller, D. (2002). Fasciocutaneous flap reconstruction of the tongue and floor of mouth: Outcomes and techniques. *Archives of Otolaryngology- Head & Neck Surgery, 128*(12), 1388–1395.

Hind, J. A., Nicosia, M. A., Roecker, E. B., Carnes, M. L., & Robbins, J. (2001). Comparison of effortful and noneffortful swallows in healthy middle-aged and older adults. *Archives of Physical Medicine and Rehabilitation, 82*(12), 1661–1665. https://doi.org/10.1053/apmr.2001.28006

Hutcheson, K. A., Barrow, M. P., Plowman, E. K., Lai, S. Y., Fuller, C. D., Barringer, D. A., ... Lewin, J. S. (2017). Expiratory muscle strength training for radiation-associated aspiration after head and neck cancer: A case series. *The Laryngoscope.* https://doi.org/10.1002/lary.26845

Hutcheson, K. A., Bhayani, M. K., Beadle, B. M., Gold, K. A., Shinn, E. H., Lai, S. Y., & Lewin, J. (2013). Eat and exercise during radiotherapy or chemoradiotherapy for pharyngeal cancers: Use it or lose it. *JAMA Otolaryngology- Head & Neck Surgery, 139*(11), 1127–1134. https://doi.org/10.1001/jamaoto.2013.4715

Hutcheson, K. A., Lewin, J. S., Holsinger, F. C., Steinhaus, G., Lisec, A., Barringer, D. A., ... Kies, M. S. (2014). Long-term functional and survival outcomes after induction chemotherapy and risk-based definitive therapy for locally advanced squamous cell carcinoma of the head and neck. *Head & Neck, 36*(4), 474–480. https://doi.org/10.1002/hed.23330

Hutcheson, K. A., Yuk, M. M., Holsinger, F. C., Gunn, G. B., & Lewin, J. S. (2015). Late radiation-associated dysphagia with lower cranial neuropathy in long-term oropharyngeal cancer survivors: Video case reports. *Head & Neck, 37*(4), E56–E62. https://doi.org/10.1002/hed.23840

Jaruchinda, P., Jindavijak, S., & Singhavarach, N. (2012). Radiation-related vocal fold palsy in patients with head and neck carcinoma. *Journal of the Medical Association of Thailand, 95*(Suppl 5), S23–S28.

Jesse, R. H., & Sugarbaker, E. V. (1976). Squamous cell carcinoma of the oropharynx: Why we fail. *American Journal of Surgery, 132*(4), 435–438.

Kahrilas, P. J., Logemann, J. A., Krugler, C., & Flanagan, E. (1991). Volitional augmentation of upper esophageal sphincter opening during swallowing. *American Journal of Physiology, 260*(3 Pt 1), G450–G456.

Kong, L., Lu, J. J., Liss, A. L., Hu, C., Guo, X., Wu, Y., & Zhang, Y. (2011). Radiation-induced cranial nerve palsy: A cross-sectional study of nasopharyngeal cancer patients after definitive radiotherapy. *International Journal of Radiation Oncology, Biology, Physics, 79*(5), 1421–1427. https://doi.org/10.1016/j.ijrobp.2010.01.002

Kotz, T., Federman, A. D., Kao, J., Milman, L., Packer, S., Lopez-Prieto, C., … Genden, E. M. (2012). Prophylactic swallowing exercises in patients with head and neck cancer undergoing chemoradiation: A randomized trial. *Archives of Otolaryngology-Head & Neck Surgery, 138*(4), 376–382. https://doi.org/10.1001/archoto.2012.187

Kulbersh, B. D., Rosenthal, E. L., McGrew, B. M., Duncan, R. D., McColloch, N. L., Carroll, W. R., & Magnuson, J. S. (2006). Pretreatment, preoperative swallowing exercises may improve dysphagia quality of life. *The Laryngoscope, 116*(6), 883–886. https://doi.org/10.1097/01.mlg.0000217278.96901.fc

Langmore, S. E., & Pisegna, J. M. (2015). Efficacy of exercises to rehabilitate dysphagia: A critique of the literature. *International Journal of Speech-Language Pathology, 17*(3), 222–229. https://doi.org/10.3109/17549507.2015.1024171

Lazarus, C. L. (2000). Management of swallowing disorders in head and neck cancer patients: Optimal patterns of care. *Seminars in Speech and Language, 21*(4), 293–309.

Llewellyn, C. D., McGurk, M., & Weinman, J. (2006). How satisfied are head and neck cancer (HNC) patients with the information they receive pre-treatment? Results from the satisfaction with cancer information profile (SCIP). *Oral Oncology, 42*(7), 726–734. https://doi.org/10.1016/j.oraloncology.2005.11.013

Logemann, J. A. (1999). Behavioral management for oropharyngeal dysphagia. *Folia Phoniatrica et Logopaedia, 51*(4–5), 199–212. https://doi.org/10.1159/000021497

Logemann, J. A., Pauloski, B. R., Rademaker, A. W., & Colangelo, L. A. (1997). Speech and swallowing rehabilitation for head and neck cancer patients. *Oncology (Williston Park, N.Y.), 11*(5), 651–656, 659; discussion 659, 663–654.

Luryi, A. L., Chen, M. M., Mehra, S., Roman, S. A., Sosa, J. A., & Judson, B. L. (2015). Treatment factors associated with survival in early-stage oral cavity cancer: Analysis of 6830 cases from the National Cancer Data Base. *JAMA Otolaryngology- Head & Neck Surgery, 141*(7), 593–598. https://doi.org/10.1001/jamaoto.2015.0719

Martin-Harris, B., McFarland, D., Hill, E. G., Strange, C. B., Focht, K. L., Wan, Z., … McGrattan, K. (2015). Respiratory-swallow training in patients with head and neck cancer. *Archives of Physical Medicine and Rehabilitation, 96*(5), 885–893. https://doi.org/10.1016/j.apmr.2014.11.022

McConnel, F. M., Logemann, J. A., Rademaker, A. W., Pauloski, B. R., Baker, S. R., Lewin, J., … Collins, S. (1994). Surgical variables affecting postoperative swallowing efficiency in oral cancer patients: A pilot study. *The Laryngoscope, 104*(1 Pt 1), 87–90. https://doi.org/10.1288/00005537-199401000-00015

Miloro, K. V., Pearson, W. G., & Langmore, S. E. (2014). Effortful pitch glide: A potential new exercise evaluated by dynamic MRI. *Journal of Speech, Language, and Hearing Research, 57*(4), 1243–1250. https://doi.org/10.1044/2014_JSLHR-S-13-0168

O'Connell, D. A., Rieger, J., Harris, J. R., Dziegielewski, P., Zalmanowitz, J., Sytsanko, A., … Seikaly, H. (2008). Swallowing function in patients with base of tongue cancers treated with primary surgery and reconstructed with a modified radial forearm free flap. *Archives of Otolaryngology- Head & Neck Surgery, 134*(8), 857–864. https://doi.org/10.1001/archotol.134.8.857

Ohmae, Y., Logemann, J. A., Kaiser, P., Hanson, D. G., & Kahrilas, P. J. (1996). Effects of two breath-holding maneuvers on oropharyngeal swallow. *Annals of Otology, Rhinology and Laryngology, 105*(2), 123–131. https://doi.org/10.1177/000348949610500207

Ohmae, Y., Ogura, M., Kitahara, S., Karaho, T., & Inouye, T. (1998). Effects of head rotation on pharyngeal function during normal swallow. *Annals of Otology, Rhinology and Laryngology, 107*(4), 344–348. https://doi.org/10.1177/000348949810700414

Palmer, J. B., Hiiemae, K. M., Matsuo, K., & Haishima, H. (2007). Volitional control of food transport and bolus formation during feeding. *Physiology & Behavior, 91*(1), 66–70. https://doi.org/10.1016/j.physbeh.2007.01.018

Pauloski, B. R. (2008). Rehabilitation of dysphagia following head and neck cancer. *Physical Medicine and Rehabilitation Clinics of North America, 19*(4), 889–928, x. https://doi.org/10.1016/j.pmr.2008.05.010

Pauloski, B. R., Logemann, J. A., Rademaker, A. W., McConnel, F. M., Heiser, M. A., Cardinale, S., et al. (1993). Speech and swallowing function after anterior tongue and floor of mouth resection with distal flap reconstruction. *Journal of Speech and Hearing Research, 36*(2), 267–276.

Pauloski, B. R., Logemann, J. A., Rademaker, A. W., McConnel, F. M., Stein, D., Beery, Q., et al. (1994). Speech and swallowing function after oral and oropharyngeal resections: One-year follow-up. *Head & Neck, 16*(4), 313–322.

Pauloski, B. R., Rademaker, A. W., Logemann, J. A., & Colangelo, L. A. (1998). Speech and swallowing in irradiated and nonirradiated postsurgical oral cancer patients. *Otolaryngology- Head and Neck Surgery, 118*(5), 616–624.

Raynor, E. M., Williams, M. F., Martindale, R. G., & Porubsky, E. S. (1999). Timing of percutaneous endoscopic gastrostomy tube placement in head and neck cancer patients. *Otolaryngology- Head and Neck Surgery, 120*(4), 479–482. https://doi.org/10.1053/hn.1999.v120.a91408

Robbins, J., Gangnon, R. E., Theis, S. M., Kays, S. A., Hewitt, A. L., & Hind, J. A. (2005). The effects of lingual exercise on swallowing in older adults. *Journal of American Geriatrics Society, 53*(9), 1483–1489. https://doi.org/10.1111/j.1532-5415.2005.53467.x

Robbins, J., Kays, S. A., Gangnon, R. E., Hind, J. A., Hewitt, A. L., Gentry, L. R., & Taylor, A. J. (2007). The effects of lingual exercise in stroke patients with dysphagia. *Archives of Physical Medicine and Rehabilitation, 88*(2), 150–158. https://doi.org/10.1016/j.apmr.2006.11.002

Rogus-Pulia, N. M., Pierce, M. C., Mittal, B. B., Zecker, S. G., & Logemann, J. A. (2014). Changes in swallowing physiology and patient perception of swallowing function following chemoradiation for head and neck cancer. *Dysphagia, 29*(2), 223–233. https://doi.org/10.1007/s00455-013-9500-y

Rosenthal, D. I., Lewin, J. S., & Eisbruch, A. (2006). Prevention and treatment of dysphagia and aspiration after chemoradiation for head and neck cancer. *Journal of Clinical Oncology, 24*(17), 2636–2643. https://doi.org/10.1200/JCO.2006.06.0079

Schoppy, D. W., Rhoads, K. F., Ma, Y., Chen, M. M., Nussenbaum, B., Orosco, R. K., … Divi, V. (2017). Measuring institutional quality in head and neck surgery using hospital-level data: Negative margin rates and neck dissection yield. *JAMA Otolaryngology-Head & Neck Surgery., 143*, 1111–1116. https://doi.org/10.1001/jamaoto.2017.1694

Shaker, R., Kern, M., Bardan, E., Taylor, A., Stewart, E. T., Hoffmann, R. G., … Bonnevier, J. (1997). Augmentation of deglutitive upper esophageal sphincter opening in the elderly by exercise. *American Journal of Physiology, 272*(6 Pt 1), G1518–G1522.

Smith, J. E., Suh, J. D., Erman, A., Nabili, V., Chhetri, D. K., & Blackwell, K. E. (2008). Risk factors predicting aspiration after free flap reconstruction of oral cavity and oropharyngeal defects. *Archives of Otolaryngology- Head & Neck Surgery, 134*(11), 1205–1208. https://doi.org/10.1001/archotol.134.11.1205

Solomon, N. P., Clark, H. M., Makashay, M. J., & Newman, L. A. (2008). Assessment of orofacial strength in patients with dysarthria. *Journal of Medical Speech-Language Pathology, 16*(4), 251–258.

Stenson, K. M., MacCracken, E., List, M., Haraf, D. J., Brockstein, B., Weichselbaum, R., & Vokes, E. E. (2000). Swallowing function in patients with head and neck cancer prior to treatment. *Archives of Otolaryngology- Head & Neck Surgery, 126*(3), 371–377.

Thompson, J., Divyak, E., Zielinski, J., & Rogus-Pulia, N (2016, November). *Swallowing-related outcomes following oropharyngeal strengthening for patients with head and neck cancer*. Presented at the meeting of the American Speech-Language-Hearing Association, Pittsburgh, PA.

Toma, A. G., Blanshard, J., Eynon-Lewis, N., & Bridger, M. W. (1995). Post-tonsillectomy pain: The first ten days. *The Journal of Laryngology and Otology, 109*(10), 963–964.

van der Molen, L., van Rossum, M. A., Burkhead, L. M., Smeele, L. E., Rasch, C. R., & Hilgers, F. J. (2011). A randomized preventive rehabilitation trial in advanced head and neck cancer patients treated with chemoradiotherapy: Feasibility, compliance, and short-term effects. *Dysphagia, 26*(2), 155–170. https://doi.org/10.1007/s00455-010-9288-y

Van Nuffelen, G., Van den Steen, L., Vanderveken, O., Specenier, P., Van Laer, C., Van Rompaey, D., … De Bodt, M. (2015). Study protocol for a randomized controlled trial: Tongue strengthening exercises in head and neck cancer patients, does exercise load matter? *Trials, 16*, 395. https://doi.org/10.1186/s13063-015-0889-5

Villa, A., & Sonis, S. (2016). Toxicities associated with head and neck cancer treatment and oncology-related clinical trials. *Current Problems in Cancer, 40*(5–6), 244–257. https://doi.org/10.1016/j.currproblcancer.2016.06.001

Virani, A., Kunduk, M., Fink, D. S., & McWhorter, A. J. (2015). Effects of 2 different swallowing exercise regimens during organ-preservation therapies for head and neck cancers on swallowing function. *Head & Neck, 37*(2), 162–170. https://doi.org/10.1002/hed.23570

Part III

Special Factors in Head and Neck Cancer

Acute and Long-Term Effects of Chemoradiation Therapy in Head and Neck Cancer

20

Ann Kearney and Patricia W. Cavanagh

Introduction

Oropharyngeal cancers involving the base of tongue, tonsil, posterior pharyngeal wall, and soft palate have been steadily rising since 1973; further, these sites are projected to account for half the incident of all head and neck cancers (HNC) by 2030 (Chaturvedi, Engels, Anderson, & Gillison, 2008). One of the factors associated with this increase is the occurrence of human papillomavirus (HPV)-associated oropharyngeal cancers (Theurer, Chap. 4). For those diagnosed with HPV-related oropharyngeal malignancies, an additional challenge has emerged. Namely, it appears that treatment for such cancers may be highly successful. However, this positive treatment outcome has led to long-term HNC survivors who are younger and who have the potential of living decades with the side effects of treatment (Chaturvedi et al., 2011).

According to the Centers for Disease Control and Prevention (CDC, 2017), each year there are approximately 3200 new cases of human papil-

lomavirus (HPV)-associated oropharyngeal cancers diagnosed in women, and nearly 13,200 cases diagnosed in men in the United States (Viens et al., 2016). This chapter presents information related to the use of radiation therapy (RT) and chemotherapy (CT) for treating these cancers. However, the discussion to follow addresses the topic of side effects resulting from treatment in those diagnosed with HNC. This will include information related to acute, chronic, and late-stage side effects of RT and CRT treatment. Regardless of when side effects of treatment occur in time, they can be highly debilitating. Thus, the resultant disability of an array of side effects secondary to treatment for HNC is addressed.

Treatment of Advanced Laryngeal Cancer: Pre- and Post-Circa 1990

Prior to 1991, the conventional treatment for stage III and stage IV squamous cell carcinoma of the larynx was total laryngectomy or a combination of total laryngectomy and postoperative adjuvant RT. In 1991, the Department of Veterans Affairs published landmark preliminary results of a multi-institutional, randomized clinical trial (Wolf et al., 1991). The aim of the trial sought to determine whether induction chemotherapy and definitive radiation represented a better initial

A. Kearney (✉)
Stanford Voice and Swallowing Center, Department of Otolaryngology, Head and Neck Surgery, Stanford University Hospital, Stanford, CA, USA
e-mail: annkearney@stanford.edu

P. W. Cavanagh
Speech Pathology Section, San Francisco Veterans Affairs Medical Center, San Francisco, CA, USA

© Springer Nature Switzerland AG 2019
P. C. Doyle (ed.), *Clinical Care and Rehabilitation in Head and Neck Cancer*,
https://doi.org/10.1007/978-3-030-04702-3_20

treatment approach for patients with stage III or IV laryngeal cancer when compared to total laryngectomy and postoperative radiation (Wolf et al., 1991). The VA cooperative study involved 332 patients who were randomly assigned to one of three groups; one group received three cycles of CT and the others received either RT or combined surgery and RT.

The major finding from this seminal study revealed that the larynx could be preserved in 64% of patients who received induction chemotherapy and definitive radiation therapy. Further, larynx preservation was obtained without reducing the estimated 2-year survival rate when compared to survival for the conventional treatment of laryngectomy and postoperative radiation (Wolf et al., 1991). However, despite organ preservation in the CRT group, current data suggest that the functional capacity of the chemoradiation therapy (CRT) can be severely impaired. This treatment-related side effect has been shown to cause significant, debilitating, and many times irreversible long-term effects on both communication and swallowing (Hutcheson et al., 2012; Hutcheson, Bhayani, & Lewin, 2013; Rosenthal et al., 2008). Specific effects on swallowing may emerge as a chronic deficit or in the late stages postradiation therapy. Both result in considerable challenges to the patient with a concomitant influence on quality of life.

The Emergence of Chemoradiation Therapy (CRT) for Head and Neck Cancer

The use of RT for the treatment of HNC has a long-standing presence in the treatment literature related to HNC with reports of chemotherapy (CT) as a viable treatment alternative first appearing in the 1970s (Cognetti, Weber, & Lai, 2008). Chemoradiation therapy (CRT) became the treatment of choice in those with HNC following the publication of a landmark cooperative study conducted by the Department of Veterans Affairs (Wolf et al., 1991) and a report provided in 1996 by the European Organization for Research and Treatment of Cancer (EORTC). If CT is given

before RT starts, this type of treatment as known as *induction CT*. If the CT is presented at the same time as RT, it is referred to as *concurrent CT*. This temporal sequence related to treatment for HNC has important implications specific to the potential for side effects and their impact on the patient.

Toxicity refers to negative side effects of a chemotherapeutic drug or, in this case, that which occurs because of treatment with either CT or RT. When these negative effects occur during treatment, they are graded in their severity in order to document change over time. In fact, standardized toxicity assessment scales are typically used to evaluate the treatment effects in those with HNC. A typical toxicity grading scale for cancer treatment ranges from grade 1 to grade 4, with the higher grade having a more toxic and potentially life-threatening impact (Trotti et al., 2000). Forastiere et al. (2003) were the first authors to report on the acute toxicities associated with induction and concurrent treatments groups. These researchers found that those who received concurrent CT exhibited a higher percentage of severe toxicities (grade 3–4) than did those individuals in either the induction CT or the radiation-alone groups. In the HNC population, toxicities are generally classified and discussed in relation to whether they are acute, chronic, and late-onset events. For this reason, each distinct category of toxicities will be presented in subsequent sections of this chapter.

Acute Toxicities Associated with the Treatment of HNC

The most common types of acute toxicities associated with CRT are reported to be mucositis, xerostomia, dysphagia, odynophagia, and an altered sense of smell and taste. Unfortunately, oral complications from cancer and cancer therapy (Table 20.1) are often underreported and under-recognized and as a result are often left undertreated (Epstein et al., 2012). Because of the unique nature of these acute toxicities, each will be described briefly in the following sections.

Table 20.1 Acute oral complications associated with treatment of head and neck cancer

Symptoms	Complication
Swollen mouth and gums, blood in the mouth, sores on mouth gums or tongue, difficulty swallowing or talking, mild burning or pain when eating, whitish patches or pus in the mouth or tongue	Mucosal; mucositis
Saliva changes, thick saliva, volume changes	Salivary glands; inflammation
Taste alteration, taste loss, neuropathic pain	Neurosensory
Pain with swallowing, coughing with meals, poor oral intake	Dysphagia

Mucositis

Oral mucositis is one of the most debilitating acute complications of cancer treatment. Mucositis results from tissue damage which occurs as a direct side effect of CRT. CT and RT have a direct influence at the cellular level. Both CT and RT serve to disrupt and breakdown the rapidly dividing epithelial cells which line the gastrointestinal tract (i.e., mouth to anus). As a direct result of this type of cellular breakdown, there also exists an increased chance of infection, as well as the potential for ulceration of tissue. Because the oral mucosa is particularly sensitive to the effects of CT and RT, the oral cavity is the most common location for mucositis to occur, in part as a result of disruptions to cytokine release by cells. Briefly, cytokines are small cellular proteins that allow cells to communicate with each other. Therefore, a locoregional breakdown of cytokines secondary to CT and RT within the gastrointestinal tract mucositis has systemic effects (Epstein et al., 2012). The most direct effects involve inflammation of tissue and tissue breakdown within the oral cavity.

Unfortunately, the details of these reactive cellular processes underlying mucositis are not entirely understood. It is known that both CT and RT can lead to direct deoxyribonucleic acid (DNA) injury and that this damage is not clinically visible or recognized until it reaches the tissue ulceration phase (Sonis, 2004). Vera-Llonch,

Oster, Hagiwara, and Sonis (2006) reported on risk factors for mucositis, such as radiation fraction size, radiated volume-area-diameter, overall treatment time, and cumulative radiation dosage. Epstein et al. (2012) have reported that chemotherapeutic agents, most notably antimetabolites and alkylating agents, resulted in a higher incidence and severity of mucositis. Similarly, Naidu, Ramana, Rani, Suman, and Roy (2004) reported that CT drugs such as etoposide and methotrexate are secreted in saliva which subsequently may increase mucosal toxicity leading to significant cellular changes.

In general, the severity of mucositis in association with CT is impacted by a low white blood cell count. With RT, the severity of mucositis is affected by the extent of cell death (necrosis) and associated inflammation. Regardless of the cause of mucositis, the tissue damage that emerges can lead to pain, increased risk of infection, open sores in the mouth, and the associated inability to eat due to these negative changes. Mucositis can become so severe in some cases that it can lead to a reduction or cessation of treatment. The mucositis severity rating scale developed by the World Health Organization (see Köstler, Hejna, Wenzel, & Zielinski, 2001; Sonis et al., 1999; World Health Organization, 1979) is widely used, and the measure incorporates assessment of functional impact as an indicator for intervention (Table 20.2).

Although full prevention of oral mucositis may not be possible, there are suggestions that may help to alleviate or lessen symptoms (see Table 20.3). The first step in managing mucositis is to consult a dentist who specialized in individuals undergoing cancer treatment (Cardosa &

Table 20.2 Mucositis severity scale: grading categories

Grade 0	No signs and symptoms
Grade 1	Painless ulcers, edema, or mild soreness
Grade 2	Pain and ulcers but can maintain ability to eat
Grade 3	Ulcers, unable to eat due to mucositis
Grade 4	Ulcers, need for parenteral or enteral support

Used with permission of World Health Organization (1979, pp. 14–18)

Table 20.3 Management of acute oral symptoms following treatment for head and neck cancer

Pain	Debris	Infection and inflammation	Dryness/ xerostomia	Oral hygiene
Ice chips, ice water, or ice pops	Baking soda and salt (1 teaspoon of table salt in 8 ounces of warm water). Rinse, gargle, and spit as needed throughout the day	Non-alcohol 0.12% chlorhexidine gluconate (NDC 52386–021-02)	Water	Frequent brushing of teeth (soft head quality)
Lidocaine	Waterpik	Paroex	Sprays, liquids, gels (Biotene, Oasis)	Brush tongue in addition to teeth
Doxepin		Orajel	Sugarless gum	Prevident toothpaste
Consider use of acetaminophen, ibuprofen, systemic narcotics, gabapentin		Fluoride – gels, rinses, toothpaste (discuss with your dentist)	Saliva stimulants (pilocarpine, cevimeline)	Floss picks (Reach Access Flosser, Oral-B Advantage)
		Antifungal (Miconazole 7)	Mucolytics (Guaifenesin, Mucinex)	Flossing with Q-tips if sensitive gumline
		Mycostatin (nystatin) *Non-premixed suspension to avoid added sugar*	Acupuncture	
		Fluconazole	Baking soda and salt	

Chambers, Chap. 21). Indications for any dental work such as tooth extractions or refitting of dentures ideally should be completed at least 1 month before starting cancer treatment. Doing so can help to increase the likelihood that the oral cavity has completely healed, thus, helping to prevent further damage to existing teeth, gums, or the mandible. Additionally, a proper, systematic oral care protocol may help prevent or decrease the severity of mucositis and subsequently help to prevent the development of infection through open sores within the oral cavity (see Cardoso & Chambers, Chap. 21; Roberts, 2016).

Additionally, RT planning and delivery via the application of intensity-modulated radiation therapy (IMRT) can help to limit a more widespread cellular damage in the radiation field (Nutting et al., 2011; Sanguineti, Endres, Gunn, & Parker, 2006). IMRT is an advanced type of radiation therapy used to treat both malignant and nonmalignant tumors. Briefly, IMRT uses advanced technology to manipulate photon and proton beams of radiation to conform to the shape of a

tumor, therefore, reducing the direct impact of radiation to healthy, non-cancerous organs, tissues, and muscle. In a small study reported by Sanguineti et al. (2006), their findings concluded that IMRT could potentially provide more mucosal sparing than do traditional approaches to radiation treatment.

At present, pharmaceutical intervention for prevention of mucositis has not been definitively identified. As an example, chlorhexidine has not been shown to prevent oral mucositis, and its use is not recommended by the Multinational Association of Supportive Care in Cancer (MASCC) or by the assessments by the Cochrane Collaboration (Keefe & Schubert, 2007; Worthington et al., 2010). According to Keefe and Schubert (2007), commercial forms of chlorhexidine rinses contain alcohol; the presence of alcohol may be poorly tolerated by patients with mucositis due to its potential for initiating further tissue irritation. However, there is a non-alcohol version of the rinse, chlorhexidine gluconate (0.12%), which can be used as a substitute, and in the United States, it does not require a prescription.

Mucositis also results in pain for many patients. Pain can be the most significant problem related to mucositis, and if present, it warrants early intervention in an effort to reduce it as much as possible. Intervention most frequently depends on the severity of the pain experienced. Pain management can range from the simple use of ice chips to large doses of gabapentin (see Table 20.3). For some, it is not uncommon for the pain to be of such severity that it may require opiates for control. However, the use of narcotics for pain control can also cause additional side effects such as constipation, and should this occur, appropriate stool softeners will need to be taken concurrently.

In a study reported by Starmer et al. (2014), it was found that gabapentin was effective in reducing pain intensity associated with mucositis. The effectiveness of its use was reported by Starmer et al. (2014) and colleagues to also lead to a decreased use of a feeding tube (FT) and to earlier FT removal. It is, however, important to note that mucositis is transient during the treatment phases, and the need for its relief can also be temporary as well. Thus, in patients who report substantial pain due to mucositis, they should not be allowed to experience pain and suffer in an effort to avoid using narcotics. For this reason, careful monitoring and management by the head and neck team provides the opportunity for timely intervention in those who suffer from mucositis.

Hyposalivation and Xerostomia

Saliva is an essential component of efficient eating and swallowing. During eating and swallowing, saliva mixes with food creating a bolus, the first step in the oral and oropharyngeal stages of swallowing; saliva also serves to trigger the digestive process. Normal stimulation of the muscarinic M3 receptors sends afferent nerve signals to the salivatory nuclei in the medulla. This nerve signal, mediated by acetylcholine, stimulates salivary glandular epithelial cells and subsequently increases salivary secretions. Saliva

is also a critical factor in normal oral health. Diminished saliva results in the risk of dental demineralization and caries and increases the risk of oral infections, mucositis, tongue fissures, dysgeusia (i.e., changes in taste), dysarthria, halitosis, oral soreness, oral burning, dysphagia, and the inability to wear dentures (Cardoso & Chambers, Chap. 21). The collective risks associated with changes in saliva volume and its chemical properties also can lead to a decreased quality of life (Duncan et al., 2005; Epstein et al., 2012; Hopcraft & Tan, 2010). Thus, a patient who reports experiencing a dry mouth over the course of treatment may be at greater risk for much broader influences on functioning over the period of treatment.

As noted, oral saliva has many critical functions specific to eating and swallowing; however, it also influences speech. Saliva is the viscous fluid secreted from the parotid, submaxillary, sublingual, and smaller mucosal glands of the oral cavity. Proteins, digestive enzymes, ions, antimicrobial constituents, and lubricating aids are found in saliva (Epstein & Scully, 1992). The most important functions of saliva include its antimicrobial activity, mechanical cleansing action, control of pH levels, removal of food debris from the oral cavity, lubrication of the oral cavity, remineralization, and maintaining the integrity of the oral mucosa (see Cardosa & Chambers, Chap. 21). The antimicrobial factors found in saliva are active against many bacteria and fungi, buffering the oral pH via bicarbonate and phosphate (Brosky, 2007; Epstein & Scully, 1992). Dental enamel integrity also is dependent upon the calcium and phosphate substrates found in saliva. Thus, a reduction in or loss of saliva production will have direct influences on eating, swallowing, and speech.

Xerostomia is the subjective complaint of a "dry mouth" that usually reflects the decreased presence of saliva (Brosky, 2007). This condition is the result of reduced or absent saliva flow secondary to treatment. Although it is not classified as a disease, it can be clinically documented, and the diminished production of saliva, or hyposalivation, can be objectively measured. This is done by placing collection devices over secretory glands and in oral orifices which are then stimulated with citric acid and measured with sialography and salivary scintigraphy. The identification of the presence of xerostomia may be based on objective measures or, more commonly, by evidence obtained from the patient's self-report and history or through a direct examination of the oral cavity.

Xerostomia is the most commonly reported acute and late-effect toxicity noted by patients treated for HNC (Murphy et al., 2010). As noted, salivary tissue is sensitive to RT, and cumulative doses greater than 30Gy can cause permanent salivary gland dysfunction (Cassolato & Turnbull, 2003). When the salivary glands are within the RT fields, there can be a dramatic impact on salivary function. RT causes xerostomia due to indirect damage to epithelial and connective tissue elements of the salivary glands, including blood vessels and nerves, or via direct injury to salivary acini and ducts, all of which affect saliva production and secretion (Baum et al., 1985; Epstein et al., 2012; Lin, Jen, Chang, & Lin, 2008). Xerostomia leads to thicker, stickier saliva, and it is often first reported around the third week of RT. Unfortunately, xerostomia will progressively worsen as the cumulative doses of radiation increases over the course of treatment.

Xerostomia and salivary gland hypofunction have been shown to strongly affect the quality of life (QOL) related to daily activities including disruption in sleep and emotional functioning, as well as those noted previously (Ettinger, 1981; Jensen et al., 2010; Sasportas et al., 2013). Acute xerostomia from radiation is due to an inflammatory reaction, while late xerostomia, a problem which can occur up to 1 year after radiation therapy, results from fibrosis of the salivary gland(s), a change that is usually permanent. Certain CT drugs can also change the composition and flow of saliva, but these changes are usually reported to be temporary (Epstein et al., 2012). It is, however, important to note that those with xerostomia run the increased risk of acquiring opportunistic infections with fungal organisms, such as candida (Epstein et al., 2012).

Because of the deficits created by xerostomia, minimizing damage to the salivary glands is a vital component of pre-treatment consideration for those undergoing treatment for HNC. The use of three-dimensional RT planning or IMRT, pharmacologic agents, and specific surgical approaches may allow for sparing of normal anatomical structures from exposure to high-dose RT (Epstein et al., 2012; Koukourakis & Danielidis, 2005; Sasportas et al., 2013). Prevention of xerostomia in the HNC population can be quite challenging and, unfortunately, may often be unsuccessful because the salivary glands are frequently so closely located to the primary tumor or lymph nodes that will be the target of treatment.

Unfortunately, at this time, there is no definitive treatment for xerostomia. A multifocal palliative care approach is frequently used today. Oral health preventive measures and palliative care suggestions are outlined in Table 20.4. Sasportas et al. (2013) have effectively provided an illustration to display the cost-effectiveness of current and emerging solutions to address xerostomia (Fig. 20.1). As the table demonstrates, there is a clear need for a low-cost, effective treatment.

Changes in Taste and Smell

A generic term *dysgeusia* is used to denote an alteration in taste perception. Historically, dysgeusia in the HNC population has been under-investigated. Dysgeusia is said to be an early complication of RT and often precedes the onset of mucositis (Denham et al., 1999; Denham & Hauer-Jensen, 2002; Irune, Dwivedi, Nutting, & Harrington, 2014; Vissink, Burlage, Spijkervet, Jansma, & Coppes, 2003). Taste alterations are frequently noted in the acute stages of treatment for HNC patients, and such changes have been reported to occur in 75% to 90% of those undergoing CRT (Irune et al., 2014; Rose-Ped et al., 2002). The cause of alterations in taste may be multifactorial, including the presence of oral infection, surgical interventions, medications, and/or RT damage to the taste buds and/or salivary glands. Malignant diseases in the head and neck also can cause taste changes due to postsurgical wounds, oral bleeding, and tissue necrosis.

Table 20.4   Guidelines for xerostomia and maintenance of oral health

Oral health	Palliative care	Others
Meticulous oral hygiene	Drink and oral rinse with *tap* water (contains fluoride)	Low-sugar diet
Multiple daily brushing with compact soft head power brush	Xylitol gum	Low-acid diet
Multiple daily flossing with flossing tool	Sugarless candy	Reduce or eliminate medications, when possible, that could exacerbate xerostomia (antianxiety, antidepressants, antihypertensives, or opioid analgesics)
Use cotton swabs to clean sensitive areas	OTC and prescription saliva substitutes	Well-fitting dentures
Antibacterial rinses (*alcohol-free*)	Moisturizing agents (Biotene, Oasis)	Avoid caffeine
Fluoride rinse (alcohol-free) or gels	Room humidification	Avoid citrus and spicy foods
Frequent dental appointments with dentist familiar with cancer patients	Use of personal steam inhaler	Tobacco cessation
		Reduce or eliminate mouth breathing
		Acupuncture specific to xerostomia
		Avoid sugar-containing soft drinks and snacks between meals

In contrast, CT may similarly affect taste, but this may be the result of the treatment directly impacting taste receptor stimulation due to secretions in saliva or gingival crevice fluid. Thus, taste changes may persist after drug clearance due to damage to receptors of taste buds (Bergdahl & Bergdahl, 2002; Epstein et al., 2012; Hauer-Jensen, Fink, & Wang, 2004). As an additional note, it is not uncommon for patients to report a perception of a metallic or chemical taste at the time when CT is being delivered.

Taste buds can be found in all areas of the tongue, in the epithelia of the pharynx, and near laryngeal surfaces of the upper aerodigestive tract. The five primary taste qualities are sweet, sour, bitter, salty, and umami (savoriness). Direct cytotoxic and anti-proliferation effects on tissues during RT are the likely cause of a loss of taste buds during the acute stage of treatment (Irune et al., 2014). Additionally, damage to the nerves necessary to process taste function also may be a factor in treatment-related dysgeusia (Mossman, 1986). Hyposalivation has also been implicated in the development of dysgeusia as decreased saliva secretion alters the number of chemicals released by foods which can then subsequently alter taste perception (Wasserman, 2012).

Regardless of pathophysiology, dysgeusia is based on a subjective report by the patient and it is rare that an objective examination is performed. Unfortunately, dysgeusia is seldom mentioned or reported unless the health-care provider specifically asks whether the patient is experiencing such problems (Bernhardson, Tishelman, & Rutqvist, 2007, 2008) or if such a concern is offered without request. Thus, seeking information about changes in taste in general or in relation to eating through direct questioning over the course of treatment is essential. Steinbach et al. (2009) found most food aversions secondary to perceived changes in taste were related to consumption of meat, followed by chocolate, fruit, and coffee. Taste sensations are also varied, with some patients reporting chemosensory changes in taste that are described as perceptions of the taste of "saw dust," "toilet paper," and "metal" (Bernhardson et al., 2008).

The onset of taste impairment for CRT patients also can be variable, but it has been reported to occur as early as 3 weeks from the start of

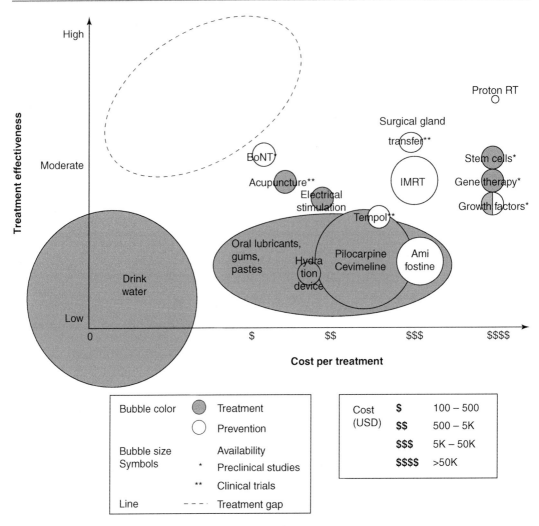

Fig. 20.1 Treatment gap analysis. Synthesis of the solutions for addressing xerostomia in H&N cancer patients undergoing RT. The solutions are summarized in a graph showing the effectiveness of the solution at treating or preventing xerostomia versus the cost per treatment. The solutions are categorized according to the following criteria: treatment versus prevention and preclinical versus clinical stage. Relative clinical availability is also estimated and represented as bubble size. Highlighted by the dashed circle is the treatment gap, which corresponds to the area of greatest innovation opportunity. (From Sasportas et al. (2013), Fig. 1, with permission of Elsevier)

treatment (Irune et al., 2014; Sandow, Hejrat-Yazdi, & Heft, 2006). All qualities of taste can be affected, but bitter and salt receptors tend to be affected earliest and to the most significant extent (Irune et al., 2014). Improvements in taste have been observed as early as 6–8 weeks after treatment has ended, and complete recovery has been reported to occur within 1-year posttreatment (Tomita & Osaki, 1990). However, it is of interest that the loss of umami may have the strongest correlation with decreased QOL (Shi et al.,

2004). There is, nevertheless, a general paucity of research in this area of sensory loss and its recovery, and many of the studies in the literature report on only a limited number of participants.

The treatment for dysgeusia is limited to patient education and non-pharmacologic management, but the negative effects of such changes should not be undervalued. Taste alterations can lead to food aversion, decreased oral intake, weight loss, and ultimately malnutrition (Irune et al., 2014; Lynch, Theurer, & Doyle, 2018;

Table 20.5 Summary of suggestions for dysgeusia

Chewing gum or sucking on candy may mask unpleasant tastes
Adding seasoning and spices to foods, especially umami flavoring
Add small amounts of sugar to decrease salty or bitter tastes
Add fats and sauces to foods
Mild flavor protein (eggs, tofu, turkey, chicken)
Cold or room temperature foods
Increase water intake throughout the day to rinse away bad taste
Smaller meals throughout the day
Marinate meats to change the taste
Avoid bitter or metallic tasting foods such as coffee, chocolate, and red meat
Avoid the use of metallic silverware
Zinc supplementation

McLaughlin, 2013). Therefore, as part of comprehensive cancer care, health professionals working with those treated for HNC should be encouraged to actively seek to identify the problem and offer supportive measures as needed. A list of suggestions that may be of benefit to clinicians and patients is provided Table 20.5.

Dysphagia

Dysphagia, by definition, means merely a difficulty in swallowing. Although it has been addressed more comprehensively in this volume (see Starmer, Chap. 18, and Arrese & Shieve, Chap. 19), oropharyngeal dysphagia is an underestimated problem that occurs in those treated for HNC patients (Pignon, le Maitre, Maillard, & Bourhis, 2009; Feng et al., 2010). Acute dysphagia is often less concerning given that it can be transient; however, should it persist without resolution, it can lead to malnutrition that can lead to morbidity with associated decreases in QOL and in some instances mortality. Acute dysphagia also may increase late effects such as fibrosis and lymphedema which may result in increased dysphagia severity (Smith, Chap. 22; Trotti et al., 2003). During the acute phase of CRT, mucositis, xerostomia, and dysgeusia can contribute further to difficulties in swallowing. Additionally,

fatigue, reduced appetite, nausea/vomiting, edema, and odynophagia can all contribute to the inability "to swallow" with an additional impact on overall perceived QOL.

In the last few years, active efforts to limit RT exposure to those structures essential for swallowing, mastication, and salivation have been pursued. Several studies have sought to identify the dysphagia/aspiration-related structures such as the pharyngeal constrictors, tongue base, and larynx (Eisbruch et al., 2004). It is clear that efforts to reduce the amount of radiation exposure via dosimetric constraints may reduce the impact of RT on swallowing ability (Goldstein, Maxymiw, Cummings, & Wood, 1999; Nutting, 2012). Similarly, information from reports of RT techniques that seek to spare key swallowing structures have suggested that doing so results in improved judgments of overall QOL (see Cardoso & Chambers, Chap. 21; Nutting et al., 2011).

Understanding the etiology of acute swallowing changes that occur during or in the early period following treatment is essential. Treatment recommendations can vary from those directed at managing pain to specific swallowing facilitation techniques. A common mistake of speech pathologists who are not as familiar with the HNC population is to recommend non-oral nutrition or tube feedings without any oral stimulation or oral trials. The practice of feeding tube use varies considerably from center to center for those treated for HNC. When safe oral feeding is not possible, non-oral nutrition is essential for the maintenance of hydration and calorie needs; however, oral trials and oral nutrition should continue as much as tolerated by patients, even if only an intake of ice chips is possible (Table 20.6). Active use and stimulation of the oropharyngeal swallow also may be of benefit in reducing late-stage dysphagia. Finally, the active clearance of residual debris in the oral cavity is a major component of oral management during the early period of treatment when acute deficits begin to emerge. However, acute problems can also persist over time, and in some instances, chronic and late-stage changes will occur in those treated for HNC. Aspects of chronic and late-

Table 20.6 Multifactorial suggestions for management of acute dysphagia

Hydration/calories
Fluids most important/water throughout the day
"Grazers"
Scandishakes
Dinner in a bag
Benecalorie
Water
Ice chips
Warm/cold
Pedialyte popsicles
Lubrication
Steam inhalation
Moist and slippery
Sponges
Oral hygiene
Tube feedings→ still swallow as tolerated

stage toxicities will be addressed in the subsequent portion of this chapter.

Chronic and Late Toxicities

Chronic Versus Late Radiation-Associated Dysphagia

Chronic effects of RT are identified to occur at 6 months to 5 years post-treatment, whereas late effects are described as the development or progression of dysphagia in disease-free HNC patients after 5 years (Hutcheson et al., 2013). Perhaps the most concerning issue that negatively affects swallowing at both the chronic and late stages is that of tissue fibrosis. Fibrosis is an insidious and irreversible problem, the effects of which may cause dysphagia. For this reason, fibrosis warrants some detailed discussion in the section to follow.

Fibrosis

Radiation fibrosis is characterized by a loss of vascularity and disorganization of the complex tissue meshwork called the extracellular matrix. The extracellular matrix fills the space between cells and provides structural support for the cells

within tissue. Extracellular matrix also guides cell division and growth. Thus, the loss of tissue vascularity and disorganization of the extracellular matrix will disrupt well-defined, compartmentalized structures (King, Dunlap, Tennant, & Pitts, 2016). This in turn will affect tissue structure and function. When relating information about radiation fibrosis to those treated for HNC, we find that using the term "scar tissue" often facilitates the patient's understanding of the condition.

Fibrosis can affect any human tissue including the skin, muscle, blood vessels, ligaments, tendons, nerve, and bone (Stubblefield, 2011). In the case of HNC, small blood vessels in the radiation field are more susceptible to damage and can become sclerotic or less pliable, causing areas of tissue that will no longer receive an adequate blood supply. This devascularization of the radiated field makes tissues more "friable" or brittle, placing the patient at risk for tissue breakdown and the potential development of a fistula(s) among other complication sequelae from reduced tissue integrity. Changes of this type have the potential to negatively influence both speech and swallowing with a resultant impact on long-term rehabilitation outcomes.

As noted, fibrosis is a chronic to late complication of RT. However, it must be acknowledged that fibrosis can manifest clinically from many months to many years after treatment has been completed. As mentioned previously, fibrosis is usually insidious, but when it does manifest, it may progress rapidly. Unlike lymphedema (Smith, Chap. 22), it is important to note that in all cases, fibrosis is an irreversible problem (Johansson, Svensson, & Denekamp, 2000, 2002). Although the underlying mechanism causing fibrosis is not well understood, a disturbance to normal cellular behavior is thought to be the primary factor in its development, a change that may lead to dysfunction in both speech communication and swallowing (Lin, Jen, & Lin, 2002). Despite the lack of a clear underlying mechanism of tissue change, fibrosis is the result of specific pathologic features that include progressive collagen accumulation, permanent fiber disorganization of any tissue, altered microvasculature, production of pro-fibrotic growth factors, and loss of tissue elasticity (Martin, Lefaix, Pinton, Crechet, & Daburon, 1993; Remy, Wegrowski, Crechet, Martin, & Daburon, 1991). When the pathologic processes that underlie fibrotic changes in the chronic stage continue over time, abnormalities can expand over multiple anatomical areas and compartments such as those related to the base of tongue, valleculae, and epiglottis, which may result in entrapment of underlying muscle and nerves (Remy et al., 1991).

For example, when the primary site of cancer is the base of the tongue and RT is employed, the pharyngeal constrictor muscles will be in the radiation field. Due to the side effects of RT, some individuals may initially demonstrate reduced bolus propulsion when swallowing, an observation that may be due to swelling in the region. However, if chronic and late-stage fibrosis develops in these same areas, there may be entrapment of the muscles and limitations in strength and range of motion, resulting in profoundly impaired swallowing. For a dysphagia therapist, when a patient is at the point of oropharyngeal late-stage fibrosis, there is to date very little evidence-based treatment that can be provided to restore the oropharyngeal swallow. Thus, if late-stage fibrosis develops in the pharynx and larynx, the patient's ability to propel a bolus and protect the airway from aspiration can be profoundly impaired. If this is observed, an instrumental swallowing evaluation will typically reveal that there is no range of motion for the critical anatomy required for swallowing or airway protection. In such circumstances, it is possible that the fibrosis has progressed to the point of what is referred to as "radiation fibrosis syndrome" (Stubblefield, 2011).

The term radiation fibrosis syndrome refers to a multitude of clinical manifestations that can occur secondary to the development of progressive fibrosis (Stubblefield, 2011). As noted previously, radiation fibrosis can affect any tissue (skin, muscle, nerve, and bone). For this reason, those in the HNC population are at very high risk for developing radiation fibrosis syndrome because of the high doses of radiation required for tumor treatment and the very close proximity

of various tissues to the radiation field (Marcus & Tishler, 2010). Conformal radiation is a technique in which the exact shape of the tumor is programmed into a computer and used to plan the radiation treatment. This type a radiation treatment can reduce dose/effects on surrounding normal tissues and to some extent reduce risk of a fibrotic change.

Radiation to surrounding normal tissues, known as a "bystander dose," may impact key swallowing structures such as the base of tongue, pharyngeal constrictor muscles, and the larynx and is frequently an unavoidable consequence of RT. Additionally, this increased risk is also the result of radiation fields that must adequately cover the primary treatment targets (Rosenthal et al., 2008; Stubblefield, 2011). While the primary goal of RT is to eliminate the cancer cells, there is an effort to minimize exposure to other areas and structures during the treatment process. However, in the case of HNC, the close proximity of many anatomical structures and their relationship to the site of the primary tumor increases the possibility that normal tissue in the region can inadvertently receive a significant dose of radiation. Once radiated, this otherwise "normal" tissue is subject to the same potential side effects as are those tissues that comprise the cancer itself.

Late Radiation-Associated Dysphagia

Late radiation-associated dysphagia (late-RAD) was defined by Hutcheson et al. (2013) as a distinct clinical disorder. This disorder is described as "dysphagia that develops or progresses in disease-free HNC survivors 5 or more years after completion of radiation therapy" (Hutcheson et al., 2013, p. 1127). Hutcheson et al. found that there was physiologic impairment in 100% of late-RAD head and neck cancer patients. This impairment involved deficits in laryngeal elevation, epiglottis retroflexion, base of tongue retraction, and pharyngeal wall contraction. Due to these changes, Hutcheson et al. (2013). reported that those with late-RAD exhibited poor propulsive forces to move a bolus efficiently through the pharynx, profound likelihood of exhibiting pharyngeal residue, frequent silent aspiration, and trismus. These impairments are likely to contribute to dysphagia in those who present with late-RAD. Because of the physiologic deficits identified, information related to impairments at the neuromuscular and musculoskeletal levels will be reviewed in the sections to follow.

Neuromuscular: Sensory Loss and Weakness in HNC

Neuromuscular control of head and neck structures is an essential component of normal functioning for speech, eating, and swallowing. Sensory deprivation and weakness are commonly observed clinical features of dysphagia when there is peripheral nerve or nerve root involvement due to radiation. Sensory input specific to bolus size, taste, consistency, and temperature can be reduced when neuromuscular changes occur; such changes subsequently place the patient at risk for aspiration (Arrese & Schieve, Chap. 19). Disruption of these intricate sensory pathways that influence structures of the head and neck causes hyposensitivity, and the resultant minimum sensory thresholds will be insufficient to signal the pattern generators to trigger a swallow or a cough (Stubblefield, 2011). The post-radiation deficit of hyposensitivity is likely responsible for the increased incidence of silent aspiration in those treated for HNC. That is, when neural signals cannot be processed in a normal fashion, a variety of deficits to the larger control mechanisms of this complex system are likely to be influenced.

Motor weakness is a common side effect of radiation-induced abnormalities in the oropharyngeal system. These changes can be caused by treatment-related damage to a peripheral nerve(s) and the muscle(s) that such nerves innervate. Radiation-induced myelopathy in late-RAD is almost always progressive and permanent (Giglio & Gilbert, 2010). When muscle weakness involves structures that serve the base of tongue or the pharyngeal constrictors, bolus propulsion will be significantly reduced, thus, placing the patient at risk of aspiration both during and after the swallowing process.

A cricopharyngeal stricture or narrowing at the cricopharyngeus (CP) muscle is a known complication of RT to the area. A stricture can impede the bolus from moving from the pharynx to the esophagus. However, it is important for the dysphagia therapist working with the HNC patient to pay close attention to all the parameters that may serve to facilitate opening of the CP muscle before diagnosing a stricture at this level. For normal CP opening, the following must occur: (1) CP relaxation, (2) adequate anterior movement of the hyoid bone, and (3) adequate propulsive forces of the bolus to distend the CP. Once these three events occur in sequence, the CP will be wide enough for the bolus to pass through into the esophagus without backflow of material into the pyriform sinuses. If radiation fibrosis is present and results in muscular weakness and limited range of motion, the hyoid bone may not be able to move anteriorly. Should this lack of anterior hyoid movement occur, there will be insufficient traction placed on the CP which serves to widen its lumen, an action which is necessary for normal swallowing. Furthermore, the propulsive forces on the bolus from the base of tongue and pharyngeal constrictors may not be enough to distend the CP. In this case, if the dysphagia therapist recommends a dilation procedure, it will have little if any effect on the patient's swallowing ability since the propulsive forces are poor.

Musculoskeletal: Loss of Elasticity and Range of Motion in HNC

The clinical effect of radiation on ligaments and tendons in the late stages is progressive fibrosis with loss of elasticity, shortening, and contracture, resulting in loss of function and range of motion (Stubblefield, 2011). For those treated for HNC, this can lead to functional changes in a variety of areas including deficits in speech articulation, vocal changes or dysphonia, and/or trismus. Trismus is the impaired ability to open the mouth beyond an intrinsic measurement distance of 35 cm. Surgery and radiation are the primary causes of trismus (Bensadoun et al.,

2010), and its prevalence is reported to occur in up to 45% of patients who receive curative doses of radiotherapy (Jeremic et al., 2011; Kent et al., 2008). Depending on its severity, trismus can reduce one's ability to place and manipulate a bolus of food in the mouth, masticate food, receive dental care, maintain regular oral hygiene, and receive required oral examinations as part of regular cancer surveillance (see Cardoso & Chambers, Chap. 21).

Radiation damage to the vascular system including the small arteries that carry nutrients and oxygen to the bone can also cause osteoradionecrosis (ORN) (Leeper, Gratton, Lapointe, & Armstrong, 2005; Stubblefield, 2011). With ORN, the bone will eventually become brittle and weak which carries additional risks (Cardoso & Chambers, Chap. 21). This is the reason why all patients who are to receive CRT where the mandible will be in the radiation field are recommended to have all unsalvageable teeth extracted before treatment. If tooth extraction is done after RT in a patient with ORN of the mandible, there can be serious complications (Teng & Futran, 2005). Finally, ill-fitting dentures that are worn after RT further increases the risk of ORN, and thus, wearing them should be avoided (Mendenhall, 2004).

Hyperbaric oxygenation (HBO) therapy is the primary treatment for ORN. Exposure to pure oxygen at increased pressures of 2–4.5 ppsi is typical. The increased pressure allows for increased circulation and oxygen uptake by the cells which theoretically enhance healing of bone necrosis (Bennett, Feldmeier, Hampson, Smee, & Milross, 2012). Fritz, Gunsolley, Abubaker, and Laskin (2010) completed a systematic review of 696 articles which appeared in the literature between January 1948 and March 2008 and concluded there is insufficient evidence to support the belief that the use of HBO reduces ORN in patients requiring tooth extraction. Similarly, Annane et al. (2004) reported that the efficacy of HBO is based almost exclusively on uncontrolled studies. Annane et al. (2004). reported on a prospective randomized trial that compared HBO to a placebo in 68 patients. Their study "failed to show any beneficial effect of HBO in patients

with overt mandibular radionecrosis" (p. 4896). Additionally, Annane et al. (2004, p. 4896) reported that "HBO failed to slow the progression of the disease and to accelerate pain relief."

Given the unknown efficacy of HBO and calls for further investigation of this treatment approach in the literature, the post-irradiated HNC patient should be fully educated and aware of the risks of developing ORN. Unfortunately, some risk factors are not under the patient's control, including the stage of the primary tumor, the proximity of tumor to the bone, dentition, and type of treatment. According to Mendenhall (2004), factors such as nutritional status and continued tobacco or alcohol abuse probably influence an increased likelihood of developing ORN. If the patient's dentition is determined to be healthy before radiation, however, it is important to ensure regular dental care and excellent oral/dental hygiene to reduce the potential for radiation caries (see Cardoso & Chambers, Chap. 21).

Radiation Caries

When salivary glands, oral mucosa, and the mandible are in the radiation field, hyposalivation and xerostomia can occur. Irradiated patients are at an increased risk for the development of a rapid and rampant carious process called radiation caries (Aguilar, Jham, Magalhaes, Sensi, & Freire, 2009; Cardoso & Chambers, Chap. 21). Radiation caries is defined as tooth decay that results from radiation-induced xerostomia. The lack of normal saliva which serves to destroy oral bacteria reduces the patient's ability to remineralize the tooth enamel following RT. Xerostomia decreases the pH balance within the oral cavity, which in turn significantly increases plaque and tooth decay (Aguilar et al., 2009). Therefore, the development of radiation caries indicates that there are more bacteria in the oral cavity due to the tooth decay. If oral bacteria are aspirated as the patient swallows saliva, eats, or drinks, it can place them at an increased risk for an aspiration pneumonia. Given the potential for swallowing deficits described earlier in this chapter and elsewhere

(Arrese & Schieve, Chap. 19), this risk cannot be understated. Therefore, it is important to educate all who undergo treatment for HNC regarding oral hygiene and the need for regular dental visits as part of overall postradiation health care (Cardoso & Chambers, Chap. 21).

Lymphedema

Lymphedema is defined as swelling caused by impaired tissue drainage when the lymphatic load exceeds the transport capacity of the lymphatic system. Lymphedema is due to either vascular malformation or acquired damage to the lymphatic system (Foldi & Foldi, 2006; Smith, Chap. 22). This inadequate drainage of fluid from tissues of the head and neck results in an overload of high protein lymphatic fluid within the interstitial tissues. Chronic tissue lymphostasis causes tissue inflammation that increases tissue fibrosis, which can subsequently increase functional impairment (Foldi & Foldi, 2006). The effects of lymphedema are not just cosmetic (Smith, Chap. 22). Lymphedema of the face, mouth, and neck can cause significant functional deficits in both communication and swallowing (Lewin, Hutcheson, Smith, Barringer, & Alvarez, 2009; Smith & Lewin, 2010). For this reason, *complete decongestive therapy* (CDT) is widely accepted as the best current treatment of lymphedema. Additional and detailed information on CDT is provided by Smith (Chap. 22).

Evaluation and Treatment of Dysphagia

Assessment and management of dysphagia requires multidisciplinary input including that of the physician/surgeon, dentist, and SLP. A recurrence of cancer or another medical condition must be excluded as the etiology of the dysphagia, and the status of the patient's dentition will also affect their diet level. The SLP's evaluation is likely to include a cranial nerve exam, oral motor speech exam, trismus screening, and clinical swallowing assessment (see Arrese & Shieve,

Chap. 19; Hutcheson et al., 2013; Starmer, Chap. 18). Given that the anatomy and physiology in those with HNC are likely to be altered significantly regardless of the modality of treatment, imaging studies such as a video fluoroscopic swallowing study (VFSS), flexible endoscopic evaluation of swallowing (FEES), and videostroboscopy are informative components of the evaluation.

The results of the swallowing evaluation are likely to provide the SLP with a detailed analysis of swallowing function, and several compensatory techniques may be employed in therapy to mitigate dysphagia symptoms. Given what is known about fibrosis in late radiation-associated dysphagia, therapists will often require more information to provide evidence-based treatment to facilitate improved swallowing function. Some of the many questions that arise include whether swallow and non-swallow exercises are effective, whether treatment should start before, during, or after CRT, whether ordinary swallowing is an exercise, and if a patient has undergone a percutaneous endoscopic gastrostomy (PEG) and is PEG dependent, how much swallowing therapy will be helpful? Currently, there is no definitive swallowing paradigm for restorative dysphagia therapy. There is some evidence suggesting that eating and exercising during CRT decreases the duration of PEG dependence and disuse atrophy (Crary, Carnaby, Lagorio, & Carvajal, 2012), but further confirmation of these data is necessary. Data related to PEG dependence in individuals who did not eat during CRT have demonstrated a longer duration of PEG dependence; the longest duration of dependence was observed in those who did not eat or exercise (Hutcheson et al., 2013).

Impaired strength and range of motion (ROM) for musculature comprising the base of the tongue, pharynx, and hyolaryngeal complex are the primary factors contributing to the dysphagia in late-RAD. The impaired strength and ROM are due to the underlying fibrotic process, and any dysphagia program must target these areas of impairment (Hutcheson et al., 2013). Progressive resistance exercise protocols report functional gains among patients with refractory dysphagia many years after completion of CRT (Crary et al., 2012). Additional information on dysphagia is provided by Starmer (Chap. 18) and Arrese and Schieve (Chap. 19).

Based on existing data, beginning swallowing treatment before CRT is initiated may have some benefit. Normal muscles display significant plasticity with exercise. Muscles must have efficient antioxidant capabilities to combat the effects of RT that lead to fibrosis (De Lisio et al., 2011). Other fields have demonstrated that preconditioning was shown to increase antioxidant enzymes in the tissue (Citrin et al., 2010). For this reason, pre-radiation prophylactic dysphagia therapy could be used to increase antioxidant capabilities which may increase muscle fatigue resistance attributed to the oxidative stress during radiation therapy (Adhihetty, Irrcher, Joseph, Ljubicic, & Hood, 2003; Hood, 2001). Irradiation inhibits the energy capacity and contractile mechanism needed for the muscle to make gains from repetitive, strength-based exercises; therefore, starting swallowing exercises before CRT may be more useful for improved swallowing outcomes.

The challenge with any potential application of pre-radiation exercises and this type of prophylactic treatment paradigm will be influenced by compliance (see Starmer, Chap. 24). In a study of 98 participants on their adherence to preventative exercises in postradiated HNC, Shinn et al. (2013) reported that only 13% were adherent, 32% were partially adherent, and 55% were non-adherent. The reasons for non-compliance were a general lack of understanding about the importance of the exercises, limited information on radiation side effects which may interfere with the ability to complete the exercises, and, unfortunately, simply forgetting to do the exercises. Further information on the general issue of adherence to treatment regimes in those with HNC is addressed by Starmer (Chap. 18).

Finally, in those who receive CRT, dysphagia can occur at any stage of cancer treatment, and it may continue throughout the healing stages and for many years afterward. Some patients may only report minimal dysphagia during the early stages of treatment but then report significant impairments in the chronic stages; this may also occur in reverse order in some instances. With what is currently known about swallowing and CRT, the goal is to keep the patient eating by mouth or per oris (PO) during treatment in order minimize disuse atrophy. Disuse of swallowing is likely to lead to rapid and irreversible functional decline, especially in patients with fibrosis (King et al., 2016). In such instances, the patient may require instruction related to compensatory techniques so that they can learn to swallow without aspiration. This may require a lifelong use of the techniques; therefore, keeping compensations to a minimum while insuring that they are effective is important. If successfully employed, such an approach may be of value in maintaining the most natural swallow for long-term use. Restorative swallowing therapy research is ongoing. More information is certainly needed to identify the exact paradigm, frequency, and intensity that is effective for improving an impaired swallow after CRT. Intensive outpatient training with a progressive resistance exercise protocol may be helpful and likely most beneficial if begun before CRT commences.

Conclusions

The side effects of both RT and CRT can occur in the acute, chronic, and/or late stages post-treatment. The most common acute side effects include mucositis, xerostomia, dysphagia, odynophagia, and an altered sense of smell and taste. These acute effects are often less concerning given the transient nature in the overall treatment of the oropharyngeal cancer. However, if not identified, these problems can lead to malnutrition and can impact morbidity, mortality and perceived quality of life. Chronic effects of CRT occur from 6 months to 5 years post-treatment, and late effects occur after 5 years in a disease-free HNC survivor. Tissue fibrosis in the chronic and late stages is perhaps the most concerning issue causing dysphagia. Research to mitigate fibrosis is ongoing, but currently there is no ability to reduce fibrosis once it has occurred. When oral feeding is not safe or sufficient due to treatment-related dysphagia, tube feeding may be necessary to assure nutrition and hydration. The authors stress the importance of patient education and encouragement of continued oral trials and oral nutrition as much as tolerated; consistent and active use and stimulation of the oropharyngeal swallow may be of benefit in reducing late-stage dysphagia. Current research suggests that the goal is to keep the patient eating by mouth throughout treatment and during the healing stages to minimize disuse atrophy. The patient may require lifelong use of techniques to swallow safely, so minimizing compensations while assuring they are effective is important. Finally, restorative swallowing therapy research continues in that clinical area, and it is anticipated that an effective treatment paradigm, as well as the frequency and intensity of therapy will be determined in hopes of improving impaired swallowing after CRT.

References

Adhihetty, P. J., Irrcher, I., Joseph, A. M., Ljubicic, V., & Hood, D. A. (2003). Plasticity of skeletal muscle mitochondria in response to contractile activity. *Experimental Physiology, 88*(1), 99–107.

Aguilar, G. P., Jham, B. C., Magalhaes, C. S., Sensi, L. G., & Freire, A. R. (2009). A review of the biological and clinical aspects of radiation caries. *The Journal of Contemporary Dental Practice, 10*(4), 1–11.

Annane, D., Depondt, J., Aubert, P., Villart, M., Géhanno, P., Gajdos, P., & Chevret, S. (2004). Hyperbaric oxygen therapy for radionecrosis of the jaw: A randomized, placebo-controlled, double-blind trial from the ORN96 study group. *Journal of Clinical Oncology, 22*(24), 4893–4900.

Baum, B. J., Bodner, L., Fox, P. C., Izutsu, K. T., Pizzo, P. A., & Wright, W. E. (1985). Therapy-induced dysfunction of salivary glands: Implications for oral health. *Special Care in Dentistry, 5*(6), 274–277.

Bennett, M. H., Feldmeier, J., Hampson, N., Smee, E., & Milross, C. (2012). Hyperbaric oxygen therapy for late radiation tissue injury. *Cochrane Database of Systematic Reviews, 5.* https://doi.org/10.1002/14651858.CD005005.pub3

Bensadoun, R. J., Riesenbeck, D., Lockhart, P. B., Elting, L. S., Spijkervet, F. K., & Brennan, M. T. (2010). A systematic review of trismus induced by cancer therapies in head and neck cancer patients. *Supportive Care in Cancer, 18*(8), 1033–1038.

Bergdahl, M., & Bergdahl, J. (2002). Perceived taste disturbance in adults: Prevalence and association with oral and psychological factors and medication. *Clinical Oral Investigations, 6*(3), 145–149.

Bernhardson, B.-M., Tishelman, C., & Rutqvist, L. E. (2007). Chemosensory changes experienced by patients undergoing cancer chemotherapy: A qualitative interview study. *Journal of Pain and Symptom Management, 34*, 403–411. https://doi.org/10.1016/j.jpainsymman.2006.12.010

Bernhardson, B.-M., Tishelman, C., & Rutqvist, L. E. (2008). Self-reported taste and smell changes during cancer chemotherapy. *Supportive Care in Cancer, 16*, 275–283. https://doi.org/10.1007/s00520-007-0319-7

Brosky, M. E. (2007). The role of saliva in oral health: Strategies for prevention and management of xerostomia. *Journal of Supportive Oncology, 5*(5), 215–225.

Cassolato, S. F., & Turnbull, R. S. (2003). Xerostomia: Clinical aspects and treatment. *Gerodontology, 20*(2), 64–77.

Centers for Disease Control (CDC). (2017). *HPV-related oropharyngeal cancers by race and ethnicity in the United States.* Retrieved 6/2/2017 from https://www.cdc.gov/cancer/hpv/statistics/headneck.htm.

Chaturvedi, A. K., Engels, E. A., Anderson, W. F., & Gillison, M. L. (2008). Incidence trends for human papillomavirus-related and unrelated oral squamous cell carcinomas in the United States. *Journal of Clinical Oncology, 24*(4), 612–619.

Chaturvedi, A. K., Engels, E. A., Pfeiffer, R. M., Hernandez, B. Y., Xiao, W., Kim, E., & Gillison, M. L. (2011). Human papillomavirus and rising oropharyngeal cancer incidence in the United States. *Journal of Clinical Oncology, 29*(32), 4294–4301.

Citrin, D., Cotrim, A. P., Hyodo, F., Baum, B. J., Krishna, M. C., & Mitchell, J. B. (2010). Radioprotectors and mitigators of radiation-induced normal tissue injury. *The Oncologist, 15*(4), 360–371.

Cognetti, D. M., Weber, R. S., & Lai, S. Y. (2008). Head and neck cancer. *Cancer, 113*(S7), 1911–1932.

Crary, M. A., Carnaby, G. D., Lagorio, L. A., & Carvajal, P. J. (2012). Functional and physiological outcomes from an exercises-based dysphagia therapy: A pilot investigation of the McNeill Dysphagia Therapy Program. *Archives of Physical Medicine and Rehabilitation, 93*(7), 1173–1178.

De Lisio, M., Kaczor, J. J., Phan, N., Tarnopolsky, M. A., Boreham, D. R., & Parise, G. (2011). Exercise training enhances the skeletal muscle response to radiation-induced oxidative stress. *Muscle & Nerve, 43*(1), 58–64.

Denham, J. W., & Hauer-Jensen, M. (2002). The radiotherapeutic injury – a complex "wound". *Radiotherapy Oncology, 63*(2), 129–145.

Denham, J. W., Peters, L. J., Johansen, J., Poulsen, M., Lamb, D. S., Hindley, A., … Williamson, S. (1999). Do acute mucosal reactions lead to consequential late reactions in patients with head and neck cancer? *Radiotherapy and Oncology, 52*(2), 157–164.

Duncan, G. G., Epstein, J. B., Tu, D., Sayed, S. E., Bezjak, A., Ottaway, J., & Pater, J. (2005). Quality of life, mucositis, and xerostomia from radiotherapy for head and neck cancers: A report from the NCIC CTG HN2 randomized trial of an antimicrobial lozenge to prevent mucositis. *Head & Neck, 27*(5), 421–428.

Eisbruch, A., Schwartz, M., Rasch, C., Vineberg, K., Damen, E., van As, C. J., … Balm, A. J. (2004). Dysphagia and aspiration after chemoradiotherapy for head-and-neck cancer: Which anatomic structures are affected and can they be spared by IMRT? *International Journal of Radiation Oncology, Biology, and Physics, 60*(5), 1425–1439.

Epstein, J. B., & Scully, C. (1992). The role of saliva in oral health and the causes and effects of xerostomia. *Journal of the Canadian Dental Association, 58*(3), 217–221.

Epstein, J. B., Thariat, J., Bensadoun, R. J., Barasch, A., Murphy, B. A., Kolnick, L., … Maghami, E. (2012). Oral complications of cancer and cancer therapy. *CA: A Cancer Journal for Clinicians, 62*(6), 400–422.

Ettinger, R. L. (1981). Xerostomia—a complication of aging. *Australian Dental Journal, 26*(6), 365–371.

Feng, F. Y., Kim, H. M., Lyden, T. H., Haxer, M. J., Worden, F. P., Feng, M., … Bradford, C. R. (2010). Intensity-modulated chemoradiotherapy aiming to reduce dysphagia in patients with oropharyngeal cancer: Clinical and functional results. *Journal of Clinical Oncology, 28*(16), 2732–2738.

Foldi, M., & Foldi, E. (2006). Lymphostasis diseases. In R. H. Strossenrither & S. Kubix (Eds.), *Foldi's textbook of Lymphology for physicians and lymphedema therapists* (pp. 224–240). New York: Elsevier.

Forastiere, A. A., Goepfert, H., Maor, M., Pajak, T. F., Weber, R., Morrison, W., … Peters, G. (2003). Concurrent chemotherapy and radiotherapy for organ preservation in advanced laryngeal cancer. *New England Journal of Medicine, 349*(22), 2091–2098.

Fritz, G. W., Gunsolley, J. C., Abubaker, O., & Laskin, D. M. (2010). Efficacy of pre- and postirradiation hyperbaric oxygen therapy in the prevention of postextraction osteoradionecrosis: A systematic review. *Journal of Oral and Maxillofacial Surgery, 68*(11), 2653–2660.

Giglio, P., & Gilbert, M. R. (2010). Neurologic complications of cancer and its treatment. *Current Oncology Reports, 12*, 50–59.

Goldstein, M., Maxymiw, W. G., Cummings, B. J., & Wood, R. E. (1999). The effects of antitumor irradiation on mandibular opening and mobility: A prospective study of 58 patients. *Oral Surgery, Oral Medicine, Oral Pathology, Oral Radiology, and Endodontology, 88*(3), 365–373.

Hauer-Jensen, M., Fink, L. M., & Wang, J. (2004). Radiation injury and the protein C pathway. *Critical Care Medicine, 32*(5), 325–330.

Hood, D. A. (2001). Invited review: Contractile activity-induced mitochondrial biogenesis in skeletal muscle. *Journal of Applied Physiology, 90*(3), 1135–1157.

Hopcraft, M. S., & Tan, C. (2010). Xerostomia: An update for clinicians. *Australian Dental Journal, 55*(3), 238–244.

Hutcheson, K. A., Bhayani, M. K., & Lewin, J. (2013). Use it or lose it: Eat and exercise during radiotherapy or chemoradiotherapy for pharyngeal cancers. *JAMA Otolaryngology – Head & Neck Surgery, 139*(11), 1127–1134.

Hutcheson, K. A., Lewin, J. S., Barringer, D. A., Lisec, A., Gunn, G. B., Moore, M. W., & Holsinger, F. C. (2012). Late dysphagia after radiotherapy-based treatment of head and neck cancer. *Cancer, 118*(23), 5793–5799.

Irune, E., Dwivedi, R. C., Nutting, C. M., & Harrington, K. J. (2014). Treatment-related dysgeusia in head and neck cancer patients. *Cancer Treatment Reviews, 40*(9), 1106–1117.

Jensen, S. B., Pedersen, A. M. L., Vissink, A., Andersen, E., Brown, C. G., Davies, A. N., … Mello, A. L. (2010). A systematic review of salivary gland hypofunction and xerostomia induced by cancer therapies: Prevalence, severity, and impact on quality of life. *Supportive Care in Cancer, 18*(8), 1039–1060.

Jeremic, G., Venkatesan, V., Hallock, A., Scott, D., Hammond, A., Read, N., … Fung, B. (2011). Trismus following treatment of head and neck cancer. *Journal of Otolaryngology, 40*(4), 323–329.

Johansson, S., Svensson, H., & Denekamp, J. (2000). Time scale of evolution of late radiation injury after postoperative radiotherapy of breast cancer patients. *International Journal of Radiation Oncology, Biology, and Physics, 48*, 645–750.

Johansson, S., Svensson, H., & Denekamp, J. (2002). Dose-response and latency for radiation-induced fibrosis, edema, and neuropathy in breast cancer patients. *International Journal of Radiation Oncology, Biology, and Physics, 52*, 1207–1219.

Keefe, D. M., & Schubert, M. M. (2007). Mucositis Study Section of the Multinational Association of Supportive Care in Cancer and the International Society for Oral Oncology. Updated clinical practice guidelines for the prevention and treatment of mucositis. *Cancer, 109*, 820–831.

Kent, M. L., Brennan, M. T., Noll, J. L., Fox, P. C., Burri, S. H., Hunter, J. C., & Lockhart, P. B. (2008). Radiation-induced trismus in head and neck cancer patients. *Supportive Care in Cancer, 16*(3), 305–309.

King, S. N., Dunlap, N. E., Tennant, P. A., & Pitts, T. (2016). Pathophysiology of radiation-induced dysphagia in head and neck cancer. *Dysphagia, 31*, 339–351.

Köstler, W. J., Hejna, M., Wenzel, C., & Zielinski, C. C. (2001). Oral mucositis complicating chemotherapy and/or radiotherapy: Options for prevention and treatment. *CA: A Cancer Journal for Clinicians, 51*(5), 290–315.

Koukourakis, M. I., & Danielidis, V. (2005). Preventing radiation-induced xerostomia. *Cancer Treatment Reviews, 31*(7), 546–554.

Leeper, H. A., Gratton, D. G., Lapointe, H. J., & Armstrong, J. E. A. (2005). Maxillofacial rehabilitation for oral cancer. In P. C. Doyle & R. L. Keith (Eds.), *Contemporary considerations in the treatment and rehabilitation of head and neck cancer* (pp. 261–313). Austin: ProEd.

Lewin, J. S., Hutcheson, K. A., Smith, B. G., Barringer, D. A., & Alvarez, C. P. (2009). *Early experience with head and neck lymphedema after treatment for head and neck cancer*. Paper presented at the Multidisciplinary Head & Neck Cancer Symposium, Chandler, AZ.

Lin, S. C., Jen, Y. M., Chang, Y. C., & Lin, C. C. (2008). Assessment of xerostomia and its impact on quality of life in head and neck cancer patients undergoing radiotherapy, and validation of the Taiwanese version of the xerostomia questionnaire. *Journal of Pain and Symptom Management, 36*(2), 141–148.

Lin, Y. S., Jen, Y. M., & Lin, J. C. (2002). Radiation-related cranial nerve palsy in patients with nasopharyngeal carcinoma. *Cancer, 95*(2), 404–409.

Lynch, M. J. P., Theurer, J., & Doyle, P. C. (2018). Assessment of nutritional status in outpatient head and neck cancer survivors. Unpublished manuscript, Western University, London, ON, Canada.

Marcus, K. J., & Tishler, R. B. (2010). Head and neck carcinomas across the age spectrum: Epidemiology, therapy and late effects. *Seminars in Radiation Oncology, 20*, 53–57.

Martin, M., Lefaix, J. L., Pinton, P., Crechet, F., & Daburon, F. (1993). Temporal modulation of TGF-beta 1 and beta-actin gene expression in pig skin and muscular fibrosis after ionizing radiation. *Radiation Research, 134*(1), 63–70.

McLaughlin, L. (2013). Taste dysfunction in head and neck cancer survivors. *Oncology Nursing Forum, 40*(1), E4–E13. https://doi.org/10.1188/13.onf.e4-e13

Mendenhall, W. M. (2004). Mandibular osteoradionecrosis. *Journal of Clinical Oncology, 22*(24), 4867–4868.

Mossman, K. L. (1986). Gustatory tissue injury in man: Radiation dose-response relationships and mechanisms of taste loss. *The British Journal of Cancer. Supplement, 7*, 9.

Murphy, B. A., Dietrich, M. S., Wells, N., Dwyer, K., Ridner, S. H., Silver, H. J., … Yarbrough, W. G. (2010). Reliability and validity of the Vanderbilt head and neck symptom survey: A tool to assess symptom burden in patients treated with chemoradiation. *Head & Neck, 32*(1), 26–37.

Naidu, M. U. R., Ramana, G. V., Rani, P. U., Suman, A., & Roy, P. (2004). Chemotherapy-induced and radiation therapy-induced oral mucositis-complicating the treatment of cancer. *Neoplasia, 6*(5), 423–431.

Nutting, C. M. (2012). Intensity modulated radiotherapy (IMRT) in head and neck cancers – an overview. *The Gulf Journal of Oncology*, (12), 17–26.

Nutting, C. M., Morden, J. P., Harrington, K. J., Urbano, T. G., Bhide, S. A., Clark, C., … Adab, F. (2011). Parotid-sparing intensity modulated versus conventional radiotherapy in head and neck cancer (PARSPORT): A phase 3 multi-centered randomized controlled trial. *The Lancet Oncology, 12*(2), 127–136.

Pignon, J. P., le Maitre, A., Maillard, E., & Bourhis, J. (2009). Meta-analysis of chemotherapy in head and neck cancer (MACH-NC): An update on 93 ran-domised trials and 17,346 patients. *Radiotherapy Oncology, 7*(92), 4–1.

Remy, J., Wegrowski, J., Crechet, F., Martin, M., & Daburon, F. (1991). Long-term overproduction of collagen in radiation-induced fibrosis. *Radiation Research, 124*(1), 14–19.

Roberts, G. (2016). *Oral care and management of the head and neck cancer patient*. Paper presented at the Stanford/Harvard Tracheoesophageal Puncture Voice Restoration Course, Stanford, CA.

Rosenthal, D. I., Chambers, M. S., Fuller, C. D., Rebueno, N. C., Garcia, J., Kies, M. S., & Garden, A. S. (2008). Beam path toxicities to non-target structures during intensity-modulated radiation therapy for head and neck cancer. *International Journal of Radiation Oncology, Biology, and Physics, 73*(3), 747–755.

Rose-Ped, A. M., Bellm, L. A., Epstein, J. B., Trotti, A., Gwede, C., & Fuchs, H. J. (2002). Complications of radiation therapy for head and neck cancers: The patient's perspective. *Cancer Nursing, 25*(6), 461–467.

Sandow, P. L., Hejrat-Yazdi, M., & Heft, M. W. (2006). Taste loss and recovery following radiation therapy. *Journal of Dental Research, 85*(7), 608–611.

Sanguineti, G., Endres, E. J., Gunn, B. G., & Parker, B. (2006). Is there a "mucosa-sparing" benefit of IMRT for head-and-neck cancer? *International Journal of Radiation Oncology, Biology, and Physics, 66*(3), 931–938. https://doi.org/10.1016/j.ijrobp.2006.05.060

Sasportas, L. S., Hosford, A. T., Sodini, M. A., Waters, D. J., Zambricki, E. A., Barral, J. K., … Sirjani, D. (2013). Cost-effectiveness landscape analysis of treatments addressing xerostomia in patients receiving head and neck radiation therapy. *Oral Surgery, Oral Medicine, Oral Pathology, and Oral Radiology, 116*(1), e37–e51.

Shi, H. B., Masuda, M., Umezaki, T., Kuratomi, Y., Kumamoto, Y., Yamamoto, T., & Komiyama, S. (2004). Irradiation impairment of umami tastes in patients with head and neck cancer. *Auris Nasus Larynx, 31*(4), 401–406.

Shinn, E. H., Basen-Engquist, K., Baum, G., Steen, S., Bauman, R. F., Morrison, W., … Lewin, J. S. (2013). Adherence to preventative exercises and self-reported swallowing outcomes in post-radiated head and neck cancer patients. *Head & Neck, 35*(12), 1707–1712.

Smith, B. G., & Lewin, J. S. (2010). The role of lymphedema management in head and neck cancer. *Current Opinions in Otolaryngology & Head and Neck Surgery, 18*(3), 153–158.

Sonis, S. T. (2004). A biological approach to mucositis. *Journal of Supportive Oncology, 2*(1), 21–32.

Sonis, S. T., Eilers, J. P., Epstein, J. B., LeVeque, F. G., Liggett, W. H., Mulagha, M. T., … Wittes, J. P. (1999). Validation of a new scoring system for the assessment of clinical trial research of oral mucositis induced by radiation or chemotherapy. *Cancer, 85*(10), 2103–2113.

Starmer, H. M., Yang, W., Raval, R., Gourin, C. G., Richardson, M., Kumar, R., … Quon, H. (2014).

Effect of gabapentin on swallowing during and after chemoradiation for oropharyngeal squamous cell cancer. *Dysphagia, 29*(3), 396–402.

Steinbach, S., Hummel, T., Bohner, C., Berktold, S., Hundt, W., Kriner, M., … Harbeck, N. (2009). Qualitative and quantitative assessment of taste and smell changes in patients undergoing chemotherapy for breast or gynecologic malignancies. *Journal of Clinical Oncology, 27*, 1899–1905. https://doi.org/10.1200/JCO.2008.19.2690

Stubblefield, M. D. (2011). Radiation fibrosis syndrome: Neuromuscular and musculoskeletal complication in cancer survivors. *American Academy of Physical Medicine and Rehabilitation, 3*, 1041–1054.

Teng, M. S., & Futran, N. D. (2005). Osteoradionecrosis of the mandible. *Otolaryngology Head & Neck Surgery, 13*(4), 217–221.

Tomita, Y., & Osaki, T. (1990). Gustatory impairment and salivary gland pathophysiology in relation to oral cancer treatment. *International Journal of Oral and Maxillofacial Surgery, 19*(5), 299–304.

Trotti, A., Byhardt, R., Stetz, J., Gwede, C., Corn, B., Fu, K., … Curran, W. (2000). Common toxicity criteria. version 2.0. an improved reference for grading the acute effects of cancer treatment impact on radiotherapy. *International Journal of Radiation Oncology Biology Physics, 47*(4), 13–47.

Trotti, A., Bellm, L. A., Epstein, J. B., Frame, D., Fuchs, H. J., & Gwede, C. K. (2003). Mucositis incidence, severity and associated outcomes in patients with head and neck cancer receiving radiotherapy with or without chemotherapy: A systematic literature review. *Radiotherapy Oncology, 66*(3), 253–262.

Vera-Llonch, M., Oster, G., Hagiwara, M., & Sonis, S. (2006). Oral mucositis in patients undergoing radiation treatment for head and neck carcinoma. *Cancer, 106*(2), 329–336.

Viens, L. J., Henley, S. J., Watson, M., Markowitz, L. E., Thomas, C. C., Thompson, T. D., … Saraiya, M. (2016). Centers for Disease Control and Prevention (CDC). Human papillomavirus-associated cancers—United States 2008–2012. *Morbidity and Mortality Weekly Report, 65*(26), 661–666.

Vissink, A., Burlage, F. R., Spijkervet, F. K. L., Jansma, J., & Coppes, R. P. (2003). Prevention and treatment of the consequences of head and neck radiotherapy. *Critical Reviews in Oral Biology & Medicine, 14*(3), 213–225.

Wasserman, A. E. (2012). *Management of chemotherapy-induced dysgeusia.* University of Pennsylvania School of Nursing. http://www.online.org/resources/article.cfm.

Wolf, G. T., Fisher, S. G., Hong, W. K., Hillman, R., Spaulding, M., Laramore, G. E., … Henderson, W. G. (1991). Induction chemotherapy plus radiation compared with surgery plus radiation in patient with advanced laryngeal cancer. *New England Journal of Medicine, 324*(24), 1685–1690.

World Health Organization. (1979). *WHO handbook for reporting results of cancer treatment.* Geneva, Switzerland: World Health Organization. http://www.who.int/iris/handle/10665/37200.

Worthington, H. V., Clarkson, J. E., Bryan, G., Furness, S., Glenny, A. M., Littlewood, A., … Khalid, T. (2010). Interventions for preventing oral mucositis for patients with cancer receiving treatment. *Cochrane Database of Systematic Review,* (4), CD000978.

Oral Considerations for the Head and Neck Cancer Patient

Richard C. Cardoso and Mark S. Chambers

Introduction

There is a link between person's overall health and the oral cavity, a relationship that is often underestimated (Haumschild & Haumschild, 2009). Oral challenges such as periodontal disease, dental caries, poorly restored dentition, iatrogenic dentistry, as well as poor nutrition and general hygiene neglect can have a systemic impact on patient's overall health and, at times, a psychologic impact. There are several systemic conditions that can reflect in the oral cavity and similarly; there are oral conditions that can have systemic consequences (Haumschild & Haumschild, 2009). This is of particular importance for patients with head and neck cancer (HNCa). Cancer treatments can have substantial oral and dental sequelae that, if left untreated, may not only delay/complicate treatment but also result in systemic, and even morbid, effects (Store, Eribe, & Olsen, 2005). Acute side effects, such as pain and mucositis and chronic side effects, such as xerostomia, dental caries, and osteoradionecrosis, can be reduced or eliminated with a thorough oral dental evaluation, simple elimination of foci of infection, and patient education session (see Kearney & Cavanagh, Chap. 20).

Minimizing or reducing oral challenges associated with head and neck cancer therapy becomes increasingly important as the survivability of these cancers improves, particularly those of the oropharynx. For decades, a large emphasis was placed on prevention of head and neck malignancies by controlling risk factors such as smoking and alcohol consumption, behaviors which are associated with carcinogenic tissue changes (Gritz, 1988; Peterson & D'Ambrosio, 1994; Rankin, Jones, & Redding, 2008). While there has been an overall decrease in most HNCa sites, oropharyngeal cancers have continued to rise in spite of these efforts (Sturgis & Cinciripini, 2007). This is thought to be related to infection by human papilloma virus (HPV) (Panwar, Batra, Lydiatt, & Ganti, 2014). HPV-related head and neck cancers are thought to be more responsive to therapy. With this increased treatment response and decreased recurrence rates, there is a larger population of survivors who now live with long-term effects of therapy, including treatment impacts to oral mucosa, bone, and salivary glands, in essence creating a population of survivors (Pezzuto et al., 2015; Pytynia, Dahlstrom, & Sturgis, 2014; Simard, Torre, & Jemal, 2014). Patients with HPV-related disease are also diagnosed at a younger age, thus, increasing the likelihood of

R. C. Cardoso (✉) · M. S. Chambers
Head and Neck Surgery – Section of Oral Oncology
& Maxillofacial Prosthodontics, The University of
Texas, MD Anderson Cancer Center,
Houston, TX, USA
e-mail: rcardoso@mdanderson.org

© Springer Nature Switzerland AG 2019
P. C. Doyle (ed.), *Clinical Care and Rehabilitation in Head and Neck Cancer*,
https://doi.org/10.1007/978-3-030-04702-3_21

long-term complications from therapy. Therefore, the prevention and resolution of oral dental complications related to cancer therapy becomes a critical aspect of the care or these patients.

Oral oncology/maxillofacial prosthodontics is a branch of dentistry with advanced education in the care of the patient with cancer. These specialists fabricate prostheses (i.e., obturators and palatal augmentation prostheses) to enable and facilitate speech and swallowing, as well as providing services to prevent and treat the oral morbidities associated with cancer care. Complex case management of advanced HNCa involves multidisciplinary care including that by head and neck surgeons, radiation oncologists, medical oncologists, plastic surgeons, oral oncologists, speech pathologists, and nutritionists, each providing unique expertise. Toward this end, collaboration is critical for improved outcomes, and thus, team efforts among these specialists should be cultivated. Miscommunication or a lack of communication among the treatment team can cause posttreatment complications related to the rehabilitation and/or increase the likelihood of complications following therapy (Barnhart, 1960). Patients should be referred to the oral oncologist/maxillofacial prosthodontist early in the diagnostic phase of a patient's care for evaluation of oral/dental status, discussion of oral morbidities associated with cancer care, as well as prosthetic options for rehabilitation should an oral/dental prosthesis be needed. The primary treatment physician can then integrate the results of this evaluation into the overall treatment plan.

This chapter describes the scope and integration of oral oncology and maxillofacial prosthodontic concepts in the treatment of patients with HNCa. This includes the presentation of general and specific aspects of oral morbidities associated with cancer care. Further, practical approaches for preventing, recognizing, and treating the oral sequelae associated with cancer care will also be outlined. Finally, the prosthetic management of this patient population will also be presented.

Oral/Dental Evaluation

The primary objective of a pre-treatment, oral/dental evaluation is the elimination of foci of infection in an effort to prevent oral morbidities such as mucositis, oral infection, and osteoradionecrosis (ORN). The initial examination will document pre-existing acute and chronic oral conditions (e.g., dental abscesses, periodontal compromised teeth, non-restorable or poorly restored teeth, and ill-fitting oral prostheses) and related problems (Chambers, Toth, Martin, Fleming, & Lemon, 1995). The dental clinician should obtain the appropriate diagnostic radiographs which commonly include panoramic, periapical, and bitewing radiographs. The panoramic radiograph (Figs. 21.1 and 21.2) provides an overall picture of the dentition, maxilla, mandible, and temporomandibular joint (Langland, Langlais, Morris, & Preece, 1980). A periapical or a bitewing radiograph will provide more detailed information regarding a specific tooth or area. A cone beam computed tomography (CBCT) has also become an invaluable tool in not only the diagnosis oral pathology but also in a three-dimensional planning for endosteal implants. Using this technology, the restoring dentist has the ability to establish the dimensions of the potential implant sites, with great accuracy, facilitating surgical placement and predictability (Bertram, Bertram, Rudisch, & Emshoff, 2018).

Extraction of Troublesome Teeth

To date, there are no universally accepted *evidence-based guidelines* for pre-radiation dental extractions; most decisions are based on practitioner experience (Brennan et al., 2017). The following are recommendations to identify potentially troublesome teeth that may require intervention and, thus, minimizing the risk of ORN. The dentition should be evaluated with respect to its periodontal, restorative, and hygiene status. Every effort should be made to eradicate foci of infection associated with the dentition prior to cancer therapy. Teeth that are deemed non-restorable should be extracted prior to

Fig. 21.1 Panoramic radiograph showing the condition of all remaining teeth. As can be seen, there are no periapical radiolucencies, evidence of gross caries, or substantial bone loss surrounding the teeth

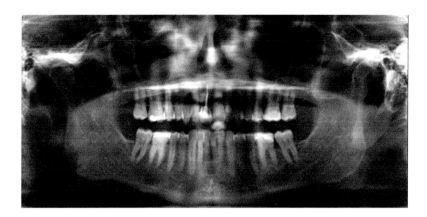

Fig. 21.2 In contrast, this radiograph reveals substantial bone loss, periapical radiolucenies, and multiple missing teeth

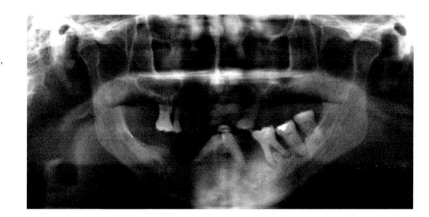

treatment, possibly at the time of tumor ablative surgery if indicated. Teeth with moderate to severe periodontal disease (bone loss), advanced dental caries, or periapical pathology should be extracted at least 2 weeks prior to radiation therapy (RT), particularly when those teeth that are within the volume of tissue radiated. Figure 21.3 provides an example of failing dentition requiring full mouth dental extraction prior to RT.

Healthy teeth that are not well maintained or difficult to maintain, such as those that are partially impacted, should also be extracted. Fully bony impacted or deeply partially impacted third molars should not be extracted due to the potential need for extended healing time or the risk of permanent damage to inferior alveolar nerve. Teeth, however, should not be removed indiscriminately, not only for their potential to retain an eventual oral prosthesis but also to maintain patient's quality of life (QOL). In the general population, it has been shown that a

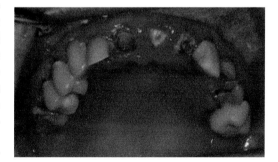

Fig. 21.3 Patient dentition showing substantial dental caries, missing/unacceptable restorations, multiple missing teeth, and severe periodontal disease. If this patient were to undergo radiation therapy without oral surgical intervention, the patient would be at substantial increased risk for oral morbidities, including ORN

decreased number of teeth is associated with an lower overall quality of life (Gerritsen, Allen, Witter, Bronkhorst, & Creugers, 2010). A similar finding has been found in HNCa patients undergoing pre-radiation extractions; specifically, patients who had greater than eight teeth extracted prior to RT showed a statistically significant decrease in quality of life (Beech, Porceddu, & Batstone, 2016).

Patient Education

The best treatment for any oral morbidities associated with treatment for HNCa is prevention. Arguably, the most important part of the pre-radiation evaluation is the patient education component. Oral hygiene procedures, designed to reduce plaque and oral contamination, should be reinforced. The oral care regimen should be personalized to the patient. Similarly, the need for the daily use of fluoride should be stressed at this appointment. Oral care, in general, should include brushing twice daily with a fluoride toothpaste and flossing once a day. Sodium bicarbonate rinses or chlorhexidine gluconate mouth rinses can be beneficial to reduce oral contaminates (Ciancio, 1994). Figure 21.4 shows the distinct differences between a healthy periodontium and an inflamed periodontium.

The main goal of oral hygiene is to reduce and minimize the formation of plaque—a proteinaceous, adherent, biofilm which accumulates on the teeth, restorations, and dental prostheses (i.e., dentures). This material is so adherent, in fact, that it can only be mechanically removed with an instrument such as a scaler, toothbrush, or floss

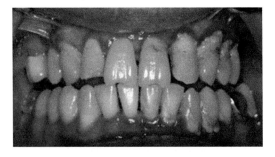

Fig. 21.4 Patient after professional dental cleaning on the patient's right side of the mouth. Notice the difference in health of the gingiva; on the patient's right side, the gingiva is pink, stippled which is a sign of minimal inflammation; on the patient's left, the gingiva is red, inflamed, and there is gross plaque and calculus accumulation

(Mariotti, 1999). Plaque formation begins with the formation of a pellicle, a layer of saliva, composed mostly of glycoproteins (Costerton, Stewart, & Greenberg, 1999; Darveau, Tanner, & Page, 1997). This layer provides a surface to which bacteria can adhere, usually Gram-positive cocci, such as *Streptococcus mutans*. These bacteria begin to proliferate, form microcolonies, and create a protective polysaccharide layer to which other, more pathogenic bacteria can attach. As plaque matures, it provides an environment for anaerobic bacteria, a microorganism that can survive without the presence of oxygen, as well as providing protection from immune host responses and exogenous bactericidal agents (Costerton et al., 1999; Darveau et al., 1997).

Accumulation of plaque is the root cause of almost all dental conditions, beginning with gingivitis, inflammation of the gingiva, which can progress to periodontal disease, and a pathologic loss of tooth-supporting bone (Chambers et al., 1995). As bone loss progresses, the teeth can become loose and eventually require extraction. An overgrowth of bacteria can also lead to dental caries, the softening of the tooth structure as a result of acids produced by bacteria. As caries progress, it can impact the dental nerve subsequently forming a periapical abscess and, thus, increase the risk of osteoradionecrosis (ORN) in the region (Chambers et al., 1995; Lindquist, Hickey, & Drane, 1978; Toth, Chambers, & Fleming, 1996; Toth, Chambers, Fleming, Lemon, & Martin, 1995).

Effective removal of plaque is dependent on different factors including patient's knowledge, motivation, and dexterity (Yaacob et al., 2014). Several techniques for toothbrushing have been recommended, including but not limited to simple techniques the horizontal scrub technique or Fone's technique to more complex techniques such as the modified bass technique (Poyato-Ferrera, Segura-Egea, & Bullon-Fernandez, 2003). Technique selection is often practitioner dependent and limited by patient ability, for example, complex techniques cannot be given to patients with decreased manual dexterity or children. There is no universally accepted method for toothbrushing, and several techniques have been recommended in the literature (Harnacke, Mitter, Lehner, Munzert, & Deinzer, 2012). This is where personalization plays a critical role; the dental practitioner must select an appropriate toothbrushing technique that the patient is able to complete.

Similarly, there are a several products on the market aimed at improving oral hygiene. Several studies suggest that powered tooth-brushes are superior to manual toothbrushes in regard to reduction of plaque and gingivitis (Yaacob et al., 2014); however, it has been sug-gested that with proper instruction, a manual toothbrush can be equally effective (Schmalz et al., 2018). While powered toothbrushes are generally discouraged during cancer therapy, they can be an effective tool for patients with dexterity issues, in particular, or those that are less motivated.

Clinical trials specifically looking at superior-ity of different toothbrushing techniques or tooth-brush types are confounded by the Hawthorne effect, in which study subjects modify behavior in response to the awareness of being observed (Monahan & Fisher, 2010). In simpler terms, any improvement seen in oral hygiene could be related to the fact that subjects are aware that oral status is being closely monitored. A conclusion that can be drawn indirectly from these studies is that oral hygiene habits can be influenced simply by placing importance on that habit (Harnacke et al., 2012; Poyato-Ferrera et al., 2003). The actual technique is less important than stressing the importance of oral hygiene.

Radiation Stents

A radiation stent is an intraoral device that is used to reduce the side effects of radiation by moving normal tissue away from the treatment field with-out compromising the total dose to the target. Patients whose primary tumor is in the oral cav-ity, oropharynx, paranasal/maxillary sinus, or salivary glands benefit the most by repositioning critical tissue away from the beam of radiation. For example, in those patients with a base of tongue carcinoma, the tongue and mandible can be depressed. This will reduce not only the acute effects by moving the maxillary arch away from the radiation treatment volume and decreasing mucositis but also chronic effects reducing the number of salivary glands radiated and decreas-ing the risk of osteoradionecrosis (Kearney & Cavanagh, Chap. 20).

These fully customizable stents are easily fabricated using simple dental procedures. Impressions of the maxillary and mandibular arches are made using a relatively inexpensive material such as irreversible hydrocolloid. Casts that are fabricated from these impressions are mounted on a simple hinge articulator using a simple interocclusal record. The interocclusal distance is dependent upon the type of radiation stent needed. Traditionally, a mouth-opening tongue-depressing stent requires about 2 cm of inter-incisal opening, while the mouth-opening tongue-deviating stent would require about 5 mm of inter-incisal opening. A customizable "bite block" also can be attached to the radiation stent. This bite block attaches to the aquaplast radiotherapy mask to ensure repeatable position-ing, thus, ensuring a therapy of exactness that reduces error.

There are two basic types of radiation stents that can be modified to accommodate most cir-cumstances. The mouth-opening, tongue-deviating radiation stent will direct the tongue to the contralateral side during treatment. This type of stent is used when treatment is given unilater-ally, such as tumors of the parotid gland or early tonsil cancers. The mouth-opening, tongue-depressing (MOTD) radiation stent is mostly used for cancers of the nasopharynx, most areas of the oropharynx, and oral cavity. An example of this stent is shown in Fig. 21.5. In circumstances which require irradiation to the floor of mouth or anterior oral cavity is needed, the MOTD can be modified by replacing the horizontal tongue blade portion with an inclined ramp. This ramp is used to lift and retract the tongue away from the volume of tissue radiated.

A further modification can be made if the patient has a history of maxillectomy, a proce-dure that results in an oronasal communication. In these situation, a portion of the maxilla and

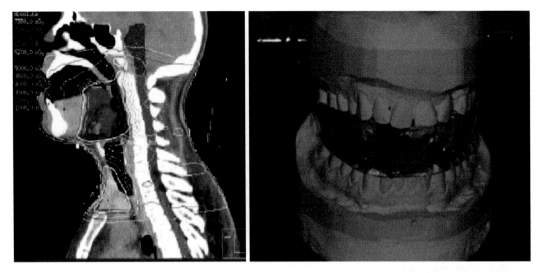

Fig. 21.5 Dosimetry for patient with an oropharyngeal cancer. As can be seen, a radiation stent was fabricated to depress the tongue even with the lower teeth and open the mouth, thus making it possible to spare the upper jaw

usually contents of the nose are removed due to disease. A tissue-equivalent material, usually saline, is placed into the defect to eliminate the air gap and allow for more homogenous energy distribution (Zemnick, Woodhouse, Gewanter, Raphael, & Piro, 2007). A second blade is added to the superior portion of the stent to support a latex balloon (Faultless Balloon Rubber Co., Ashland, Ohio).

Proton Therapy Radiation Stent

Oral morbidities associated with RT are often a direct result of irradiation to uninvolved tissues of the head and neck such as salivary gland and muscles of mastication. By targeting the tumor more precisely, the dose to critical structures can be reduced and, thus, help reduce coordinating oral morbidities. This is accomplished by the proton energy itself. By eliminating radiation exit dose and decreasing entrance dose through a phenomenon known as Bragg peak, the dose to normal tissue can be reduced without compromising total dose to the tumor site (Gunn & Frank, 2013). Figure 21.6 depicts a comparison of dosimetries of standard intensity-modulated radiation therapy (IMRT) and intensity-modulated photon therapy (IMPT).

Randomized, blinded clinical trials comparing IMRT and IMPT are currently underway to assess quality of life and specific oral morbidities, including deficits in salivary flow and oral opening. The largest difference between a traditional IMRT radiation stent and the IMPT radiation stent is the addition of an anterior bite block. This bite block eventually attaches to the aquaplast mask, further improving treatment accuracy.

Oral Morbidities Associated with Radiation Therapy

Oral morbidity associated with RT is generally divided into two phases: acute (i.e., mucositis and pain) and chronic effects (i.e., osteoradionecrosis, xerostomia, caries, trismus). The acute effects can be treatment limiting if they are not managed appropriately, and the chronic, late effects can be debilitating and lead to an overall decreased QOL. Prevention of these oral morbidities and maintenance of QOL is an integral goal of the multidisciplinary team, second only to curing the cancer. While there are no effective means to completely eliminate these morbidities, there are methods to either reduce or mitigate the effects. The following sections will

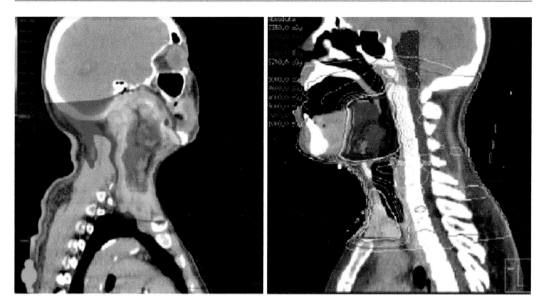

Fig. 21.6 Comparison of dosimetries of protons and photons. As can be seen, the anterior oral cavity is spared. This reduction is irradiation to normal tissue which is thought to reduce oral morbidities associated with cancer therapy

describe some of the most common oral morbidities associated with cancer therapy as well as methods of prevention/mitigation.

Radiation-Induced Mucositis

Oral mucositis is an unavoidable consequence of RT. Oral mucosa that is within the volume of tissue radiated will be impacted during treatment; it is, however, dependent upon dose (Buglione et al., 2016). The etiology for radiation-induced mucositis is predicated on cell death of the rapidly dividing epithelial cell layer by DNA damage (Sonis, 2009). Sonis has described mucositis in five phases: initiation (damage), upregulation of inflammation, signaling and amplification, ulceration, and wound healing (Sonis, 2007, 2009). During the ulceration phase of mucositis, the oral tissue is prone to superinfection from oral bacteria. It has been reported that the microbiome of the oral cavity can have an impact on the severity and duration of mucositis (Zhu et al., 2017). Zhu et al. (2017) have reported that in patients with severe mucositis, difference in bacteria colonization between controls and at baseline (pre-treatment) were noted. At this point, however, it is difficult to determine if the changes are as a result of mucositis or if the severity of the mucositis was impacted by the bacteria (Kearney & Cavanagh, Chap. 20; Sonis, 2017).

Grading

The most commonly used scale to assess mucositis severity is the World Health Organization (WHO) classification system (1 = soreness, erythema; 2 = erythema, ulcers, can eat solids; 3 = confluent ulcers, requires liquid diet only; 4 = oral alimentation not possible, hemorrhage) although it has been used in less than one-half of all reported studies. The Radiation Therapy Oncology Group (RTOG) oral mucositis grading system incorporates both a patient-graded component and an assessment by a medical professional (1 = erythema; 2 = patchy mucositis; 3 = greater than one-half of the mucosa affected by a fibrinous mucositis; 4 = necrosis and hemorrhage, functional component graded by patient). However, validity and reliability has yet to be established with this grading scale which may lead to difficulty in interpreting result of clinical trials or systematic reviews. The National Cancer Institute (NCI) first created the *Common Toxicity System* (CTC v1.0) in 1983 to aid in the recognition and grading of adverse chemotherapy events. Since that time, several versions have been introduced. The CTCAE 4.0 scale is the most updated version of their adverse events (AE) (1 = erythema; 2 = patchy ulcerations or pseudomembranes; 3 = confluent ulcerations, bleeding with minor trauma; 4 = tissue necrosis, significant spontaneous bleeding, life-threatening consequences; 5 = death). Validation studies are currently being undertaken.

Prevention and Treatment

The prevention of mucositis usually involves eliminating all secondary sources of irritation such as alcohol, smoking, plaque and calculus, coarse or hot foods, alcohol- or phenol-containing mouth rinses, and sodium products that can further dehydrate oral tissues (Mallick, Benson, & Rath, 2016). Oral rinses are commonly prescribed, but baking soda rinses are the most commonly adopted practice, used by 70% of practitioners (Mallick et al., 2016). Supersaturated calcium phosphate rinses have also been recommended, yet the results have been conflicting; Quinn (2013) reported some benefits to prevention of mucositis, while others have reported no benefits (Lambrecht et al., 2013). In 2013, the Multinational Association of Supportive Care in Cancer (MASCC), in partnership with the International Society of Oral Oncology (ISOO), completed a review of the relevant literature of therapies for the treatment of oral mucositis, the most promising being low-level laser therapy (LLLT). The group was able to conclude that LLLT (wavelength of 632.8 nm) was effective for the prevention of mucositis in patients undergoing RT without concomitant chemotherapy (Migliorati et al., 2013). However, at present, LLLT is not a common practice, and therefore, treatments for mucositis consist mostly of palliation through pain reduction.

Osteoradionecrosis

Osteoradionecrosis (ORN) is generally defined as persistent exposed bone of the jaw for longer than 3 months (Epstein, Wong, & Stevenson-Moore, 1987); however, there are patients without any breach of the mucosa who develop deteriorating bone that can only be visualized radiographically (Store & Boysen, 2000). ORN has a wide spectrum of presentations, ranging from asymptomatic areas that can only be visualized radiographically to minor areas of exposed bone that heal with conservative medical management to serious non-healing, progressive areas of necrotic bone requiring mandibulectomy and reconstruction (Beadle et al., 2013). This range of presentations is most likely responsible for the wide range of incidence reported in the literature, that is, from 2% to 20% (Lyons, Osher, Warner, Kumar, & Brennan, 2014). A large population-based cohort, from SEER-Medicare data, reported an incidence of 16.1% overall, 14.0% for IMRT techniques, and 17.3% from non-IMRT techniques (Beadle et al., 2013).

Etiology and Pathophysiology

As early as 1926, there were reports of jaw challenges as a result of head and neck RT (Rivero, Shamji, & Kolokythas, 2017). Initially, ORN was thought to be a result of injury and infection, but there are several theories surrounding the etiology of ORN. One of the most widely accepted theories was presented by Marx (1983) in which ORN is posited to be the result of hypoxic, hypovascular, and hypocellular tissue which results in tissue breakdown and surface bacterial contamination. Similarly, Delanian and Lefaix (2002) proposed a radiation-induced fibroatrophic mechanism in which free radical damage leads to inflammation, thrombosis, and fibrosis, leading to remodeling and eventual necrosis. Furthermore, Lyons, Nixon, Papadopoulou, and Crichton (2013) hypothesized that allelic variation C-509 T in the TGF-B1 gene is part of the genetic basis for late radiation toxicities mediated by fibrosis. Other authors, specifically Store et al. (2005), demonstrated that bacterial contamination deep in the medullary bone played at least a role in the development of ORN, and others report that due to radiation, damage to the osteoclasts is the precipitating event in ORN (Ruggiero, Mehrotra, Rosenberg, & Engroff, 2004).

Prevention

Regardless of the actual etiology, it has been determined that there is an increased risk ORN following oral surgical procedures in an irradiated field; therefore, prevention has been targeted at reducing the need for dental extraction in the volume of tissues radiated (Beumer, Silverman, & Benak, 1972; Fleming, 1990; Marciani & Ownby, 1986; Schweiger, 1987). For this reason, elective oral surgical procedures, specifically dental extraction, within the volume of tissue radiated for risk of ORN are generally discouraged. Noninvasive dental procedures, namely, oral prophylaxis, radiography, direct restorative such as fillings, and endodontic and prosthodontic procedures such as crowns and dentures, can be performed without any risk[1] (Toth et al., 1995, 1996). Should a tooth be deemed non-restorable via conventional methods, it is generally recommended that a crown amputation be performed. In such a procedure, the tooth is endodontically treated, and the tooth structure above the gingiva is reduced to a dome, as depicted in Fig. 21.7. Once completed, the tooth is allowed to exfoliate naturally over the period of several years.

Should dental surgery be required following RT and one or more teeth was/were within the

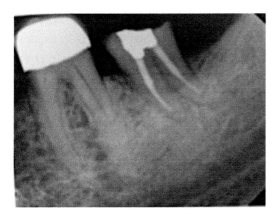

Fig. 21.7 Radiograph of tooth #18 in a patient having received radiation therapy. The tooth was deemed non-restorable, and, due to history radiation, it was decided to endodontically treat the tooth and amputate the crown

---

[1] National Institute of Dental and Craniofacial Research (2016).

volume of tissue irradiated, the clinician should discuss with the treating radiation oncologist the volume of tissue irradiated and specific treatment parameters. The treatment summary and the dosimetries should also be reviewed to assess the risk for ORN. Preoperative hyperbaric oxygen (HBO) is generally recommended to increase the potential for wound healing by promoting angiogenesis and osteogenesis (Farmer, Shelton, Angelillo, Bennett, & Hudson, 1978; Mansfield, Sanders, Heimbach, & Marx, 1981; Marx & Johnson, 1987). According to Marx and colleagues (Marx & Johnson, 1987; Marx, Johnson, & Kline, 1985), 20 treatments are recommended preoperatively followed by 10 postoperative treatments. This prescription may be altered to 20 postoperative treatments should wound healing still be compromised; however, little benefit has been found in patients who receive more than 40 total treatments. There is minimal evidence to suggest a clinical benefit to more than 40 treatments.

When compared to antibiotics alone, HBO has shown to decrease the development of ORN following dental extraction within the volume of tissue irradiated in a randomized prospective trial; specifically, 5.4% of those studied developed ORN in the HBO group, while 29.9% developed ORN in the antibiotic group (Marx et al., 1985). Others have investigated the use of HBO in a preextraction setting and have found varying ORN rates, ranging from 0% to 16.3% (Rivero et al., 2017). However, these studies are based on small population samples and have short follow-up times (Rivero et al., 2017).

Grading

Several grading systems have been proposed by several authors based on different criteria. For example, the Marx (1983) staging system is predicated on response to HBO treatment, while others classify based on extent and evidence of progression (Epstein et al., 1987; Notani et al., 2003). To date, there is no universally accepted staging classification for ORN (Rivero et al., 2017). The National Cancer Institute (NCI) has

Table 21.1 Common terminology criteria for adverse events, version 4.0 (2010)

Grade	Osteonecrosis of the jaw
1	Asymptomatic; no treatment
2	Symptomatic; minor medical intervention
3	Symptomatic; operative intervention needed
4	Life-threatening; urgent care needed
5	Death

From Duchnay et al. (2015)

published standardized definitions for adverse events, known as Common Terminology Criteria for Adverse Events (CTCAE). According to this group, osteoradionecrosis is stratified into five classifications based on severity and symptoms and impact on activities of daily life (Duchnay et al., 2015). A summary of this classification is provided in Table 21.1.

Treatment

There is no standard approach to the treatment of ORN. While some clinicians opt to treat aggressively with surgery and HBO, others opt for a more conservative approach with careful monitoring, oral decontamination regimens, and systemic antibiotics. Bacterial and fungal contamination types similar to those found in odontogenic infections are commonly found in exposed bone, and thus, broad-spectrum antibiotics can have an impact, reducing symptoms and, at times, resolving ORN completely. Complete resolution of ORN has been seen in up to 1/3 of patients with antibiotics and improved oral hygiene regimens over the period of a year (Rivero et al., 2017). ORN is polymicrobial in nature, and antibiotic selection should be dictated by culture and sensitivity results; however, a broad-spectrum antibiotics, such as penicillin or clindamycin, can be prescribed empirically while waiting for results. Also, this is most often accompanied by a debridement or sequestrectomy, a surgical procedure in which an area of non-vital bone is removed once it has separated from the vital bone.

Should conservative management of ORN fail or there is progression of the necrotic area, par-ticularly if there is an impact of patient's QOL or pathologic fracture, a segmental (partial) mandibulectomy should be considered. Without reconstruction, this procedure can be disfiguring, leading to occlusal discrepancies as the jaw will deviate to the affected side. Free tissue transfer techniques have revolutionized jaw reconstruction with improved function, predictability, and prosthetic outcomes. The most common reconstruction for mandibulectomy defects is a fibula graft mostly because of its adequate bone length and quality to repair defects of the mandible. The fibula graft is also a good choice for dental implant placement and eventual support of a mandibular resection prosthesis (Yeh, Sahovaler, & Yoo, Chap. 2; Schusterman, Reece, Miller, & Harris, 1992).

HBO therapy can also be used once ORN has occurred, particularly as an adjunct to surgery. The benefits of HBO have been reported to be improved wound healing in infected ischemic tissue, osteoclastic stimulation, the restoration of normal defense mechanisms responsible for bacterial killing, and the direct killing of anaerobes (Mansfield et al., 1981; Marx et al., 1985). While there is evidence to suggest that HBO improves outcomes, other studies have suggested the opposite. Specifically, Marx and colleagues (Marx, 1983; Marx & Johnson, 1987; Marx et al., 1985) reported that 15% of patients responded to HBO alone, 14% required minor surgical intervention such as a sequesterectomy, and 70% required major resection and reconstruction. Therefore, Marx and colleagues felt that HBO followed by major surgery and reconstruction led to the complete resolution of ORN in the entire study population. However, in a separate randomized clinical trial (Annane et al., 2004), no overt benefit was identified using HBO; specifically, 19% of those in the HBO arm of the study recovered, while 32% in the conservative approach arm were reported to recover.

The use of pentoxifylline and alpha-tocopherol (vitamin E) has recently been presented in the literature for medical management for ORN. Although the mode of action for clinical improvement is still not clearly understood, pentoxifylline induces vascular dilation and improves blood flow by increasing erythrocyte flexibility (Delanian & Lefaix, 2002). Alpha-tocopherol has a similar effect on blood flow by inhibiting platelet aggregation, but also there is an antioxidant effect which is thought to scavenge for free radical species that are involved in ORN pathogenesis (Delanian & Lefaix, 2002). Most interestingly, these two drugs have a synergistic effect as a potent anti-fibrotic agent (Delanian, Depondt, & Lefaix, 2005; Delanian & Lefaix, 2004). In small ($n = 54$), phase II trials, this combination has shown to be safe and effective in the treatment of ORN, with all patients showing complete recovery in a median of 9 months (Delanian & Lefaix, 2002). However, further randomized clinical trials are required to confirm initial findings.

Xerostomia

The importance of saliva is often underestimated; it is a complex bodily fluid with an influence on multiple functions: (1) lubrication, (2) cleansing, (3) buffering capacity, (4) remineralization, (5) antimicrobial capacity, (6) digestion, (7) taste, and (8) phonation (Deng, Jackson, Epstein, Migliorati, & Murphy, 2015; Mandel, 1989). RT can permanently decrease salivary flow. When curative radiation involves the major salivary glands, a mean decrease of salivary flow was found to be around 80% for both stimulated and unstimulated saliva (Liu, Fleming, Toth, & Keene, 1990). With the introduction of IMRT, parotid gland sparing techniques can be employed. Reducing the dose to the salivary glands to less than 26–30 Gy of radiation whenever possible also can allow for salivary function perseveration (Chambers et al., 2005; Kearney & Cavanagh, Chap. 20).

Treatment

When there is a decrease in saliva production, there are changes in oral flora. Further, there is an increase in pathologic bacteria and a decrease in non-pathologic bacteria (Chambers et al., 1995). Oral alkalization is critical to protect the oral mucosa from dehydration, mechanical lavage of food debris, and reduction of oral bacteria (Mandel, 1989). Rinsing several times each day with a solution of one teaspoon of sodium bicarbonate dissolved in one quart of water is recommended to alkalinize the oral cavity and keep the oral and oropharyngeal tissues moist (Chambers et al., 1995; Toth et al., 1995). While there are multiple salivary substitutes available on the commercial market, none which will replace the natural salivary mucin and protective salivary components (Engelmeier, 1987; Fleming, 1990). Multiple studies have shown that acupuncture is effective at reducing the symptoms associated with xerostomia; however, no significant increase in flow rates was found in most studies (Meng et al., 2012a, 2012b; Simcock et al., 2013). One study (Braga, Lemos Junior, Alves, & Migliari, 2011) in which patients were treated with acupuncture during RT reported higher stimulated and unstimulated salivary flow rates. Figure 21.8 depicts an oral cavity with profound xerostomia.

Cholinergic agonists have been shown to have some success in the relief of xerostomia symptoms. Medications, such as pilocarpine or cevimeline, have shown an effective increase in salivary flow, 0.04 ml/min, with decreased symptoms of xerostomia reported. These effects are thought to be modest and short-lived (Mercadante, Al Hamad, Lodi, Porter, & Fedele, 2017). The decision to treat patients complaining of xerostomia with these medication is, at present, practitioner dependent. The risks and benefits must be carefully considered carefully as these medications have side effects that may not be well tolerated; excessive sweating, urinary frequency, and nausea have been reported (LeVeque et al., 1993).

Dental Caries

Dental caries is a particularly challenging sequelae of RT leading to local pain, dental abscess formation, and an overall decrease in QOL. Radiation of the salivary glands causes hyposalivation which in turn leads to increased plaque/bacterial accumulation, decreased salivary pH, and an overall decrease in remineralization

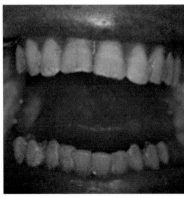
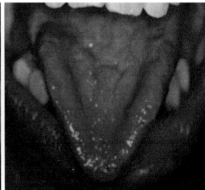

Fig. 21.8 Oral cavity of patient complaining of profound xerostomia. Notice there is a lack of saliva present. This patient is high risk for dental caries and requires fluoride therapy. The tongue is also dry, often reported as "raw."

This tongue can be painful and lead to trouble tasting food and swallowing. A dry tongue is also at increased risk for infection

of the enamel matrix of teeth. These conditions create a cariogenic oral environment, particularly in patients with a soft, sucrose-rich diet.

While there is extensive research to implicate salivary hyposalivation as the cause of dental caries (Flink, 2007; Furness, Bryan, McMillan, & Worthington, 2013; Logemann et al., 2001), there is mounting evidence to suggest that radiation has a direct impact on the dentition (Deng et al., 2015; Lieshout & Bots, 2014). Because of the multifactorial nature of caries, it is often difficult to distinguish between caries as a result of hyposalivation and increased levels of bacteria in the oral cavity versus microscopic changes to tooth structure; however, there is evidence to suggest the microhardness of the dental tissues is changed (Walker, Wichman, Cheng, Coster, & Williams, 2011). Although there is no actual difference in caries between irradiated and non-radiated teeth, all the components of the teeth, the enamel, dentin, and dentoenamel junction are affected negatively by RT (Kielbassa, Hellwig, & Meyer-Lueckel, 2006; Lieshout & Bots, 2014). Studies have shown that there is a decrease in the fracture resistance of the tooth both in the enamel and dentin, making the tooth more prone to fracture, as well as changes in the demineralization behavior of the tooth structure (Deng et al., 2015; Lieshout & Bots, 2014).

Caries Prevention

Caries formation begins with presence of caries-forming bacteria, specifically *Streptococcus mutans*. These bacteria are present in most all mouths and nearly impossible to eliminate completely from the oral cavity. Caries-forming bacteria ingest the fermentable carbohydrates (i.e., glucose and sucrose) from the diet and produce an acid. It is this acid that deteriorates teeth and subsequently causes caries. Caries prevention surrounds three main components: bacterial reduction through appropriate oral hygiene techniques (brushing and flossing), limiting exposure to fermentable carbohydrates, and finally, making the tooth structure more resistant to acid. Fluorides are well known to repair and inhibit caries by combining with the apatite in the enamel matrix to form a fluoridated apatite, which is much more resistant acids (Kutsch, 2014).

The best prevention of dental caries for a patient who has undergone radiation consists of a strict oral hygiene regimen consisting of daily flossing, toothbrushing, and fluoride therapy. A daily fluoride regimen has been shown to not only remineralize cavitated enamel matrices but also decrease postradiation dentinal sensitivity and inhibit caries-forming organisms (Chambers et al., 1995; Fleming, 1990). Topical fluoride treatments consist of a daily application of 0.4% stannous fluoride or 1.1% sodium fluoride applied to the dentition using a brush-on technique or gel-filled trays (i.e., fluoride carriers) are often used (Chambers et al., 1995; Fleming, 1990; Keene & Fleming, 1987; Toljanic & Saunders, 1984). Compared with sodium fluoride, stannous fluoride is slightly more acidic, and as a result the uptake into the enamel matrices is four times greater (Haumschild & Haumschild, 2009; Mansfield et al., 1981). While there is substantial evidence to support the use of topical fluorides in the prevention of caries, there is a lack of high-level evidence to support the superiority of any one formulation of fluoride (Marinho, 2014; Marinho, Higgins, Logan, & Sheiham, 2003; Weyant et al., 2013). Most recommendations are based on practitioner's professional judgment and patient preferences (Weyant et al., 2013).

In adults with xerostomia, fluoride leaches out of tooth enamel within 24 h, so a daily routine is imperative for optimal protection. A custom-made polypropylene fluoride carrier is highly recommended to allow for maximal surface contact of the fluoride. The carrier is to extend just beyond the surface of the tooth onto the gingiva to ensure application to the vulnerable root surface of the teeth. Patients fill the carrier approximately 1/3 full of fluoride gel and place them on the teeth for about 10 min with no eating, drinking, or rinsing for at least 30 min. This is a critical step in the process to allow absorption of fluoride into the teeth (Fleming, 1990).

Trismus

Trismus is a general term used to describe the restricted mandibular opening, regardless of etiology (Rapidis et al., 2015). Trismus can lead not only to difficulty accessing the oral cavity for examination/treatment and to decreased hygiene but also to decreased speech resonance and difficulty inserting and manipulating food (Dijkstra, Kalk, & Roodenburg, 2004). The incidence of radiation-induced trismus following treatment for head and neck malignancies can

vary widely (Davies & Epstein, 2010). This wide variation is, most likely, related to the lack of uniform criteria and threshold standards for trismus and differences in clinical assessment styles. Some authors have defined trismus as <20 mm inter-incisally, while others have defined trismus as <40 mm (Scott et al., 2008). In an attempt to standardize the definition of trismus, some authors have used QOL measures. For example, Scott, Butterworth, Lowe, and Rogers (2008) determined that an inter-incisal opening of 35 mm or less is associated with a decreased QOL.

Etiology

There are various etiologies of trismus, including infection, inflammation (e.g., as a result of dental treatment or trauma), temporomandibular joint disorder, RT, and malignancy (Dijkstra, Huisman, & Roodenburg, 2006). RT for therapeutic intervention has been implicated as the cause of trismus when the muscles of mastication are in the volume of tissue irradiated. It has been determined that radiation alone to the pterygoid region is sufficient to cause restricted mouth opening (Goldstein, Maxymiw, Cummings, & Wood, 1999). Furthermore, Kent et al. (2006) demonstrated a high prevalence of trismus (47%) in cancer patients who had received radiation doses greater than 55 Gy to the masseter and/or pterygoid musculature.

Treatment

Appropriate treatment of trismus depends upon correct diagnosis of the etiology; for example, trismus that occurs as a result of the tumor mass is treated by eradication of the malignancy, while radiation-induced trismus is treated with pain management, anti-inflammatories, and physical therapy, usually with the aid of devices. Several treatment options for trismus have been proposed; however, there is limited well-structured research on their efficacy and as such there is no standard treatment regimen that can be recommended. Most of the regimens include a device to aid in stretching. Devices as simple as tongue blades and unassisted and finger-assisted stretching exercises (Lund & Cohen, 1993; Rouse, 1970) to more complex devices, such as Jaw Dynasplint System (Shulman, Shipman, & Willis, 2008) (JDS) and TheraBite Jaw Motion Rehabilitation System® (TJMRS), have been described in the literature (Buchbinder, Currivan, Kaplan, & Urken, 1993). These devices can be generally classified into passive or active motion, depending on whether the muscles of mastication are not involved or involved in opening and stretching of the mandible, respectively.

Although limited, several studies (Buchbinder et al., 1993; Maloney et al., 2002) have shown that TJMRS showed increased range of motion when compared to tongue blades and unassisted exercise. This device uses hand strength to stretch the user's jaw, joint, and facial tissues for increased mobility. In assessments at 6 weeks in patients who had a mandibular opening of 30 mm or less, Buchbinder et al. (1993) reported that the net increase in maximum incisal opening was 13.6 mm (±1.6 mm) for the group treated with TJMRS. This is significantly greater than other groups 6.0 mm (±1.8 mm) using unassisted exercise and 4.4 mm (±2.1 mm) with tongue blades. The average inter-incisal opening for the three groups was 22.6 mm (2.2 mm standard deviation [SD]), 21.1 mm (1.5 mm SD), and 21.3 mm (1.7 mm SD), respectively (Buchbinder et al., 1993).

The JDS is a custom-fitted machine with a spring-loaded opening mechanism that is controlled by an adjustable tension system (Shulman et al., 2008). The device provides a low load, prolonged duration stretch to the head and neck muscles and tissues by directing a controlled vertical force to two custom-fitted mouthpieces. A case report (Shulman et al., 2008) using the JDS has also shown its efficacy in increasing the inter-incisal distance in the radiation-induced trismus patient. Shulman et al. (2008) presented a case series with 48 patients stratified by etiology of trismus. The mean initial maximum inter-incisal opening pre-treatment was 24.97 mm for all groups and 37.63 mm posttreatment. Following 6 months of therapy with JDS, the radiation

oncology patient showed a mean average increase in inter-incisal opening of 13.6 mm (Shulman et al., 2008).

Oral Morbidities Associated with Chemotherapy

Most patients diagnosed with HNCa receive chemotherapy, usually, in combination with RT (Krakoff, 1991; Rosenberg, 1990). Most chemotherapeutic regimens are generally cytotoxic, i.e., the agent damages mitotically active cells, both tumor cells and normal cells, and therefore, chemotherapy induces toxicity in the hematopoietic cells, skin/mucosa, and aerodigestive tract (Toth et al., 1995). It is therein that most the oral complications arise. With a decrease in hematopoietic cells, there is a decreased immunity and increased risk of infection. Oral complications associated with cancer and its therapy have been well-documented and are broadly categorized as infection/bleeding problems or mucositis (Toth et al., 1996). Today, there are targeted therapies, usually a monoclonal antibody or an immune modulator, which generally results in reduced toxicity. While targeting a specific molecule or receptor, however, these agents have been found to have oral effects including xerostomia and increased mucositis.

Oral Infection

Cytotoxic chemotherapy, specifically, can lead to multiple serious infection with varying potential to involve the oral cavity. Empirical use of an oral decontamination agents, that is, 0.12% chlorhexidine gluconate and 1.1% sodium fluoride toothpaste, may substantially lower the risk of infection of the oral cavity. Ideally the oral cavity should be evaluated prior to the beginning of therapy, and reservoirs of infections should be eliminated. Clinically, the risk of infection depends on multiple interacting factors, such as oral hygiene status, immune-myelosuppressive status, chemotherapeutic agents used, prophylactic or therapeutic antimicrobial agents used, and the degree of periodontal disease.

If patient's health and hematologic parameters allow, acute oral/dental problems found during the dental evaluation should be addressed prior to chemotherapeutic treatment or in between cycles. Chronic problems, also, should not go unattended as these can quickly become acute and delay treatment course. For example, a moderately large carious lesion can quickly invade the dental nerve and cause a pulpitis. It is equally important, however, that the dental practitioner not lose sight of the overall oncologic goal and, therefore, not implement an elaborate restorative treatment plan. Treatment plans should be simple, practical, and functional in relation to the patient's oral or dental health and should not be in the realm of cosmetic dentistry, extensive, complex fixed prosthodontics, or advanced periodontal therapy (Karr & Kramer, 1992; Toth et al., 1995).

Patients who are immune compromised as a result of chemotherapy can undergo invasive dental care (i.e., dental extraction or periodontal scaling and root planning) provided that they meet the following hematologic conditions: (1) an absolute neutrophil count of approximately 1000/mm^3 (white blood cell count times percent neutrophils equals the absolute neutrophil count), a level at which the risk of developing an infection is minimal and (2) a platelet count above 50,000/mm^3 with a normal coagulation profile (Bodey, Buckley, Sathe, & Freireich, 1966).

Oral Care

The reinforcement of adequate daily oral hygiene is also critical in these patients. By controlling plaque accumulation, gingival inflammation can be minimized along with the bacterial load and potential for infection (Lefkoff, Beck, & Horton, 1995). Often the medical team and patients are fearful of creating complications from routine dental care such as brushing and flossing (fear that toothbrushing can cause a bacteremia). This results in suboptimal oral care and, thus, an increase in bacteria levels in the mouth which could then create further challenges. Toothbrushing and flossing should be the standard of dental care. As in the general population, how-ever, many patients with cancer either do not floss or floss only infrequently. In this situation, clinicians either may instruct these patients to not floss or stress its importance in areas where food accumulates, as these areas pose a risk for substantial inflammation and infection (Toth et al., 1996).

Patients who regularly floss should be instructed to modify their technique. First, patients should be instructed to floss gently, particularly as the lining of the oral cavity becomes thin from the suppressive effects of the chemotherapy. Secondly, the platelet count should be above 50,000/mm^3 to prevent excessive bleeding (Toth et al., 1995). Toothbrushing is also imperative in controlling plaque. In certain clinical situations, such as increased sensitivity to toothbrush bristles, irritation of gingival tissue, or profound thrombocytopenia (<20,000/mm^3), patients should be instructed to change from a soft to an ultrasoft-bristled toothbrush (Chambers et al., 1995; Toth et al., 1995, 1996; Toth, Martin, Chambers, Robinson, & Andersson, 1998).

Chemotherapy-Induced Mucositis

Mucositis, the most common acute complication of chemotherapy, has a specific, defined progression. This process is similar to that of radiation-induced mucositis in that mucosal erythema progresses to oral sensitivity and then to mucosal denudation. An important distinction must be made between stomatitis and mucositis; identifying the appropriate etiology will provide insight into the appropriate treatment (Chambers et al., 1995; Epstein, Ransier, Lunn, & Spinelli, 1994; Toth et al., 1995). A diagnosis of stomatitis should be made when the integrity of the mouth has been altered by a traumatic event such as ill-fitting dentures or an infectious agent such as viral, bacterial, or fungal contamination. In contrast, mucositis is oral tissue changes directly resulting from the cytotoxic effects of chemotherapy. Misdiagnosis of the appropriate etiology of the oral condition can lead to treatment delays and increased patient discomfort (Toth et al., 1995). Stomatitis is often preventable assuming the condition is corrected with antimicrobial agents or dental intervention, for example, smoothing of a sharp cusp causing frictional irritation on the tongue with subsequent ulceration and discomfort.

Prevention and Treatment

Patients vary considerably in their tolerance of chemotherapy agents and the development of mucositis. There is no standard therapy for the reduction or prevention of oral mucositis. In 2013, MASCC, in partnership with the ISOO, extensively reviewed the literature on treatments for the chemotherapy-induced mucositis. Multiple treatments were reviewed including cryotherapy, keratinocyte growth factor-1 (KGF-1), and amifostine. While amifostine did not have sufficient evidence for the prevention of oral mucositis (Nicolatou-Galitis et al., 2013), cryotherapy (Raber-Durlacher et al., 2013) using ice chips seems to be effective for agents with short half-lives, and KGF-1 is effective at prevention of oral mucositis in patients undergoing autologous stem cell transplant if given 3 days before the conditioning regimen (Peterson et al., 2013).

Diet should always be taken into consideration when seeking to prevent oral mucositis. The oral mucosa thins as a direct result of chemotherapy, and therefore, the diet should consist of non-traumatizing, soft foods to reduce the risk of increased abrasion. Hard or abrasive foods can lead to increased pain, infection, or episodes of bleeding (Chambers et al., 1995). Similarly, abrasive toothpastes, such as those containing whitening agents, should also be avoided.

Oral Effects of Targeted Therapy

As cancer care becomes more personalized, new targeted agents are available, and head and neck cancers are no exception. Multiple drugs have been developed that either target specific receptors on cancer cells or stimulate the immune to react toward cancer cells. Because of their specificity, the myelosuppression associated with traditional cytotoxic chemotherapy are practically

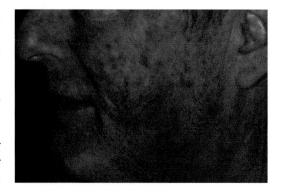

Fig. 21.9 Acne-form rash associated with concurrent cetuximab with radiation therapy for tonsil cancer. This rash is often managed by topical antibiotic cream

eliminated; however, there are often other side effects associated with these therapies. The best example of this is epidermal growth factor receptor (EGFR) inhibitors commonly referred to as *cetuximab*. This medication is often given in combination with RT for locally advanced head and neck cancers, often causing an acne-form rash as seen in Fig. 21.9; this side effect would be unexpected in a patient undergoing cytotoxic chemotherapy (Gold, Neskey, & William, 2013). There is some discrepancy regarding the incidence of mucositis when EGFR inhibitors are administered concurrently versus treatment with radiation alone. Several authors have reported no significant increase in incidence of mucositis with EGFR inhibitors, while others have indicated a higher incidence of high-grade mucositis when given in combination with RT (Magrini et al., 2016; Tejwani et al., 2009; Vigarios, Epstein, & Sibaud, 2017).

In regard to immune checkpoint inhibitors (commonly referred to as immunotherapy), some authors believe that there is a decrease in the overall systemic effects when compared to traditional cytotoxic therapy; however, there are some very substantial oral effects associated with immunotherapy, such as mucositis, stomatitis, and xerostomia, which can adversely affect patients and lead to treatment interruptions (Vigarios et al., 2017). Due to the novelty of these medications, little is known about their oral effects; hence, further studies are required.

Prosthetic Rehabilitation After Treatment for Head and Neck Cancer

Dental rehabilitation with oral prostheses following treatment for HNCa is not only recommended but often required. For example, patients that undergo maxillectomy require placement of an obturator prosthesis to allow for more intelligible speech and adequate, efficient swallowing. The overall goal of these prostheses is to restore function and provide esthetics, while adhering to strict prosthodontic principles and avoiding trauma to fragile tissue previously subjected to RT or surgery. RT impairs the healing capacity of the treated tissue, and therefore, every effort should be made to reduce any level of trauma to the easily friable tissue. Areas of excess pressure should be identified with the appropriate disclosing medium (i.e., pressure indicating paste) at the time of delivery in an effort to prevent oral wounds that can then progress to ORN. Furthermore, tissues that have been subjected to surgery or RT can readily change in contour. A regular recall schedule is highly recommended for these patients to evaluate tissue changes and maintain adequate prosthesis fit.

Maxillary Defects

Malignancies of the maxilla or the maxillary sinus are often surgically resected. Should the resection create a communication between the mouth and nose, complications such as unintelligible speech, impaired swallowing, and nasal regurgitation can be expected (Constantinescu & Rieger, Chap. 16). These can be reduced, or eliminated, by reestablishing the oral-nasal partition. This can be accomplished in one of two ways: (1) prosthetically with an obturator prosthesis or (2) surgically with a flap reconstruction. An obturator prosthesis is a removable prosthesis that replaces the missing portion of the palate.[2] The primary function of this prosthesis is to recreate the necessary partition between the mouth and

the nose and, secondarily, to recreate the palatal contours for appropriate speech sound production (Aramany, 1978a, 1978b; Okay, Genden, Buchbinder, & Urken, 2001). As the size of the defect increases, the amount of residual palate and number of teeth is decreased which then in turn can reduce the stability, retention, and support of the prosthesis (Okay et al., 2001). This, then, can decrease overall functionality and potentially patient satisfaction.

An alternative method of management would be reconstruction with a microvascular free flap in which tissue is transposed from a different part of the body into the oral cavity. These flaps are effective in restoring general function and cosmetics; however, at times it may preclude placement of the prosthesis due to the bulk of the tissue, the type of graft, and/or position of the reconstruction. For example, in order to establish appropriate esthetics and function, there is a limited area within which teeth can be placed; if the flap invades this space, it may be difficult to place teeth without substantial revision. An osseous (bony) element is often necessary for successful prosthetic rehabilitation. The vertical height of an average fibula has been found to range from 13.1 to 16.7 mm which is ideal for implant placement. The anatomy of the fibula bone is such that dense cortical bone surrounds a marrow space. In order to achieve adequate implant stability, the superior most cortex must be engaged along with the inferior cortex. This is called bicortical stabilization. The fibula bone provides support for the prosthetic but also adequate bone stock for placement of endosteal implants providing retention for the prosthetic making it the most well-suited bone graft for this type of restoration.

Currently, there is no gold standard for the restoration of these types of maxillary defects. Several factors are always taken into account during the process of treatment planning for these defects. Factors such as patient health, size of proposed defect, extent of disease, and patient expectations should factor into the treatment planning decision. While there have been reports that patients restored with an obturator prosthesis have a lower overall QOL (Wang et al., 2017), there are others who have reported that the quality

---

[2] The glossary of prosthodontic terms (2005).

of the data is poor. This difference suggests that further study using standardized questionnaires and validated objective tests may be of benefit in understanding such outcomes (Wijbenga, Schepers, Werker, Witjes, & Dijkstra, 2016). To date, either flap reconstruction or conventional obturator placement continues to represent viable treatment options, and both can lead to a reasonable posttreatment QOL.

Phases of Prosthetic Rehabilitation

Patients who undergo maxillectomy and will undergo prosthetic rehabilitation with an obturator prosthesis will require three distinct phases of treatment: the surgical phase, interim phase, and definitive phase of obturator rehabilitation. In the surgical phase, a surgical obturator prosthesis is placed immediately at the time of surgery. The primary objective of this prosthesis is to restore palatal continuity and support the surgical packing, thus, reducing the risk for postsurgical bleeding. These prostheses most often obviate the need for a feeding tube and decrease overall surgical time. Additionally, the ability to eat and speak almost immediately postoperatively has been reported to improve patients' psychological status (Fukuda, Takahashi, Nagai, & Iino, 2004; Teichgraeber, Larson, Castaneda, & Martin, 1984). This prosthesis is secured using an interdental wrought wire for the dentate patient and using titanium screws for the edentulous patient. These prostheses remained fixed in place for approximately 5–10 days but can remain in place for up to 14 days without challenge.

Once the surgical obturator is removed, an interim obturator must immediately be placed to maintain speech and swallowing. This prosthesis is removable, and it has prosthetic teeth added to establish appropriate lip/cheek support (Fukuda et al., 2004; Teichgraeber et al., 1984). During normal healing, the maxillectomy defect will continue to change, and at times, this will lead to challenges with nasal regurgitation and hypernasality. The interim obturator is periodically modified with a resilient polymethyl methacrylate material to improve the intimacy of the fit of the prosthesis to the tissue. This prosthesis is used throughout the cancer treatment phase.

Once cancer treatment has been completed and the defect is dimensionally stable, a definitive obturator can be fabricated. This process typically usually occurs 3–4 months following the completion of treatment. These prostheses can be designed with a metal framework, fabricated from chrome cobalt, or it can be made of polymethyl methacrylate. As with any maxillofacial prosthesis, preserving the remaining dentition is critical for maximal functionality, and every effort should be made to maintain the dentition (Martin, Austin, Chambers, Lemon, & Toth, 1994).

Hygiene of Maxillary Defect

Once the surgical obturator and packing are removed, the patient is required to clean the defect. Using a bulb irrigator, the patient is instructed to rinse and debride the defect three times a day using a salt and sodium bicarbonate solution. The solution is made by adding 1 tsp. of salt and 1 tsp. of sodium bicarbonate to 16 oz. of water. The patient is expected to return to routine dental hygiene (i.e., brushing and flossing) once the surgical obturator is removed. Most patients are apprehensive about dental and defect hygiene mostly due to concerns of harming the surgical site; however, they must be specifically instructed and encouraged to resume regular hygiene. Oral hygiene is one of the most important aspects of the postoperative phase (Martin et al., 1994).

Following some healing of the surgical defect (approximately 4 weeks), a 1:1 mixture of 3% hydrogen peroxide and water can be added to the hygiene routine to loosen the dried crust and debris from the site. This should be completed just prior to the irrigation with salt and sodium bicarbonate solution. A piece of gauze or a washcloth can be wrapped around the index finger to cleanse the borders of the defect. A sponge-tipped applicator can also be used for purpose. Once the defect is cleaned, the entire oral cavity is rinsed for overall decontamination.

Mandibular Defects

Mandibular defects secondary to tumor ablation create a functional and esthetic challenge. Due to the nature of the mandible, a non-reconstructed mandible will deviate to the side of the defect. This will lead to dental malocclusion, decreased speech intelligibility, lip incompetence, and poor bolus control. A mandibular resection prosthesis can help with most of these issues. Free tissue transfers, most commonly from the fibula, has revolutionized mandibular resections due to their predictability and the improved prosthetic and functional outcome. Similar to that of maxillary reconstructions, the fibula graft appears to be in the most adaptable in relation to mandibular reconstruction (Schusterman et al., 1992).

Osteointegrated Implant Following Radiation Therapy

The incorporation of osteointegrated implants for retention and support of oral prosthesis have revolutionized dental practice. Osteointegrated implants can provide support and retention of a prosthesis that otherwise would be difficult to use (McCord & Michelinakis, 2004). Factors such as fixture and abutment length and appropriate selection of implant sites are critical to the success of any prosthetic rehabilitation. However, patients that have undergone RT pose a substantial risk of ORN, and therefore, radiation dose to the proposed implant site requires special consideration (Tumerdem-Ulug et al., 2011). As the dose of radiation increases to an implant site, so does the risk for developing ORN. Although it remains controversial, hyperbaric oxygen therapy has been suggested to reduce this risk and is actively being studied (Tumerdem-Ulug et al., 2011).

Because of the nature of flap reconstructions, it is often difficult to retain a prosthesis due to flap thickness and lack of a vestibule without the use of implants. These patients often undergo RT which, for most practitioners, is a relative contraindication for implants. With the aid of computer-aided design and three-dimensional printing, implants can be placed at the time of the primary fibula reconstruc-

tion. These digital techniques not only result in decreased overall time to prosthetic delivery as well as overall higher utilization of implants but also are thought to reduce the risk of ORN as implants are placed prior to RT (Chuka et al., 2017). This is a relatively new technique and, therefore, long-term, multicenter, data are not yet available.

Palatal Augmentation Prosthesis

Speech and swallowing dysfunction are common problems for patients following glossectomy or with lingual nerve dysfunction. Articulation is accomplished, in part, by precise positioning of the tongue against the palate and teeth. Similarly, deglutition requires maximum tongue contact with the palate (Marunick & Tselios, 2004). Reduced contact with the palate, either as result of resection or decreased mobility, will result in speech and swallowing challenges. A palatal augmentation prosthesis will modify the contours of the palate, based on the contours of the tongue, to allow for adequate tongue contact during speech and swallowing.

A direct correlation has been established between the amount of lingual tissue removed and impairment of articulation. That is, patients with 50% or more of the tongue missing will have speech/swallowing challenges postoperatively (Marunick & Tselios, 2004). This is mostly related to a lack of tissue volume, but free flap reconstructions have improved this problem. However, these patients may still have impaired mobility and still require a palatal augmentation prosthesis. A review of studies has shown that patients with severe restrictions in tongue-palate contact following resection had an improvement in speech (86%; 36 of 42 subjects) and swallowing (86%; 32 of 37 subjects) in those assessed (Marunick & Tselios, 2004).

Conclusions

Evaluation of the oral cavity is a critical aspect of the initial diagnostic evaluation for every patient diagnosed with HNCa. Pre-treatment interventions such as pre-treatment evaluation, daily fluoride, and judicious dental extractions can reduce most the morbidities associated with cancer therapy, such as osteoradionecrosis, post-radiation dental caries, and alike. By reducing or eliminating the oral complications associated with cancer care, we can improve outcomes and overall quality of life. This becomes increasingly important as the survivability of these sort of cancer improves particularly in the oropharynx. The oral oncologist can play a key role in the management of these morbidities should they develop. Oral prostheses such as obturators and mandibular resection prostheses play key roles in speech and swallowing and thus maintaining quality of life following tumor ablative surgery. Maintaining quality of life is a critical aspect of cancer care and is a concerted effort of the multidisciplinary team.

References

Annane, D., Depondt, J., Aubert, P., Villart, M., Gehanno, P., Gajdos, P., & Chevret, S. (2004). Hyperbaric oxygen therapy for radionecrosis of the jaw: A randomized, placebo-controlled, double-blind trial from the ORN96 study group. *Journal of Clinical Oncology, 22*(24), 4893–4900. https://doi.org/10.1200/JCO.2004.09.006

Aramany, M. A. (1978a). Basic principles of obturator design for partially edentulous patients. Part I: Classification. *Journal of Prosthetic Dentistry, 40*(5), 554–557.

Aramany, M. A. (1978b). Basic principles of obturator design for partially edentulous patients. Part II: Design principles. *Journal of Prosthetic Dentistry, 40*(6), 656–662.

Barnhart, G. W. (1960). A new material and technic in the art of somato-prosthesis. *Journal of Dental Research, 39*, 836–844. https://doi.org/10.1177/00220345600390041001

Beadle, B. M., Liao, K. P., Chambers, M. S., Elting, L. S., Buchholz, T. A., Kian Ang, K., … Guadagnolo, B. A. (2013). Evaluating the impact of patient, tumor, and treatment characteristics on the development of jaw complications in patients treated for oral cancers: A SEER-Medicare analysis. *Head & Neck, 35*(11), 1599–1605. https://doi.org/10.1002/hed.23205

Beech, N., Porceddu, S., & Batstone, M. D. (2016). Preradiotherapy dental extractions and health-related quality of life. *Oral Surgery, Oral Medicine, Oral Pathology, and Oral Radiology, 122*(6), 672–679. https://doi.org/10.1016/j.oooo.2016.07.020

Bertram, F., Bertram, S., Rudisch, A., & Emshoff, R. (2018). Assessment of location of the mandibular canal: Correlation between panoramic and cone beam computed tomography measurements. *International Journal of Prosthodontics.* https://doi.org/10.11607/ijp.5430

Beumer, J., Silverman, S. J., & Benak, S. B. (1972). Hard and soft tissue necroses following radiation therapy for oral cancer. *Journal of Prosthetic Dentistry, 27*(6), 640–644.

Bodey, G. P., Buckley, M., Sathe, Y. S., & Freireich, E. J. (1966). Quantitative relationships between circulating leukocytes and infection in patients with acute leukemia. *Annals of Internal Medicine, 64*(2), 328–340.

Braga, F. P., Lemos Junior, C. A., Alves, F. A., & Migliari, D. A. (2011). Acupuncture for the prevention of radiation-induced xerostomia in patients with head and neck cancer. *Brazilian Oral Research, 25*(2), 180–185.

Brennan, M. T., Treister, N. S., Sollecito, T. P., Schmidt, B. L., Patton, L. L., Mohammadi, K., … Lalla, R. V. (2017). Dental disease before radiotherapy in patients with head and neck cancer: Clinical registry of dental outcomes in head and neck Cancer patients. *Journal of the American Dental Association, 148*(12), 868–877. https://doi.org/10.1016/j.adaj.2017.09.011

Buchbinder, D., Currivan, R. B., Kaplan, A. J., & Urken, M. L. (1993). Mobilization regimens for the prevention of jaw hypomobility in the radiated patient: A comparison of three techniques. *Journal of Oral and Maxillofacial Surgery, 51*(8), 863–867.

Buglione, M., Cavagnini, R., Di Rosario, F., Maddalo, M., Vassalli, L., Grisanti, S., … Magrini, S. M. (2016). Oral toxicity management in head and neck cancer patients treated with chemotherapy and radiation: Xerostomia and trismus (Part 2). Literature review and consensus statement. *Critical Reviews in Oncology/Hematology, 102*, 47–54. https://doi.org/10.1016/j.critrevonc.2016.03.012

Chambers, M. S., Garden, A. S., Rosenthal, D., Ahamad, A., Schwartz, D. L., Blanco, A. I., … Weber, R. S. (2005). Intensity-modulated radiotherapy: Is xerostomia still prevalent? *Current Oncology Reports, 7*(2), 131–136.

Chambers, M. S., Toth, B. B., Martin, J. W., Fleming, T. J., & Lemon, J. C. (1995). Oral and dental management of the cancer patient: Prevention and treatment of complications. *Supportive Care in Cancer, 3*(3), 168–175.

Chuka, R., Abdullah, W., Rieger, J., Nayar, S., Seikaly, H., Osswald, M., & Wolfaardt, J. (2017). Implant utilization and time to prosthetic rehabilitation in conventional and advanced fibular free flap reconstruction of the maxilla and mandible. *International Journal of Prosthodontics, 30*(3), 289–294. https://doi.org/10.11607/ijp.5161

Ciancio, S. (1994). Expanded and future uses of mouthrinses. *Journal of the American Dental Association, 125*(Suppl 2), 29S–32S.

Costerton, J. W., Stewart, P. S., & Greenberg, E. P. (1999). Bacterial biofilms: A common cause of persistent infections. *Science, 284*(5418), 1318–1322.

Darveau, R. P., Tanner, A., & Page, R. C. (1997). The microbial challenge in periodontitis. *Periodontology 2000, 14,* 12–32.

Davies, A., & Epstein, J. (2010). *Oral complications of Cancer and its management.* Oxford, U.K.: OUP Oxford.

Delanian, S., Depondt, J., & Lefaix, J. L. (2005). Major healing of refractory mandible osteoradionecrosis after treatment combining pentoxifylline and tocopherol: A phase II trial. *Head & Neck, 27*(2), 114–123. https://doi.org/10.1002/hed.20121

Delanian, S., & Lefaix, J. L. (2002). Complete healing of severe osteoradionecrosis with treatment combining pentoxifylline, tocopherol and clodronate. *British Journal of Radiology, 75*(893), 467–469. https://doi.org/10.1259/bjr.75.893.750467

Delanian, S., & Lefaix, J. L. (2004). The radiation-induced fibroatrophic process: Therapeutic perspective via the antioxidant pathway. *Radiotherapy and Oncology, 73*(2), 119–131. https://doi.org/10.1016/j.radonc.2004.08.021

Deng, J., Jackson, L., Epstein, J. B., Migliorati, C. A., & Murphy, B. A. (2015). Dental demineralization and caries in patients with head and neck cancer. *Oral Oncology, 51*(9), 824–831. https://doi.org/10.1016/j.oraloncology.2015.06.009

Dijkstra, P. U., Huisman, P. M., & Roodenburg, J. L. (2006). Criteria for trismus in head and neck oncology. *International Journal of Oral and Maxillofacial Surgery, 35*(4), 337–342. https://doi.org/10.1016/j.ijom.2005.08.001

Dijkstra, P. U., Kalk, W. W., & Roodenburg, J. L. (2004). Trismus in head and neck oncology: A systematic review. *Oncology, 40*(9), 879–889. https://doi.org/10.1016/j.oraloncology.2004.04.003

Duchnay, M., Tenenbaum, H., Wood, R., Raziee, H. R., Shah, P. S., & Azarpazhooh, A. (2015). Interventions for preventing osteoradionecrosis of the jaws in people receiving head and neck radiotherapy. *Cochrane Database of Systematic Reviews,* (2), CD011559. https://doi.org/10.1002/14651858

Engelmeier, R. L. (1987). A dental protocol for patients receiving radiation therapy for cancer of the head and neck. *Special Care in Dentistry, 7*(2), 54–58.

Epstein, J., Ransier, A., Lunn, R., & Spinelli, J. (1994). Enhancing the effect of oral hygiene with the use of a foam brush with chlorhexidine. *Oral Surgery, Oral Medicine, and Oral Pathology, 77*(3), 242–247.

Epstein, J. B., Wong, F. L., & Stevenson-Moore, P. (1987). Osteoradionecrosis: Clinical experience and a proposal for classification. *Journal of Oral and Maxillofacial Surgery, 45*(2), 104–110.

Farmer, J. C., Jr., Shelton, D. L., Angelillo, J. D., Bennett, P. D., & Hudson, W. R. (1978). Treatment of radiation-induced tissue injury by hyperbaric oxygen. *The Annals of Otology, Rhinology, and Laryngology, 87*(5 Pt 1), 707–715. https://doi.org/10.1177/000348947808700517

Fleming, T. J. (1990). Oral tissue changes of radiation-oncology and their management. *Dental Clinics of North America, 34*(2), 223–237.

Flink, H. (2007). Studies on the prevalence of reduced salivary flow rate in relation to general health and dental caries, and effect of iron supplementation. *Swedish Dental Journal, 192,* 3–50. 52.

Fukuda, M., Takahashi, T., Nagai, H., & Iino, M. (2004). Implant-supported edentulous maxillary obturators with milled bar attachments after maxillectomy. *Journal of Oral and Maxillofacial Surgery, 62*(7), 799–805.

Furness, S., Bryan, G., McMillan, R., & Worthington, H. V. (2013). Interventions for the management of dry mouth: Non-pharmacological interventions. *Cochrane Database of Systematic Reviews, 8,* CD009603. https://doi.org/10.1002/14651858.CD009603.pub2

Gerritsen, A. E., Allen, P. F., Witter, D. J., Bronkhorst, E. M., & Creugers, N. H. (2010). Tooth loss and oral health-related quality of life: A systematic review and meta-analysis. *Health and Quality of Life Outcomes, 8,* 126. https://doi.org/10.1186/1477-7525-8-126

The glossary of prosthodontic terms. (2005). *Journal of Prosthetic Dentistry, 94*(1), 10–92.

Gold, K. A., Neskey, M., & William, W. N., Jr. (2013). The role of systemic treatment before, during, and after definitive treatment. *Otolaryngologic Clinics of North America, 46*(4), 645–656. https://doi.org/10.1016/j.otc.2013.04.005

Goldstein, M., Maxymiw, W. G., Cummings, B. J., & Wood, R. E. (1999). The effects of antitumor irradiation on mandibular opening and mobility: A prospective study of 58 patients. *Oral Surgery, Oral Medicine, Oral Pathology, Oral Radiology and Endodontology, 88*(3), 365–373.

Gritz, E. R. (1988). Cigarette smoking: The need for action by health professionals. *CA: A Cancer Journal for Clinicians, 38*(4), 194–212.

Gunn, G. B., & Frank, S. J. (2013). Advances in radiation oncology for the management of oropharyngeal tumors. *Otolaryngologic Clinics of North America, 46*(4), 629–643. https://doi.org/10.1016/j.otc.2013.04.004

Harnacke, D., Mitter, S., Lehner, M., Munzert, J., & Deinzer, R. (2012). Improving oral hygiene skills by computer-based training: A randomized controlled comparison of the modified bass and the Fones techniques. *PLoS One, 7*(5), e37072. https://doi.org/10.1371/journal.pone.0037072

Haumschild, M. S., & Haumschild, R. J. (2009). The importance of oral health in long-term care. *Journal of the American Medical Directors Association, 10*(9), 667–671. https://doi.org/10.1016/j.jamda.2009.01.002

Karr, R. A., & Kramer, D. C. (1992). You can treat the chemotherapy patient. *Texas Dental Journal, 109*(6), 15–20.

Keene, H. J., & Fleming, T. J. (1987). Prevalence of caries-associated microflora after radiotherapy in patients with cancer of the head and neck. *Oral Surgery, Oral Medicine, and Oral Pathology, 64*(4), 421–426.

Kent, M. L., Brennan, M. T., Noll, J. L., Fox, P. C., Burri, S. H., Hunter, J. C., & Lockhart, P. B. (2006). Radiation-induced trismus in head and neck cancer patients. *Oral Surgery, Oral Medicine, Oral Pathology, Oral Radiology, and Endodontology, 102*(3), 305–309.

Kielbassa, A. M., Hellwig, E., & Meyer-Lueckel, H. (2006). Effects of irradiation on in situ remineralization of human and bovine enamel demineralized in vitro. *Caries Research, 40*(2), 130–135. https://doi.org/10.1159/000091059

Krakoff, I. H. (1991). Cancer chemotherapeutic and biologic agents. *CA: A Cancer Journal for Clinicians, 41*(5), 264–278.

Kutsch, V. K. (2014). Dental caries: An updated medical model of risk assessment. *Journal of Prosthetic Dentistry, 111*(4), 280–285. https://doi.org/10.1016/j.prosdent.2013.07.014

Lambrecht, M., Mercier, C., Geussens, Y., & Nuyts, S. (2013). The effect of a supersaturated calcium phosphate mouth rinse on the development of oral mucositis in head and neck cancer patients treated with (chemo)radiation: A single-center, randomized, prospective study of a calcium phosphate mouth rinse + standard of care versus standard of care. *Supportive Care in Cancer, 21*(10), 2663–2670. https://doi.org/10.1007/s00520-013-1829-0

Langland, O. E., Langlais, R. P., Morris, C. R., & Preece, J. W. (1980). Panoramic radiographic survey of dentists participating in ADA health screening programs: 1976, 1977, and 1978. *Journal of the American Dental Association, 101*(2), 279–282.

Lefkoff, M. H., Beck, F. M., & Horton, J. E. (1995). The effectiveness of a disposable tooth cleansing device on plaque. *Journal of Periodontology, 66*(3), 218–221. https://doi.org/10.1902/jop.1995.66.3.218

LeVeque, F. G., Montgomery, M., Potter, D., Zimmer, M. B., Rieke, J. W., Steiger, B. W., … Muscoplat, C. C. (1993). A multicenter, randomized, double-blind, placebo-controlled, dose-titration study of oral pilocarpine for treatment of radiation-induced xerostomia in head and neck cancer patients. *Journal of Clinical Oncology, 11*(6), 1124–1131. https://doi.org/10.1200/JCO.1993.11.6.1124

Lieshout, H. F., & Bots, C. P. (2014). The effect of radiotherapy on dental hard tissue--a systematic review. *Clinical Oral Investigations, 18*(1), 17–24. https://doi.org/10.1007/s00784-013-1034-z

Lindquist, S. F., Hickey, A. J., & Drane, J. B. (1978). Effect of oral hygiene on stomatitis in patients receiving cancer chemotherapy. *Journal of Prosthetic Dentistry, 40*(3), 312–314.

Liu, R. P., Fleming, T. J., Toth, B. B., & Keene, H. J. (1990). Salivary flow rates in patients with head and neck cancer 0.5 to 25 years after radiotherapy. *Oral Surgery, Oral Medicine, and Oral Pathology, 70*(6), 724–729.

Logemann, J. A., Smith, C. H., Pauloski, B. R., Rademaker, A. W., Lazarus, C. L., Colangelo, L. A.,

… Newman, L. A. (2001). Effects of xerostomia on perception and performance of swallow function. *Head & Neck, 23*(4), 317–321.

Lund, T. W., & Cohen, J. I. (1993). Trismus appliances and indications for use. *Quintessence International, 24*(4), 275–279.

Lyons, A., Osher, J., Warner, E., Kumar, R., & Brennan, P. A. (2014). Osteoradionecrosis--a review of current concepts in defining the extent of the disease and a new classification proposal. *British Journal of Oral and Maxillofacial Surgery, 52*(5), 392–395. https://doi.org/10.1016/j.bjoms.2014.02.017

Lyons, A. J., Nixon, I., Papadopoulou, D., & Crichton, S. (2013). Can we predict which patients are likely to develop severe complications following reconstruction for osteoradionecrosis? *British Journal of Oral and Maxillofacial Surgery, 51*(8), 707–713. https://doi.org/10.1016/j.bjoms.2013.08.017

Magrini, S. M., Buglione, M., Corvo, R., Pirtoli, L., Paiar, F., Ponticelli, P., … Grisanti, S. (2016). Cetuximab and radiotherapy versus Cisplatin and radiotherapy for locally advanced head and neck cancer: A randomized Phase II trial. *Journal of Clinical Oncology, 34*(5), 427–435. https://doi.org/10.1200/JCO.2015.63.1671

Mallick, S., Benson, R., & Rath, G. K. (2016). Radiation induced oral mucositis: A review of current literature on prevention and management. *European Archives of Oto-Rhino-Laryngology, 273*(9), 2285–2293. https://doi.org/10.1007/s00405-015-3694-6

Maloney, G. E., Mehta, N., Forgione, A. G., Zawawi, K. H., Al-Badawi, E. A., & Driscoll, S. E. (2002). Effect of a passive jaw motion device on pain and range of motion in TMD patients not responding to flat plane intraoral appliances. *Cranio, 20*(1), 55–66.

Mandel, I. D. (1989). The role of saliva in maintaining oral homeostasis. *Journal of the American Dental Association, 119*(2), 298–304.

Mansfield, M. J., Sanders, D. W., Heimbach, R. D., & Marx, R. E. (1981). Hyperbaric oxygen as an adjunct in the treatment of osteoradionecrosis of the mandible. *Journal of Oral Surgery, 39*(8), 585–589.

Marciani, R. D., & Ownby, H. E. (1986). Osteoradionecrosis of the jaws. *Journal of Oral and Maxillofacial Surgery, 44*(3), 218–223.

Marinho, V. C. (2014). Applying prescription-strength home-use and professionally applied topical fluoride products may benefit people at high risk for caries - the American Dental Association (ADA) 2013 clinical practice guideline recommendations. *The Journal of Evidence-Based Dental Practice, 14*(3), 120–123. https://doi.org/10.1016/j.jebdp.2014.07.011

Marinho, V. C., Higgins, J. P., Logan, S., & Sheiham, A. (2003). Topical fluoride (toothpastes, mouthrinses, gels or varnishes) for preventing dental caries in children and adolescents. *Cochrane Database of Systematic Reviews*, (4), CD002782. https://doi.org/10.1002/14651858.CD002782

Mariotti, A. (1999). Dental plaque-induced gingival diseases. *Annals of Periodontology, 4*(1), 7–19. https://doi.org/10.1902/annals.1999.4.1.7

Martin, J. W., Austin, J. R., Chambers, M. S., Lemon, J. C., & Toth, B. B. (1994). Postoperative care of the maxillectomy patient. *ORL-Head and Neck Nursing, 12*(3), 15–20.

Marunick, M., & Tselios, N. (2004). The efficacy of palatal augmentation prostheses for speech and swallowing in patients undergoing glossectomy: A review of the literature. *Journal of Prosthetic Dentistry, 91*(1), 67–74. https://doi.org/10.1016/S0022391303007352

Marx, R. E. (1983). Osteoradionecrosis: A new concept of its pathophysiology. *Journal of Oral and Maxillofacial Surgery, 41*(5), 283–288.

Marx, R. E., & Johnson, R. P. (1987). Studies in the radiobiology of osteoradionecrosis and their clinical significance. *Oral Surgery, Oral Medicine, and Oral Pathology, 64*(4), 379–390.

Marx, R. E., Johnson, R. P., & Kline, S. N. (1985). Prevention of osteoradionecrosis: A randomized prospective clinical trial of hyperbaric oxygen versus penicillin. *Journal of the American Dental Association, 111*(1), 49–54.

McCord, J. F., & Michelinakis, G. (2004). Systematic review of the evidence supporting intra-oral maxillofacial prosthodontic care. *The European Journal of Prosthodontic and Restorative Dentistry, 12*(3), 129–135.

Meng, Z., Garcia, M. K., Hu, C., Chiang, J., Chambers, M., Rosenthal, D. I., … Cohen, L. (2012a). Randomized controlled trial of acupuncture for prevention of radiation-induced xerostomia among patients with nasopharyngeal carcinoma. *Cancer, 118*(13), 3337–3344. https://doi.org/10.1002/cncr.26550

Meng, Z., Garcia, M. K., Hu, C., Chiang, J., Chambers, M., Rosenthal, D. I., … Cohen, L. (2012b). Sham-controlled, randomised, feasibility trial of acupuncture for prevention of radiation-induced xerostomia among patients with nasopharyngeal carcinoma. *European Journal of Cancer, 48*(11), 1692–1699. https://doi.org/10.1016/j.ejca.2011.12.030

Mercadante, V., Al Hamad, A., Lodi, G., Porter, S., & Fedele, S. (2017). Interventions for the management of radiotherapy-induced xerostomia and hyposalivation: A systematic review and meta-analysis. *Oral Oncology, 66*, 64–74. https://doi.org/10.1016/j.oraloncology.2016.12.031

Migliorati, C., Hewson, I., Lalla, R. V., Antunes, H. S., Estilo, C. L., Hodgson, B., … Mucositis Study Group of the Multinational Association of Supportive Care in Cancer/International Society of Oral, Oncology. (2013). Systematic review of laser and other light therapy for the management of oral mucositis in cancer patients. *Supportive Care in Cancer, 21*(1), 333–341. https://doi.org/10.1007/s00520-012-1605-6

Monahan, T., & Fisher, J. A. (2010). Benefits of "observer effects": Lessons from the field. *Qualitative Research, 10*(3), 357–376. https://doi.org/10.1177/1468794110362874

National Institute of Dental and Craniofacial Research. (2016). *Oral complications of cancer treatment: What the dental team can do.* http://www.nidcr.nih.gov/oralhealth/Topics/CancerTreatment/OralComplicationsCancerOral.htm. Accessed 5 Oct 2016.

Nicolatou-Galitis, O., Sarri, T., Bowen, J., Di Palma, M., Kouloulias, V. E., Niscola, P., … Mucositis Study Group of the Multinational Association of Supportive Care in Cancer/International Society of Oral, Oncology. (2013). Systematic review of anti-inflammatory agents for the management of oral mucositis in cancer patients. *Supportive Care in Cancer, 21*(11), 3179–3189. https://doi.org/10.1007/s00520-013-1847-y

Notani, K., Yamazaki, Y., Kitada, H., Sakakibara, N., Fukuda, H., Omori, K., & Nakamura, M. (2003). Management of mandibular osteoradionecrosis corresponding to the severity of osteoradionecrosis and the method of radiotherapy. *Head & Neck, 25*(3), 181–186. https://doi.org/10.1002/hed.10171

Okay, D. J., Genden, E., Buchbinder, D., & Urken, M. (2001). Prosthodontic guidelines for surgical reconstruction of the maxilla: A classification system of defects. *Journal of Prosthetic Dentistry, 86*(4), 352–363. https://doi.org/10.1067/mpr.2001.119524

Panwar, A., Batra, R., Lydiatt, W. M., & Ganti, A. K. (2014). Human papilloma virus positive oropharyngeal squamous cell carcinoma: A growing epidemic. *Cancer Treatment Reviews, 40*(2), 215–219. https://doi.org/10.1016/j.ctrv.2013.09.006

Peterson, D. E., & D'Ambrosio, J. A. (1994). Nonsurgical management of head and neck cancer patients. *Dental Clinics of North America, 38*(3), 425–445.

Peterson, D. E., Ohrn, K., Bowen, J., Fliedner, M., Lees, J., Loprinzi, C., … Mucositis Study Group of the Multinational Association of Supportive Care in Cancer/International Society of Oral Oncology. (2013). Systematic review of oral cryotherapy for management of oral mucositis caused by cancer therapy. *Supportive Care in Cancer, 21*(1), 327–332. https://doi.org/10.1007/s00520-012-1562-0

Pezzuto, F., Buonaguro, L., Caponigro, F., Ionna, F., Starita, N., Annunziata, C., … Tornesello, M. L. (2015). Update on head and neck cancer: Current knowledge on epidemiology, risk factors, molecular features and novel therapies. *Oncology, 89*(3), 125–136. https://doi.org/10.1159/000381717

Poyato-Ferrera, M., Segura-Egea, J. J., & Bullon-Fernandez, P. (2003). Comparison of modified bass technique with normal toothbrushing practices for efficacy in supragingival plaque removal. *International Journal of Dental Hygiene, 1*(2), 110–114. https://doi.org/10.1034/j.1601-5037.2003.00018.x

Pytynia, K. B., Dahlstrom, K. R., & Sturgis, E. M. (2014). Epidemiology of HPV-associated oropharyngeal cancer. *Oral Oncology, 50*(5), 380–386. https://doi.org/10.1016/j.oraloncology.2013.12.019

Quinn, B. (2013). Efficacy of a supersaturated calcium phosphate oral rinse for the prevention and treatment of oral mucositis in patients receiving high-dose cancer therapy: A review of current data. *European Journal of Cancer Care (Engl), 22*(5), 564–579. https://doi.org/10.1111/ecc.12073

Raber-Durlacher, J. E., von Bultzingslowen, I., Logan, R. M., Bowen, J., Al-Azri, A. R., Everaus, H., … Mucositis Study Group of the Multinational Association of Supportive Care in Cancer/International Society of Oral, Oncology. (2013). Systematic review of cytokines and growth factors for the management of oral mucositis in cancer patients. *Supportive Care in Cancer, 21*(1), 343–355. https://doi.org/10.1007/s00520-012-1594-5

Rankin, K. V., Jones, D. L., & Redding, S. W. (2008). *Oral health in cancer therapy. A guide for health care professionals* (3rd ed.). Dallas, TX/Austin, TX: Baylor Oral Health Foundation/Cancer Prevention and Research Institute of Texas.

Rapidis, A. D., Dijkstra, P. U., Roodenburg, J. L., Rodrigo, J. P., Rinaldo, A., Strojan, P., … Ferlito, A. (2015). Trismus in patients with head and neck cancer: Etiopathogenesis, diagnosis and management. *Clinical Otolaryngology, 40*(6), 516–526. https://doi.org/10.1111/coa.12488

Rivero, J. A., Shamji, O., & Kolokythas, A. (2017). Osteoradionecrosis: A review of pathophysiology, prevention and pharmacologic management using pentoxifylline, alpha-tocopherol, and clodronate. *Oral Surgery, Oral Medicine, Oral Pathology, and Oral Radiology, 124*(5), 464–471. https://doi.org/10.1016/j.oooo.2017.08.004

Rosenberg, S. W. (1990). Oral care of chemotherapy patients. *Dental Clinics of North America, 34*(2), 239–250.

Rouse, P. B. (1970). The role of physical therapists in support of maxillofacial patients. *Journal of Prosthetic Dentistry, 24*(2), 193–197.

Ruggiero, S. L., Mehrotra, B., Rosenberg, T. J., & Engroff, S. L. (2004). Osteonecrosis of the jaws associated with the use of bisphosphonates: A review of 63 cases. *Journal of Oral and Maxillofacial Surgery, 62*(5), 527–534.

Schmalz, G., Kiehl, K., Schmickler, J., Rinke, S., Schmidt, J., Krause, F., … Ziebolz, D. (2018). Correction to: No difference between manual and different power toothbrushes with and without specific instructions in young, oral healthy adults-results of a randomized clinical trial. *Clinical Oral Investigations, 22*(*3*), 1609. https://doi.org/10.1007/s00784-017-2200-5

Schusterman, M. A., Reece, G. P., Miller, M. J., & Harris, S. (1992). The osteocutaneous free fibula flap: Is the skin paddle reliable? *Plastic and Reconstructive Surgery, 90*(5), 787–793. discussion 794-788.

Schweiger, J. W. (1987). Oral complications following radiation therapy: A five-year retrospective report. *Journal of Prosthetic Dentistry, 58*(1), 78–82.

Scott, B., Butterworth, C., Lowe, D., & Rogers, S. N. (2008). Factors associated with restricted mouth opening and its relationship to health-related quality of life in patients attending a maxillofacial oncology clinic. *Oral Oncology, 44*(5), 430–438.

Shulman, D. H., Shipman, B., & Willis, F. B. (2008). Treating trismus with dynamic splinting: A cohort, case series. *Advances in Therapy, 25*(1), 9–16. https://doi.org/10.1007/s12325-008-0007-0

Simard, E. P., Torre, L. A., & Jemal, A. (2014). International trends in head and neck cancer incidence rates: Differences by country, sex and anatomic site. *Oral Oncology, 50*(5), 387–403. https://doi.org/10.1016/j.oraloncology.2014.01.016

Simcock, R., Fallowfield, L., Monson, K., Solis-Trapala, I., Parlour, L., Langridge, C., … Committee, A. S. (2013). ARIX: A randomised trial of acupuncture v oral care sessions in patients with chronic xerostomia following treatment of head and neck cancer. *Annals of Oncology, 24*(3), 776–783. https://doi.org/10.1093/annonc/mds515

Sonis, S. T. (2007). Pathobiology of oral mucositis: Novel insights and opportunities. *Journal of Supportive Oncology, 5*(9 Suppl 4), 3–11.

Sonis, S. T. (2009). Mucositis: The impact, biology and therapeutic opportunities of oral mucositis. *Oral Oncology, 45*(12), 1015–1020. https://doi.org/10.1016/j.oraloncology.2009.08.006

Sonis, S. T. (2017). The chicken or the egg? Changes in oral microbiota as cause or consequence of mucositis during radiation therapy. *eBioMedicine, 18*, 7–8. https://doi.org/10.1016/j.ebiom.2017.03.017

Store, G., & Boysen, M. (2000). Mandibular osteoradionecrosis: Clinical behaviour and diagnostic aspects. *Clinical Otolaryngology and Allied Sciences, 25*(5), 378–384.

Store, G., Eribe, E. R., & Olsen, I. (2005). DNA-DNA hybridization demonstrates multiple bacteria in osteoradionecrosis. *International Journal of Oral and Maxillofacial Surgery, 34*(2), 193–196. https://doi.org/10.1016/j.ijom.2004.06.010

Sturgis, E. M., & Cinciripini, P. M. (2007). Trends in head and neck cancer incidence in relation to smoking prevalence: An emerging epidemic of human papillomavirus-associated cancers? *Cancer, 110*(7), 1429–1435. https://doi.org/10.1002/cncr.22963

Teichgraeber, J., Larson, D. L., Castaneda, O., & Martin, J. W. (1984). Skin grafts in intraoral reconstruction. A new stenting method. *Archives of Otolaryngology, 110*(7), 463–467.

Tejwani, A., Wu, S., Jia, Y., Agulnik, M., Millender, L., & Lacouture, M. E. (2009). Increased risk of high-grade dermatologic toxicities with radiation plus epidermal growth factor receptor inhibitor therapy. *Cancer, 115*(6), 1286–1299. https://doi.org/10.1002/cncr.24120

Toljanic, J. A., & Saunders, V. W., Jr. (1984). Radiation therapy and management of the irradiated patient. *Journal of Prosthetic Dentistry, 52*(6), 852–858.

Toth, B. B., Chambers, M. S., & Fleming, T. C. (1996). Prevention and management of oral complications associated with cancer therapies: Radiotherapy/chemotherapy. *Texas Dental Journal, 113*(6), 23–29.

Toth, B. B., Chambers, M. S., Fleming, T. J., Lemon, J. C., & Martin, J. W. (1995). Minimizing oral complications of cancer treatment. *Oncology (Williston Park), 9*(9), 851–858. discussion 858, 863-856.

Toth, B. B., Martin, J. W., Chambers, M. S., Robinson, K. A., & Andersson, B. S. (1998). Oral candidiasis: A morbid sequela of anticancer therapy. *Texas Dental Journal, 115*(6), 24–29.

Tumerdem-Ulug, B., Kuran, I., Ozden, B. C., Mete, O., Kemikler, G., Aktas, S., & Calik, B. (2011). Does hyperbaric oxygen administration before or after irradiation decrease side effects of irradiation on implant sites? *Annals of Plastic Surgery, 67*(1), 62–67. https://doi.org/10.1097/SAP.0b013e3181e6cfa4

Vigarios, E., Epstein, J. B., & Sibaud, V. (2017). Oral mucosal changes induced by anticancer targeted therapies and immune checkpoint inhibitors. *Supportive Care in Cancer, 25*(5), 1713–1739. https://doi.org/10.1007/s00520-017-3629-4

Walker, M. P., Wichman, B., Cheng, A. L., Coster, J., & Williams, K. B. (2011). Impact of radiotherapy dose on dentition breakdown in head and neck cancer patients. *Practical Radiation Oncology, 1*(3), 142–148. https://doi.org/10.1016/j.prro.2011.03.003

Wang, F., Huang, W., Zhang, C., Sun, J., Qu, X., & Wu, Y. (2017). Functional outcome and quality of life after a maxillectomy: A comparison between an implant supported obturator and implant supported fixed prostheses in a free vascularized flap. *Clinical Oral Implants Research, 28*(2), 137–143. https://doi.org/10.1111/clr.12771

Weyant, R. J., Tracy, S. L., Anselmo, T. T., Beltran-Aguilar, E. D., Donly, K. J., Frese, W. A., … American Dental Association Council on Scientific Affairs Expert Panel on Topical Fluoride Caries Preventive, A. (2013). Topical fluoride for caries prevention: Executive summary of the updated clinical recommendations and supporting systematic review. *Journal of the American Dental Association, 144*(11), 1279–1291.

Wijbenga, J. G., Schepers, R. H., Werker, P. M., Witjes, M. J., & Dijkstra, P. U. (2016). A systematic review of functional outcome and quality of life following reconstruction of maxillofacial defects using vascularized free fibula flaps and dental rehabilitation reveals poor data quality. *Journal of Plastic, Reconstructive & Aesthetic Surgery, 69*(8), 1024–1036. https://doi.org/10.1016/j.bjps.2016.05.003

Yaacob, M., Worthington, H. V., Deacon, S. A., Deery, C., Walmsley, A. D., Robinson, P. G., & Glenny, A. M. (2014). Powered versus manual toothbrushing for oral health. *Cochrane Database of Systematic Reviews,* (6), CD002281. https://doi.org/10.1002/14651858.CD002281.pub3

Zemnick, C., Woodhouse, S. A., Gewanter, R. M., Raphael, M., & Piro, J. D. (2007). Rapid prototyping technique for creating a radiation shield. *Journal of Prosthetic Dentistry, 97*(4), 236–241. https://doi.org/10.1016/j.prosdent.2007.02.005

Zhu, X. X., Yang, X. J., Chao, Y. L., Zheng, H. M., Sheng, H. F., Liu, H. Y., … Zhou, H. W. (2017). The potential effect of oral microbiota in the prediction of mucositis during radiotherapy for nasopharyngeal carcinoma. *eBioMedicine, 18*, 23–31. https://doi.org/10.1016/j.ebiom.2017.02.002

Lymphedema in Head and Neck Cancer

Brad G. Smith

Introduction

Speech pathologists working in a general medical setting may encounter swelling (edema) of the face, neck, oral cavity, or upper airway. In both adult and pediatric populations, neck and facial edema is often due to either allergic reactions (anaphylaxis) or angioedema (a rapid swelling of deep levels of the skin or mucosa). In severe cases, anaphylaxis is a rapidly emergent problem which will require prompt medical treatment with epinephrine to avoid life-threatening airway restrictions; in some instances, this may necessitate tracheotomy or intubation. In contrast, in the case of angioedema, when there is an intact lymphatic drainage system to aid in the reduction of tissue edema, swelling should reduce quickly without residual deficits. Reduction of angioedema may also be achieved following proper medical intervention with anti-inflammatory medications like antihistamines or steroids. It is, however, critical to acknowledge that management of lymphedema of the head and neck is different than treatment of either angioedema or anaphylaxis since epinephrine, antihistamines, steroids, and other medical treatments are inappropriate in the long-term reduction of

lymphedema. Therefore, proper evaluation by a physician is essential to identify the nature of the problem and determine the appropriate intervention.

Treatment for head and neck cancer with radiation often reduces the contractility of lymphatic vessels, while oncologic surgery frequently involves removal of lymph nodes and severing of lymphatic vessels, disrupting the lymphatic drainage pathways. This type of damage specifically can result in head and neck lymphedema (HNL) which is swelling that occurs in the skin when the lymphatic system of the head and neck region can no longer accommodate the increased levels of fluid. Inadequate drainage results in fluid collection and dispersal throughout the soft tissues in an affected area. Over time, congested lymph fluid can thicken, increasing tissue firmness. With the rates of human papilloma virus (HPV) positive oropharynx cancers increasing at an alarming rate over the past 20 years and with continued increases projected (Theurer, Chap. 4), it is anticipated that more patients will require treatment for HNC. As a result, the potential for development of lymphedema in the head and neck region will also increase. Since many of these patients will require posttreatment rehabilitation, it is reasonable to assume there will be an increased number of speech pathologists exposed to patients with HNL in the coming years.

HNL can be a devastating and debilitating condition when it becomes severe and persistent.

B. G. Smith (✉)
Sammons Cancer Center, Baylor Scott & White Insitute of Rehabilitation, Dallas, TX, USA
e-mail: bgsmith@bswrehab.com

© Springer Nature Switzerland AG 2019
P. C. Doyle (ed.), *Clinical Care and Rehabilitation in Head and Neck Cancer*,
https://doi.org/10.1007/978-3-030-04702-3_22

It can affect vision, speech, swallowing, and respiration, and even mild or moderate lymphedema can impede communication and swallowing function (Smith & Lewin, 2010). The intent of this chapter seeks to introduce the speech pathologist to HNL; this objective may serve to enhance their clinical awareness of the condition and provide a general guide regarding the processes involved in its evaluation and management. This chapter *is not* intended as an instruction manual so that you can treat the patient without additional education. Lymphedema management requires specialized training, and improper treatment can worsen the condition or cause injury to the patient. Appropriate treatment may sufficiently reduce both the size and firmness of edematous tissues and potentially result in a complete resolution of the edema (Smith et al., 2014). However, it is important to note that many patients will experience a more chronic condition that can be particularly challenging to treat. Whether or not you elect to pursue/receive training in lymphedema management, your ability to recognize HNL and make appropriate recommendations to the patient's medical team is an important aspect of posttreatment rehabilitation for patients with HNC. As a starting point, this will require a brief orientation to the blood and lymphatic circulatory systems which are directly related to the development of lymphedema. For this reason, the following portions of this chapter will provide a brief orientation to the blood and lymphatic circulatory systems, which are directly related to the development of lymphedema.

Lymphedema Defined

What is lymphedema and why should you care about it as a speech pathologist? Lymphedema is the abnormal accumulation of protein-rich lymphatic fluid in the interstitial (between the cells) spaces of the soft tissues of the body. Depending on the site and severity of the swelling, lymphedema can create a substantial degree of both cosmetic and functional impairment, affecting performance of daily activities. Lymphedema can be classified as either *primary* or *secondary*. Primary lymphedema typically is related to a malformation of the lymphatic system; this may be characterized by either an excessive or insufficient number of lymphatic vessels in an area or a lymphatic system that is functioning abnormally without obvious reason. Primary lymphedema may be seen at birth, during childhood or adolescence, or even during adulthood, but, typically, it is not associated with a traumatic injury (Földi & Földi, 2006a, b). However, a trauma such as a twisted ankle can sometimes be sufficient to trigger the onset of chronic and progressive swelling in patients with primary lymphedema. Primary lymphedema does occur in the head and neck region, but it is much less common than primary lymphedema of the extremities that typically is associated with genetic disorders such as Hennekam syndrome, Turner syndrome, Milroy disease, and Apert syndrome (Feely, Olsen, Gamble, Davis, & Pittelkow, 2011). It is, however, important to note that primary lymphedema of the head and neck is rare.

In contrast, secondary lymphedema develops following some form of direct trauma to the lymphatic system. Examples include blunt force injury to soft tissues, chronic constriction of vessels via the long-term application of a tourniquet, chronic cellulitis infections, vessel obstruction, and cancer treatment with surgery and/or radiation (Földi & Földi, 2006a). Those who work in cancer care may have encountered someone with lymphedema of the arm after treatment for breast cancer, which is the most common presentation of lymphedema in the United States (Maclellan et al., 2015). However, most speech pathologists working with patients treated for head and neck cancer (HNC) will encounter lymphedema of the neck (Fig. 22.1) and/or face (Fig. 22.2) following radiation and/or surgery.

A Brief Review of Lymphatics

The Circulatory System. In order to understand lymphedema, one first must have a basic understanding of the human cardiovascular (circulatory)

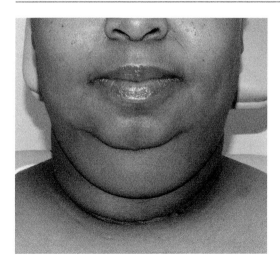

Fig. 22.1 Example of patient exhibiting submental edema. (Photo courtesy of B. Smith)

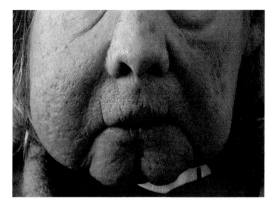

Fig. 22.2 Example of patient exhibiting facial edema. (Photo courtesy of B. Smith)

system. The cardiovascular system is dynamic and can increase or decrease its speed of performance upon demand with changes in physical activity, stress, fear, etc. The circulatory system transports oxygen and nutrients to the body's tissues, is involved in fighting infections, and assists with blood clotting in times of injury. The three primary components of the cardiovascular system are the heart, the blood vessels, and the blood itself.

The heart contains four chambers that consist of muscle tissue called myocardium, an organ which contracts continuously and rhythmically to pump the blood throughout the body. Blood nor-

mally flows between these chambers in a specific order, with deoxygenated blood entering the right atrium of the heart from the superior and inferior vena cava, large veins that receive blood from the upper and lower parts of the body. As the right atrium contracts, the blood moves into the right ventricle. As the ventricle contracts, blood travels through the pulmonary artery into the lungs for oxygenation. Oxygen-rich blood returns to the left atrium via the pulmonary vein. It is then delivered to the left ventricle, from which it exits via the aorta to be delivered to all the tissues of the body (except the lungs).

Blood is composed of three types of cells, each with specific functions: red blood cells that carry oxygen and other nutrients, white blood cells (lymphocytes) that battle infection, and platelets that aid with clotting. All of these cells are contained in plasma, a fluid that is composed of water, salts, proteins, vitamins, minerals, hormones, dissolved gases, and fats. Blood plasma is transported through a series of blood vessels to deliver the nutrients throughout the body (Zuther & Norton, 2017).

Blood vessels include arteries, veins, and capillaries. Arteries serve to transport oxygenated blood away from the heart, and these vessels are thicker than veins, a feature that serves to withstand increased intravascular pressures created by pumping of the heart. The arteries are lined with increased amounts of smooth muscle that contracts to assist with the propulsion of blood through the arterial system to reach all the body's tissues. The multiple branches of the arterial system gradually decrease in size as the vessels get further away from the primary arteries. Capillaries are the smallest blood vessels and can only be seen under a microscope, being much smaller than a human hair. A comprehensive capillary network exists, merging the tiny arterioles of the arterial system with the smallest venules of the venous system. At this conversion of vessels, essential nutrients and oxygen are delivered to all tissues of the body, though the cellular waste is retrieved by the lymphatic capillaries so that it then can be transported and filtered through multiple lymph nodes before being returned to the bloodstream and eventually to the kidneys for elimination. After this transition, the veins, which also have many different branches and gradually increase in size as they approach the heart, carry the deoxygenated blood from all parts of the body back to the heart. Vein walls also have smooth muscle, but they are thinner than arteries. As a result, blood flows with much less pressure after leaving the arteries, being diffused through the smaller capillary network. Since the veins must transport blood back to the heart against gravity, they contain one-way valves that prevent backflow and the excess collection of blood within them. When working properly, venous blood flow is enhanced by the contraction of surrounding muscle tissues in the calf, arm, and other areas that serve as a pump, constricting the veins and forcing the blood from one section of the vein to the next, eventually returning the blood to the heart. However, when the veins are not working properly and are unable to prevent backflow for some reason, they can engorge, dilate, and eventually become dysfunctional, resulting in varicose veins, ulcerations, and other complications like edema, which is excessive fluid collection in the interstitial spaces of the soft tissues (Kubik & Kretz, 2003; Zuther & Norton, 2017).

You may be asking "What does this have to do with the lymphatic system?" The answer to this question is critical. Remember the capillaries? The thin walls of the capillaries are porous and allow dissolved oxygen and nutrients from the blood to be diffused in interstitial fluid, which is found between the cells of tissues or organs and delivered to the cells by diffusion across the cell membranes. In a similar fashion, carbon dioxide and other waste products leave the cell through the diffusion process via the interstitial fluid. Certain wastes cross through the capillary walls and enter the blood. In this way, the bloodstream itself delivers nutrients and removes waste without leaving the capillary tube. It is at this level that the lymphatic system becomes involved by collecting the waste material that is not carried by the blood (Kubik & Kretz, 2003; Zuther & Norton, 2017).

The Lymphatic System

The lymphatic system is a separate vascular system that is heavily involved in the body's immune and fluid regulatory systems. It features lymphatic organs such as the spleen, thymus, tonsils, bone marrow, and Peyer's patches, as well as a hierarchy of lymphatic vessels to transport lymphatic fluid (lymph) to the body's approximately 700 lymph nodes for cleaning and then eventually return into the bloodstream (Kubik & Kretz, 2003; Zuther & Norton, 2017). What is lymph? Remember the capillary network and the diffusion process that occurred in the interstitial spaces when the blood traveled from the arterial to the venous systems? During that exchange of nutrients and wastes, not all fluid components were delivered to the venous system. Certain substances that are present in the interstitial fluid cannot be fully absorbed by the venous system. This includes proteins, water, fatty acids, white blood cells, some red blood cells, and other cellular debris. These substances are absorbed through lymphatic capillaries that are intertwined with the venous and arterial capillaries. Once this fluid is absorbed into the lymphatic capillary, it is called lymph (Kubik & Kretz, 2003; Zuther & Norton, 2017). Additional details on the functional relationship between the lymphatic system and blood circulation can be found in the work of Zuther and Norton (2017). This now leads us to the lymphatic vessels which will be addressed in the following section.

Lymphatic Vessels Like the venous and arterial systems, the lymphatic system is comprised of several different vessel types that are multilayered, have many branches, and vary in size. Each type of lymphatic vessel performs a slightly different task. From smallest to largest, the lymphatic vessels are termed capillaries, pre-collectors, lymph collectors, trunks, and ducts. Similar to veins, all the lymphatic vessels except the "initial lymphatics" (capillaries and pre-collectors) have interior, one-way valves to prevent backflow (Kubik & Kretz, 2003; Zuther & Norton, 2017). Interestingly, it is the absence of the one-way valves in the initial lymphatics that allows a therapist to effectively treat lymph-edema. "How does that work," you ask? This question will be addressed in the subsequent section.

Nestled among the venous and arterial capil-laries are the slightly larger lymphatic capillaries, which are the most superficial lymphatic vessels. Lymphatic capillaries feature fingerlike projec-tions like "dead-end tubes" with small gatelike valves on the outer walls. These valves open and close, allowing the capillaries to absorb a portion of the interstitial fluid that does not reenter the venous system. Since there are no one-way valves inside them to prevent backflow, lymph can move freely within the capillary system. This is an important feature, since the capillary network covers the surface of the entire body, much like a web of tightly knit lace. Effective lymphedema management requires movement of lymph away from a damaged drainage area to an adjacent area that is working properly. This is accomplished with a very lightweight, superficial skin stretch-ing technique called manual lymph drainage (MLD) that moves lymph through the capillary network. This will be discussed in more detail later in this chapter.

Based on information provided to this point, you may ask "Ok. Lymph can be absorbed and move laterally within the capillary network, but if there are no valves to control flow, how does it travel to the deeper lymphatic vessels to return to the lymph nodes for cleaning?" Good question. Even if you weren't asking, let me tell you. The web of "lace" (lymphatic capillaries) serves to absorb lymph from the superficial skin layer. The capillaries are vertically connected to "pre-collectors," which tie into larger lymphatic "col-lectors," which are the first, "valved" lymphatic vessels. There is then a progression in vessel size as lymph flows to the lymphatic trunks and ducts. As previously noted, all the lymphatic vessels, except the initial lymphatics, contain a series of one-way valves to prevent backflow. However, unlike veins, these valves serve to divide the lymph vessel into contractile sections known as lymphangions, which will be described in the next section (Kubik & Kretz, 2003; Zuther & Norton, 2017).

Lymphangions and Lymphangiomotoricity The cardiovascular system requires the heart to pump the blood through the arteries, and the muscle pump effect associated with muscle contraction of the legs, arms, etc. assists the veins in returning the blood to the heart. However, the lymphatic system does not fea-ture a central "pump" similar to the heart – a mechanism to propel lymph throughout the body. Lymphatic vessels are segmented into separate, valved sections called lymphangions. Each lymphangion contracts independently, pumping the lymph from one section of the ves-sel into the next until it reaches its structural destination. This sequential contraction of the lymphangions is known as lymphangiomotoric-ity, and it occurs approximately once every 5–6 seconds (Földi & Földi, 2006b; Zuther & Norton, 2017). Lymphatic fluid is pumped from the smaller vessels such as the pre-collectors and collectors through numerous lymph nodes for filtering before traveling through the larger lymphatic ducts and trunks to be returned into the bloodstream (Kubik & Kretz, 2003; Zuther & Norton, 2017).

While there are differences in orientation of drainage patterns in different regions of the body, the basic mechanics of this system are the same, regardless of the location. For example, in the head and neck region, superficial lymphatic drainage begins in the surface of the skin of the face and neck or the mucosal linings of the throat, oral cavity, larynx, and other associated regions. Lymph then is pumped through the gradually enlarging network of lymph vessels, through many lymph nodes in the face and neck for filter-ing, and eventually to the deeper right and left lymphatic ducts before entering the juncture of the subclavian and jugular veins, an area known as the venous angle. Similarly, lymph from the lower extremities is directed through large lum-bar trunks toward the abdomen, where the lymph is transferred to the largest lymph vessel in the body, the thoracic duct. This vessel begins in the abdomen and drains vertically, emptying its lymphatic contents into the left venous angle. Approximately 75% of the lymphatic drainage in the body is directed to the left venous angle, since lymph from both lower extremities, a majority of the trunk, the left chest and arm, and the left side of the neck and head, are routed there. The remaining 25% of the body (right arm, upper right quadrant of the trunk, right neck, and head) are channeled into the right lymphatic duct and eventually drained into the bloodstream via the right venous angle. In a normal lymphatic system, this provides a very efficient drainage process, preventing the accumulation of excessive interstitial fluid, regardless of body position, activity level, or other external factors. However, there are factors that can impact the extent and location of edema when it occurs, as well as how we can reduce the swelling with treatment (Kubik & Kretz, 2003; Zuther & Norton, 2017).

Lymphatic Watersheds and Drainage Territories The lymphatic vessels discussed previously create various drainage pathways that are organized regionally across the body. Although they are not visible from the surface, there are several linear "boundaries" in the skin known as lymphatic "watersheds." These watersheds represent areas with very few lymphatic collectors, so drainage of excess fluid along a watershed is not as efficient as that found in other areas. Lymphatic watersheds essentially divide the body into several different sections or drainage territories, each draining toward the nearest regional lymph node beds that contain heavier concentrations of lymph nodes. Commonly referred to as the sagittal–median watershed, this vertical division separates the body into left and right sides, forcing each side to drain unilaterally. There is the superior horizontal (clavicular) watershed that occurs near the level of the clavicle on the chest and the back, separating the drainage from the head and neck from the drainage of the trunk. There is also the more inferior transverse watershed that runs diagonally across the abdomen at the level of the navel and posteriorly across the back at approximately the level of lower rib cage. Finally, there is the "chaps" watershed area that divides the posterior gluteal region and legs. These lymphatic watersheds are important, as they impact the natural lymphatic drainage pathways (Kubik & Kretz, 2003; Zuther & Norton, 2017).

The separation of lymphatic drainage territories becomes evident whenever there is damage to the lymphatic system, resulting in lymphedema. For example, a patient who develops lymphedema in the upper extremity after treatment for breast cancer may develop swelling in the arm and possibly the breast of the affected side. If only one side is involved with treatment, swelling is typically limited to the treated side with no significant contralateral swelling. While the watersheds typically help contain edema in the immediate region, there are areas along the watersheds with increased concentrations of lymphatic vessels. These areas are known as "anastomoses," and they allow for improved drainage across the lymphatic watershed. The presence of these anastomoses is what allows MLD to effectively direct fluid from a swollen region to an area that is functioning more effectively (Kubik & Kretz, 2003; Zuther & Norton, 2017).

Lymph Nodes

Just as there is a well-defined system of vascular and lymphatic vessels designed and organized for maximum effectiveness for transportation of the blood and lymph, there is also a complex system of approximately 700 lymph nodes situated along the lymphatic vessels and veins throughout the body. While some areas of the body have relatively few lymph nodes, there are several specific regions in which lymph nodes are more heavily concentrated. These areas of heavier nodal concentrations may be called drainage basins or lymph node beds and are typically considered the axilla, groin, abdomen, chest, and neck (Kubik & Kretz, 2003). These basin areas serve as destinations for lymph that is draining from adjacent lymphatic territories. For example, the right chest and arm drain to the right axillary lymph nodal basin, and the left lower extremity will drain to the lymph nodes in the left groin. However, more relevant to your field of interest are the cervical lymph nodes which will be described subsequently.

Cervical Lymph Nodes

Lymphatics of the head and neck region drain into a very complex system of approximately 300 cervical lymph nodes (Kubik & Kretz, 2003); this system can be divided into seven different and more specific levels of drainage (Som, Curtin, & Mancuso, 2000). It is, therefore, possible to predict the drainage pattern for most structures within the head and neck. This may assist the clinician to determine which group or groups of lymph nodes are most likely to be affected by a given head and neck tumor. This is of critical importance since cancer treatment involves not only management of the primary tumor but also the lymphatic drainage basins associated with a given tumor site. Cancer typically originates in one area and can metastasize via the lymphatic system or the blood system to another region. Commonly, lymph nodes will swell as an indicator of infection or, in the case of malignancy, metastatic disease associated with HNC. In fact, a swollen lymph node in the neck may be the first indication that there is a cancer present elsewhere in the head and neck region. In addition to the need for accurate identification of a primary tumor, the ability to identify and predict which lymph nodes may be involved with a particular tumor site allows surgeons and radiation oncologists to accurately plan their treatments for maximum cure, least chance for recurrence, and minimal morbidity. This also may allow the lymphedema therapist to anticipate areas of potential damage to a given lymphatic region. This becomes important during preoperative planning and education, as well as in postoperative evaluation and treatment planning since lymphedema treatment is based on the ability to redirect lymph from areas of edema to more functional lymph drainage regions.

Nodal Classification

Within the head and neck region, cervical lymph nodes have been described in several ways. They may be named according to the adjacent structure such as "jugular lymph nodes" or the "supraomo-

hyoid nodal chain," depending on adjacent structures in the region; the relationship of these structures and the evolution of cervical lymph node classification can be found in several excellent sources (Robbins et al., 1991, 2002). Som, Curtin, and Mancuso (2000) also have provided classification for metastatic neck adenopathy based on imaging. This system grouped cervical lymph nodes into seven different levels to facilitate better identification and description of lymph groupings by physicians.[1]

For example, a typical classification for cervical lymph nodes involves levels one (I) through seven (VII). Using this classification, it begins beneath the chin with Level I, progressively traveling down the neck to the area just below the mandible, or Level II. Further progression inferiorly down the lateral neck will lead to Levels III and IV. Level V involves the posterior lateral neck and posterior scalp, while Level VI is found just below the larynx. Finally, Level VII involves the mediastinal region. These designations are commonly used during descriptions of surgical procedures like neck dissections, and they may also be referenced during radiation treatment planning. For these reasons, it is important for speech pathologist to be aware of the cervical lymphatic system and its associated classification.

The type of cervical lymph node classification outlined reflects the geographic connection between certain structures and the lymph nodes to which they will drain. There are, however, differences between systems, with some being more detailed than others. Typically, structures will drain to the group of lymph nodes that are closest to their geographic region, but depending on the classification system, certain levels may be divided in to more specific groups. For example, Level I lymph nodes drain the oral cavity. However, Level I can be further divided into Level Ia, a system that drains more anterior structures of the oral cavity, while Level Ib extends more posteriorly beneath the mandible and drains

---

[1] A comprehensive review of these levels can be found at the following website: https://radiopaedia.org/articles/lymph-node-levels-of-the-neck

the more posterior portions of the oral cavity. Level II and level V are also divided into two separate zones (see Som et al., 2000). This classification also has relevance to the overall incidence and patterns of metastatic spread of cancer via the lymphatic system (Cracchiolo & Wong, 2017).

Within the head and neck region, there is significant redundancy in the lymphatic drainage pattern. This overlap of lymphatic drainage allows for great resiliency when recovering from various types of trauma to the region, like the damage that follows surgery or radiation treatment for HNC. For example, structures within the posterior oral cavity and oropharynx drain to levels two, three, and/or four, rather than just to a single group. As a result, a patient who has an oropharyngeal tumor and requires a neck dissection may have lymph nodes removed from levels II, III, and IV on the affected side to achieve a more comprehensive resection and reduce the risk of nodal metastasis or recurrence. Thus, patterns of lymphatic drainage can be clearly defined (e.g., drainage of the tongue to levels I, II, III, and IV, as well as other patterns) (Gray, 2017). Since there is also the possibility of contralateral drainage within the cervical lymph nodes, those with advanced disease may also require a bilateral neck dissection involving these same levels. Lymphedema may occur when radiation or surgical treatment results in severe damage to multiple levels of lymph nodes and the associated lymphatic vessels. When patients undergo a neck dissection as part of treatment for HNC, it is not uncommon to remove greater than 40 lymph nodes (Smith, 2013). In fact, with some advanced cases of HNC, the removal of over 100 lymph nodes may occur. However, due to the redundant drainage in the head and neck region, it is sometimes difficult to predict which patients will develop lymphedema and how severe it will be. Some patients who have undergone extensive resections never develop any lymphedema, while others develop swelling after removal of only a few lymph nodes. Consequently, information provided in the next sections will discuss HNL, its etiology, and its clinical management.

Edema Versus Lymphedema

As mentioned previously, both venous and lymphatic vessels feature one-way valves with the purpose of preventing backflow of fluid within their respective systems. If there is excessive production of fluid and the venous system has been overloaded due to a trauma, poor cardiac performance, poor vessel contraction, or faulty valve performance, fluid can back up within the veins. This can create increased intravascular pressure, resulting in vessel engorgement, dilation, and eventual spillage of fluid through the vein walls into the surrounding tissues. The mechanical result is soft tissue swelling that is known as edema (Zuther & Norton, 2017). Due to the low protein content of fluids found in these tissues, swelling associated with injury or that related to early stage of venous edema may be reduced more readily. That is, in such instances, tissues typically remain soft, and fluids can be quickly reduced when the lymphatic system is intact. In this circumstance, the lymphatic system works in conjunction with the venous system, increasing its rate of contraction to decrease the swelling in the tissues. This is evident in cases when there is immediate swelling with quick resolution, like that of a twisted ankle or similar soft tissue injury.

However, when the swelling that arises is due to a malfunctioning lymphatic system, the lymph backs up within the lymphatic vessels, creating vessel dilation, engorgement, and eventual leakage of lymph into the interstitial spaces of the soft tissues. The collection of thick, high-protein lymph in the soft tissues results in swelling known as lymphedema. Left untreated, the fluid in the interstitial spaces can increase, creating increased swelling and tissue thickness. Over time as edema worsens, this fluid can thicken since it is not being drained adequately, and this results in increased tissue firmness, which is itself an indicator in increased severity. Without proper intervention, ongoing tissue changes can occur, creating increased tissue firmness and progressive fibrosis that can worsen functional performance over time (Földi & Földi, 2006a, b; Zuther & Norton, 2017).

Etiology of Lymphedema

Lymphedema can occur anywhere in the body, but it most commonly develops in the extremities. Worldwide, the most common etiology for lymphedema is filariasis (lymphatic filariasis), a parasitic infestation within the lymphatics that occurs most often in equatorial countries with warm, moist climates that foster uncontrolled mosquito populations (Taylor, Hoerauf, & Bockarie, 2010). The parasite is commonly transmitted through repeated mosquito bites. Where individuals do not wear mosquito repellent or walk barefoot in wet fields, etc., there is an increased risk of multiple exposures, increasing the risk of infestation. Once the parasite is present, it nests within the lymphatic vessels and creates an obstruction that often results in massive edema of the lower extremities, genitalia, or other areas (Zuther & Norton, 2017). In North America, the most common cause of lymphedema is treatment for breast cancer with surgery and/or radiation (Maclellan et al., 2015), which commonly results in swelling of the upper extremity or breast region. Lower extremity edema occurs after cancer treatment, but it is also commonly encountered in cases of chronic obesity where the venous system has become dysfunctional and the increased load on the lymphatics eventually results in lymphedema (Shallwani, Hodgson, & Towers, 2017). Lymphedema can develop in other parts of the body, as well, including the abdomen, trunk, and genitalia (Földi & Földi, 2006a, b; Zuther & Norton, 2017). However, the remainder of this chapter will focus on HNL.

Head and Neck Lymphedema

As noted earlier, HNL most commonly presents as a secondary lymphedema due to injury of the lymphatic tissues. In addition to the sources of injury mentioned previously, facial edema can also result from allergic reactions and other sources of inflammation. Inflammatory causes of facial lymphedema include severe rosacea (including rhinophyma and otophyma), acne vulgaris, Melkersson–Rosenthal syndrome, and other dermatologic conditions (Smith, 2013). Facial edema is also a potential complication of certain cosmetic and dermatologic procedures. Even though chronic HNL is not commonly reported as a side effect of those treatments, MLD treatments are commonly provided to reduce postoperative edema after facelift procedures. Interestingly, tissue orientation is often altered with surgery, forcing the use of atypical facial drainage pathways to accommodate the postoperative changes (Mottura, 2002). Recovery in these cases is typically good, however, since the lymphatic system generally suffers minimal damage with these procedures and full recovery of lymphatic function is seen within 3–6 months (Meade, Teotia, Griffeth, & Barton, 2012). Interestingly, chronic HNL is uncommon after surgery of the face or neck that is non-cancer related. One possible explanation for this discrepancy is that lymph nodes are typically not removed during head and neck surgeries for non-cancerous conditions, allowing for continuation of good lymphatic drainage postoperatively.

However, as with facelifts, postoperative facial and neck edema is very common during the acute recovery phase of many surgeries. In cases of blunt facial trauma, edema can be substantial and create substantial impairments of speech, swallowing, and vision when severe. While there is no current literature describing its use, the author is aware of several programs in the United States that are treating facial trauma patients with MLD and achieving good results. This is a logical treatment choice, since MLD has been found to be very relaxing (Shim & Kim, 2014; Shim, Yeun, Kim, & Kim, 2017) and is known to facilitate improved lymphatic drainage. It has been theorized that MLD combined with traditional orthopedic rehabilitation would improve recovery of limb function after orthopedic injury, but current literature is lacking high-level evidence (Vairo, Miller, Rier, & Uckley, 2009). One recent article discusses the regeneration of lymphatic channels after facial transplant, suggesting that MLD could be a useful tool to promote lymphatic drainage in that population as well (Sosin, Mundinger, Drachenberg, & Rodriguez, 2017). Unfortunately, even though the most common etiology of HNL is treatment for HNC, literature related to HNL and its management are limited. For that reason, the remainder of this chapter will discuss HNL, its impact on patients, and effective treatment.

How is HNL Different than Lymphedema Elsewhere?

Head and neck lymphedema (HNL) is particularly concerning for both patients and their families. When severe, there can be both functional and cosmetic complaints associated with HNL. For example, functional complaints may include impairment of vision when eyelids are swollen. This not only affects visual acuity and peripheral vision but may also disrupt other tasks that require adequate vision such as reading, writing, walking, and driving. Similarly, speech, mastication, swallowing, and respiration can be impaired when the lips, tongue, and upper airway are swollen. In severe cases of HNL, a tracheotomy or a feeding tube may be required. Dysphagia also has been associated with lymphedema of the external neck tissues and supraglottic edema (Murphy & Gilbert, 2009; Smith, 2013; Smith et al., 2014; Smith & Lewin, 2010). Severe submental and anterior neck edema may be chronic and severe; if this occurs, it can occlude the tracheostoma, potentially interfering with efficient breathing after a total laryngectomy. This may mandate use of an intraluminal device like a laryngectomy tube or laryngectomy button to maintain a patent airway. Severe facial edema also can be quite disfiguring which may result in decreased socialization and increased social anxiety. Even when the edema is relatively minor and does not create a significant functional impairment, patients often report cosmetic concerns that can affect psychosocial and emotional issues since HNL cannot be easily hidden. Thus, the larger impact of HNL on individuals and members of their family may be substantial (Deng et al., 2012; Deng et al., 2015; Deng, Ridner, Aulino, & Murphy, 2015; Smith, 2013; Smith & Lewin, 2010; Smith et al., 2014).

Despite its obvious presentation, HNL has often been overlooked, misdiagnosed, or dismissed as an expected side effect of cancer treatment without effective treatment options (Smith, 2013; Smith et al., 2014). Other times, a clinician may identify HNL but have minimal experience with the condition, creating a lack of confidence or inadequate skills to effectively treat the patient. This is in stark contrast to management of the more common presentations of lymphedema, since most lymphedema therapists are adequately prepared to treat edema in the trunk and limbs after being trained to do so during their basic certification coursework. Management of HNL, however, requires advanced training that is not mandatory, so many lymphedema therapists do not feel it is essential for their practice.

There has been increased interest in the management of HNL in recent years. It is presumed this could be related to the continued increase in the number of patients diagnosed with oropharyngeal cancer related to the human papilloma (HPV) virus over the past 20 years (Tanakka & Alawi, 2018; Theurer, Chap. 4). Since HPV+ cancers typically are being diagnosed in a younger population and there is a higher rate of survival after treatment (Deng et al., 2012a), we are now being presented with patients who wish to return to work and maintain an active lifestyle posttreatment. Since HNL is typically quite visible and is often associated with functional deficits, its presence often prompts requests for intervention. With the increased numbers of cancer survivors who are now dealing with the aftereffects of treatment, including HNL, more therapists are encountering patients with HNL and are requesting advanced training to adequately treat this population. The ability to effectively evaluate and treat HNL is crucial to reducing the edema and improving the patient's quality of life (Deng, et al., 2012; Smith, 2013).

Cancer Treatment and HNL

As noted previously, HNL occurs most frequently in patients who have undergone surgery and/or radiotherapy for cancer and seems to be most severe after receiving a combination of both treatments (Deng, Murphy, et al., 2015; Deng, et al., 2012a; Deng, Ridner, et al., 2015; Smith et al., 2014). The impact of chemotherapy on the development of HNL is not known. HNL has been reported in patients who received both chemotherapy and radiotherapy (Deng, Murphy, et al., 2015; Deng, Ridner, et al., 2015; Smith et al., 2014; Smith & Lewin, 2010), and taxane-based chemotherapy has been linked to lymphedema of the extremities (Cariati et al., 2015; Zhu et al., 2017). However, even though taxane-based chemotherapy is sometimes used in management of HNC, there have been no published accounts of HNL following chemotherapy in isolation for HNC. There has been a publication documenting pemetrexed-induced edema of the eyelid and periorbital region when used for with lung cancer treatment (Charfi, Kastalli, Sahnoun, & Lakhoua, 2016; Mangla, Carlson, Wakil, Wu, & Wladis, 2015). Currently, sufficient data do not exist to suggest a causative relationship between most current chemotherapy regimens and chronic HNL.

HNL has been documented in up to 75% of patients treated with surgery or radiotherapy to the head and neck (Buntzel, Glatzel, Mucke, Micke, & Bruns, 2007; Deng et al., 2012b). It is not surprising that radiotherapy contributes to development of HNL, since the primary tumor, adjacent soft tissues, bony structures, and relevant lymphatic drainage pathways may all be irradiated in an effort to shrink existing tumors, treat persistent microscopic disease, and prevent metastasis. Tissue fibrosis also is a common complication of radiotherapy (Deng, et al., 2012a; Kim, Shin, Kim, Yoon, & Kim, 2015), and it can impair tissue drainage by decreasing tissue elasticity and constricting vascular flow (Deng, et al., 2012a; Patel & McGurk, 2017; Smith, 2013), subsequently decreasing lymphangiomotoricity. Patients who receive radiation to the head and neck often develop chronic edema of tissues within the irradiated field, which commonly encompasses the lower face, neck, and supraclavicular fossa. When re-irradiation is required to treat cancer recurrence, further tissue damage occurs which in turn

increases the severity of tissue fibrosis and associated HNL. It is not uncommon for patients to experience mild edema in the treatment field during radiotherapy. This type of tissue inflammation typically reduces within a few weeks of treatment completion, and, in many cases, no subsequent lymphedema develops. However, it is also typical for HNL to develop 8–12 weeks after treatment has been completed (Deng, et al., 2012a; Smith, 2013). In such circumstances, it is hypothesized that 2–3 months may be required for the diffuse postradiation tissue changes that occur to substantially affect lymph transport and create visible edema in the tissue of the head and neck. Thus, the onset of observable changes specific to HNL may be delayed in some instances.

Surgery as a treatment modality for HNC is a common contributor to lymphedema (Deng, et al., 2012a, 2012b; Smith, 2013; Smith et al., 2014; Smith & Lewin, 2010). Its occurrence is due to direct anatomic disruption of the lymphatic and/or venous drainage systems. Cancer surgery typically requires the removal of the tumor and some of the surrounding soft tissues for reasons of oncologic safety. Further, the bone may be removed if there is tumor invasion or severe damage to the bone from radiotherapy (osteoradionecrosis) (Smith, 2013). More extensive surgeries also may require microvascular reconstruction if the surgical defect is too large to leave unrepaired. Sometimes, these "flaps" are large, and the boundaries that are sutured in place create barriers to drainage (Yeh, Sahovaler & Yoo, Chap. 2). In these cases, the use of reconstructive "flap" procedures may also be considered as a contributor to HNL.

Two common reconstruction techniques include pedicled flaps or free tissue transfer (Hanasono, 2014; Hanasono, Matros, & Disa, 2014). Pedicled flaps typically involve a local tissue transfer or "rotational" flap, a procedure that involves surgical release of skin, fat, and/or fascia from one area, while keeping the other end intact to retain the original vascular supply. Using this technique, the surgeon repositions the unattached end of the "flap" into the surgical defect and reattaches the arteries and veins to ensure adequate blood flow. An example of a pedicled flap is the use of a pectoralis major flap. Free tissue transfers, commonly referred to as free flaps, involve transplanting tissue from one part of the body to another. For example, tissue from the forearm or thigh may be used to replace a portion of the tongue or pharynx. The skill of the surgeon, the extensiveness of the surgical defect, and the availability of an adequate donor site will typically determine if a free flap can be performed. Depending on the type of reconstruction and surgery performed, HNL may be an expected complication. However, lymphedema management may be delayed, allowing adequate time for tissue healing before any active manipulation of tissues to reduce edema is initiated.

One of the most common surgical procedures in the treatment of HNC is a neck dissection (lymphadenectomy), which is the surgical removal of lymph nodes. Depending on the extensiveness of the disease, cervical, facial, mediastinal, paratracheal, or supraclavicular lymph nodes may be included in a neck dissection. It is not uncommon for greater than 30 lymph nodes to be removed, though often there may be more than 50 nodes involved (Smith, 2013). In cases where there is tumor involvement or severe radiation scarring of the jugular vein(s), the disruption of the venous drainage system in the head and neck increases the risk of HNL. This lymphatic and venous disruption results in a lympho-venous or "mixed edema," which is typically less responsive to treatment than a pure lymphedema that may be present in an area where radiotherapy was not delivered. Additionally, surgical scarring can directly impact the development of HNL due to a "trapdoor effect" (Szolnoky, Mohos, Dobozy, & Kemény, 2006). That is, with such an effect, a scar prevents drainage through the lymphatic channels of the skin, resulting in edema above the scar, but not below it. Therefore, multimodality cancer treatment creates a unique environment for the development of lymphedema in the face and neck that can be challenging to evaluate and treat.

Speech Pathology and Head and Neck Lymphedema

Currently, the evaluation and treatment of lymphedema does not typically fall within the responsibilities of speech pathologists. While rehabilitation of communication and swallowing has long been within the scope of practice for medical speech pathologists, HNL management has typically been relegated to other rehabilitation disciplines. Therapists who have completed the requisite specialty training in the evaluation and management of lymphedema may be referred to as "certified lymphedema therapists" or CLTs ("How to Locate a Certified Lymphedema Therapist in Your Area,", n.d.). This has not traditionally been a specialty pursued by speech pathologists, despite their often significant and active participation in the rehabilitation of patients with HNC. However, over the past decade, there has been an increased overall awareness and interest in HNL within the medical community who serve those treated for HNC. This may be partially due to the increased number of younger patients being diagnosed with HPV-positive oropharyngeal cancer, as mentioned previously. Regardless of the reason, more therapists are now learning to manage HNL, including increasing numbers of speech pathologists. Since HNL often accompanies deficits in swallowing and communication following HNC treatment (Deng, et al., 2012; Murphy & Gilbert, 2009; Smith et al., 2014; Smith & Lewin, 2010), speech pathologists may be among the first to identify HNL. As such, SLPs should be instrumental in referring the patient for lymphedema evaluation and treatment and, with proper training, may also become a practitioner of HNL management techniques.

Clinical Evaluation for Head and Neck Lymphedema

As a speech pathologist who is not trained in management of lymphedema, you will not be performing formal assessments of patients with HNL. However, it is likely that you will be seeing these patients for other issues, and, as their clinician, you may be the first to observe potential lymphedema. In that capacity, the clinician should be aware of the signs of lymphedema and be able to perform an assessment screening; doing so will identify the need for a referral for lymphedema assessment and treatment. Further, there are a number of symptoms that typically may be observed with HNL. When present, many of these symptoms can serve to differentiate HNL from other types of swelling. Most commonly, the patient will present with fullness in the face, neck, or oral cavity that is not associated with fever, tissue irritation, or pain. Some patients may report that the condition developed slowly after insult to the system, most likely associated with the completion of radiation or surgery. Edema may be bilateral or unilateral, and tissues may be either soft and "doughy" or, in contrast, firm to touch. The observed edema may be generalized, for example, in an area such as the central anterior neck or lower face. However, edema may be more focal, such as that which occurs in the area around a scar, one half of the tongue, or an eyelid. In either case, the degree and extent of HNL will depend on the area treated and the amount of damage potential sustained as a result of treatment. In cases of lymphedema, the color and general appearance of the edematous area are usually consistent with the surrounding tissues, and the skin is not painful. In contrast, however, swelling associated with tissue redness, reports of pain, drainage of pus, or a sensation of heat is more consistent with an infection, and, as such, the patient should be referred to a physician for further medical assessment and management (Földi & Földi, 2006a; Smith, 2013; Zuther & Norton, 2017).

As part of the general clinical evaluation, and since swelling can occur for many different reasons, it is important to determine whether or not the patient has experienced some specific event that may underlie the development of lymphedema. For example, your patient may present with arm swelling that developed after suffering a stroke. This commonly is the result of poor circulation, and swelling may occur when the arm is not properly supported. The color of the arm and hand should be normal and there should not be pain at rest. Management of this scenario typically involves elevating the arm to an appropriate level and providing support to the limb ("Upper Limb Management After Stroke Fact Sheet," 2017). Management of swelling that results from venous obstruction related to a blood clot, which can be a medical emergency, is much different. To elaborate, swelling related to a deep vein thrombosis (DVT) or blood clot can be painful, warm, and discolored. If you observe those signs, medical attention should be obtained immediately so the patient can undergo imaging and begin medical treatment, typically with anticoagulants, but possibly surgical intervention (Barclay, n.d.). Development of a DVT is a serious condition that cannot be disregarded.

The same type of discernment is important when evaluating patients with possible edema of the head and neck since facial edema can result from a wide variety of causes (Miest et al., 2017). Some cases of facial edema are related to an allergic reaction, requiring urgent medication administration (Pope & Pillai, 2014). Other urgent medical conditions may include superior vena cava syndrome (Pope & Pillai, 2014), where there is an obstruction of the superior vena cava, typically related to compression of the vessel by a large mass. Postoperative swelling within a surgical bed (seroma) is not uncommon, and it is treated by draining the fluid from the affected region (Liu, Gullane, Brown, & Irish, 2001). Other reasons for facial swelling include trauma, hypothyroidism, or growths such as benign tumors, cysts, etc., so it is important to ask questions to account for the areas of concern before making a referral back to the physician. Doing so can help to ensure that appropriate referrals and potential interventions can be provided. However, when the clinical presentation and medical history do not support the diagnosis of lymphedema, referral to the patient's physician for further evaluation is appropriate.

Once the patient is referred for a lymphedema evaluation by a certified lymphedema therapist, assessment should include a thorough medical history and evaluation of cervical and upper extremity range of motion, general communication and swallowing function, and documentation of the patient's appearance with photographs and tape measurements (Smith, 2013). Depending on the sophistication of the lymphedema program, the evaluation process may be very simple or could be quite extensive. More comprehensive levels of the evaluation may include instrumental assessment with ultrasound, 3-D photography, or advanced imaging assessments to achieve a more detailed profile of the patient's lymphatic functioning and severity of impairment. While there is a well-defined assessment protocol for lymphedema of the extremities, evaluation of HNL has been less standardized (Smith, 2013). This limitation is due to the inconsistency of head and face shapes among individuals, making it much more difficult to establish a reliable measurement protocol that can be easily and uniformly applied to all patients. In general, measurements should be obtained in a consistent, repeatable fashion so that sequential assessments will reflect changes over time. Tape measurements are subject to human error due to differences in the pressure application during the measurement process, so care must be taken to ensure accuracy and consistency over time. As with any measurement process, efforts that seek to "standardize" procedures will be of great benefit relative to the documentation of outcomes. Despite several publications outlining specific measurement protocols and rating scales, assessment of HNL remains inconsistent among clinicians (Deng, Murphy, et al., 2015; Deng, Ridner, et al., 2015; Smith, 2013; Smith et al., 2014; Smith & Lewin, 2010).

In most cases, assessment of HNL has addressed only the external skin of the neck and face, as well as the structures that can be easily visualized within the oral cavity. It is also possible to endoscopically assess the laryngeal and pharyngeal mucosa, which may also become edematous and create significant functional impairments affecting respiration, voice, and swallowing (Deng, et al., 2012b; Jackson et al., 2016; Murphy & Gilbert, 2009; Smith et al., 2014). In high-volume HNC centers where a large number of patients with HNL are seen, endoscopic assessments may be performed to document the extent of the "inter-

nal edema." However, at present, this type of clinical documentation is uncommon in most centers.

Currently, there are no established guidelines to determine what defines the "normal" face or neck, aside from an expectation of relative symmetry. In fact, several studies have shown that most people's facial appearance is not identical when compared side by side and most facial measurements are not symmetrical, even in the "normal" population (Jackson et al., 2013). However, asymmetry of the neck, face, or oral cavity can be determined through careful visual observation (Taylor et al., 2014). Nevertheless, the subjective nature of visual assessment alone is inadequate to document change. More objective methods like tape measurements can reflect differences in one side of the face or neck when compared to the other, but, at present, there is not an agreed-upon degree of difference used to indicate that one side is edematous and the other is normal. As a result, most assessment protocols used to evaluate facial or neck edema utilize a longitudinal comparison of measurements to evaluate changes in neck or facial size over time (Deng, Murphy, et al., 2015; Deng, Ridner, et al., 2015; Smith, 2013; Smith et al., 2014; Smith & Lewin, 2010). Subjective lymphedema rating scales are also used to assess and document the texture of the edematous tissues, attempting to rate the severity of edema based on tissue firmness, pliability, etc. (Deng, Ridner, Dietrich, Wells, & Murphy, 2013; Smith, 2013; Smith et al., 2014; Smith & Lewin, 2010). As tissues become less elastic secondary to HNL and increase in terms of firmness, thickness, and fibrosis (scarring), the degree of edema is rated as more severe. Thus, a comprehensive assessment is required to adequately determine the severity of the edema and the potential for improvement with treatment and to develop an appropriate treatment plan. However, there remains a substantial need for development of more sensitive assessment methodologies that are both clinically friendly and affordable. The development of such evaluative methodologies may offer advantages of a more accurate and comprehensive diagnosis of HNL, as well as better identifying its impact on patient performance.

HNL Treatment

Like a formal lymphedema evaluation, treatment of HNL should not be performed by therapists without specialized training. In recent years, more speech pathologists who work with HNC patients have received training in HNL management. This is appropriate for therapists who see HNC patients frequently, and, since some disciplines other than speech pathology may be less comfortable with the HNC population, it may make sense for the SLP to provide this treatment. However, evaluation and management by a skilled physical or occupational therapist is always of benefit when addressing the other physical needs of the patient, like limitations in cervical range of motion, upper extremity impairment, mobility, posture, etc. In some locations, there is not a CLT available, prompting speech pathologists to pursue training in HNL management and, in some cases, pursue full CLT certification. Thus, the purpose of the section to follow seeks to discuss general treatment considerations, rather than specific treatment techniques.

Complete Decongestive Therapy

Lymphedema management typically features four major components that, when combined together, are referred to as complete decongestive therapy (CDT) (Strossenreuther, 2006; Zuther & Norton, 2017). These four components include MLD, compression wrapping or bandaging, exercise, and wound/skin care. Each component of the CDT process is designed to achieve a particular treatment goal. Thus, for each patient, one component may be used with increasing frequency over another. Not everyone has significant wound or skin issues, for example. However, MLD is a very gentle, skin stretching style of massage that uses a particular sequence of lateral skin manipulations. These manipulations are done in a slow, rhythmic fashion to improve lymph transport, a function that is a key component of treatment for almost all patients with lymphedema, regardless of the edema location. The use of compression bandages or similar garments is an equally important component of CDT. The use of compression approaches enhances the longevity of the MLD effects, allowing a greater period time between the emptying and refilling of the tissues once treatment is complete. Exercise combined with compression can magnify the treatment effect even further, so for patients with HNL, the two most common interventions are MLD and compression, followed by exercise and skin care, as needed (Smith, 2013).

A typical approach for MLD is to decongest the deeper lymphatic vessels first, and then decongest the superficial system beginning in the trunk, gradually moving to the distal portion of the limbs, and then reversing the sequence to move the fluid away from the congested hand, arm, foot, or leg back to the body and across the midline (watershed) to an unaffected lymph node bed (Strossenreuther, 2006; Zuther & Norton, 2017). This process can be quite effective, but, without the use of compression wrapping or a compression garment, the fluid will refill the limb somewhat quickly. This process must be repeated on a daily basis and also may be required for months or years in order to maintain the size of the limb that is at an acceptable level. In severe cases, the affected limb can swell to enormous proportions, creating terrible consequences for the patients in terms of mobility, completion of activities of daily living (ADLs), socialization, and overall health, since a large immobile limb with poor lymphatic function is more prone to infection.

Treatment for HNL can often be quite effective, and, anecdotally, it appears that patients with HNL have a gravitational advantage over patients with edema in other locations (Smith, 2013; Smith et al., 2014). It is not uncommon for patients with HNL to display increased edema when they first arise in the morning, but since the head is at the top of the body, there is improved drainage when the patient is upright and becomes more mobile during the day. This is in opposition to edema in the limbs where it may frequently be observed to worsen over the day due to the dependent (downward) position of the feet and hands.

When Should Treatment Occur?

Postsurgery Treatment timeframes vary according to the patient's treatment history and medical complexity. In an acute setting with trauma cases where lymphatics are not compromised, MLD treatment may be provided very soon after surgery to reduce postoperative edema, and results may be observed quite rapidly. With patients who have undergone surgery for HNC, however, there is often compromise of the cervical lymphatics and the major blood vessels of the neck. These types of patients may be able to receive MLD to the face and trunk within the first 2 weeks of surgery if judged medically appropriate, but, in many cases, acute management of the neck is often not possible due to complex microvascular reconstructions (Smith, 2013). Diaphragmatic breathing and manual lymph drainage of the trunk may be perfectly safe and can usually be used to facilitate improved lymph drainage even if the most edematous areas cannot be directly addressed. In most postoperative situations for patients with HNC, unless the edema is severe enough to create substantial visual or breathing deficits, direct treatment is usually not provided for 4 weeks to allow adequate healing of reconstructions and to allow reduction of general postoperative edema.

Postradiation As noted earlier, radiation treatment is another common contributor to development of HNL. Following radiotherapy to the head and neck, it is not uncommon to see HNL appear between 8 and 12 weeks after the completion of treatment. If the skin is intact and the patient can tolerate the manipulation of their skin with MLD, treatment of postradiation-induced HNL can usually begin immediately upon identification. In patients who have undergone surgery and have postoperative edema, but who will be receiving postsurgical radiotherapy, it is possible to treat them before and during the early stages of radiation treatment. However, treatment may need to be discontinued when their skin becomes too sensitive. However, it has been observed that patients who experience edema reductions, while performing MLD during radiotherapy can lose their progress once they stop treatment due to skin breakdown (Fig. 22.3). This delay in treatment typically results in refilling of tissues, and lymphedema management essentially starts over once their skin is healed adequately to resume MLD and begin wearing a compression garment. Another complicating factor is the poor tolerance of compression garments during radiotherapy, which also results in more rapid refilling of tissues, as mentioned previously. As a result, many patients and/or therapists elect to minimize treatment before radiotherapy and focus their efforts on the postirradiation developments that arise after treatment (Smith, 2013).

Palliation Finally, in addition to traditional lymphedema management following radiation or surgery, HNL can also be treated on a palliative basis. Massive facial and neck edema (Fig. 22.4) can occur when a patient develops a large tumor in the neck or chest that is creating an obstruction of lymphatic vessels, veins, or both. This has been called "malignant lymphedema" since it

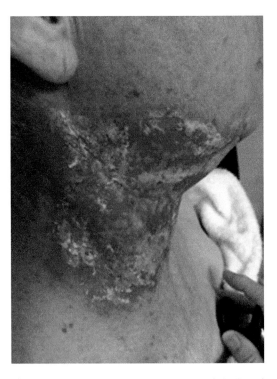

Fig. 22.3 Radiation damage on the skin of the lateral neck. (Photo courtesy of B. Smith)

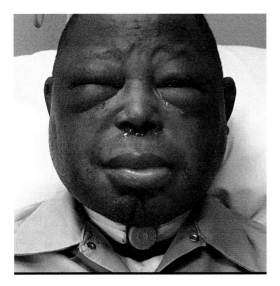

Fig. 22.4 Example of patient with extensive facial edema. (Photo courtesy of B. Smith)

arises due to a malignancy (Földi & Földi, 2006a, b). It may be present before treatment if the tumor has grown quite large, but more often this occurs with recurrent disease after surgical, radiation, and /or chemotherapy treatment have been provided. Palliative treatment is often provided near the patient's end of life and intended as a comfort measure, without expectation of resolving the edema long-term.

MLD is very soothing and can improve the patient's quality of life by decreasing discomfort, increasing relaxation, and temporarily improving function as swollen tissues are reduced. In some instances, the results of MLD may be relatively short. This is a direct result of the lymphatic drainage system being severely impaired which then allows tissues to refill more quickly. However, although the results of MLD may be short in some instances, the positive impact of treatment in terms of quality of life can be substantial to many. Swollen eyes being opened can allow someone to write or see, and reduction of swollen lips or a swollen tongue may allow improved speech or swallowing, even if only for a short time before the tissue refill again. Palliative treatment is usually a worthwhile effort and should be encouraged if it appears that treat-

ment can be provided with no immediate risk of harm, but it must be noted that treatment is not appropriate in all cases (Smith, 2013).

Contraindications for Lymphedema Management

Clinicians need to be aware that not all patients are appropriate candidates for lymphedema management due to medical contraindications. Consequently, evaluation by a physician and qualified lymphedema therapist is essential to prevent inappropriate treatment. Examples of contraindications include but are not limited to upper-quadrant deep vein thrombosis (DVT), severe cerebrovascular disease with multiple cerebrovascular accidents (CVA) or transient ischemic attacks (TIA) related to carotid disease, severe carotid artery occlusion, congestive heart failure (CHF), renal failure, acute infection, and/or hyperthyroidism. Treatment provided in the face of these conditions may create substantial complications; therefore, lymphedema management should not be provided until one is medically cleared to do so (Strossenreuther, 2006).

Summary

This chapter has provided information related to the basic anatomy and physiology of the cardiovascular and lymphatic systems, various etiologies of facial edema, differences between venous edema and HNL, treatment precautions and contraindications, and general management strategies. Most importantly, this chapter has outlined the relevance of HNL for the speech pathologist who may be treating patients with a history of HNC treatment. With increasing rates of head and neck cancer expected in the years to come, understanding HNL becomes of even greater importance to clinicians. While HNL management may never be your direct responsibility, understanding how it occurs and how it can be managed is essential. However, if you are working with HNC patients who receive surgery or radiation treatment, it is likely that you will encounter at least one patient with HNL. Whether or not you ever receive training to directly provide lymphedema management, your ability to recognize HNL and refer those who present with this problem for proper treatment is of substantial value. By doing so, access to treatment may result in substantial functional improvement secondary to the reduction of HNL, as well as increasing their subsequent potential to maximize quality of life.

References

Barclay, L. (n.d.). Management of upper extremity deep-vein thrombosis reviewed. Retrieved 13 Nov, 2017, from https://www.medscape.com/viewarticle/738886

Buntzel, J., Glatzel, M., Mucke, R., Micke, O., & Bruns, F. (2007). Influence of amifostine on late radiation-toxicity in head and neck cancer: a follow-up study. *Anticancer Research, 27*, 1953–1956.

Cariati, M., Bains, S. K., Grootendorst, M. R., Suyoi, A., Peters, A. M., Mortimer, P., … Purushotham, A. D. (2015). Adjuvant taxanes and the development of breast cancer-related arm lymphoedema. *British Journal of Surgery, 102*(9), 1071–1078. https://doi.org/10.1002/bjs.9846

Charfi, O., Kastalli, S., Sahnoun, R., & Lakhoua, G. (2016). Eyelid and feet edema induced by pemetrexed. *Indian Journal of Pharmacology, 48*(6), 741. https://doi.org/10.4103/0253-7613.194862

Cracchiolo, J. R., & Wong, R. J. (2017). Management of the lateral neck in well differentiated thyroid cancer. *European Journal of Surgical Oncology, 44*(3), 332–337.

Deng, J., Murphy, B. A., Dietrich, M. S., Sinard, R. J., Mannion, K., & Ridner, S. H. (2015). Differences of symptoms in head and neck cancer patients with and without lymphedema. *Supportive Care in Cancer, 24*(3), 1305–1316. https://doi.org/10.1007/s00520-015-2893-4

Deng, J., Murphy, B. A., Dietrich, M. S., Wells, N., Wallston, K. A., Sinard, R. J., … Ridner, S. H. (2012). Impact of secondary lymphedema after head and neck cancer treatment on symptoms, functional status, and quality of life. *Head & Neck, 35*(7), 1026–1035. https://doi.org/10.1002/hed.23084

Deng, J., Ridner, S. H., Aulino, J. M., & Murphy, B. A. (2015). Assessment and measurement of head and neck lymphedema: State-of-the-science and future directions. *Oral Oncology, 51*(5), 431–437. https://doi.org/10.1016/j.oraloncology.2015.01.005

Deng, J., Ridner, S. H., Dietrich, M. S., Wells, N., & Murphy, B. A. (2013). Assessment of external lymphedema in patients with head and neck cancer: A comparison of four scales. *Oncology Nursing Forum, 40*(5), 501–506. https://doi.org/10.1188/13.onf.501-506

Deng, J., Ridner, S. H., Dietrich, M. S., Wells, N., Wallston, K. A., Sinard, R. J., … Murphy, B. (2012a). Factors associated with external and internal lymphedema in patients with head-and-neck cancer. *International Journal of Radiation Oncology, Biology, and Physics, 84*(3), e319.

Deng, J., Ridner, S. H., Dietrich, M. S., Wells, N., Wallston, K. A., Sinard, R. J., … Murphy, B. A. (2012b). Prevalence of secondary lymphedema in patients with head and neck cancer. *Journal of Pain and Symptom Management, 43*(2), 244–252. https://doi.org/10.1016/j.jpainsymman.2011.03.019

Feely, M. A., Olsen, K. D., Gamble, G. L., Davis, M. D., & Pittelkow, M. R. (2011). Cutaneous lymphatics and chronic lymphedema of the head and neck. *Clinical Anatomy, 25*(1), 72–85. https://doi.org/10.1002/ca.22009

Földi, M., & Földi, E. (2006a). Lymphostatic diseases. In M. Földi & E. Földi (Eds.), *Földi's textbook of lymphology for physicians and lymphedema therapists* (2nd ed., pp. 224–319). Munich, Germany: Urban & Fischer.

Földi, M., & Földi, E. (2006b). Physiology and pathophysiology of the lymphatic system. In M. Földi & E. Földi (Eds.), *Földi's textbook of lymphology for physicians and lymphedema therapists* (2nd ed., pp. 180–222). Munich, Germany: Urban & Fischer.

Gray, H. *Anatomy of the Human Body*. Retrieved 12 Nov, 2017 from http://www.bartleby.com/107/illus605.html

Hanasono, M. M. (2014). Reconstructive surgery for head and neck cancer patients. *Advances in Medicine, 2014*, 1–28. https://doi.org/10.1155/2014/795483

Hanasono, M. M., Matros, E., & Disa, J. J. (2014). Important aspects of head and neck reconstruction. *Plastic and Reconstructive Surgery, 134*(6), 968e–980e. https://doi.org/10.1097/prs.0000000000000722

How to Locate a Certified Lymphedema Therapist in Your Area. (n.d.). Retrieved November 13, 2017, from http://www.lymphedemablog.com/2010/09/16/how-to-locate-a-certified-lymphedema-therapist-in-your-area/

Jackson, T. H., Mitroff, S. R., Clark, K., Proffit, W. R., Lee, J. Y., & Nguyen, T. T. (2013). Face symmetry assessment abilities: Clinical implications for diagnosing asymmetry. *American Journal of Orthodontics and Dentofacial Orthopedics, 144*(5), 663–671. https://doi.org/10.1016/j.ajodo.2013.06.020

Jackson, L. K., Ridner, S. H., Deng, J., Bartow, C., Mannion, K., Niermann, K., … Murphy, B. A. (2016). Internal lymphedema correlates with subjective and objective measures of dysphagia in head and neck cancer patients. *Journal of Palliative Medicine, 19*(9), 949–956. https://doi.org/10.1089/jpm.2016.0018

Kim, J., Shin, E. S., Kim, J. E., Yoon, S. P., & Kim, Y. S. (2015). Neck muscle atrophy and soft-tissue fibrosis after neck dissection and postoperative radiotherapy for oral cancer. *Radiation Oncology Journal, 33*(4), 344. https://doi.org/10.3857/roj.2015.33.4.344

Kubik, S., & Kretz, O. (2003). Anatomy of the lymphatic system. In M. Földi, E. Földi, & P. Kubik (Eds.), *Textbook of lymphology: For physicians and lymphedema therapists* (pp. 2–149). Munich, Germany: Urban & Fischer.

Liu, R., Gullane, P., Brown, D., & Irish, J. (2001). Pectoralis major myocutaneous pedicled flap in head and neck reconstruction: Retrospective review of indications and results in 244 consecutive cases at the Toronto General Hospital. *The Journal of Otolaryngology, 30*(01), 034. https://doi.org/10.2310/7070.2001.21011

Maclellan, R. A., Couto, R. A., Sullivan, J. E., Grant, F. D., Slavin, S. A., & Greene, A. K. (2015). Management of primary and secondary lymphedema. *Annals of Plastic Surgery, 75*(2), 197–200. https://doi.org/10.1097/sap.0000000000000022

Mangla, N., Carlson, A., Wakil, A., Wu, N., & Wladis, E. J. (2015). Pemetrexed-associated eyelid edema. *Ophthalmic Plastic and Reconstructive Surgery, 31*(6). https://doi.org/10.1097/iop.0000000000000186

Meade, R. A., Teotia, S. S., Griffeth, L. K., & Barton, F. E. (2012). Facelift and patterns of lymphatic drainage. *Aesthetic Surgery Journal, 32*(1), 39–45. https://doi.org/10.1177/1090820x11430683

Miest, R. Y., Bruce, A. J., Comfere, N. I., Hadjicharalambous, E., Endly, D., Lohse, C. M., & Rogers, R. S. (2017). A diagnostic approach to recurrent orofacial swelling: A retrospective study of 104 patients. *Mayo Clinic Proceedings, 92*(7), 1053–1060. https://doi.org/10.1016/j.mayocp.2017.03.015

Mottura, A. A. (2002). Face lift postoperative recovery. *Aesthetic Plastic Surgery, 26*(3), 172–180. https://doi.org/10.1007/s00266-001-0029-3

Murphy, B. A., & Gilbert, J. (2009). Dysphagia in head and neck cancer patients treated with radiation: Assessment, sequelae, and rehabilitation. *Seminars in Radiation Oncology, 19*(1), 35–42. https://doi.org/10.1016/j.semradonc.2008.09.007

Patel, V., & McGurk, M. (2017). Use of pentoxifylline and tocopherol in radiation-induced fibrosis and fibroatrophy. *British Journal of Oral and Maxillofacial Surgery, 55*(3), 235–241. https://doi.org/10.1016/j.bjoms.2016.11.323

Pope, C., & Pillai, S. K. (2014). Intermittent facial swelling. *British Medical Journal Case Reports*. https://doi.org/10.1136/bcr-2013-202355

Robbins, K. T., Clayman, G., Levine, P. A., Medina, J., Sessions, R., Shaha, A., ... Wolf, G. T. (2002). Neck dissection classification update: revisions proposed by the American Head and Neck Society and the American Academy of Otolaryngology–Head and Neck Surgery. *Archives of Otolaryngology–Head & Neck Surgery, 128*(7), 751–758.

Robbins, K. T., Medina, J. E., Wolfe, G. T., Levine, P. A., Sessions, R. B., & Pruet, C. W. (1991). Standardizing neck dissection terminology: Official report of the Academy's Committee for Head and Neck Surgery

and Oncology. *Archives of Otolaryngology–Head & Neck Surgery, 117*(6), 601–605.

Shallwani, S. M., Hodgson, P., & Towers, A. (2017). Comparisons between cancer-related and noncancer-related lymphedema: An overview of new patients referred to a specialized hospital-based center in Canada. *Lymphatic Research and Biology, 15*(1), 64–69. https://doi.org/10.1089/lrb.2016.0023

Shim, J., & Kim, S. (2014). Effects of manual lymph drainage of the neck on EEG in subjects with psychological stress. *Journal of Physical Therapy Science, 26*(1), 127–129. https://doi.org/10.1589/jpts.26.127

Shim, J., Yeun, Y., Kim, H., & Kim, S. (2017). Effects of manual lymph drainage for abdomen on the brain activity of subjects with psychological stress. *Journal of Physical Therapy Science, 29*(3), 491–494. https://doi.org/10.1589/jpts.29.491

Smith, B. G. (2013). Head and neck lymphedema. In J. E. Zuther & S. Norton (Eds.), *Lymphedema management: The comprehensive guide for practitioners* (3rd ed., pp. 191–208). New York, NY: Thieme.

Smith, B. G., Hutcheson, K. A., Little, L. G., Skoracki, R. J., Rosenthal, D. I., Lai, S. Y., & Lewin, J. S. (2014). Lymphedema outcomes in patients with head and neck cancer. *Otolaryngology-Head and Neck Surgery, 152*(2), 284–291. https://doi.org/10.1177/0194599814558402

Smith, B. G., & Lewin, J. S. (2010). Lymphedema management in head and neck cancer. *Current Opinion in Otolaryngology & Head and Neck Surgery, 18*(3), 153–158. https://doi.org/10.1097/moo.0b013e3283393799

Som, P. M., Curtin, H. D., & Mancuso, A. A. (2000). Imaging-based nodal classification for evaluation of neck metastatic adenopathy. *American Journal of Roentgenology, 174*(3), 837–844. https://doi.org/10.2214/ajr.174.3.1740837

Sosin, M., Mundinger, G. S., Drachenberg, C. B., & Rodriguez, E. D. (2017). Lymphatic reconstitution and regeneration after face transplantation. *Annals of Plastic Surgery, 79*(5), 505–508. https://doi.org/10.1097/sap.0000000000001222

Strossenreuther, R. H. K. (2006). Practical instructions for therapists-manual lymph drainage according to Dr E. Vodder. In M. Földi & E. Földi (Eds.), *Földi's textbook of lymphology for physicians and lymphedema therapists* (2nd ed., pp. 526–546). Munich, Germany: Urban & Fischer.

Szolnoky, G., Mohos, G., Dobozy, A., & Kemény, L. (2006). Manual lymph drainage reduces trapdoor effect in subcutaneous island pedicle flaps. *International Journal of Dermatology, 45*(12), 1468–1470. https://doi.org/10.1111/j.1365-4632.2006.03165.x

Tanakka, T. I., & Alawi, F. (2018). Human papilloma virus and oropharyngeal cancer. *Dental Clinics of North America, 62*(1), 111–120. https://doi.org/10.1016/j.cden.2017.08.008. Epub 2017 Oct 7.

Taylor, M. J., Hoerauf, A., & Bockarie, M. (2010). Lymphatic filariasis and onchocerciasis. *The Lancet, 376*(9747), 1175–1185.

Taylor, H. O., Morrison, C. S., Linden, O., Phillips, B., Chang, J., Byrne, M. E., … Forrest, C. R. (2014). Quantitative facial asymmetry. *Journal of Craniofacial Surgery, 25*(1), 124–128. https://doi.org/10.1097/scs.0b013e3182a2e99d

Upper limb management after stroke fact sheet — Stroke Foundation - Australia. (n.d.). Retrieved 13 Nov, 2017., from https://strokefoundation.org.au/About-Stroke/Help-after-stroke/Stroke-resources-and-fact-sheets/Upper-limb-management-after-stroke-fact-sheet

Vairo, G. L., Miller, S. J., Rier, N. M., & Uckley, W. B. (2009). Systematic review of efficacy for manual lymphatic drainage techniques in sports medicine and rehabilitation: An evidence-based practice approach. *Journal of Manual & Manipulative Therapy, 17*(3). https://doi.org/10.1179/jmt.2009.17.3.80e

Zhu, W., Li, D., Li, X., Ren, J., Chen, W., Gu, H., … Wang, D. (2017). Association between adjuvant docetaxel-based chemotherapy and breast cancer-related lymphedema. *Anti-Cancer Drugs, 28*(3), 350–355. https://doi.org/10.1097/cad.0000000000000468

Zuther, J. E., & Norton, S. (2017). *Lymphedema management: The comprehensive guide for practitioners* (4th ed.). New York, NY: Thieme.

Shoulder Dysfunction and Disability Secondary to Treatment for Head and Neck Cancer

23

Angelo Boulougouris and Philip C. Doyle

Introduction

The shoulder complex is the most mobile joint in the human body (Veeger & van der Helm, 2007), and the complex is composed of three bones that join together to form four articulations (joints). These articulations occur between the humerus, clavicle, and scapula which collectively allow for a tremendous amount of mobility in the upper extremity. Functional demands of daily living such as putting on socks, pushing to open a door, or even brining food to our mouth rely on the shoulder complex to operate in a coordinated fashion. Thus, normal shoulder functioning allows for a range of activities that have a direct impact on common, everyday activities. Changes in shoulder function is a commonly reported side effect of treatment for many cancers of the head and neck where neck dissection will be undertaken for cancer control (Ahlberg et al., 2012; Bradley et al., 2011). Thus, having a clinical awareness of the disability that may result from treatment for cancers arising from the head and neck region will serve to enhance the comprehensive rehabilitation efforts (Moukarbel et al., 2010). This is of particular importance to the speech-language pathologist (SLP) who will serve this population.

In order to achieve the wide range of mobility required for such activities in the shoulder complex, there is a corresponding sacrifice in joint stability. Stated more simply, stability is sacrificed for mobility. The shoulder complex lacks bony congruency especially at the glenohumeral (GH) joint with its large spherical end resting upon a small "platform" (this is analogous to a golf ball resting on a tee-tipped sideways). The shoulder complex has only a single attachment to the axial skeleton through the clavicle, a long thin bone with small articulations at the acromioclavicular (AC) and sternoclavicular (SC) joints. Furthermore, the scapula "floats" upon the thorax and acts as a stable base for numerous muscle attachments, as well as serving as a "perch" for the humeral head to be supported upon.

Although the shoulder complex does have a number of passive supports to stability such as ligaments, the labrum, and the joint capsule, it relies substantially on a tremendous amount of muscular coordination to prevent movement dysfunction from occurring. The rotator cuff and the muscles that control the scapula are extremely important in maintaining coordination among the joints of the shoulder complex and, thus, serve to

A. Boulougouris (✉)
Fowler-Kennedy Sports Medicine Clinic, Western University, London, ON, Canada

P. C. Doyle
Voice Production and Perception Laboratory & Laboratory for Well-Being and Quality of Life, Department of Otolaryngology – Head and Neck Surgery and School of Communication Sciences and Disorders, Western University, Elborn College, London, ON, Canada

© Springer Nature Switzerland AG 2019
P. C. Doyle (ed.), *Clinical Care and Rehabilitation in Head and Neck Cancer*,
https://doi.org/10.1007/978-3-030-04702-3_23

maintain functional mobility. However, because the shoulder must rely on such a complex system of controlled movement due to the lack of joint congruency, it is susceptible to injury and subsequently can result in a detrimental loss of function. However, a restriction or loss of shoulder function can occur due to a variety of circumstances.

Any injury to the muscular control of the shoulder complex can result in a significant loss of joint mobility. Consequently, this can lead to difficulty in performing activities of daily living and pain symptoms resulting from tissue irritation. This is the case when patients are undergoing neck dissection for the treatment of head or neck cancer. As a consequence of the procedure, there is a possibility for injury to the spinal accessory nerve (SAN) which innervates the trapezius and is an important muscle affecting control of the scapula. This chapter endeavors to describe the structure and function of the shoulder complex and the possibility of dysfunction as a consequence of postsurgical neck dissection (Leipzig, Suen, English, Barnes, & Hooper, 1983), with some options for postsurgical interventions.

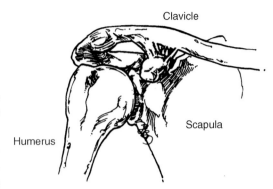

Fig. 23.1 Bony anatomy of the shoulder complex. (Reprinted with permission from Terry and Chopp (2000), Fig. 1, *J Athl Train*)

Table 23.1 Active range of motion of the shoulder complex

Abduction	170°–180°
Forward flexion	160°–180°
External rotation	80°–90°
Internal rotation	60°–100°
Extension	50°–60°
Adduction	50°–75°
Horizontal adduction/abduction	130°

Adapted from Magee (2002, p. 223)
°Degrees

Anatomy and Joint Articulations

Bony Anatomy

The humerus is considered a long bone and the site of many muscle attachments (see Fig. 23.1); it has a spherical end that forms an articulation with the glenoid fossa of the scapula (Biel, 2010, p. 48). This joint is commonly referred to as a "ball and socket" joint. The clavicle (Fig. 23.1) is also classified as a long bone, and it provides the only bony connection between the scapula and humerus to the axial skeleton. The clavicle also serves as a site for muscle attachments and provides support for any load bearing that may occur over the extended shoulder complex when the arm is elevated. The scapula (Fig. 23.1) is triangular in appearance and is classified as a flat bone. Interestingly, it does not form a typical

joint with any other bones but rather "floats" upon the thorax between ribs 2 and 7 (Culham & Peat, 1993). The scapula is also the site for many muscular attachments and acts as a "perch" for the spherical end of the humeral head. The ranges (in degrees) available for the shoulder complex are provided in Table 23.1.

Glenohumeral Joint

The glenohumeral (GH) joint is inherently unstable, with only 25–30% of the surface area of the spherical end of the humerus making contact with the glenoid fossa at any one point in time (Culham & Peat, 1993; Terry & Chopp, 2000). The GH joint is supported by the position of the glenoid fossa that faces forward, outward, and upward (Kisner & Colby, 2012). Furthermore, several structures, both passive, such as the capsule that surrounds the GH joint, ligaments, and the labrum, and dynamic control from the rotator cuff muscles, contribute to GH joint stability (Culham & Peat, 1993). Thus, although unstable from a boney "fit" perspective, the GH joint relies on positioning and several static and dynamic structures to work together in a coordinated fashion to produce functional pain-free movement.

As described by Kendall, McCreary, Provance, Rodgers, and Romani (2005, p. 305), the GH joint has three degrees of freedom, meaning that it can achieve movements of flexion/extension, abduction/adduction, and internal/external rotation. That is, we can lift the arm in front of us in order to reach for an object off a high shelf (flexion) or reach behind us as we pull a suitcase (extension). We can lift the arm to the side and lean against the wall (abduction) or reach across our body to buckle our belt (adduction). Furthermore, we can rotate through the shoulder to reach into our back pocket (internal rotation) or to scratch behind our head (external rotation). The total range of motion achieved through the shoulder complex is achieved through the combined movements of the GH joint, scapulothoracic (ST) joint, and both the acromioclavicular (AC) and sternoclavicular (SC) joints. However, the total range of motion available to the GH joint when elevating the arm is approximately 90–120° (Culham & Peat, 1993). The remaining range of motion available to the shoulder complex is achieved through the movement of the ST joint. Additional details on the dynamic nature of this system have been provided by several authors (Ludewig & Reynolds, 2009; McClure, Michener, Sennett, & Karduna, 2001; Poppen & Walker, 1976; and others). Therefore, the function of the ST joint will be further discussed in the following section.

Scapulothoracic Joint

The scapulothoracic (ST) joint is not a "true" joint but rather refers to the connection between the concave surface of the scapula and the convex surface of the thorax (Hislop & Montgomery, 2002). The motions that are facilitated at the ST joint are elevation, abduction, adduction, downward rotation, and upward rotation. To achieve full elevation (raising) of the shoulder complex, the scapula must have the ability to rotate through both the sternoclavicular (SC) and acromioclavicular (AC) joints. That is, movement at these joints must allow for the clavicle to move upward, downward, forward, and backward and to rotate (Marieb, Mallatt, & Wilhelm, 2005; Paine & Voight, 2013). Try placing your hand on the SC joint (where your collar bone meets your sternum), and shrug your shoulders, and then lower your shoulders. Reach forward with your arm, and then squeeze your shoulder blades together, and appreciate the movement that occurs through this joint.

The scapula provides a stable base for the entire shoulder complex and, by doing so, allows for greater ranges in shoulder elevation beyond the 90–120° available at the GH joint (Terry & Chopp, 2000). Generally speaking, during elevation of the shoulder complex, it is suggested that for every two degrees of GH joint elevation, there is one degree of ST joint elevation (Culham & Peat, 1993; Terry & Chopp, 2000). Stated slightly differently, when measuring the total range of motion available at the shoulder complex when one elevates the arm, two-thirds of the change in range comes from the GH joint and one-third from the ST joint.

In order for the scapula to be positioned to optimize both mobility and stability, the muscular control for the scapula requires the appropriate activation and inhibition of the 17 muscles that attach or originate off the scapula (Culham & Peat, 1993; Mottram, 1997). Of those muscles that control scapular movement, the trapezius (Fig. 23.2a) and the serratus anterior (Fig. 23.2b) are two of the most important "dynamic" movers and stabilizers to functioning (Terry & Chopp, 2000). These muscles help maintain the position of the scapula against the thorax and also to provide the rotational movement necessary to create a stable base at the GH joint throughout elevation of the shoulder complex (Culham & Peat, 1993; Mottram, 1997). The term "scapular setting" refers to the most "ideal" position of the scapula

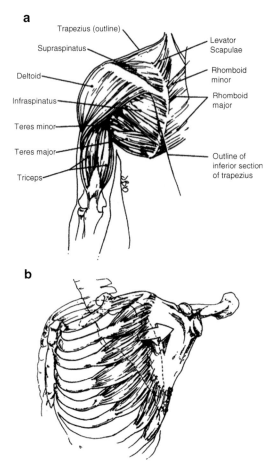

a

Trapezius (outline)

Supraspinatus

Deltoid

Infraspinatus

Teres minor

Teres major

Triceps

Levator Scapulae

Rhomboid minor

Rhomboid major

Outline of inferior section of trapezius

b

Fig. 23.2 Muscles of the shoulder complex (**a**) and associated movement (**b**). (Reprinted with permission from Terry and Chopp (2000), Fig. 9A/B, *J Athl Train*)

for the GH joint to be elevated while continuously being positioned on a moving scapula, such that it maintains the humeral head in an optimally stable position (Mottram, 1997). Thus, the capacity for rhythmic movement of this joint permits a level of stability without significant restriction in functional movement.

In summary, the ST joint provides approximately one-third of the total range of motion that is available at the shoulder complex when elevating the arm. The serratus anterior and the trapezius are also important muscles with respect to controlling the movement of the scapula when elevating the arm. During shoulder elevation, scapulohumeral rhythm allows for the optimal GH joint position through the coordinated effort of those muscles that move the shoulder complex. Therefore, it cannot be stressed enough that shoulder function is highly dependent on muscular control when attempting to maintain a delicate balance between mobility and stability (Veeger & van der Helm, 2007); further, it has long been acknowledged that changes to the trapezius muscle may carry significant functional importance secondary to neck dissection (Harris & Dickey, 1965; Nahum, Mullally, & Marmor, 1961).

Muscular Control of the Shoulder Complex

Although very mobile, the shoulder complex lacks the structural congruency providing stability, especially at the GH joint during shoulder elevation. Fortunately, the motor control necessary for stability during movement stems from the coordinated interaction of numerous muscles that act on the shoulder complex. This coordination permits one to produce motion while also allowing the shoulder to maintain stability. The subsequent section will focus on some of the more important muscular supports of the shoulder complex; however, it is not meant to be an exhaustive review of the multifaceted interactions of all the dynamic supports of the shoulder complex during movement.

during movement of the shoulder complex. In other words, the ideal is defined by the position that the scapula must be set in to optimize both mobility and stability at the GH joint (Mottram, 1997). It should, however, be stated that there are some controversy and debate regarding the most "ideal" position of the scapula during its movement (Mottram, 1997).

The rotational movement of the scapula during shoulder elevation allows for the GH joint to be rotated upward, thus, providing a stable "perch" for the humeral head (Culham & Peat, 1993). This coordination during shoulder elevation between the GH and ST joints is referred to as "scapulohumeral rhythm" (Codman, 1934). More specifically, scapulohumeral rhythm allows

Rotator Cuff

The rotator cuff (RC) consists of four muscles that originate from the scapula (Biel, 2010). These muscles are the subscapularis, supraspinatus, infraspinatus, and teres minor (Fig. 23.3). Independently, the supraspinatus generates a force that abducts the arm. Both the infraspinatus and teres minor muscles provide the primary external rotation force at the GH joint. Finally, the subscapularis functions as an internal rotator at the GH joint (Huegel, Williams, & Soslowsky, 2015; Terry & Chopp, 2000). These four muscles "wrap" around the humeral head and are integral to GH joint stability from a dynamic standpoint.

The main function of the RC is to provide stability to the GH joint in a coordinated effort that maintains the humeral head firmly in the glenoid fossa of the scapula. To clarify this, it may be illustrative to imagine that the GH joint is somewhat similar to a golf ball resting on a tee. Now, imagine trying to rotate the golf ball on the tee using a system of pulleys without having it fall off. If you wanted to rotate the ball to the left, you would require a pulley pulling in the opposite direction (to the right) on the other side of the ball with a similar force. By doing this, you could maintain the golf ball on the tee during rotation – if both forces were not present, you would risk it falling off. The muscles of the RC, therefore, act on the GH joint to produce a rotational force without allowing a translational movement. Thus, the RC is an important group of muscles that surround the humeral head, serving to support its orientation against the scapula.

When relating movement to the shoulder complex, imagine elevating the arm into abduction (lifting your arm to the side); without the action of the RC, the deltoid muscle would end up working in a manner that would translate (i.e., lift) the humeral head upward and off of the glenoid socket. In this instance, the supraspinatus acts as a compressor which pulls the humeral head into the glenoid socket. The infraspinatus, teres minor, and subscapularis exert a downward pull that serves to counteract the upward pull of the deltoid. Thus, the humeral head is able to rotate in the joint without allowing the humeral head to translate out of its position on the glenoid. Consequently, the RC is designed to maintain the humeral head centered in the scapula when elevating the shoulder complex. Weakness of the RC can lead to dysfunctional movement and a number of pathological conditions causing pain and loss of function.

Fig. 23.3 Muscles and attachments to the head of the humerus for shoulder range of motion. (Reprinted with permission from Terry and Chopp (2000), Fig. 6, *J Athl Train*)

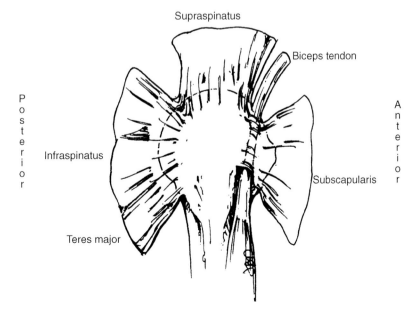

Dynamic Control of the Scapula

As discussed in the previous section, the scapula has the ability to elevate, abduct, adduct, and rotate both upward and downward (Hislop & Montgomery, 2002). However, one of the most important functions is the ability for the scapula to upwardly rotate. This capacity allows for the shoulder complex to achieve greater ranges of motion than what would be available only at the GH joint. As stated by Schenkman and Rugo De Cartaya (1987), in order to accomplish this increase in range, the serratus anterior and the trapezius are two important muscles that act together to provide the upward rotation of the scapula. The serratus anterior muscle functions to upwardly rotate and depress the scapula, while the upper trapezius upwardly rotates and elevates the scapula (Schenkman & Rugo De Cartaya, 1987).

The shoulder complex requires the coordination of several muscles in order to effectively elevate and rotate the scapula. Again, this ability results in increased range of motion for the upper extremity. Therefore, a loss of muscular control leads to movement dysfunction which can then impact functional movements through the loss of range available to the shoulder complex (Schenkman & Rugo De Cartaya, 1987). Elevation of the shoulder complex against gravity is necessary in order to perform a variety of activities of daily living such as reaching, dressing, eating, and grooming (Schenkman & Rugo De Cartaya, 1987). When shoulder mobility is compromised due to dysfunction of the muscular systems that control its movement, the result is a detrimental decline in function. However, loss of function may also be associated with symptoms of pain which may subsequently affect one's overall quality of life (QoL).

Shoulder Dysfunction After Surgical Neck Dissection for Head and Neck Cancer

Spinal Accessory Nerve

Neck dissection broadly involves a surgical procedure that is performed during the treatment of

head and neck cancer (HNCa). Because of the anatomical relationship between critical structures specific to HNCa and the neural supply to the shoulder, the potential for loss of upper extremity function does exist. Of particular importance is the course of the spinal accessory nerve (cranial nerve XI) within the neck. Some reports suggest that injury to the spinal accessory nerve (SAN) may occur in as many as 67% of HNCa cases (McGarvey, Hoffman, Osmotherly, & Chiarelli, 2015; Short, Kaplan, Laramore, & Cummings, 1984). The SAN is the primary motor supply to the trapezius muscle (Marieb et al., 2005, p. 410); loss of the nerve supply to this muscle can result in significant dysfunction in the shoulder complex (see Fig. 23.4). If the nerve supply to the trapezius muscle is compromised due to neck dissection, the result is muscle weakness and decreased scapular control. Furthermore, damage to the surrounding tissue can lead to neuropathic pain in the neck and shoulder region (El Ghani et al., 2002; Garzaro et al., 2015; Van Wilgen, Dijkstra, Van der Laan, Plukker, & Roodenburg, 2004). The reader is encouraged to peruse an excellent review of SAN palsy and its signs and symptoms that have been provided by Kelley, Kane, and Leggin (2008).

Additionally, it is important to note that adjuvant treatments for HNCa after surgery such as

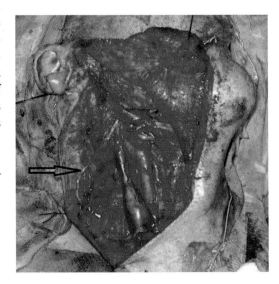

Fig. 23.4 Neck dissection with course of the spinal accessory nerve (CN XI). (Photo courtesy of Dr. K. Fung)

radiation therapy can result in further physical deconditioning that will negatively impact shoulder function. Furthermore, several authors suggest that QoL post neck dissection is related to shoulder and neck pain itself, more so than as the physical result of the actual surgical procedure (Kuntz & Weymuller, 1999; Laverick, Lowe, Brown et al., 2004; Terrell et al., 2000; Van Wilgen et al., 2004). Regardless of the underlying mechanism, it is well recognized that the influence of shoulder disability secondary to the treatment of HNCa can have a significant, negative impact on one's perceived quality of life (Weymuller et al., 2000; and others).

If you recall from the previous section of this chapter, the trapezius muscle is very important when it comes to the motor control of the scapula during arm elevation (Magee, 2002). As a consequence of any injury to the SAN and the resulting loss of muscle control, the scapula ends up being downwardly rotated and in a depressed (lower) position. Because of this altered posture, GH joint mobility becomes impaired, and total ROM of the shoulder complex is reduced, most notably in ranges of abduction and flexion. Reductions in ROM of this type will significantly limit the overall functional capacity of this system complex when compared to the normal system. Furthermore, and perhaps most critical to the present discussion, is the fact that these ROM changes can have debilitating effects on function especially with respect activities of daily living.

Imagine all the tasks that one performs each day which require lifting your arms (e.g., washing your hair, putting on or taking off clothing, applying deodorant, or even putting on eyeglasses; then imagine if such arm movements lead the person to experience painful symptoms. Furthermore, activities that may not even require movement of the shoulder such as sleeping or prolonged sitting may lead to painful symptoms a result of tissue irritation to prolonged postures. Thus, it is quite important that treatment of shoulder dysfunction focuses on managing pain symptoms and improving shoulder mechanics. In the case of those who have undergone total laryngectomy, critical issues such as maintaining hygiene of the tracheostoma may be altered due to upper limb restrictions. Similarly, the ability to use an artificial electrolarynx, clean a tracheoesophageal puncture voice prosthesis in situ, and change and maintain a heat and moisture exchange device may be negatively influenced. Further details on these types of issues will be outlined in later sections of this chapter.

Treatment of Shoulder Dysfunction

Treatment of shoulder dysfunction after surgical injury to the SAN should attempt to address the loss of motor control to the scapula. Several studies (McGarvey et al., 2015; McNeely et al., 2008; Nibu et al., 2010) have evaluated the use of physiotherapy to address the lack of strength and pain symptoms postoperatively. Specifically, exercise regimens that emphasize progressive scapular strengthening exercises in patients with functional limitations due to the lack of postoperatively shoulder ROM due to SAN injury demonstrated improvements in both pain and function (McGarvey et al., 2015; McNeely et al., 2004, 2008). Nibu et al. (2010) demonstrated improved QoL upon assessment in patients with SAN injury who attended postoperatively physiotherapy. As a result of injury to the SAN, a rehabilitation program focused on a progressive scapular strengthening regimen prescribed by a physiotherapist may be beneficial in controlling pain, improving mobility, and optimizing QoL.

Strengthening the muscles that control the scapula may not be the only muscles that will require consideration during treatment. If you recall, the muscles comprising the rotator cuff are extremely important in controlling the position of the humeral head against the glenoid fossa. As a result of HNCa surgical procedures and the subsequent immobilization due to pain or postsurgical restrictions, these muscles would likely be compromised due to deconditioning. Loss of strength will then results in poor positioning of the humeral head during movement and can lead to painful movement patterns. Treatment should likely focus on general strengthening for the RC group of muscles that demonstrate significant weakness. Physiotherapists and other rehabilitation specialists commonly treat weakness of the

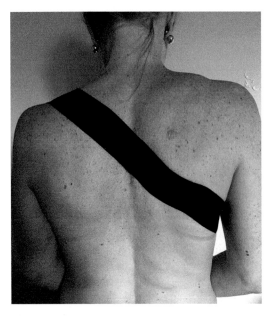

Fig. 23.5 Scapular support taping technique. (Photo courtesy of Dr. A. Boulougouris)

RC muscle group and would be able to provide a tailored exercise regimen to address this postoperatively.

Other treatments' considerations that target the poor postural positioning of the scapula after injury to the SAN may include therapeutic taping techniques. As a result of trapezius inhibition due to SAN injury, the scapula develops a downward and depressed position. Using tape to support, an elevated and upwardly rotated position (Fig. 23.5) may be helpful in managing pain symptoms and may even provide an increase in shoulder mobility. Therapeutic taping is a common practice in physiotherapy as well as other rehabilitation professions, and its application may provide some early support while working on a strengthening program.

Relationship of Shoulder Dysfunction to Airway Changes and Voice and Speech Rehabilitation

In prior sections of this chapter, the information provided outlines the structural complexities of the shoulder. Evolving from this complexity,

functional concerns have also been raised. Because head and neck cancers are located in the region where critical neural structures which supply the muscles of the shoulder exist, disruptions to shoulder function are often observed and reported posttreatment. However, it is important to note that negative changes to the functional integrity of the shoulder complex may result from combined influences of treatment which includes anatomical, physiologic, and neurophysiologic changes to this rather complex mobile motor system. While the direct effects of changes secondary to surgery for HNCa in general and for neck dissection should be obvious, it is equally important to acknowledge that other modalities of treatment, either alone or in combination, can have a negative influence on shoulder functioning.

Information addressed previously clearly outlines that changes in shoulder mobility, stability, and control can be physically disabling (Taylor et al., 2004). This not only includes a reduction in functional limitations but perhaps more importantly, a potential for the presence of pain and discomfort. Although the impact on shoulder function secondary to treatment for HNCa is widely acknowledged with a particular focus on limitations specific to activities of daily living, one area of impact that has often been directly omitted pertains to the impact of shoulder disability on the use of alaryngeal voice and speech. That is, for two alaryngeal methods, electrolaryngeal speech and tracheoesophageal (TE) speech, shoulder function may be a critical component of communication rehabilitation. Further, in the case of total laryngectomy, a permanent tracheostoma will be created, and the ability to maintain daily hygiene is necessary; this process will require action of the upper limb, and if one is unable to perform such duties, difficulties may be encountered (e.g., excessive crusting, difficulty removing mucus from the airway, etc.). In the sections to follow, information on the importance of the upper extremity during the process of alaryngeal speech will be presented. Because of the unique nature of both of these alaryngeal methods, each will be addressed separately.

Electrolaryngeal Speech

The use of the electronic artificial larynx, often referred to as the electrolarynx (EL), will require considerable manual dexterity for its successful use. This involves aspects of both fine control of the hand and gross movements of the arm. The inability to meet the basic requirements of correct positioning of the device is essential. In fact, it has long been known that failure to successfully acquire and use any type of EL is often related to the user's inability to position the device appropriately (Deidrich & Youngstrom, 1966; Doyle, 1994). In the vernacular of the speech pathologist, instruction related to correct positioning of an EL device seeks to identify and consistently place the device in the "sweet spot" (Doyle, 1994; Hillman et al., 2005). In addition to positioning the device correctly, the EL user also needs to initiate relatively fine control of an on-off button to generate the signal that will ultimately be articulated into speech.

Despite a need for accurate control of multiple movements for EL use, consistent positioning is the key element to successful acquisition of the requisite skills that will underlie successful speech production. This is true regardless of whether the alaryngeal speaker uses a *transcervical* (neck-type) or *intraoral* EL device. But, with that said, unique issues are of importance to each type of device in the context of shoulder functioning and the potential presence of pain. Details specifying the potential influence of shoulder disability on the use of neck-type devices and those associated with intraoral devices will be addressed in the subsequent sections.

Use of a Transcervical EL Device

As the name implies, transcervical or neck-type EL devices are most frequently placed in contact with some region of the postlaryngectomy neck. It should, however, also be noted that some speakers are able to position an EL directly under the chin (without contact with the anterior mandible) or similarly on either cheek while avoiding substantial manual contact pressure so that teeth

behind the cheek do not impede the signal. Through a careful and systematic process of assessing EL sound production in the early stages of training, the speech pathologist will ideally be able to identify the sweet spot (see Nagle, Chap. 9). The location of this sweet spot is highly individualized and must be determined with considerations of potential scar lines and scar tissue, general neck thickness, and proximity to bony structures such as the mandible, as well as other factors. However, the ability to move to the sweet spot and maintain control of the device will require adequate movement and control of the upper extremity to position the device correctly.

The ideal location for positioning the EL is identified as that contact point (vibrating head of the EL and neck skin) where the EL generates the strongest signal when transmitted into the vocal tract (Fig. 23.6). This is typically confirmed when the EL signal is determined by the ear to be at its greatest resonance; that is, the transmitted signal is passed into the vocal tract at its greatest acoustic strength. When this objective is achieved, the articulation of speech in the oral cavity holds its greatest potential for the "fullest" sound to the

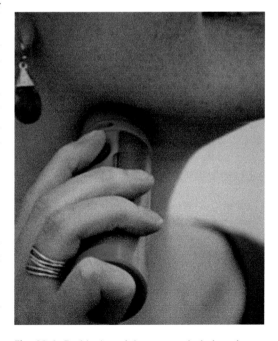

Fig. 23.6 Positioning of the transcervical electrolarynx on the lateral neck. (Photo courtesy of Dr. P.C. Doyle)

listener. While details concerning the process of determining the sweet spot and the clinical process associated with incrementally training use of the EL are addressed elsewhere in this volume (Nagle, Chap. 9) and in other sources (Doyle, 1994, 2005), the present discussion will focus on finer considerations related to the training process in the context of shoulder function.

Most importantly, the postlaryngectomy speaker's ability to generate the strongest EL sound during speech can only be achieved if they are able to accurately and consistently place to device at the sweet spot. Any inability in correctly positioning the EL will result in a weakened signal because signal transmission through neck tissues will be reduced or, potentially, will be problematic because the vibrating head of the EL will not be flush to the skin. In such instances, the EL signal will "leak" because flush contact with the skin is incomplete; this in turn will provide a competing sound source to that which moves into the vocal tract for speech purposes. Stated differently, a flush contact between the EL and neck skin will permit the full signal to be passed into the vocal tract.

Based on the prior information related to the shoulder and its functioning, it should be recognized that the ability to accurately position an EL device on any area of the neck requires substantial demand on the shoulder complex. Although the majority of this movement is gross in nature, control is nevertheless required. Further, information discussed previously indicates that any level of shoulder dysfunction secondary to treatment (i.e., neck dissection) may place an additional challenge on the EL training process. Reductions in shoulder movement will almost certainly add to the user's capacity to efficiently move to the sweet spot and do so consistently. Training use of any type of EL, whether a neck-type or intraoral device, will necessitate a process of motor learning and associated motor memory.

The exceptional speech clinician must understand that "triggering" onset of the EL is important, but it serves a little purpose if the user cannot acquire a consistent placement (Doyle, 2005; Nagle, Chap. 9). Thus, those who train EL must acknowledge the potential limitations in one's

capacity to move and carefully position their upper extremity in an effort to approximate their sweet spot. Practice will make perfect, but clinicians must be aware that in some individuals, specific movements of the arm may not be possible due to physical restrictions, as well as being painful. Clinical common sense would suggest that any training demand that exceeds the individual's functional capacity or one that results in discomfort or pain is likely to be highly problematic with a resultant impact on one's ability to successfully acquire the use of the EL.

In such circumstances where the ideal neck placement proves problematic, the clinician may wish to identify a secondary sweet spot which may more easily facilitate consistent and perhaps, most importantly, a less painful movement of the shoulder and upper extremity for EL usage. Such decisions are made with knowledge that speech production may be less than ideal because the "best" point of neck contact cannot be achieved. As such, the "first-choice" sweet spot as determined by the clinician may be sacrificed for consistency of EL positioning. This sacrifice may, however, be overcome to some extent through direct instruction for common EL training goals including over-articulation, slowing of speech rate, and careful phrasing and pauses during the speech process. Adaptations in the clinical training process will often be necessary in an effort to facilitate the best possible EL speech as early on in the process as possible.

It is essential that the clinician realizes that learning to use an EL device is influenced by multiple factors. Given that substantial changes do occur with treatment of HNCa (e.g., the characteristics of the posttreatment neck) and that secondary physical changes are also likely, a careful and comprehensive approach to training is required. In this regard, the clinician must consider the functional capacity of the upper extremity, as well as any pain that may coexist with requests for a particular movement necessary for EL use. This may involve consideration of both gross and fine motor aspects of the EL speech process. Because of such considerations, the following section will address issues that may impact training of an intraoral EL device.

Use of an Intraoral EL Device

Intraoral or mouth-type EL devices have existed for many years for postlaryngectomy speech rehabilitation. The most widely recognized intraoral EL version is that manufactured by Cooper-Rand (the "old and still gold" device[1]). Further, in many instances an intraoral EL is the preferred method of speech rehabilitation for those in the very early stages of postlaryngectomy speech rehabilitation.[2] Although the Cooper-Rand EL is the only truly dedicated intraoral device, many if not all neck-type EL devices can be modified into intraoral devices with the use of a simple adaptor cap which fits onto the vibrating head of device; this adapter is then designed to accommodate an intraoral tube for speech production (Doyle, 2005).

Regardless of whether a stand-alone device such as the Cooper-Rand is used, or if a neck-type device has been converted, the process of training postlaryngectomy speech production remains relatively consistent in that correct placement is the most important task to acquire. Once an intraoral sweet spot has been determined, the speaker is trained to over-articulate and slow their overall speech rate. In many respects, regardless of what type of EL is used, the generalized requirements for movements of the upper extremity are similar. But the unique challenge often encountered with training use of the intraoral EL relates to an increasing demand on the individual specific to fine control issues. That is, the tube of the intraoral device must be finely and consistently directed into the appropriate region of the oral cavity. This positioning involves not only the ability to maneuver the upper arm to a specific location in the oral cavity but also to ori-

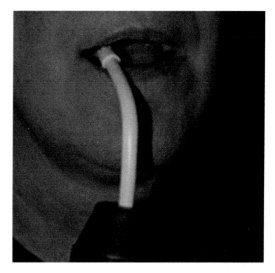

Fig. 23.7 Positioning of the intraoral electrolarynx within the oral cavity. (Photo courtesy of Dr. P.C. Doyle)

ent the tube to the correct depth and to make sure that the tube is directed slightly upward in that location (see Fig. 23.7).

The combined influence of making sure that all of these "placement" goals are met not only helps to ensure that the resonance of the signal is maximized, but to avoid placing the tube in a position that will collect saliva. If saliva occludes the intraoral tube, the signal propagated through the tube will be impeded with negative impact on speech produced. With this set of considerations presented, the clinician must realize that not only are gross motor skills with the upper extremity required, but fine motor skills must also be employed. As was noted for training with the neck-type device in the previous section, any change in shoulder mobility and/or the presence of pain or discomfort will result in greater challenges in learning to efficiently use the intraoral EL.[3]

---

[1] Tom Lennox, Luminaud Inc., Mentor, OH, personal communication.

[2] Because the postlaryngectomy neck wound is fresh with sutures/staples and may have included some type of flap reconstruction, in additional to potential swelling of the neck postsurgery and lymphedema, pain or tenderness, etc., neck-type EL devices are seldom introduced to individuals until sufficient healing has occurred. Hence, intraoral EL devices are the preferred option of choice early in the rehabilitation process.

[3] One of the simplest approaches to understanding the demands associated with the acquisition of speech with either a neck-type or intraoral EL is for the clinician to learn the behavior themselves. When one who is likely to have normal shoulder mobility, no pain, and adequate fine motor skills for positioning a device and activating it requires substantial practice, the impact of shoulder deficits is often very well understood.

Clinicians should also be mindful that the simple age demographic of those typically diagnosed with and treated for head and neck cancers, particularly for laryngeal malignancies, frequently may be older adults. Therefore, additional age-related physical changes, as well as the potential for past injuries and subsequent levels of disability, may also influence EL use. Of specific importance to the present discussion would be changes in fine motor control of the hand and fingers. When coupled with a change in shoulder function secondary to cancer treatment, the combined limitations may require additional training time. However, the if client-clinician relationship is developed with care, new strategies for overcoming shoulder disabilities that effect the training and use of an EL can be overcome. While such efforts may require additional therapy sessions and individualized refinements in training task structure, these types of cooperative approaches to acquiring the necessary skills for successful EL use may be optimized.

Tracheoesophageal Voice Restoration

One area of postlaryngectomy clinical voice and speech rehabilitation that is potentially influenced by shoulder disability pertains to tracheoesophageal (TE) voice restoration. Since its introduction more than 35 years ago (Singer & Blom, 1980), the TE voice restoration method has become widely used worldwide. However, while one of the important criteria for potential application of TE voice restoration is "good manual dexterity," larger concerns related to upper extremity function have seldom been noted. The primary focus of the "dexterity" concern has related to issues of voice prosthesis insertion and its necessary maintenance (e.g., cleaning of the device and associated tracheostoma). Larger considerations that relate to manually closing the tracheostoma for speech production, regardless of whether or not a heat and moisture exchange (HME) device is used, have not been common areas of clinical concern.

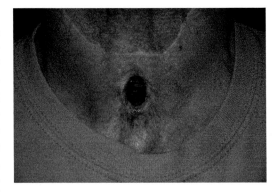

Fig. 23.8 Location of the postlaryngectomy tracheostoma at the anterior midline neck. (Photo courtesy of Dr. P.C. Doyle)

Should one choose to manually occlude the tracheostoma for speech production, dexterity of the upper arm will be required.[4] Given the location of the tracheostoma (Fig. 23.8), movement of the arm and hand to the midline of the lower neck will be required. The inability to easily and completely seal the tracheostoma or to depress the internalized component of an HME cartridge for TE speech will prove to be a major obstacle for this alaryngeal rehabilitation method. Thus, clinicians must be able to carefully assess any limitations in the function of the shoulder and the individual's ability to achieve a reasonable range of motion for TE speech production. Ideally this type of assessment should be done jointly between an SLP and a physical therapist. Working together, these two professionals can work to identify options and to potentially engage in therapeutic tasks that over time may further assist in using the TE prosthesis and when employing HMEs most effectively.

One of the questions that emerges within the present discussion is that of eliminating the need for digital closure of the tracheostoma/HME through the use of "hands-free" valves (see Graville, Palmer & Bolognone, Chap. 11 and

---

[4] It is also important to point out that in some instances, the use of the non-dominant hand may be required, and consequently, additional challenges to achieving desired positioning of the arm and hand may be observed.

Lewis, Chap. 8). Briefly, these devices are designed to close in response to a particular level of respiratory flow through the stoma. When this hands-free closure occurs, the airway is sealed upon expiration, and pulmonary air is directed into the esophageal reservoir just as it would have occurred with digital closure. Although some individuals who have undergone total laryngectomy and chose to use TE speech may use a hands-free device quite successfully, that does not eliminate all of the potential problems that may occur due to shoulder immobility. For example, and as noted previously, some daily maintenance of the region and the devices use is required. If limitations in shoulder function do exist, the ability to remove and change housings, withdraw cartridges, etc. will be disrupted. Changes of this type will then result in potential hygiene considerations, as well as holding the potential for reductions in one's speech ability. Consequently, the assumption that TE voice restoration will eliminate any potential negative impact due to limitations in the functional integrity of the shoulder complex is incomplete. For this reason, careful assessment of what an individual can and cannot do relative to movement and range of the upper extremity is an important first step in TE voice restoration and the daily self-management of the products that are involved in this rehabilitation method.

In summary, the impact of shoulder dysfunction must extend beyond a singular consideration of "activities of daily living." Speech production using an artificial laryngeal device or TE speech with or without the presence of an HME device will require actions of the upper extremity to varying degrees. Although the primary demand on shoulder function relates to movements that are gross in nature, both EL use and TE speech will require degrees of fine motor control. Thus, clinicians who work with those who undergo total laryngectomy must be aware of the potential impact of shoulder disability on speech production for these two alaryngeal groups. Increasing awareness of these potential impacts will provide clinicians with the ability to be proactive in their

evaluation, monitoring, and long-term follow-up with this complex clinical population.

Conclusion

The shoulder complex is the most mobile joint in the human body, however, that comes at the cost of joint stability. The passive and dynamic systems that control shoulder movements are complex and require a tremendous amount of coordination to ensure that tasks such as reaching, lifting, and bringing food to our mouth can be accomplished without dysfunction. However, when injury or weakness does occur, the resulting loss of motor control and the resulting pain symptoms have a detrimental impact on overall QoL. These types of changes hold the potential to create challenges for some methods of postlaryngectomy alaryngeal speech. More specifically, those who use an artificial electrolarynx (both neck-type devices and those that are intraoral) or those who have chosen to use tracheoesophageal speech may exhibit challenges in the use and maintenance of these methods of communication. Further, the use of heat and moisture exchange (HME) systems or non-hands-free systems may also be problematic if one experiences limitations in upper extremity mobility.

Injury to the SAN as a result of surgical treatment for neck cancer, and more directly secondary to neck dissection, can severely impact shoulder mobility due to its innervation of the trapezius muscle. Consequently, poor postural positioning and the inability to elevate and rotate the scapula result in a loss of functional movement leading to difficulties performing activities of daily living. These types of complaints are not uncommon in those who are treated for HNCa. However, there is evidence that supports the referral of patients who undergo surgical neck dissection to be assessed by a physiotherapist postoperatively in order to develop a treatment regimen for the dynamic supports of the shoulder complex. Furthermore, seeking professional rehabilitation guidance can provide the appropriate client-centered care regarding education of the movement dysfunction, pain management strategies, and general activity advice. If positive changes in upper extremity mobility and reductions in pain can be realized, both may have a positive impact on the overall rehabilitation outcome for these patients. Finally, if mobility can be enhanced and pain and discomfort can be reduced in those who utilize the electrolarynx, tracheoesophageal puncture voice prosthesis, and/or HME devices, longer-term communication and breathing outcomes may also be improved.

References

Ahlberg, A., Nikolaidis, P., Engström, T., Gunnarsson, K., Johansson, H., Sharp, L., & Laurell, G. (2012). Morbidity of supraomohyoidal and modified radical neck dissection combined with radiotherapy for head and neck cancer. A prospective longitudinal study. *Head & Neck, 34*(1), 66–72.

Biel, A. (2010). *Trail guide to the body* (4th ed.). Boulder, CO: Books of Discovery.

Bradley, P. J., Ferlito, A., Silver, C. E., Takes, R. P., Woolgar, J. A., Strojan, P., ... Rinaldo, A. (2011). Neck treatment and shoulder morbidity: Still a challenge. *Head & Neck, 33*(7), 1060–1067.

Codman, E. A. (1934). *The shoulder.* Boston, MA: Thomas Todd Co.

Culham, E., & Peat, M. (1993). Functional anatomy of the shoulder complex. *The Journal of Orthopaedic & Sports Physical Therapy, 18*(1), 342–350.

Deidrich, W., & Youngstrom, K. (1966). *Alaryngeal speech.* Springfield, IL: Thompson.

Doyle, P. C. (1994). *Foundations of voice and speech rehabilitation following laryngeal cancer.* San Diego, CA: Singular Publishing Group.

Doyle, P. C. (2005). Clinical procedures for training use of the electronic artificial larynx. In P. C. Doyle & R. L. Keith (Eds.), *Rehabilitation following treatment for head and neck cancer: Voice, speech, and swallowing.* Austin, TX: Pro-Ed Publishers.

El Ghani, F., Van Den Brekel, M. W. M., De Goede, C. J. T., Kuik, J., Leemans, C. R., & Smeele, L. E. (2002). Shoulder function and patient well-being after various types of neck dissections. *Clinical Otolaryngology and Allied Sciences, 27*(5), 403–408.

Garzaro, M., Riva, G., Raimondo, L., Aghemo, L., Giordano, C., & Pecorari, G. (2015). A study of neck and shoulder morbidity following neck dissection: The benefits of cervical plexus preservation. *Ear, Nose, & Throat Journal, 94*(8), 330–344.

Harris, H. H., & Dickey, J. R. (1965). LXXIII nerve grafting to restore function of the trapezius muscle after radical neck dissection: A preliminary report. *The Annals of Otology, Rhinology, and Laryngology, 74*(3), 880–886.

Hislop, H. J., & Montgomery, J. (2002). *Muscle testing: Techniques of manual examination* (7th ed.). Philadelphia, PA: Saunders Company.

Huegel, J., Williams, A. A., & Soslowsky, L. J. (2015). Rotator cuff biology and biomechanics: A review of normal and pathological conditions. *Current Rheumatology Reports, 17,* 476–484.

Kelley, M. J., Kane, T. E., & Leggin, B. G. (2008). Spinal accessory nerve palsy: Associated signs and symptoms. *The Journal of Orthopaedic and Sports Physical Therapy, 38*(2), 78–86.

Kendall, F. P., McCreary, E. K., Provance, P. G., Rodgers, M. M., & Romani, W. A. (2005). *Muscles testing and function with posture and pain* (5th ed.). Philadelphia, PA: Lippincott Williams & Wilkins.

Kisner, C., & Colby, L. A. (2012). *Therapeutic exercise.* Philadelphia, PA: F.A. Davis Company.

Kuntz, A. I., & Weymuller, E. A. (1999). Impact of neck dissection on quality of life. *Laryngoscope, 109*(8), 1334–1338.

Laverick, S., Lowe, D., Brown, J. S., Vaughan, E. D., & Rogers, S. N. (2004). The impact of neck dissection on healthrelated quality of life. *Archives of Otolaryngology–Head & Neck Surgery, 130*(2), 149–154.

Leipzig, B., Suen, J. Y., English, J. L., Barnes, J., & Hooper, M. (1983). Functional evaluation of the spinal accessory nerve after neck dissection. *American Journal of Surgery, 146*(4), 526–530.

Ludewig, P. M., & Reynolds, J. F. (2009). The association of scapular kinematics and glenohumeral joint pathologies. *The Journal of Orthopaedic and Sports Physical Therapy, 39*(2), 90–104.

Magee, D. J. (2002). *Orthopedic physical assessment* (4th ed.). Philadelphia, PA: Elsevier Sciences.

Marieb, E. N., Mallatt, J., & Wilhelm, P. B. (2005). *Human Anatomy* (4th ed.). San Francisco, CA: Pearson Benjamin Cummings.

McClure, P. W., Michener, L. A., Sennett, B. J., & Karduna, A. R. (2001). Direct 3-dimensional measurement of scapular kinematics during dynamic movements in vivo. *Journal of Shoulder and Elbow Surgery, 10*(3), 269–277.

McGarvey, A. C., Hoffman, G. R., Osmotherly, P. G., & Chiarelli, P. E. (2015). Maximizing shoulder function after accessory nerve injury and neck dissection surgery: A multicenter randomized controlled trial. *Head & Neck, 37*(7), 1022–1031.

McNeely, M. L., Parliament, M., Courneya, K. S., Seikaly, H., Jha, N., Scrimger, R., & Hanson, J. (2004). A pilot study of a randomized controlled trial to evaluate the effects of progressive resistance exercise training on shoulder dysfunction caused by spinal accessory neurapraxia/neurectomy in head and neck cancer sur-vivors. *Head & Neck, 26*(6), 518–530.

McNeely, M. L., Parliament, M. B., Seikaly, H., Jha, N., Magee, D. J., Haykowsky, M. J., & Courneya, K. S. (2008). Effect of exercise on upper extremity pain and dysfunction in head and neck cancer survivors. *Cancer, 113*(1), 214–222.

Meltzner, G., Hillman, R. E., Heaton, J. T., Houston, K. M., Kobler, J. B., & Qi, Y. (2005). Electrolaryngeal speech: The state of the art and future directions for development. In P. C. Doyle & R. L. Keith (Eds.), *Contemporary considerations in the treatment and rehabilitation of head and neck cancer: Voice, speech, and swallowing* (pp. 571–590). Austin, TX: Pro-Ed Publishers.

Mottram, S. L. (1997). Dynamic stability of the scapula. *Manual Therapy, 2*(3), 123–131.

Moukarbel, R. V., Fung, K., Franklin, J. H., Leung, A., Rastogi, R., Anderson, C. M., & Yoo, J. H. (2010). Neck and shoulder disability following reconstruction with the pectoralis major pedicled flap. *Laryngoscope, 120*(6), 1129–1134.

Nahum, A. M., Mullally, W., & Marmor, L. (1961). A syndrome resulting from radical neck dissection. *Archives of Otolaryngology, 74*(4), 424–428.

Nibu, K. I., Ebihara, Y., Ebihara, M., Kawabata, K., Onitsuka, T., Fujii, T., & Saikawa, M. (2010). Quality of life after neck dissection: A multicenter longitudinal study by the Japanese Clinical Study Group on Standardization of Treatment for Lymph Node Metastasis of Head and Neck Cancer. *International Journal of Clinical Oncology, 15*(1), 33–38.

Paine, R., & Voight, M. L. (2013). The role of the scapula. *International Journal of Sports Physical Therapy, 8*(5), 617.

Poppen, N. K., & Walker, P. S. (1976). Normal and abnormal motion of the shoulder. *Journal of Bone and Joint Surgery (American), 58*(2), 195–201.

Schenkman, M., & Rugo De Cartaya, V. (1987). Kinesiology of the shoulder complex. *The Journal of Orthopaedic and Sports Physical Therapy, 8*(9), 438–450.

Short, S. O., Kaplan, J. N., Laramore, G. E., & Cummings, C. W. (1984). Shoulder pain and function after neck dissection with or without preservation of the spinal accessory nerve. *American Journal of Surgery, 148*(4), 478–482.

Singer, M. I., & Blom, E. D. (1980). An endoscopic technique for restoration of voice after laryngectomy. *The Annals of Otology, Rhinology, and Laryngology, 89*, 529–533.

Taylor, J. C., Terrell, J. E., Ronis, D. L., Fowler, K. E., Bishop, C., Lambert, M. T., … Duffy, S. A. (2004). Disability in patients with head and neck cancer. *Archives of Otolaryngology – Head & Neck Surgery, 130*(6), 764–769.

Terrell, J. E., Welsh, D. E., Bradford, C. R., Chepeha, D. B., Esclamado, R. M., Hogikyan, N. D., & Wolf, G. T. (2000). Pain, quality of life, and spinal accessory nerve status after neck dissection. *Laryngoscope, 110*(4), 620–626.

Terry, G. C., & Chopp, T. M. (2000). Functional anatomy of the shoulder. *Journal of Athletic Training, 35*(3), 248–255.

Van Wilgen, C. P., Dijkstra, P. U., Van der Laan, B. F. A. M., Plukker, J. T., & Roodenburg, J. L. N. (2004). Shoulder and neck morbidity in quality of life after surgery for head and neck cancer. *Head & Neck, 26*(10), 839–844.

Veeger, H. E. J., & van der Helm, F. C. T. (2007). Shoulder function: The perfect compromise between mobility and stability. *Journal of Biomechanics, 40*, 2119–2129.

Weymuller, E. A., Yueh, B., Deleyiannis, F. W. B., Kuntz, A. L., Alsarraf, R., & Coltrera, M. D. (2000). Quality of life in head and neck cancer. *Laryngoscope, 110*(S94), 4–7.

Factors Influencing Adherence to Treatment for Head and Neck Cancer

24

Heather M. Starmer

Introduction

Behavioral therapeutic intervention requires active patient participation for optimal outcomes. Speech and swallowing rehabilitation in the head and neck cancer population relies heavily on such behavioral intervention, and therefore treatment adherence is a key contributor to outcomes. In this chapter we will highlight the differences between compliance and adherence, review theoretical frameworks for thinking about treatment adherence, discuss factors that may impact patient adherence, and discuss strategies for enhancing adherence in the head and neck cancer population.

What Is Adherence?

Adherence has been defined as "the extent to which a patient continues an agreed-upon mode of treatment without close supervision" (Cramer et al., 2008). The key concept that differentiates adherence from compliance is the concept of the "agreed-upon mode of treatment." In contrast to

adherence, compliance assumes that the patient will follow through with a treatment recommendation without that shared decision-making experience. Compliance is more akin to acquiescence, whereas adherence allows the patient to be a true partner in treatment decision-making. For example, if a speech language pathologist (SLP) recommends nectar-thickened liquids but the patient indicates they have no intention of following that recommendation, we might say that patient is non-compliant with treatment recommendations. In contrast, if the patient agreed that thickening liquids was an acceptable treatment recommendation that they intended to follow, but then did not, we would say they had poor treatment adherence. Both concepts are important for a behavioral therapist like a speech pathologist to consider; however, efforts should be focused on enhancing adherence as this assumes a level of patient willingness to participate. While it is important to provide education in an attempt to make a non-compliant patient follow recommendations, efforts to intervene in a willing patient are more likely to result in success than those directed toward a non-willing patient.

Adherence to a treatment has a temporal, step-wise progression. First, there must be initiation of the behavior. In the case of a longitudinal treatment, there must then be continuation of the behavior. Finally, there may be discontinuation of the behavior when clinically indicated. Patients may fail to adhere to treatment at any point along

H. M. Starmer (✉)
Department of Otolaryngology – Head and Neck Surgery, Head and Neck Speech and Swallowing Rehabilitation, Stanford Cancer Center, Stanford, CA, USA
e-mail: hstarmer@stanford.edu

© Springer Nature Switzerland AG 2019
P. C. Doyle (ed.), *Clinical Care and Rehabilitation in Head and Neck Cancer*,
https://doi.org/10.1007/978-3-030-04702-3_24

this continuum. For example, thickened liquids may be recommended by a SLP to reduce aspiration risk. If a patient agrees to this treatment but then never starts thickening liquids, their non-adherence would be at the point of initiation. If the same patient started thickening liquids, but after a month stopped without concordance with the SLP, their non-adherence would be at the implementation or continuation phase. Finally, if the SLP recommended discontinuation of thickened liquids due to concerns regarding hydration, but the patient decided on their own to continue thickening the liquids, this would be non-adherence at the point of discontinuation.

Theories of Patient Adherence

In order to consider ways to optimize treatment adherence, the therapist should have an understanding of adherence theory. Most of the theories that we will discuss assume significant patient contributions to adherence/non-adherence. In addition to patient factors, there are a number of external factors that may also influence patient adherence. We will first discuss theory as applied to the patient and then will consider systemic and logistical barriers to treatment adherence.

The health belief model of adherence is based upon the patient's perception of illness and susceptibility to illness (Becker, 1974; Rosenstock, 1974). It is particularly salient when applied to preventative treatment recommendations. This model proposes that there are four conditions necessary for adherence to preventative treatment recommendations. First, the patient must believe there is potential that they may acquire or develop the condition. The second tenet is that the patient must believe that the risk is significant and the consequences of the condition are unacceptable. Next, the person must believe that the risk of developing the condition can be minimized if a particular behavior or treatment is applied. Finally, the patient must accept that barriers to the target behavior can be overcome. Additional considerations that have been added to this model include a patient's general health motivation, the

patient-provider relationship, perceived susceptibility to return of the illness/condition, reminders reinforcing the threat of illness, and belief in personal self-efficacy (Becker & Rosenstock, 1984). We can apply this model when considering a head and neck cancer patient undergoing radiation therapy and seeing a SLP for prophylactic swallowing exercises. In order for the patient to follow the recommendations of the SLP, they must first believe that they are at risk for developing dysphagia as a result of radiation therapy and feel that the consequences of such dysphagia (feeding tube dependence, diet modification, aspiration, etc.) are undesirable. The patient then needs to have confidence in the efficacy of the recommended exercises to minimize the risk of dysphagia. Finally, the patient must have faith that barriers to completing exercises, such as pain and fatigue, can be managed. Understanding what part of this model is not embraced by the patient may help the SLP to determine how to shape treatment to enhance adherence.

Another theory to consider in regard to patient adherence is the rational choice theory (Corrigan, Rusch, Ben-Zeev, & Sher, 2015). This theory revolves around perceived benefits versus perceived costs of a treatment. This model assumes that the patient may *choose* not to adhere for valid reasons. For example, a patient might think a treatment is not working, has excessive side effects, or that there are too many barriers to adopting the recommended treatment. Hence, the patient is deliberately choosing not to follow a recommendation because they think the costs outweigh the benefits. For example, a patient prescribed with thickened liquids may choose not to thicken their liquids because they feel that they cough the same amount with thick and thin liquids, they don't like the taste of liquids thickened, and they find the thickener inconvenient and expensive. In this example, the patient has made a clear decision that the costs (distaste, expense, inconvenience) outweigh the benefits (reduction in coughing with liquids). Some argue that this simple theory fails to account for the degree to which such decisions are made in a subconscious manner with overlying nonrational influences. However, it is worthwhile to consider the possible contribution of rational decision weighing as a component of patient adherence.

The locus of control theory suggests that the more perceived control a patient feels they have over a situation, the more likely they are to adhere to treatment recommendations (Wallston & Wallston, 1978). Individuals who feel that they have the ability to control situations are said to have an internal locus of control and therefore are more likely to believe that their actions may make a difference. In contrast, individuals who feel that situations are out of their control are said to have an external locus of control and therefore are less likely to believe their actions may impact outcomes. If we think of the patient undergoing radiation therapy for head and neck cancer again, if this individual had an internal locus of control, they might think that completing exercises is likely to lead to a better outcome. In contrast, an individual with an external locus of control may believe that whatever happens is the result of the radiation treatment being applied to them and that nothing they do will change their outcome. In comparing these two individuals, we would expect the patient with an internal locus of control to have better adherence to treatment recommendations than the patient with external locus of control.

Factors that Impact Patient Adherence

In addition to these theoretical frameworks regarding adherence, there are also a number of patient and treatment characteristics that have been linked to adherence. The World Health Organization (WHO) has classified these factors into five distinct groupings: patient-related factors, socioeconomic factors, therapy-related factors, condition-related factors, and health-care system-related factors (Sabate, 2003). It must be emphasized that there is marked overlap and co-occurrence of these factors and that each factor should not be considered an independent predictor of adherence.

Inherent patient characteristics may directly or indirectly impact adherence. Issues such as

psychiatric disorders, procrastination, forgetfulness, avoidance, denial, and lack of understanding may reduce the potential for patient adherence. A patient who has issues with forgetfulness may regularly forget to use compensatory strategies like a supraglottic swallow when eating and drinking. Thus, even if the patient understands the maneuver, accepts the risk/benefit ratio, and has the capacity to complete the maneuver, their adherence may be reduced due to their inherent tendency toward forgetfulness. Depression has been shown repeatedly to have a major impact on treatment adherence (Capoccia, Odegard, & Letassy, 2016; Law, Naughton, Ho, Roebuck, & Dabscheck, 2014) and is a common finding in the head and neck cancer population (Archer, Hutcheson, & Korszun, 2008). Thus, the SLP should be mindful of mood issues that may impact patient adherence. Patient factors associated with non-adherence have been described by Meichenbaum and Turk (1987) and are summarized in Table 24.1.

Additionally, physical patient characteristics may influence adherence to treatment recommendations. It is understood that tracheoesophageal voice prostheses (TEP) require daily care and maintenance (see Graville, Palmer & Bolognone, Chap. 11). Issues such as reduced visual acuity and manual dexterity may interfere with a patient's ability to adhere to cleaning procedures

Table 24.1 Patient factors associated with non-adherence

Type/severity of psychiatric diagnosis
Sensory disabilities
Forgetfulness
Lack of understanding
Inappropriate or conflicting health beliefs
Competing sociocultural concepts of disease and treatment
Implicit model of illness
Apathy and pessimism
Failure to recognize one is ill or in need of treatment
Previous history of non-adherence to recommendations
Characteristics of patient's social situation/support
Residential instability
Competing or conflicting demands
Lack of resources

recommended by the SLP. Similarly, a patient with back or neck problems may not be able to follow through with a recommendation to complete an exercise such as the Shaker exercise. Comorbidities such as chronic obstructive pulmonary disease (COPD), diabetes, and chronic fatigue syndrome may influence patient adherence indirectly as well through physical limitations or restrictions.

Socioeconomic characteristics that may impact patient adherence involve logistic barriers as well as interactions with family, caregivers, and the support network. A patient lacking in social support to complete a treatment may be less likely to follow through with recommendations. This may be true whether a patient is entirely lacking in support network or if the support network is not supportive of the proposed treatment. For example, when trying to rehabilitate alaryngeal speech after total laryngectomy, social support can be very important in the patient's acceptance and the use of the electrolarynx as a communication tool. If the patient does not have friends and family to talk with, they may be less engaged in treatment. Similarly, if their friends and family express dissatisfaction with the electrolarynx, the patient may be less likely to use it. The attitudes of the support network regarding a particular treatment and their expectations of the treatment can dramatically impact a patient's adherence.

Health beliefs are another social characteristic that should be considered as a potential impediment to adherence. Individuals possess social and cultural concepts of disease and treatment. When these health beliefs contradict treatment recommendations, patients are less likely to follow recommendations. For example, a SLP may desire to train a patient in how to care for their tracheostoma and TEP. The SLP wants the patient to be independent in this self-care; however, the patient and their family believe all care should be provided by trained medical staff. They may assert that home health nursing should provide this care indefinitely. In this case, the patient's social beliefs about treatment may interfere with the SLP's goal of training self-care.

Logistical issues such as competing demands and lack of resources may also negatively impact adherence. Again, using a laryngectomee patient as an example, if a patient is under or uninsured, they may not follow recommendations for the use of a heat and moisture exchanger (HME) filter due to costs even if they believe using the filter would be in their best interest (see Lewis, Chap. 8). In this case the lack of monetary resources is the primary contributor to non-adherence. Similarly, if a patient lives a distance from the treatment center and does not drive, their adherence to recommendations for weekly swallowing therapy may be poor.

Characteristics of treatment should also be considered in regard to adherence. Preparation for treatment, how the treatment is administered, and the consequences of treatment are all likely to impact adherence. A number of factors leading up to treatment have been identified as having a potential impact on adherence. These include inconvenience of clinical operations and long wait time between referral and appointment. Time between consult and first visit has been shown to have a negative correlation with adherence to voice therapy (Portone-Maira, Wise, Johns, & Hapner, 2011). If a patient is referred to a SLP for swallowing assessment but has to wait 2 months for the consult, they might think the problem is not very important to the treatment team and, therefore, will put less emphasis on the importance of following recommendations after the evaluation. Organizational features which may enhance adherence are summarized in Table 24.2 (Meichenbaum & Turk, 1987).

Treatment administration may also impact patient adherence. This refers to factors such as the complexity of treatment, duration of treatment, degree of behavioral change required, and inconvenience. In general, the more complex and lengthy a treatment is, the less likely the patient is to continue the treatment. For example, peristomal attachments used for hands-free speech in the total laryngectomy population historically required a multistep application of glue, adhesives, and the baseplate. Because of the multiple steps required, many patients would abandon the use of a hands-free valve. Advances in adhesive

Table 24.2 Organizational variables that influence patient adherence

Nature of referral process
Continuity of care/provider
Personalized care
Scheduling of appointments
Length of time between referral and appointment
Length of time waiting in waiting room prior to appointment
Provision of on-site treatment
Increased patient supervision
Established connections between inpatient and outpatient care
Positive attitude of the staff and enthusiasm toward treatment

Table 24.3 Relationship variables associated with non-adherence

Patient's perception of the approachability/friendliness of the provider
Patient's feelings of being held in esteem or treated with respect by the provider
Degree to which the patient participates in the development of the treatment regimen
Degree to which the patient feels their needs are met by the provider
Amount of supervision provided by the provider
Degree to which the provider is perceived as being considerate of the patient's feelings and needs
Degree to which provider establishes sense of trust, communicates effectively regarding treatment recommendations, and motivates patient cooperation

baseplates now require only a one-step application process; thus, more patients appear willing to consider and continue the use of a hands-free device. The reduction of complexity of the treatment appears to yield better adherence to this treatment.

An additional factor, which cannot be overstated is the relationship between the patient and the provider. Patient dissatisfaction with providers may lead to rejection of recommendations and missed appointments (Whitcher-Alagna, 1983). It is inherent that providers develop a true collaborative partnership with patients, allowing patients to express their feelings and preferences about treatment. This open dialogue facilitates provider understanding of barriers to adherence and will allow treatment recommendations to reflect these differences. For example, a patient presenting to a SLP for TEP management may have a chronically filthy prosthesis. The SLP may engage in conversation with the patient about the reason for poor cleaning of the device. Through this conversation they may learn that the patient merely forgets to clean it each day. The SLP then could tailor recommendations to pair cleaning with other daily activities such as toothbrushing to enhance the likelihood of adherence. This relational conversation is much more likely to achieve the desired goal than just lecturing to the patient why they need to clean the TEP. Relationship variables associated with adherence have been described by Meichenbaum

and Turk (1987) and are summarized in Table 24.3.

Finally, we must consider how the consequences of treatment impacts adherence. Treatments with limited consequences will be more readily adopted than those with real or potential consequences. Consequences can include physical but also social side effects. It is easy to envision how physical side effects of radiation and chemotherapy (such as pain, dry mouth, and fatigue) may impact a patient's adherence to prophylactic swallowing exercises (see Starmer, Chap. 18, and Arrese and Schieve, Chap. 19). However, we must also consider the social side effects of some of our treatments. For example, when we ask a patient to use a combined chin tuck and supraglottic swallow to minimize aspiration risk, the patient may be less willing to adopt these strategies in social situations due to stigma and embarrassment.

The condition under treatment also has the potential to impact adherence. An example of this would be the total laryngectomee who is unable to produce tracheoesophageal voice. While the care provider might encourage the patient to call the clinic if any needs arise, if the patient is unable to speak, they may not be able to communicate with their care provider. Another example of the condition impacting patient adherence would be a patient with aphagia who is physically unable to perform swallowing exercises due to complete lack of swallow ability.

Finally, there are issues related to the health-care system at large that can influence the patient's ability to adhere to treatment recommendations. In a health-care system, where insurers define what services are covered, there is potential for under-coverage from a monetary perspective. SLPs often see this in cases where patients requiring voice therapy are denied coverage for this intervention. Additionally, due to the classification of TEPs by Medicare, covered costs for a device might be significantly less than the actual costs. In a patient with limited financial resources, this may lead to leaving a problematic, leaking valve in for a longer duration than clinically recommended. In contrast, in a socialized health-care system, specialty care centers may be located a distance from the patient's home, thus adding a logistical barrier to adherence.

It is easy to see that adherence is a multifactorial concept with varied external and internal influences. This complexity ensures that interventions to enhance adherence will similarly need to be multifaceted and that practitioners need to consider factors in each patient that may contribute to adherence/non-adherence. It is unlikely that any one treatment will be equally effective across patients. Key factors that have been associated with non-adherence that should be emphasized include patient failure to understand recommendations, lack of skills or resources to complete treatment, lack of patient self-efficacy, lack of belief that the treatment may be of benefit, excessive complexity of treatment, adverse side effects of treatment, poor patient-provider relationship, lack of continuity of care, and poor clinical operations. We will consider later in the chapter how addressing these challenges may help to enhance patient adherence.

Measuring Adherence

Adherence is a complex concept with multiple influences. Additionally, adherence encompasses a wide range of behaviors such as initiating a desired behavior, continuing that behavior, and discontinuing that behavior. As a result, measuring adherence can be a challenging endeavor.

Measures may be objective (such as pill counts) or subjective (such as patient reports). Indirect, subjective measures of adherence that rely on either the patient or the care provider's reported estimation of adherence rates while simple and affordable have repeatedly been found to overestimate adherence (Daniels et al., 2011; Dunbar-Jacob & Rohay, 2016; Vik, Maxwell, & Hogan, 2004). This is likely due to a number of factors such as recall bias, confirmation bias, and social desirability bias. Recall bias refers to a tendency to under- or overestimate a past occurrence based on future knowledge. For example, if a patient did not develop dysphagia after radiation therapy and they believed this was due to swallowing exercises, they may overestimate how frequently they performed the exercises. Prospective reporting at the time of the event may be less prone to recall bias than reporting done after the fact; however, patient journals are still prone to overestimation when compared to more objective measures (Farmer, 1999). Patients may fall prey to recall bias in reporting but also to social desirability bias where they want to provide only the data that is socially acceptable (adherence) while underreporting less desirable behaviors (non-adherence). A provider may be subject to confirmation bias in that they want to believe that their patient is adhering to recommendations so only focus on patient reports that confirm adherence.

Objective measures of adherence include pill counts, electronic monitoring, and biochemical/physiologic measures. Applying such measures to SLP behavioral interventions can be more challenging as there are no existing tests to directly measure adherence as can be done in medication adherence. Using the treatment outcome (dysphagia) as a marker for adherence is problematic as a number of factors aside from adherence may influence that outcome (extent of disease, oncologic treatment, other medical comorbidities, etc.) Additionally, objective tests may be burdensome and costly. Thus, at the current time, indirect measures of adherence are the primary reported measure in regard to behavioral interventions like speech and swallowing therapy. As technologies develop, electronic monitoring also may hold a promise as a way to objectively measure adherence for behavioral therapies, particularly in the clinical trial context.

Adherence in Head and Neck Cancer

We have discussed general barriers to patient adherence that cross disease populations and interventions, however, for the purpose of the present readership, it is important to dive deeper into understanding adherence to speech and swallowing rehabilitation in the head and neck cancer population. Issues with adherence can be seen in patients receiving both operative and non-operative cancer care. Unfortunately, there is a paucity of information regarding patient adherence to SLP recommendations in this population; however, we will examine the available studies for trends that may help to inform directions for interventions, as well as future research.

Following total laryngectomy, patients are encouraged to use heat and moisture exchanger (HME) units for pulmonary rehabilitation. A recent study examining the long-term adherence with this recommendation demonstrated that nearly one-quarter of patients abandoned the use of HME filter (Pedemonte-Sarrias et al., 2013). Reasons cited for non-adherence included difficulty with HME interface. This may reflect issues in the realm of education about how to optimize interface use, logistical issues with affordability of options, and/or treatment-related effects of skin irritation and excessive mucus. Understanding these contributors to non-adherence will help the SLP to tailor treatments to minimize their impact.

Standard of care for patients receiving radiation +/− chemotherapy for head and neck tumors is referral to a speech pathologist prior to initiation of radiation for administration of prophylactic swallowing exercises. Despite the importance of these exercises in the prevention of radiation-associated dysphagia, a recent study demonstrated that only 15% of patients were fully adherent to SLP recommendations during radiation, and an additional 36% reported partial adherence (Shinn et al., 2013). As this data was clinician-reported, it likely reflects an overestimation of actual adherence rates. Thus, patient adherence to these recommendations is suboptimal at best. When these patients were queried about reasons for non-adherence, three trends emerged: lack of understanding about reason for and how to complete exercises (44%), treatment toxicity interference (38%), and logistic barriers (21%). These findings are consistent with studies of prophylactic medication regimens where adherence to recommendations is ~30% (Marston, 1970).

Enhancing Adherence

When considering ways to enhance adherence at a population level, one must understand the common barriers to adherence in the target population. Interventions to enhance adherence may focus on logistical, educational, and treatment-related barriers as discussed previously. Individual tailoring of interventions related to personal barriers should be considered by the treating clinician as well.

The patient-provider relationship should be given significant importance when considering ways to enhance adherence. It has been said that "what should be avoided is the traditional paternalistic attitude whereby the physician assumes in advance what the patient needs to know and thus makes no attempt to include the patient in the decision-making process out of fear of burdening the patient with too much information or too much responsibility" (Hanson, 1986, p. 194). The shared decision model of collaborative care should rather be adopted whenever possible. Additionally, providers should strive to avoid behaviors that have been associated with non-adherence including unfriendly/disengaged affect, distractability/disruption during clinical visits, excessive use of jargon, interruption of patients, failure to ask questions regarding understanding and agreement, and abruptly terminating the visit without ensuring the patient feels their needs have been met. Instead, the provider should engage in some nonmedical conversation to ensure the patient feels that they are being treated as a person rather than a disease, encourage the patient to discuss their goals and concerns, discuss the pros and cons of different treatment options, and elicit patient opinions about these options. Clinicians must ensure that their treatment recommendations match with those of the patient's concerns so that they are invested in following our recommendations. For example, a patient is more likely to follow through with recommendations to use a HME after laryngectomy if the clinician relates this back to the patient's concerns regarding coughing up excessive mucous. Communication skills that may contribute to a positive clinician-client relationship are summarized in Table 24.4.

Logistic barriers to adherence may include distance to the treatment site, coordination of multiple appointments, cost of care, and availability of care. In the head and neck population, we can consider clinical models as one possible intervention to enhance adherence to prehabilitation and rehabilitation. SLP participation in a multidisciplinary head and neck cancer clinic has been shown to increase the probability of patient follow-up for future SLP visits (Starmer, Sanguineti, Marur, & Gourin, 2011). Integrating the SLP into this initial team visit may facilitate less frequent visits to the medical center through coordinated care. Additionally, it is suspected that there is an educational benefit from this model as well, in that patients have a greater understanding of the SLP role on the head and neck care team. Finally, establishing a relationship between the patient and the SLP from the onset of care will help the SLP to identify any additional barriers that may need to be addressed prior to treatment in order to enhance potential for adherence.

In the medication administration adherence literature, it has been demonstrated that the number of times each day a medication is required is more closely associated with nonadherence than the actual number of pills required (Malahey, 1966). The level of intrusiveness of the recommended treatment may be a barrier to adherence. This may be applicable to therapeutic interventions in that more frequent exercise sessions may serve as a barrier to adherence. For example, one trismus treatment regimen involves the use of a TheraBite™ device, seven repetitions of a 7-second hold, 7 times daily. Such a frequent regimen may not be practical for some patients, and therefore adherence may not be achieved. Negotiating with the patient how frequent home practice is feasible and reducing the number of treatment sessions per day may help to enhance adherence to TheraBite™ use.

Education and understanding of treatment recommendations are a hallmark of each of the adherence theories discussed previously. Optimizing understanding of presented material as well as retention of that material over the treatment course is of paramount importance. Ley's cognitive model (Ley, 1982) considers how the understanding and recall of information impact adherence. This model proposes characteristics of knowledge acquisition that may strengthen learning. For example, information presented first during a learning session is more likely to be retained and recalled. Additionally, information presented in a structured manner is similarly more likely to be retained. If a learner has prior knowledge of a topic, they are more likely to understand and retain new information. Finally, this model asserts that the greater the amount of information presented, the greater the potential for information to be forgotten. A SLP engaging in patient education endeavors then should consider these tenets when planning patient education events. In general, the thera-

Table 24.4 Communication skills important for positive patient-provider relationship

Provider empathy and concern
Provider respect for patient feelings and needs
Provider sincerity and warmth during patient encounters
Provider self-disclosure of similar challenges to those the patient is experiencing
Positive provider nonverbal communication (eye contact, smiling, nodding in understanding, open body posture, etc.)
During encounter, provider sitting at the same level as patient
Provider sense of humor

pist would want to highlight the most salient information first and to provide the information in a structured format. Further, providing too much information at a single setting may be counterproductive. Regularly checking in with a patient during education and having them repeat back their understanding of the content will help the SLP to determine if the amount of material presented is too much for that point in time. Building on education sequentially may enhance both comprehension and recall. Further, providing multimodal educational content that can be reviewed at a later date/time may be of benefit in enriching knowledge and, thus, adherence. Technological advances such as web-based content and mobile applications provide new opportunities for information dissemination to increase adherence to treatment recommendations.

Finally, the head and neck care team must consider treatment factors that may influence adherence. In the case of patients undergoing radiotherapy, pain is frequently cited as the side effect most likely to impact adherence to recommendations to eat and perform swallowing exercises (Shinn et al., 2013). Thus, efforts should be centered on pain management in order to optimize adherence. Traditional pain management strategies during radiotherapy have focused on the use of narcotic analgesics. While narcotics have good efficacy for nociceptive pain, less efficacy is observed for neuropathic pain. As pain during radiation has both nociceptive and neuropathic components, attention to management of neuropathic pain is critical. Recent investigation of the role of prophylactic gabapentin during radiation demonstrated better pain control with less narcotic medication during radiation, less need for feeding tube use, and better swallowing outcomes (Starmer et al., 2014; Yang et al., 2016). It has been hypothesized that the use of prophylactic gabapentin helps to minimize pain during treatment, thus enhancing patient adherence to recommendations to maintain oral intake and complete swallowing exercises. This is one example of how considering treatment effects and their management may influence adherence.

Conclusions

Speech and swallowing therapy in the head and neck cancer population relies heavily on patient adherence to treatment recommendations. There are numerous factors inherent to the patient as well as external to the patient that may influence the potential that they will adhere to recommendations. The SLP needs to understand contributing factors and strive to minimize those factors that may enhance the potential for non-adherence. In the head and neck cancer population, integration of the SLP into the multidisciplinary clinic and pain management through the use of gabapentin have shown promise for enhancing adherence. Future efforts should continue to explore how alteration of treatment logistics, patient education, and treatment effects may enhance adherence. As adherence-enhancing interventions are identified, it is important for the clinician to remember that no single strategy is likely to apply to all patients; therefore, personalization of treatment strategies remains critical.

References

Archer, J., Hutcheson, I., & Korszun, A. (2008). Mood and malignancy: Head and neck cancer and depression. *Journal of Oral Pathology & Medicine, 37*, 255–270.

Becker, M. H. (Ed.). (1974). The health belief model and personal behavior. *Health Education Monographs, 2*, 324–373.

Becker, M. H., & Rosenstock, I. M. (1984). Compliance with medical advice. In A. Steptoe & A. Matthews (Eds.), *Health care and human behavior*. New York, NY: Academic Press.

Capoccia, K., Odegard, P. S., & Letassy, N. (2016). Medication adherence with diabetes medication: A systematic review of the literature. *Diabetes Education, 42*, 34–71.

Corrigan, P. W., Rusch, N., Ben-Zeev, D., & Sher, T. (2015). The rational patient and beyond: Implications for treatment adherence in people with psychiatric disabilities. *Rehabilitation Psychology, 59*, 85–98.

Cramer, J. A., Roy, A., Burrell, A., Fairchild, C. J., Fuldeore, M. J., Ollendorf, D. A., & Wong, P. K. (2008). Medication compliance and persistence: Terminology and definitions. *Value in Health, 11*, 44–47.

Daniels, T., Goodacre, L., Sutton, C., Pollard, K., Conway, S., & Peckham, D. (2011). Accurate assessment of adherence: Self-report and clinician report versus electronic monitoring of nebulizers. *Chest, 140*, 425–432.

Dunbar-Jacob, J., & Rohay, J. (2016). Predictors of medication adherence: Fact or artifact. *Journal of Behavioral Medicine, 39*(6), 957–968.

Farmer, K. C. (1999). Methods for measuring and monitoring medication regimen adherence in clinical trials and clinical practice. *Clinical Therapeutics, 21*, 1074–1090.

Hanson, R. W. (1986). Physician-patient communication and compliance. In K. E. Gerber & A. M. Nehemkis (Eds.), *Compliance: The dilemma of the chronically ill*. New York, NY: Springer.

Law, M., Naughton, M., Ho, S., Roebuck, T., & Dabscheck, E. (2014). Depression may reduce adherence during CPAP titration trial. *Journal of Clinical Sleep Medicine, 10*, 163–169.

Ley, P. (1982). Satisfaction, compliance, and communication. *The British Journal of Clinical Psychology, 21*, 241–254.

Malahey, B. (1966). The effects of instructions and labeling in the number of medication errors made by patients at home. *American Journal of Hospital Pharmacy, 23*, 283–292.

Marston, M. V. (1970). Compliance with medical regimens: A review of the literature. *Nursing Research, 10*, 312–323.

Meichenbaum, D., & Turk, D. C. (1987). *Facilitating treatment adherence: A practitioner's guidebook*. New York, NY: Plenum Press.

Pedemonte-Sarrias, G., Villatoro-Sologaistoa, J. C., Ale-Inostroza, P., López-Vilas, M., León-Vintró, X., & Quer-Agustí, M. (2013). Chronic adherence to heat and moisture exchanger use in laryngectomized patients. *Acta Otorhinolaryngol Espana, 64*, 247–252.

Portone-Maira, C., Wise, J. C., Johns, M. M., & Hapner, E. R. (2011). Differences in temporal variables between voice therapy completers and dropouts. *Journal of Voice, 25*, 62–66.

Rosenstock, I. M. (1974). Historical origins of the health belief model. *Health Education Monographs, 2*, 328–335.

Sabate, E. (2003). *Adherence to long-term therapies: Evidence for action*. Geneva, Switzerland: World Health Organization.

Shinn, E. H., Basen-Engquist, K., Baum, G., Steen, S., Bauman, R. F., Morrison, W., … Lewin, J. S. (2013). Adherence to preventive exercises and self-reported swallowing outcomes in post-radiation head and neck cancer patients. *Head & Neck, 35*, 1707–1172.

Starmer, H. M., Sanguineti, G., Marur, S., & Gourin, C. G. (2011). Multidisciplinary head and neck cancer clinic and adherence with speech pathology. *Laryngoscope, 121*, 2131–2135.

Starmer, H. M., Yang, W., Raval, R., Gourin, C. G., Richardson, M., Kumar, R., … Quon, H. (2014). Effect of gabapentin on swallowing during and after chemoradiation for oropharyngeal squamous cell cancer. *Dysphagia, 29*, 396–402.

Vik, S. A., Maxwell, C. J., & Hogan, D. B. (2004). Measurement, correlates, and health outcomes of medication adherence among seniors. *The Annals of Pharmacotherapy, 38*, 303–312.

Wallston, B. D., & Wallston, K. A. (1978). Locus of control and health: A review of the literature. *Health Education Monographs, 6*, 107–117.

Whitcher-Alagna, S. (1983). Receiving medical help: A psychosocial perspective on patient reactions. In A. Nadler, J. D. Fisher, & B. M. DePaulo (Eds.), *New directions in helping*. New York, NY: Academic Press.

Yang, W., McNutt, T. R., Dudley, S. A., Kumar, R., Starmer, H. M., Gourin, C. G., … Quon, H. (2016). Predictive factors for prophylactic percutaneous endoscopic gastrostomy (PEG) tube placement and use in head and neck patients following intensity-modulated radiation therapy (IMRT) treatment: Concordance, discrepancies, and the role of gabapentin. *Dysphagia, 31*, 206–213.

The Role of the Clinical Nurse Specialist in Head and Neck Oncology

25

Wendy Townsend

Introduction

Squamous cell carcinoma of the head and neck is considered a worldwide healthcare problem. These cancers represent the sixth most common malignancy worldwide (de Leeuw, 2013). Historically, the majority of patients have presented with a history of alcohol abuse and high-level tobacco consumption; however, contemporary data increasingly suggest that head and neck cancer (HNCa) is now also associated with exposure to viruses including HPV and the Epstein-Barr virus (Theurer, Chap. 4). HNCa is often considered to be the most devastating and debilitating of all cancers (Clarke, 1998) due to myriad changes that may negatively influence eating, swallowing, and speech. Unique physiologic and psychosocial needs of patients with HNCa may potentially be magnified by physical alterations of the face and/ or neck, in addition to multiple sensorimotor functional impairments associated with the effects of surgery, radiation, and/or chemotherapy (Boulougouris & Doyle, Chap. 23; Doyle & Mac-Donald, Chap. 27).

Another major problem facing HNCa patients is that their disease may be diagnosed at an advanced stage where treatment options may not be curative; subsequently, such a prognosis can have severe posttreatment consequences which include disfigurement, significant speech and swallowing impairments, isolation, and depression. Therefore, the oncology CNS serves to integrate into clinical practice an understanding of the biology of carcinogenesis and its relationship to cancer staging and treatment (Lewandowski & Adamle, 2009, p. 77). Further, the CNS will have an advanced understanding of the significant potential for disability that may be experienced posttreatment (Doyle, 1994). Advanced practice nurses are essential members of any multidisciplinary team (MDT) that provides care for oncology patients. In no other disease site is the MDT more critical than for those diagnosed and treated for head and neck cancer (HNCa). The natural progression of this disease and the treatments required result in myriad physical and psychosocial changes for these individuals both as a result of the disease and its treatment (Bornbaum et al., 2013; Bornbaum & Doyle, Chap. 5; Doyle, 1994, 2005). The patient's ability to breath, speak, and eat is potentially affected by treatment and, often times, altered irreparably which leads to varied levels of chronic disability. As stated by Scarpa (2004, p. 579) in relation to the quality of life of head and neck cancer survivors, "…these patients are directly dependent on their ability to become self-sufficient in certain areas of their care and to receive assistance from individuals who are able to cope with the demands of caring for them." For this reason, the clinical nurse specialist

W. Townsend (✉)
Head and Neck Surgical Oncology, London Health Sciences Center, London, ON, Canada
e-mail: wendy.townsend@lhsc.on.ca

© Springer Nature Switzerland AG 2019
P. C. Doyle (ed.), *Clinical Care and Rehabilitation in Head and Neck Cancer*,
https://doi.org/10.1007/978-3-030-04702-3_25

423

(CNS) is ideally suited to fill the role of assisting patients and members of their family who are facing HNCa throughout the continuum of care.

When included as part of a comprehensive multidisciplinary team, CNSs have the comprehensive skill set to support both the patient and family, as well as providing support and guidance to others within the care team. It is well acknowledged that experienced nursing care and coordination is vital to the support of HNCa patients (de Leeuw, 2013). Further, the role of the CNS can change in response to the dynamic needs of patients and family members by integrating clinical knowledge, skills, and expertise (Pan-Canadian Core Competencies for the Clinical Nurse Specialist, 2014). Consequently, the objective of this chapter seeks to provide information on the role and scope of the CNS in the care of those treated for HNCa. The discussion to follow will address issues related to nursing as a profession and its historical development and impact on patient care. Additionally, aspects of the roles and skills of the CNS as a navigator and educator of both patients and members of their family are presented. Finally, the importance of developing the CNS-patient relationship as a critical component of patient care is addressed.

Nursing as a Profession

Nursing as a profession has been defined by de Leeuw (2013, p. 11) "as one which uses clinical judgment to provide care that enables people to improve, maintain, or recover health." De Leeuw goes on to state that "nurses assist people in achieving the best quality of life, regardless of disease process until recovery or death." The International Council of Nurses (ICN) defines a nurse practitioner/advanced practice nurse as a "registered nurse who has acquired the expert knowledge base, complex decision-making skills, and clinical competencies...the characteristics of which are shaped by the context and or country in which they are credentialed to practice" (ICN Fact Sheet, 2009). According to the Canadian Nurses Association, advanced practice nursing is an "umbrella term describing an

advanced level of clinical nursing practice that maximizes the use of graduate nursing educational preparation, as well as in-depth nursing knowledge and expertise in meeting the health needs of individuals, families, groups, communities and populations" (Pan-Canadian Core Competencies for the Clinical Nurse Specialist, 2014, p. 9).

An advanced level of nursing care involves analyzing and synthesizing knowledge through understanding, interpreting, and applying nursing theory and research evidence. By demonstrating this skill set, the advanced practice nurse has the capacity to not only develop and advance nursing knowledge in general but to also advance the profession (Pan-Canadian Core Competencies for the Clinical Nurse Specialist, 2014; Staples, Ray, & Hannon, 2016). Accordingly, a master's degree is recommended for entry level to advanced practice. Further, the advanced practice nurse should have prior oncology experience and expertise; however, in some instances the acquisition of these skills may require role mentoring to develop specific oncology expertise (Gilbert, Devries-Aboud, Winquist, Waldron, & McQuestion, 2009). The Canadian Oncology Nurses Association (2012) defines two levels of oncology nursing: specialized and advanced. Both of these categories of nursing will play a role in direct patient care within the professional team charged with the care of HNCa patients. The specialized oncology nurse is one who works in a dedicated setting with their specific clinical focus on the delivery of care. Their education is more often obtained at the baccalaureate level with additional certifications in certain areas of specialized oncology skills. In contrast to the specialized nurse, and as noted, the advanced oncology nurse is prepared at the master's level but also works in a specialized setting.

The difference between the two nursing categories described above is that they are positioned to see patients throughout the continuum of care. This would include patient care that occurs in various settings such as postoperative inpatient environments, outpatient clinics, or during radiation or chemoradiation treatment(s). In some instances, these professionals may be identified as a nurse practitioner who carries a protected title or as a clinical nurse specialist. For the remaining sections of this chapter, the focus will be on the clinical nurse specialist (CNS) in the context of head and neck oncology.

CNS practice traditionally has been described using the following five component roles: expert practitioner, educator, consultant, researcher, and administrator or clinical leader (Scott, 1999, p. 2). As an advanced practice nurse, the CNS will perform a variety of duties as a part of their clinical practice. For example, the CNS utilizes the educator domain when teaching a patient about their tracheostomy. Within the cancer care environment, the CNS will frequently function "…autonomously and integrate knowledge of cancer and medical treatments into assessment, diagnosis and treatment of patients' problems and concerns" (Macmillan Cancer Support, 2014). Because of their training and education, the CNS has the advanced knowledge, skill, and judgment to recognize when each domain may or may not be applicable. Thus, the CNS demonstrates an extended skill set and range of expertise related to patient care.

According to Scarpa (2004, p. 580) "oncology advanced practice nurses are essential members of the multidisciplinary team." Further, pertaining to the nursing care of those with HNCa, it has been stated that the essential role played is in "… management of the actual and potential responses of patients to their cancer and its treatment, and of the rehabilitation of patients back into daily life" (de Leeuw, 2013, p. 10). The CNS will work in tandem with other members of the care team to ensure that the appropriate disciplines are involved as required based on the patient's healthcare needs. For example, if a patient develops dysphagia, the speech-language pathologist as well as the registered dietician should be actively involved as their input may directly impact the patient's nutrition. The type and extent of care will also change over time, potentially involving a wide range of services. As such, patients may remain in the healthcare system for extended periods of time with a need for ongoing support, surveillance, or palliation if their disease returns. Consequently, the CNS may be involved in a given patient's ongoing care throughout the continuum of their disease and survivorship. This extended level of care and the roles that have emerged the CNS have evolved over time, and this topic will be addressed in the subsequent section.

A Historical Perspective on the Role of the CNS

From a historical perspective, in 1943 the CNS was the first advanced practice role to be described, implemented, and fully evaluated in the United States. According to LaSala et al. (2007, p. 263), this type of advance practice nursing was "…introduced as a response to the growth of the health care industry and an emerging need for greater continuity in patient care." Oncology nursing was recognized as a specialty as early as 1947. Within the profession of nursing, theorist Hildegard Peplau promoted the clinical specialist as a model of expertise and, as a result, helped to shape and change nursing education to that end (Peplau, 1952, 1997). Peplau also promoted the value of interpersonal relationships as part of nursing expertise and for enhancing patient care. The first master's program designed to educate such clinical specialists was implemented in 1954; the 1960s saw a shortage of primary care providers, a deficit that resulted in the advent of the nurse practitioner (LaSala et al., 2007, p. 263).

To further delineate and distinguish the CNS role from that of the nurse practitioner, the National Association of Clinical Nurse Specialists issued a statement in 1998, clarifying the CNS role in healthcare settings. In doing so, the American Nurses Association defines the CNS as an "advanced practice nurse who integrates and applies a wide range of theoretical and evidenced-based knowledge" (Lewandowski & Adamle, 2009, p. 74). Essentially, the CNS role developed out a need to meet societal healthcare needs, improve the patient experience, and increase efficiencies within the healthcare system. Thus, advanced practice nurses work within various spheres of influence (Staples et al., 2016). This would include not only patient nursing practice but also active involvement in the development of organizational changes directed toward improving patient outcomes, the quality of care, and issues of cost-effectiveness (Lewandowski & Adamle, 2009, p. 74). Given expansions in the roles played by the CNS within the current healthcare system, the likely impact on patient care has also increased accordingly.

Roles and Responsibilities of the CNS

Multiple systematic reviews have demonstrated the effectiveness of advanced practice nursing roles for improving patient health and quality of care, as well as in reducing healthcare utilization and costs (Bryant-Lukosius et al., 2016). The aim of such specialization in nursing care was undertaken to improve patient care which encompassed advanced practice knowledge, clinical decision-making, and specialist skills, activities that have often been associated with cancer care and palliative care (Folland, 2000, p.5). The CNS role can change in response to the dynamic needs of patients (Pan-Canadian Core Competencies for the Clinical Nurse Specialist, 2014).

The CNS can also play an instrumental role in reducing costs associated with patient care. More specifically, length of hospital stays can be reduced with interventions provided by the CNS to better prepare patients and families at the time of discharge. Furthermore, ongoing assessment of health problems and care coordination has been shown to result in fewer complications for patients (Gittell et al., 2000; Wagner, Austin, & Von Korff, 1996). In fact, it has been suggested that the duration of one's stay in hospital can be reduced if a CNS is directly involved. Thus, it should be noted that the CNS may be actively involved in "…interventions to better prepare clients and their families for discharge and to strengthen client self-care abilities" (Pan-Canadian Competencies for the Clinical Nurse Specialist, 2014, p. 3).

In cancer care, CNSs are in a unique position to develop therapeutic relationships with patients,

family members, and caregivers. This is due to the fact that a CNS typically sees the patient over the entire treatment trajectory. Their skill set and educational preparation lend itself to the delivery of an integrated form of patient care. Accordingly, an overview of the CNS caregiving skills can be separated into four main functions. The first seeks to apply their knowledge of cancer treatment to oversee and coordinate care and provide complex information and supports to patients and their families. The second role is to serve as an accessible, key member of the MDT whose focus centers on the case management of patients. Thirdly, in this role the CNS provides support through empathy, knowledge, and experience to alleviate psychosocial suffering (see Doyle & MacDonald, Chap. 27). Finally, the CNS utilizes knowledge and insight to improve the patient experience while at the same time improving outcomes and reducing care costs and length of stay.

As stated previously, the first and most important function of a CNS in oncology care is to initiate a therapeutic relationship with the patient and those who form their support network. The journey of patients with HNCa often begins with a diagnosis of cancer; however, no clear treatment plan emerges until they meet with the cancer specialists (e.g., surgeons, oncologists, radiologists, dentists, etc.). The first step in the treatment of HNCa is to formally determine a diagnosis and subsequently determine staging of the tumor. This step is often completed in the multidisciplinary setting of a tumor board team consisting of key practitioners from surgery and radiation with specialized expertise in the head and neck disease site. The first meeting with the CNS often takes place after the patient has been given their diagnosis, a rationale underlying the decision-making process for a given treatment plan, and the ultimate posttreatment prognosis.

Establishing the foundation of a therapeutic relationship is the goal of the initial interactions with the patient, family members, and/or caregivers. Of significant importance in this first interaction is the ability for the clinician to recognize and adjust *what* information is presented and *how* that information is provided to the patient in accordance with factors that may interfere with their ability to absorb it. For example, if the patient is overwhelmed with emotion related to their diagnosis and/or information about their treatment, the counseling should be adjusted, shortened, or provided through another medium such as written material. Follow-up consultations may be necessary in many cases. CNSs are adept at this skill as they are trained to take a holistic approach to patient needs. They are also skilled at identifying cognitive deficits or age-related conditions that may limit the patient's ability to adjust and adapt to their change in health status. The CNS who works with those with HNCa should have an in-depth knowledge of the disease, its cause, and the outcomes of treatment, as well as complications or setbacks that may occur over the course of treatment or beyond. For this reason, additional details on such considerations are provided in the next section.

Guiding the Cancer Trajectory

Confronted with a cancer diagnosis and a variety of treatment options, the new HNCa patient may express a range of emotional reactions not withstanding fear and sadness. Patients diagnosed and treated for HNCa are observed to have a relatively high risk of developing emotional disturbances after diagnosis and treatment (Jagannathan & Juvva, 2016). During the HNCa patient journey, there are multiple stages where emotional supports can be offered. Emotional support has been shown to be of significant value in the survivorship process (List et al., 2002). For this reason, a specific professional "point of contact" should be allocated to help patients and family member navigate these emotional stages and, ideally, to deliver practical and accessible psychosocial support. This would include addressing issues such as encouraging attendance at hospital appointments, compliance with lifestyle modifications, and treatment adherence (Starmer, Chap. 24), as well as to identify if or when more advanced emotional support through access to a mental health professional might be needed. This role might be performed by a representative within the multidisciplinary healthcare team

(e.g., a nurse or social worker or psychologist). However, there is a definitive role for the CNS to serve in the role as the facilitator of comprehensive, integrated, compassionate, and holistic care of those treated for HNCa (Reich et al., 2014, p. 2116). The provision of psychological care and support to both patients and family members who are experiencing emotional difficulties as a result of their own or a loved one's HNCA is a key component of comprehensive cancer care; such care and support clearly fits within the professional role of the CNS (Skilbeck & Payne, 2003, p. 522).

CNSs also assist patients and their families in navigating the increasingly challenging healthcare system. At time of diagnosis, considerable information is provided, and many tests must be completed. In the case of head and neck oncology, a large MDT is utilized to assist patients in their treatment and rehabilitation. As suggested by McDonald-Renz and Bard (2010, p. 8), "The delivery of modern health services is a complex activity that increasingly relies on interprofessional collaboration." Patients often report feeling overwhelmed at time of diagnosis and throughout the many professional discussions related to a potential treatment plan. CNSs have advanced health assessment skills and are often recognized as first point of contact for these patients. McDonald and Sherlock (2016) concluded that the CNS model has significant benefits for both a patient's and caregiver's well-being by reducing stress and anxiety levels, which in turn is viewed to enable better decision-making.

An integral role of the CNS is to assist the patient in their processing of the information provided regarding their treatment, while also doing so in an empathetic manner. The information should be delivered with attention to both the patient's education level and cognitive status, as well as one's anxiety level or related emotional status. The CNS is frequently well versed in principles of adult learning and patient education, skills that assist them in conveying comprehensive information in a systematic fashion. In the CNS role, the advanced practice nurse may utilize other assessment tools such as cognitive screenings (Staples et al., 2016) to determine mental status, attention, orientation, etc. In the United Kingdom, the Cancer Reform Strategy (Dempsey, Orr, Lane, & Scott, 2016, p. 212) has recognized that the CNS is critical in the delivery of information, patient communication, and coordination of care. Thus, the role of the CNS is well developed in the United Kingdom, as well as throughout other parts of Europe including the Netherlands.

In 2010, the National Cancer Action Team in Britain published a position paper entitled "The Contribution of the Clinical Nurse Specialist" (Richards, Devane & Beasley, 2018). The authors of this document note that while the CNS role is varied, within the cancer care environment, there are core clinical practice functions. Additionally, there is a level of practice that could be reasonably expected of all CNS professionals in cancer care (Richards, Devane, & Beasley, 2018). Most importantly, patients often report improved understanding of information when a CNS is involved in their care. The 2014 National Cancer Patient Survey reported that 91% of patients assigned a CNS felt that they were listened to during interactions. Those who interacted directly with a CNS responded more positively to information, choices offered, and care than those who did not interact with a CNS (McDonald & Sherlock, 2016). In Britain, 74% of patients who interacted with a CNS felt they were given information about their cancer diagnosis that was easy to understand. In comparison, the figure for those who did not have contact with a CNS was just 47%. Similarly, 74% of patients who interacted with a CNS felt they had been directly involved in their treatment plan compared to 57% of those who did not have such contact (McDonald & Sherlock, 2016). Thus, information suggests that the CNS provides a valuable service in relation to facilitating the process of information provision relative to the broad issues specific to HNCA care.

The CNS as Navigator

The paramount clinical practice function of a CNS is to oversee care and coordinate services so as to individualize and personalize the cancer pathway for both patients and members of their family. The Canadian Nurses Association lists a number of competencies for the CNS. Among those competencies are the following: (1) facilitating interprofessional collaboration, (2) identifying potential and actual gaps in patient care, (3) advocating for necessary patient resources, and (4) designing care plans for patients with highly complex and often unpredictable needs (Pan-Canadian Core Competencies for the Clinical Nurse Specialist, 2014). CNSs are often one of the first members of the MDT that patients and families will meet. Establishing an early therapeutic relationship with the patient and key family members is one of the first goals upon meeting. From there, patients will work with the CNS regularly and collaboratively to identify their learning and knowledge needs, as well as working to understand their healthcare goals.

By acting as the key team member, the CNS provides information and support in addition to serving as a liaison with others to improve the cancer care process for the patient (Dempsey et al., 2016, p. 213). The *National Institute for Health and Care Excellence Improving Outcomes Guidance* recommends that the CNS must act as "gatekeeper" to a patient's cancer pathway to provide a seamless journey (Dempsey et al., 2016). The gatekeeping role is achieved by the reflective nature of the role itself. That is, the CNS working with those with HNCa has established critical thinking skills in a given oncology specialty. Those skills, along with a strong clinical knowledge base, allow the CNS to provide holistic needs assessments at different stages of the patient's cancer pathway. Through such action, the CNS will be better able to reflect the changes that most appropriately meet the patient's needs at any given time. Developing supportive nurse-patient relationships involves a complex process, one that consists of getting to "know the patient" through the effective use of open communication skills, in a variety of healthcare contexts (Skilbeck & Payne, 2003, p. 521). This level of care extends from pretreatment planning through discharge and outpatient care.

By utilizing advanced communication and advocacy skills, the CNS helps to transition patients and families through each stage of the treatment process. Upon diagnosis, a significant amount of written and oral information is often provided to the patient. The CNS begins to assist the patient in absorbing and disseminating that information. Whether the treatment involves surgery or radiation/chemotherapy, or a combined modality approach, patients and families need to be prepared for the proposed treatment and any eventualities that will likely occur (i.e., side effects of treatment). Preoperative education is a major focus prior to surgery and usually involves the entire MDT. They are well placed to support the patient at each stage of their pathway and promote integration within the team (Dempsey et al., 2016, p. 213). Beyond that, and as stated in the report "A Long and Winding Road," the CNS may coordinate a wider multidisciplinary group to ensure patient care is managed effectively (McDonald & Sherlock, 2016).

Acute Care Nursing Skills of the CNS

Once patients become inpatients for treatment, the CNS focus changes to acute care issues. Whether treatment involves radiation with or without chemotherapy or involves surgical interventions, patients require varying levels of support and information. When a patient's care needs occur unexpectedly and are acute in nature, these issues will be challenging for the patient, members of their family, and the nurses who will provide care. At the same time, however, the focus of nursing is to address the whole person and the human response rather than a particular aspect of the person or a particular pathological condition (de Leeuw, 2013, p. 12). The CNS works in partnership with patients, their relatives, and other caregivers, as well as in collaboration with other members of the MDT; where appropriate, the CNS will take the lead (de Leeuw, 2013, p. 12).

Maslow's hierarchy of needs is one theoretical model that may actively guide the CNS's assessment of patients (Maslow, 1943, 1954, 1962). Briefly, this model proposes that higher-level requirements such as the need to communicate will sometimes supersede a patient's need for basics such as food and shelter. HNCa patients often undergo profound changes in their ability to communicate effectively, and this may become a significant source of stress. The CNS role in such cases may be to liaise and advocate with the speech-language pathologist or other members of the clinical nursing staff to facilitate the patient's identified need at a specific point in their care.

In addition to the interpersonal roles they may play, the surgical CNS also has advanced skills specific to the unique care needs of HNCa patients. They are involved in the care of tracheostomy tubes, the tracheostoma following laryngectomy, advanced wound care, free tissue transfers, feeding tubes, and pain control issues, in addition to other duties. As an example, utilizing a holistic theory such as Maslow's hierarchy of needs, an ongoing process transpires as the patient rehabilitates from reconstructive surgery. A relationship will need to be developed between the healthcare practitioner, in this case the CNS, and the patient. This requires expert critical thinking skills and strong interpersonal communication on the part of the CNS. A holistic needs assessment ensures that both patients' and their caregivers' physical, emotional, and social needs are met in a timely and appropriate manner and that advice and support are available from the correct source at the right time (Dempsey et al., 2016, p. 213).

Within their scope of practice, the CNS will assist the patient to meet their goals and cope with setbacks throughout the cancer journey. The patient's needs may change daily or even hourly. As noted, education broadly defined is a significant component of the work the CNS conducts. Adult learning principles are utilized and modified based on the individual's cognitive abilities and knowledge base. Specific challenges at time may arise unexpectedly, and this will require immediate action, particularly during the inpatient phase of recovery. With such knowledge, discharge planning is orchestrated in conjunction with the other members of the MDT, as well as in partnership with the patient and family. Thus, from the beginning of any given patient's care, the CNS will play an important role in seeking to "assess the needs of and to teach, support and advocate for family members who assume caregiving roles" (Lewandowski & Adamle, 2009, p. 78).

Therapeutic Relationships with Patients

Integrated into the range of clinical skills which the CNS brings to the complexities of the HNCa population, there also must be empathy for the person and the knowledge and experience to assess and alleviate the psychosocial suffering of cancer (Doyle, 1994; Dempsey et al., 2016). The therapeutic relationship that has been established by the CNS positions them to best serve the patient in the role of trusted advocate. This is of significant importance in situations where one's ability to communicate effectively is impacted as a result of cancer and its treatment. Clearly, and as noted previously, head and neck surgery and other modalities of treatment can have a profound impact on patient's basic functions including eating, swallowing, and speaking. There can also be a significant impact on the patient's body image, particularly when visibly noticeable structures of the face, head, or neck are impacted (Dropkin, Malgady, Scott, Oberst, & Strong, 1983; Nash, Scott, Fung, Yoo, & Doyle, 2014).

Further, additional and often very challenging side effects of treatment will also require specialized care. For example, the ability to identify and correctly quantify patient alcohol and/or tobacco use is a key skill for the CNS to acquire as this preoperative assessment guides postoperative care (Scott, 1999, p. 186). Scott (1999) noted that substance abuse therapy and smoking cessation therapy were among the top 10 advanced practice nursing skills performed in the CNS role. Increasingly, the CNS may actively provide conversational interventions with seriously ill people, along with symptom control. This supportive work is seen as a primary domain of the CNS, a capacity that also may have an influence on larger advocacy concerns (Skilbeck & Payne, 2003, p. 522). Teaching themes may include postoperative self-care, advising on symptom management, clarifying the illness experience, discussing psychological responses, and preparing patients for their treatment protocols (Hughes, Hodgson, Muller, Robinson, & McCorkle, 2000, p. 25). The CNS is often called upon to evaluate a patient's ability to learn and master critical skills such as tracheostomy or laryngectomy airway care. For that reason, the critical input specific to the educational needs of the patient and potentially family members becomes of substantial importance to the HNCa care process.

The Role of the CNS in Education

Hildegard Peplau (1997) has described the clinical specialist as a "model of expertness," and this concept has been extended by others (LaSala et al., 2007). Thus, serving as a general educator also is a role that the CNS may play within the larger MDT and its functional organization. When considered in the larger context, the role of the CNS is both extensive and critical to improving patient care. The CNS may actively serve in staff development and linking professional practice to evidenced-based outcomes at the level of the patient, unit, and/or organization or facility (LaSala et al., 2007, p. 262). The CNS can, therefore, play a key role and be directly involved in identifying knowledge gaps among staff and assisting in the development of educational programs that serve to eliminate such gaps to improve patient care.

For example, those treated for HNCa often have a significantly altered airway requiring the need for a tracheotomy and the use of tracheostomy tubes. While tracheostomy tubes may not always be used, they are a key component of treatment for certain types of airway stenosis. Patients may also have complex wound healing issues that may be very challenging to address. Universally, the specialty of otolaryngology-head and neck surgery recognizes that these types of problems can be difficult to care for and that there is not a great amount of evidence specific to what constitutes "best practice" in these areas. In such circumstances, the CNS would serve as the healthcare provider who helps to educate both patients and staff, to develop protocols for such device use, and to transfer the resulting information to both patients, family members, and staff.

A further example related to the educational role the CNS may play pertains to the implementation of an alcohol withdrawal protocol. One Canadian center identified that for some patients this condition was resulting in negative postoperative outcomes that resulted in an increased length of hospitalization (LaSala et al., 2007, p. 265). The CNS liaised with pharmacy and anesthesia colleagues to develop a protocol that provided guiding orders specific to that institution. This protocol resulted in better outcomes as patients had fewer negative impacts from withdrawal. Consequently, the length of stay was as expected for these types of cases which resulted in fewer hospital days. Based on this single example, the CNS may often serve as a conduit for implementing best practice guidelines.

The CNS can play an instrumental role in reducing costs associated with the provision of acute healthcare services (Richards et al., 2018). In such a role, they can both educate and help to provide instructional expertise with the goal of instilling confidence in patients and families regarding their ongoing care. In an educator capacity, they provide the expertise to other team members regarding their care. For example, if a patient requires a tracheostomy at discharge, the education is facilitated and supported by the CNS's expertise. Lengths of hospital stays can also be reduced through CNS interventions to better prepare clients and their families for discharge and to strengthen client self-care abilities. They also assist in efforts which seek to problem solve complex care issues such as surgical site infections or difficulties that arise from poor wound healing. Readmission to hospital and emergency department visits can be avoided through ongoing assessment, early detection and management of patient problems, and care coordination (Pan-Canadian Core Competencies for the Clinical Nurse Specialist, 2014). When patients are prepared for their discharge, there are fewer risks of emergency room visits or readmissions due to lack of knowledge regarding their care requirements. For example, a patient who is independent in tracheostomy care will be better equipped to care for their airway at home and problem solve any issues that may arise. Therefore, the CNS is directly involved in the coordination of care to facilitate patient transitions to the next level of care (Lewandowski & Adamle, 2009, p. 78). As such, the CNS is involved with these complex oncology patients throughout the continuum of care.

Conclusions

This chapter has highlighted the important contribution the CNS provides to the care of patients with HNCa. The evolution of the CNS has been guided in part by a desire to facilitate greater continuity in health care, to improve system efficiencies related to health care in general, and finally to seek better patient outcomes. The advanced educational and technical knowledge acquired by the CNS adds increased levels of support to those treated for HNCa throughout the continuum of care. Thus, these specialized nurses are a key part of any comprehensive oncology treatment team. This advanced skill set has provided additional benefits to both patients and families during what is often a complex and difficult treatment regime. This includes not only direct nursing care but also a larger educational role that extends beyond the patient. Finally, advanced practice nursing by the CNS has as its ultimate goal the desire to optimize self-sufficiency, as well as to improve quality of life and well-being in those treated for HNCa.

References

Bryant-Lukosius, D., Spichiger, E., Martin, J., Stoll, H., Kellerhals, S. D., Fliedner, M., … De Geest, S. (2016). Framework for evaluating the impact of advanced practice nursing roles. *Journal of Nursing Scholarship, 48*(2), 201–209. https://doi.org/10.1111/jnu.12199

Bornbaum, C. C., Doyle, P. C., Skarakis-Doyle, E., & Theurer, J. A. (2013). A critical exploration of the International Classification of Functioning, Disability, and Health (ICF) framework from the perspective of oncology: Recommendations for revision. *Journal of Multidisciplinary Healthcare, 6,* 75.

Clarke, L. K. (1998). Rehabilitation for the head and neck cancer patient. *Oncology: Williston Park then Huntington, 12,* 81–90.

de Leeuw, J.A.M. (2013). Nurse-led follow-up care for head and neck cancer patients (Doctoral dissertation). Hertogenbosch, Netherlands: BOX Press.

Dempsey, L., Orr, S., Lane, S. & Scott, A. (2016). The clinical nurse specialist's role in head and neck cancer care: United Kingdom National Multidisciplinary Guidelines. *The Journal of Laryngology & Otology, 130(S2)*, S212-S215). https://doi.org/10.1017/S0022215116000657.

Doyle, P. C. (1994). *Foundations of voice and speech rehabilitation following laryngeal cancer*. San Diego, CA: Singular Publishing Group.

Doyle, P. C. (2005). Rehabilitation in head and neck cancer. In P. C. Doyle & R. L. Keith (Eds.), *Contemporary considerations in the treatment and rehabilitation of head and neck cancer: Voice, speech, and swallowing* (pp. 5–15). Austin, TX: Pro-Ed Publishers.

Dropkin, M. J., Malgady, R. G., Scott, D. W., Oberst, M. T., & Strong, E. W. (1983). Scaling of disfigurement and dysfunction in postoperative head and neck patients. *Head Neck, 6*(1), 559–570.

Folland, S. (2000). Palliative care. *Nursing Management, 6*(10), 5.

Gilbert, R., Devries-Aboud, M., Winquist, E., Waldron, J., & McQuestion, M. (2009). *A quality initiative of the program in evidence-based care (PEBC), Cancer Care Ontario (CCO), the Management of head and neck cancer in Ontario*. Toronto: Head and Neck Disease Site Group.

Gittell, J. H., Fairfield, K. M., Bierbaum, B., Head, W., Jackson, R., Kelly, M., … Zuckerman, J. (2000). Impact of relational coordination on quality of care, postoperative pain and functioning, and length of stay: A nine-hospital study of surgical patients. *Medical Care, 38*(8), 807–819.

Hughes, L. C., Hodgson, N. A., Muller, P., Robinson, L. A., & McCorkle, R. (2000). Information needs of elderly postsurgical cancer patients during the transition from hospital to home. *Journal of Nursing Scholarship, 32*(1), 25–30.

Jagannathan, A., & Juvva, S. (2016). Emotions and coping of patients with head and neck cancer after diagnosis: A qualitative content analysis. *Journal of Post-Graduate Medicine*, 62, 143–63, 149. https://doi.org/10.4103/0022-3859.184273

LaSala, C. A., Connors, P. M., Taylor Pedro, J., & Phipps, M. (2007). The role of the clinical nurse specialist in promoting evidenced-based practice and effecting positive patient outcomes. *The Journal of Continuing Education in Nursing, 38*(6), 262–270.

Lewandowski, W., & Adamle, K. (2009). Substantive areas of clinical nurse specialist practice. *Clinical Nurse Specialist, 23*(2), 73–90. https://doi.org/10.1097/NUR.0b013e31819971d0

List, M. A., Lee Rutherford, J., Stracks, J., Haraf, D., Kies, M. S., & Vokes, E. E. (2002). An exploration of the pretreatment coping strategies of patients with carcinoma of the head and neck. *Cancer, 95*(1), 98–104.

MacDonald-Renz, S., & Bard, R. (2010). The role for advanced practice nursing in Canada. *Nursing Leadership, 23*, 8–11. https://doi.org/10.12927/cjnl.2010.22265

Macmillan Cancer Support. (2014). Specialist adult cancer nursing in England. A census of the specialist adult cancer nursing workforce in the UK. London, UK. https://www.macmillan.org.uk/images/cns-census-report-england_tcm9-28367.

Maslow, A. H. (1943). A theory of human motivation. *Psychological Review, 50*(4), 370–396.

Maslow, A. H. (1954). *Motivation and personality*. New York, NY: Harper and Row.

Maslow, A. H. (1962). *Toward a psychology of being*. Princeton, NJ: D. Van Nostrand Company.

McDonald, A., & Sherlock, J. (2016). A long and winding road–improving communication with patients in the NHS, Marie Curie Report. Hämtad 2016-12-18, från: http://tinyurl.com/sbcoaao.

Nash, M.M., Scott, G.M., Fung, K., Yoo, J., & Doyle, P.C. (2014). An exploration of perceived body image in adults treated for head and neck cancer. Paper presented at the 5th World Congress of International Federation of Head and Neck Oncologic Society (IFNOS) Annual Meeting (AHNS), New York.

Nurse Practitioner/Advanced Practice Nurse: Definition and Characteristics (2009). Nursing Matters Fact Sheet. International Council of Nurses. Geneva, Switzerland. http://www.icn.ch/publications/fact-sheets/

Pan-Canadian Core Competencies for the Clinical Nurse Specialist (2014). Canadian Nurses Association. Ottawa. www.cna-aiic.ca

Peplau, H. E. (1952). Interpersonal relations in nursing. *AJN The American Journal of Nursing, 52*(6), 765.

Peplau, H. E. (1997). Peplau's theory of interpersonal relations. *Nursing Science Quarterly, 10*(4), 162–167.

Reich, M., Leemans, C. R., Vermorken, J. B., Bernier, J., Licitra, L., Parmar, S., … Lefebvre, J. L. (2014). Best practices in the management of the psycho-oncologic aspects of head and neck cancer patients: Recommendations from the European Head and Neck Cancer Society Make Sense Campaign. *Annals of Oncology, 25*(11), 2115–2124.

Richards, M., Devane, C., & Beasley, C. (2018). *Excellence in cancer care: The contribution of the clinical nurse specialist. National Cancer Action Team*. London, UK: Macmillan Cancer Support. https://www.macmillan.org.uk/documents/aboutus/commissioners/excellenceincancercarethecontributionoftheclinicalnursespecialist.pdf

Scarpa, R. (2004). Advanced practice nursing in head and neck cancer: Implementation of five roles. *Oncology Nursing Forum, 31*, 579–583.

Scott, R. A. (1999). A description of the roles, activities, and skills of clinical nurse specialists in the United States. *Clinical Nurse Specialist, 13*(4), 183–190.

Skilbeck, J., & Payne, S. (2003). Emotional support and the role of the clinical nurse specialists in palliative care. *Journal of Advanced Nursing, 43*(5), 521–530. https://doi.org/10.1046/j.1365-2648.2003.02749

Staples, E., Ray, S., & Hannon, R. (2016). *Canadian perspectives in advanced practice nursing*. Toronto, ON: Canadian Scholars Press.

Wagner, E. H., Austin, B. T., & Von Korff, M. (1996). Organizing care for patients with chronic illness. *The Milbank Quarterly, 74*, 511–544.

The Acquisition of Practice Knowledge in Head and Neck Cancer Rehabilitation

26

Philip C. Doyle

Introduction

All health-care professionals will likely agree that the provision of comprehensive clinical care demands a wide range of knowledge and skills, many of which are developed in the context of direct patient service. Increasingly, the demand for such knowledge is often specialized and in many instances, highly reliant on an enhanced level of technical skills. In speech-language pathology (SLP), those who provide clinical services to individuals treated for head and neck cancer (HNCa) will need a broad-based yet highly specialized knowledge base. More explicitly, knowledge is required across multiple functional areas including eating, swallowing, and speaking. For this reason, the shear extent of required knowledge and one's access to information on current practice standards will necessitate that one's breadth of proficiency is substantial.

If academic exposure to issues related to HNCa rehabilitation are to be adequately provided or if the development of advanced practice skills is desired, unique educational options will be required. This is particularly important given the limited time available within many existing academic curricula today. Therefore, expanded opportunities for students and clinicians to gather relevant knowledge must be fostered in a creative manner. However, the highest quality patient care also demands that the clinician exhibits the capacity to understand the intricacies and interrelationships of multiple areas of functioning. When these concerns are viewed together, efforts to expand the scope of academic exposure to this ever-increasing clinical population are encouraged.

Over the past 40 years, formal and dedicated classroom exposure specific to HNCa rehabilitation for those enrolled in speech and language pathology or communication sciences and disorders programs has diminished considerably. However, over the most recent 15 years, epidemiological data on the incidence of HNCas has indicated a substantial increase in this clinical population; it is also anticipated that this trend will continue to grow in the years to come. This is particularly true for those cancers that arise from structures of the oral cavity and oropharynx, an increase that has primarily been ascribed to the consequences of exposure to the human papilloma virus (HPV). In an earlier chapter, Theurer (Chap. 4) outlined the reasons behind this dramatic increase, the expectations for its continued expansion in the future, and the impact that emerges when such cancers occur.

P. C. Doyle (✉)
Voice Production and Perception Laboratory & Laboratory for Well-Being and Quality of Life, Department of Otolaryngology – Head and Neck Surgery and School of Communication Sciences and Disorders, Western University, Elborn College, London, ON, Canada
e-mail: pdoyle@uwo.ca

© Springer Nature Switzerland AG 2019
P. C. Doyle (ed.), *Clinical Care and Rehabilitation in Head and Neck Cancer*,
https://doi.org/10.1007/978-3-030-04702-3_26

This chapter provides an overview of the changes that have occurred in academic instruction related to HNCa rehabilitation. Initially, a discussion related to HNCa and professional scope of practice is provided. Next, information on the evolution of academic coursework and the reduction of clinical training hours specific to knowledge related to this special population is described. This is followed by a discussion on the continuing need to identify opportunities to facilitate learning specific to HNCa rehabilitation given the emerging increase in these types of cancer. Finally, the potential utility of several approaches for developing and providing educational opportunities while considering academic time restrictions will be briefly outlined. Beyond the obvious desire to facilitate continued self-directed learning, the value of other educational options including continuing education programs, problem-based instruction, competency-based training, clinical simulation, and self-reflection is presented.

Scope of Practice

Disorders secondary to the diagnosis and treatment of HNCa are clearly acknowledged to be appropriate for SLP relative to their documented scope of practice (American Speech-Language-Hearing Association, 2016). While increased awareness of HNCa rehabilitation as a "specialty" practice began to emerge more prominently in the early 1980s following introduction of surgical-prosthetic voice restoration (Singer & Blom, 1980), the specialty did exist before that time. Perusal of the literature related to post-cancer voice and speech disorders suggests that postlaryngectomy rehabilitation was well recognized and established beginning in the 1950s. This was also mirrored in work related to swallowing disorders that occurred as a result of cancer and its treatment, results of which were reported in some of the earliest work by Logemann and colleagues (Logemann & Bytell, 1979; McConnel, Mendelsohn, & Logemann, 1986, and others). In fact, clinical and research reports related to rehabilitation following treatment of laryngeal cancer, or malignancies that

affected structures of the oral cavity or pharynx, were readily noted in prominent journals.

Because there was early professional acknowledgment of specialty practice in speech pathology secondary to cancer treatment, instruction related to laryngectomy rehabilitation in particular comprised a long-standing and core component of the curricula of many university programs in the 1950s and 1960s (see Doyle, 1997). However, in the current era, academic exposure to such information is increasingly rare and often quite limited in many programs. With exception of several large educational programs where access to a large medical center is possible, formal academic offerings and instruction related to HNCa rehabilitation have certainly changed. This is not only a function of its omission in required coursework, but it extends to elective academic offerings as well. An informal polling of many of the largest SLP clinical training programs in North America suggests that more extensive, formal coursework in "communication disorders secondary to head and neck cancer" is uncommon.

The Evolution of Curricula in Communication Disorders

A historical perspective. Historically, five of the most widely utilized and referenced textbooks common to speech pathology curricula in the United States during the period between 1955 and 1980 were those explicitly directed toward clinical intervention related to HNCa (DiCarlo, Amster, & Herer, 1955; Diedrich & Youngstrom, 1966; Gardner, 1971; Skelly, 1973; Snidecor, 1968). The clinical populations represented in these textbooks formed a core component of many SLP curricula during that era. As the general discipline of communication sciences and disorders and the profession of speech (and language) pathology evolved, many new areas of clinical interest and expertise expanded as a consequence of the disabilities movement in the United States and the signing of the Rehabilitation Act of 1973,[1] later expanded as the Americans

---

[1] United States Access Board. https://www.access-board.gov/the-board/laws/rehabilitation-act-of-1973

with Disabilities Act (ADA) in 1990.[2] However, this also coincided with a shift in terminology that sought to partition some instructional and practice areas of the profession into binary disorder categories such as child vs. adult, developmental vs. acquired, speech vs. language, etc.

Relative to disorders in adults, the primary training sites for students have frequently been found in medical centers in large urban areas and through the Veterans Administration hospital system. Over the past 30 years, expansion in the types of disorders seen by SLPs often emerged relative to a medical model, whether those types of disorders occurred in children or adults. This shift led in part to the advent of academic/clinical curricula that was directed toward "medical speech pathology." This expansion in medically related communication problems grew to some extent with an increasing demand for "new" services for those individuals who were then identified as requiring initial and/or extended levels of clinical service.

In part, the passage of the ADA led to a process that necessitated reevaluation of the populations of interest to those in communication disorders (e.g., those with cerebral palsy) and, subsequently, how coursework was structured. It should also be acknowledged that during this time there was a concomitant increase in public awareness and subsequent advocacy for the disabled,[3] and a variety of funding considerations were often guided by this advocacy. Accordingly, university programs saw the need to reevaluate and modify the structure of academic coursework and related clinical training. Based on the simple determination of the potential demand for services given the possible inclusion of new clinical populations, coursework was adjusted accordingly. This often included the need to restrict exposure to coursework that addressed what might be identified as "smaller" populations. With this historical reference outlined, it is essential to note that in the most recent year of reporting (2015) by the Centers for Disease Control (CDC), they identified that 44,000 new cases of oral or oropharyngeal cancer and 12,000 new cases of laryngeal cancer were diagnosed in the United States.[4] Clearly, a population of more than 50,000 new individuals presenting with communication disorders secondary to cancer and its treatment each year is not insignificant.

In many respects, the changes observed in SLP programs are consistent with long-standing the evolution of medical education and training (Cooke, Irby, Sullivan, & Ludmerer, 2006). More complex or more frequently occurring health problems may understandably garner more direct instructional attention. However, within SLP training programs, individuals with HNCa also would seem to overlap many of the classification dichotomies identified previously (i.e., adult, acquired, speech). Further, the knowledge demands relating to the clinical care for those treated for HNCa also would seem to provide an ideal teaching model that links so many foundational areas underlying verbal communication (i.e., anatomy, physiology, speech acoustics, phonetics, proxemics, etc.). Yet there has been little effort directed toward the ongoing utilization and transfer of theory and knowledge-driven instruction, in combination with "learner-centered" education and training, in communication disorders or other professional areas (Frank et al., 2010; McWilliam, 2007). It is not unreasonable to suggest that many clinical "competencies" associated with communication disorders and intervention could be achieved with exposure to those treated for HNCa.

From the strict perspective of a "required clinical hours" justification for professional certification or licensing, one could argue that communication rehabilitation in those with HNCa may in fact cross multiple areas. Given the anticipated increases in the number of new cases of HNCa (CDC, 2019) and the very real potential that voice, speech, and/or swallowing deficits will occur as a result of treatment, there would appear to be an increasing need for formal educational coverage in this important and often underserved clinical population. At

---

[2]National Network: Information, Guidance, and Training on the Americans with Disabilities Act: https://adata.org/factsheet/ADA-overview

[3]This was the terminology used at that time.

[4]https://gis.cdc.gov/Cancer/USCS/DataViz.html

present, however, the opportunity for undergraduate or graduate students in SLP, or for that matter working clinicians, to acquire specialty skills in HNCa rehabilitation through accredited academic programs is diminishing. This does not discount the value of information obtained from professional conferences; but, accessing foundational knowledge and skills in this educational setting is often limited because programs are geared to provide continuing education units (CEUs) for professional clinicians who are mandated to acquire such hours. In this case, instruction assumes that foundational knowledge has been learned.

The current era With exception of academic coursework that addresses swallowing and swallowing disorders (dysphagia), in many instances today, formal education related to HNCa rehabilitation is either nonexistent or is contained in partial form within some other curricular content areas (e.g., as a component of a voice course). Typically, this may involve a single lecture related to laryngectomy and/or oral or oropharyngeal cancers. In these circumstances, the information provided may succinctly address basic terminology, the anatomic and physiologic consequences of treatment, and/or primary concepts underlying total laryngectomy (e.g., the change in one's airway and loss of normal voice) or the functional consequences of oral and oropharyngeal resections (e.g., glossectomy). Such information is important, but it is often incomplete.

Interestingly, one might argue that the range of speech deficits that may emerge as a result of treatment for tumors of the oral cavity, tongue, palate, mandible, etc. might be well served within coursework curricula that addresses motor speech disorders, namely, content specific to the dysarthrias. When this is considered relative to both undergraduate and graduate curricula, concerns specific to the comprehensiveness of one's education prior to practice may be raised. Although ideal, it is understood that it is very unlikely that any student will have a full range of educational exposure, either via the formal academic classroom or through clinical

practica, to all areas of communication disorders. For that reason, superficial instruction may be the best and only solution available in curricula today. Nevertheless, it is increasingly apparent that for many institutions, direct academic content related to HNCa is not addressed. In fact, more frequently, it is reported to come from special, external clinical placements – the proverbial "on-the-job training" – in those fortunate circumstances where a high-quality, high volume clinical placement can be accessed. However, these types of clinical placements are also quite limited which creates further challenges to the educational process relating to HNCa rehabilitation.

Clinical practica The benefits of direct exposure to patient care provide the richest of learning environments (Martin, Stark, & Jolly, 2000). As noted, the above-cited coursework-based challenges for students may be further compounded due to limitations in practicum opportunities. The inability of many academic training programs to access high-quality clinical placements that can provide exposure to those treated for HNCa is problematic. While no explicit data exist, it is not unreasonable to assume that the greatest likelihood for a student to access one of these types of clinical training environments will frequently be improved if the university is located in a large metropolitan center.

Within smaller population centers, if a student clinician desires to work with the head and neck population, not only might their access to coursework be limited, but their opportunities for training through direct patient exposure also may be restricted due to travel, potential costs, or other factors. Thus, both educational and practicum training gaps related to HNCa rehabilitation may be common. It has been suggested that practica may be influenced by external influences. More specifically, some have suggested that advancements in learning may be impeded due to the mismatch between "high standards but sometimes prescriptive expectations" (McAllister, 2005) that are dictated by professional associations or other certification/registration bodies.

Educational Training in SLP and Specialization

Learning foundational knowledge and the skills necessary to provide a high-quality clinical service to those with HNCa is multidimensional, and it represents a developmental process (Leach, 2002). In addition to the more discrete areas of fundamental academic knowledge that impact services to those with HNCa (e.g., anatomy, physiology, speech acoustics, etc.), areas that are common to all accredited university educational programs, there is also a frequent need for the development of unique and specialized technical expertise (e.g., endoscopic evaluation), as well as instruction on specific therapeutic approaches (e.g., teaching esophageal speech, fitting a tracheoesophageal puncture voice prosthesis, etc.). Despite the fact that education related to HNCa rehabilitation, most notably related to laryngectomee rehabilitation, historically formed a clinical mainstay of instruction, the breadth of a student's academic education specific to this practice area today has changed markedly. In fact, in many academic programs, exposure to this disorder area is at best often significantly limited. This does not, however, reduce the learner's responsibility to uncover knowledge on their own (Benner, 1983).

Traditional and Nontraditional Approaches to Instruction

It is widely agreed that the acquisition of clinical practice knowledge and the requisite skills required for competent clinical practice are ideally developed from both formal, traditional sources of instruction and information and through direct experience. Thus, aspects of education and training are idealized to be seamless in their evolution. Regardless of the area of clinical practice, gaining knowledge to enhance clinical proficiency or competency represents a multidimensional process. But it is becoming more apparent that nontraditional methods of instruction may also need to be developed and exploited. This is particularly true within health-care settings where patient care is a priority and where necessary knowledge may grow at an exceptional pace. It is, however, also understood that clinical knowledge is not static; hence, the dynamic and continuing nature of obtaining such knowledge and opportunities for its application is critical. This provides potential opportunities for new, creative, and nontraditional methods of instruction to be developed and instituted, yet, unfortunately, resistance to this type of change from the traditional (the presently existing) model is often observed (Sheepway, Lincoln, & Togher, 2011).

Over the past three decades, speech (and language) pathology has become a discipline/profession that has increasingly been characterized by specialization in many subareas of practice. This would include areas such as developmental speech and language disorders, acquired disorders of speech (dysarthrias) and language (aphasia), fluency, voice disorders, etc. Instruction in SLP is increasingly observed to be influenced by population-based changes and associated needs. For example, increasing instruction has emerged over the past several decades in those areas that impact older adults; this includes expanded inclusion in curricula that addresses the dementias, general age-related cognitive decline, and some progressive, neurologically based disorders. Similarly, these types of changes have also emerged in association with childhood disorders, perhaps most notably those in the area of autism and autism spectrum disorders, attention deficit disorders, etc. In fact, this level of specialized professional compartmentalization has also been encouraged through the development of Special Interest Groups by the American Speech-Language-Hearing Association (ASHA, 2016).[5] However, beyond the relatively uniform educational exposure of current students to normal processes and basic sciences underlying voice, speech, language, hearing, and swallowing,[6] the variety of "disorder" coursework that is either

---

[5]At present, ASHA is represented by 19 Special Interest Groups (SIGS).

[6]Accreditation by certification and/or licensing bodies does dictate that a minimum number of course hours specific to normal process is undertaken.

required or potentially selected as an elective for smaller clinical populations may be quite inconsistent.

Because clinicians working in the area of HNCa frequently do not have significant exposure to this demanding clinical area coming out of their academic training programs, the question that naturally arises pertains to "how" knowledge and skills can be acquired and developed. The process of knowledge acquisition specific to the clinical care of those with HNCa also exists in the circumstances of what is a rapidly evolving and demanding clinical environment. Of direct importance to this topic are the educational challenges that new clinicians confront and how they might meet these needs.

Meeting Educational Needs

With very few exceptions, the new HNCa clinician will be charged with considerable personal responsibility to grow their skill set. Although some new clinicians will experience the good fortune to work on established teams in major, comprehensive cancer centers, most students or SLPs who will work in HNCa rehabilitation may need to gather information as independent learners. It is without question that ethical, well-reasoned, and thoughtful clinical practice will be guided by ongoing efforts to extend one's knowledge and directly transfer that information to practice. This also requires that clinicians volitionally pursue the process of self-evaluation and self-reflection as skill sets evolve over time. Consequently, understanding the active process of acquiring comprehensive knowledge forms the foundation and one's ability to develop exceptional clinical skills.

Meeting Educational Needs Specific to HNCa Rehabilitation

Based on information provided in the preceding chapters of this text, comprehensive clinical care of those who are treated for HNCa is contingent upon a wide range of knowledge and skills.

Despite the recognition that formal didactic classroom instruction by one who is highly trained remains an ideal means of "first exposure" to this important practice area, it is also increasingly rare to see students exposed to HNCa clinical opportunities in many university-based educational training environments. Rather, it is increasingly common that new clinicians may gain their knowledge via direct "hands-on" exposure to the population. This can be an excellent and very productive learning experience, but acquiring clinical knowledge without prior foundational knowledge may be limiting in some instances.

In the current context, this type of exposure is ideally suited to clinical placements, and experiences are most often fostered within a hospital-based setting. However, it is equally clear that the level, range, and, unfortunately, the quality of such experiences can vary from center to center. This is also confounded by the fact that many of these patients may have complex, coexisting medical histories and comorbidities which will demand even greater foundational knowledge (McAllister, 2005). Along with that, those with more complex health concerns may also carry additional practice risks that may then limit the learning opportunity for an unexperienced clinician. In fact, some supervisors are reticent to allow students to perform some tasks in the HNCa clinical setting, opting instead for observational learning. Unless there is exceptional supervisor in these circumstances, the novice or less inexperienced clinician may be unable to integrate multiple bits of information, with a reduced level of practical learning. Though explorations related to clinical medicine have been reported (Teunissen et al., 2007), additional work to determine commonalities in approaches to clinical learning in speech-language pathology would be of value.

More explicitly, practice standards, approaches, protocols, and yes, personal or institutional biases differ across clinical settings. For example, clinical training in a small center with limited general resources and less extensive access to the widest range of technology and necessary products will provide an additional educational limitation. Smaller centers will almost certainly pale in comparison to that which takes place in major centers or those institutions that have comprehensive cancer care center status. Regardless of the type of setting, acquiring practice knowledge involves the clinician's capacity to actively access and verify not only formal sources of information from the literature but to place that information within a dynamic clinical process that extends from inpatient to outpatient service. The adage that "learning never ceases" is an underlying premise that frequently characterizes not only those who are excellent students, but those who go on to be identified as "master" clinicians.

Exploring Educational Options

As previously outlined, in many instances formal academic training programs for students in speech-language pathology may only provide cursory exposure to issues specific to HNCa as a clinical practice area. Thus, additional responsibility is expected of the learner involved in such practica in order to become more informed during clinical sessions. Practical opportunities also may be limited which further exacerbates the problem of students obtaining at least a minimum level of exposure to this patient population. These limitations may lead to the suggestion that academic training programs that do not have sufficient classroom instruction related to HNCa rehabilitation should consider developing other types of educational options to address the needs of this special clinical population. Regardless of method, there is likely to be wide agreement that promoting critical thinking and self-assessment is essential to the learning process (Maudsley & Strivens, 2000).

Fortunately, a range of potential options may be viable alternatives to more formal classroom, curricular-based instruction. As stated by Leach (2002, p. 243), the most successful method of providing clinical information to the learner will be based on "…a model of knowledge and skill acquisition that is simple, elegant and relevant." It is also important to acknowledge that establish-

ing such opportunities requires time and resources in order to increase the likelihood of both the success and relevance of instruction. Although all may come at some financial cost to institutions, it is not unreasonable to assume that many could be structured as a cost-neutral endeavor through direct cost recovery.

This also requires that the level of skill and competencies of those who will provide the instruction are of the highest quality and that such preceptors are current in their knowledge. Given the all-too-common and continuing complaints of shrinking budgets to cover the material or personnel costs associated with such endeavors, the challenges become even more substantial (Rodger et al., 2008). The greatest and certainly most significant challenge in this area would appear to be related to insuring that: (1) the information presented in any format is timely and accurate and (2) that the information provided is continuously updated so that it is consistent with standards of practice. For these reasons, the most promising nontraditional options for improved instruction related to HNCa rehabilitation are presented in the subsequent sections.

Continuing education opportunities Based on the previously noted concerns, the most obvious consideration for learning an array of topics specific to HNCa rehabilitation would be that of continuing education (CE) programs. As a method of learning, CE is a standard requirement of all health-care professions. While CE as an education opportunity emerged as a standard specific to medicine (i.e., continuing medical education or CME), it is now generalized to all health professions. The primary objective of CE/CME is viewed as a way to acquire new knowledge in a situation where information is rapidly changing, and consequently, there is a critical need for continuous and easily accessed opportunities for updating one's knowledge. CME in medicine refers to "any and all the ways by which doctors learn after formal completion of their training" (Davis, 1998). Despite questions regarding whether CE provides the desired learning outcome (Cantillon & Jones, 1999), this model has transferred to and is uniformly applied to other professions today.

CE has proven to be an excellent method of educating professionals. However, by strict definition CE carries one major limitation relative to the present concern of students or inexperienced clinicians not having acquired information on HNCa rehabilitation as part of their classroom training. That is, the underlying assumption for CE/CME initiatives is that the learner already has a sound preparatory level of foundational knowledge; CE is structured to facilitate advanced learning. In this regard, CE activities may involve aspects of both "education" (acquiring new information) and "training" (the integration and application of that knowledge). It is clear that CE activities offer valuable information which is usually presented in an approachable and efficient fashion, but CE programs may also have inherent limitations for less experienced learners. For example, CE-type endeavors that do not have a true practice or "hands-on" component may be of limited value specific to developing the types of skills and competencies that are required in HNCa rehabilitation. This limitation may support the notion that problem-based approaches to learning may better meet the needs of those who have no, or very limited, foundational knowledge in HNCa rehabilitation.

Problem-based learning The next education approach is that related to what has been identified as "problem-based learning" (PBL). Though PBL tasks hold substantial potential for facilitating learning that is driven by specific concerns, needs, or interests, and as a pedagogical approach is certainly applicable to the clinical process, it does have limitations (Norman & Schmidt, 2000). PBL does find great merit in that it can be undertaken on an individual basis or it can be done with others. The opportunity to interact with others in such problem-solving tasks may provide the added dividend of fostering professional collaboration and interaction (Morison, Boohan, Jenkins, & Moutray, 2003). However, one criticism of PBL is that at times it may become a learning approach that may be narrow in its point of view. This may be appropriate with problems that are narrow in scope, but this

becomes more challenging when one deals with more complex problems. Thus, care must be taken with the PBL model to ensure that the breadth of options and solutions to solve a given problem are as comprehensive as possible when different solutions may exist for the same problem.

For example, opportunities to work through clinical problems, whether they be relatively simple or more commonly, those that are complex and unpredictable, may create difficulty in the comprehensive evaluation of one's decision-making process (McAllister, Lincoln, Ferguson, & McAllister, 2010). Not surprisingly, the assessment of learner outcomes in these educational scenarios subsequently may be difficult to document. It is suspicioned that the limitations for PBL are more directly related to the inherent lack of integration and the potential "moving parts" that may be unique to any clinical problem posed. As with most non-didactic methods of instruction that involve clinical reasoning and problem solving, finding qualified teachers/preceptors may be difficult, not to mention the general logistics specific to the PBL process (Lenchus, 2010). This challenge may also have a direct impact on the comprehensiveness of the learner's assessment and related feedback.

Competency-based learning Competency-based learning (CBL) is a learning process common to training in medicine. However, the terminology of "competency-based medical education" (CBME) has been extended over the years, and it has increasingly become an instructional option. In fact, some residency programs are now looking to adopt this strategy for training of physicians in particular specialties and subspecialties. The CBL type of model allows for direct observation by the instructor, with the learner performing a given task or procedure. Not surprisingly, this type of training for those in medicine is somewhat of a natural but more formalized progression of the "see one, do one, teach one" instructional approach (Spencer, 2003). In situations of this type, great care is required relative to instructor oversight. In such situations, the instructor has increasing responsibility in evaluating whether competency is sufficient in order to independently and successfully perform what has been termed an "entrustable professional activity" (ten Cate, 2005).

One of the great advantages of the more contemporary CBL/CBME model is that it demands that the instructor and the student are jointly involved in the instructional and learning process. As stated by Holmboe and colleagues, "faculty work side by side with trainees on a daily basis and are therefore in an excellent position to provide real-time evaluation and feedback" (Holmboe et al., 2010). This type of training model is, however, demanding and dependent upon the procedure or task at hand. Because of the variation in the gradient of skill acquisition for any given task, this may place considerable stress on the learner and provide challenges for measuring change (Hawk & Shah, 2007). Yet it must also be noted that when the CBL model is considered fully, it is equally clear that it will place substantial demands (skill and time) on the instructor to insure learner competency. As a result, the instructor's level of responsibility increases significantly. As described by ten Cate (2013), the instructor's capacity to carefully balance the demands associated with "…an elaborate framework of competencies, subcompetencies, and milestones" can be overwhelming.

Clinical simulation   Another educational area that has been increasingly noted as an important adjunct to the acquisition of clinical skills is that of simulation. This type of instruction has most often been associated with the learning of more procedurally oriented clinical tasks (Weller, 2004). This approach to teaching and learning has been widely used in many areas of specialty training in medicine including otolaryngology. However, the ultimate "driver" underlying simulation-based education is typically the desire to replace traditional didactic instruction with a highly structured, "close to real" type of teaching.

While this approach to education has been shown to be valuable through both low- and high-fidelity methods of instruction, it still requires time within the learner's curriculum, as well as requiring an instructor's consistent demonstration and direct guidance, careful monitoring, and systematic measurement of the learner's skill, and feedback (Rodriguez-Paz et al., 2009). Similarly, although simulation-based approaches to learning may hold substantial promise, it is recognized that simulation also carries real and substantial limitations based on a systematic review of the literature (McGaghie, Issenberg, Petrusa, & Scalese, 2006).

While some ethical considerations may exist with simulated activities (as well as other nontraditional methods of instruction), those concerns relate to the need for rigorous scrutiny by instructors (Frank et al., 2010). Similarly, others have noted the important, coexisting need to provide confirmation that competency can be confirmed via simulation tasks. As noted by Rodriguez-Paz et al. (2009), with careful planning and design, a new paradigm of simulation-oriented, as well as other types of learning, can be achieved when attitudinal and behavioral expectations of the learner are also included in the required learning expectations.

The careful point of balance in such arguments centers around a need to provide exposure to learners while at the same time avoiding any unnecessary clinical risk to the patient in the first exposure situations of actual practice (Ziv, Wolpe, Small, & Glick, 2006). According to Ziv et al., simulation serves to mitigate such risk. Regardless of the fidelity of simulation, it is clearly recognized that in most instances, simulation will remain an incomplete training paradigm for many aspects of clinical rehabilitation of those treated for HNCa. Ideally, if simulation can be systematically moved forward to the training of actual procedures, the ability to evaluate competency and the accurate and direct transfer of knowledge becomes more feasible.

Learning from reflection   Reflective practice refers to the notion that one actively seeks to reflect on the process of their clinical practice (Schoen, 1983). As a strategic approach to learning, reflective practice may best define the process of knowledge acquisition that is most pertinent to active clinical practice. This does not, however, suggest that such an approach is unique to clinical practice in head and neck care, but that situational events will dictate learning in this manner. It is of equal importance to highlight that situational learning is advanced considerably in the context of a process referred to as reflection (Sandars, 2009).

Work conducted by Caty and her colleagues has demonstrated that reflective processes serve to foster improved knowledge and that such practice directly influences enhanced levels of clinical problem solving (Caty, Kinsella, & Doyle, 2009, 2015, 2016a, 2016b). Through the process of reflection, Caty et al. (2015) have demonstrated that one's approach to practice is altered and that such learning provides for better future care when similar clinical issues emerge. Further, reflection on clinical practice is a complex and multi-tiered process that grows with each new clinical contact (Caty et al., 2016a, 2016b). In this regard, the reflective process provides an ongoing opportunity to reevaluate and recontextualize the clinical process, with one's knowledge being expanded with every new clinical experience.

Therefore, one of the most important aspects of reflection centers on the notion of a willingness to look back on a given clinical experience with the learner's desire being to improve subsequent experiences (Smith & Irby, 1997). While the work of Caty and colleagues has direct relevance to HNCa rehabilitation and the associated clinical process, other factors may also be considered and integrated in the knowledge acquisition process (Leinhardt, Young, & Merriman, 1995). This is particularly true when a clinician's decision was done with hindsight of unknown but potentially serious risks to the patient. The essential issue of importance to the present discussion centers on the learner's/clinician's ability to not only look back in evaluating any given clinical process or interaction, but to allow that information to inform "real-time" decision-making during one's clinical practice. It also should permit informed anticipation for clinical decisions in the future. The process of reflection is likely the most

instructive process associated with learning, a process that can be further enhanced with direct external feedback, and the associated acknowledgment of responsibility and personal accountability (Caty et al., 2016a, 2016b).

Conclusions

Despite the anticipated increase of HNCa in the future and the communication disorders that are likely to emerge as a consequence of treatment, there appears to be very little formal exposure to educating and training students in HNCa rehabilitation. The exclusion of instruction in HNCa rehabilitation is likely not done for punitive reasons, but rather in the context of ever-expanding curricular areas of demand while at the same time seeking to address persistent limitations in the time available for such instruction. This chapter has presented information on the potential utility of nontraditional methods of exposure to the clinical area of HNCa. In doing so, an overview of several approaches to learning have been outlined. This includes continuing education activities, problem-based learning, competency-based learning, clinical simulation, and reflective practice. Although no single option provides the ideal educational approach, nor are the present options exhaustive, components of all methods may provide a viable and valuable strategy that seeks to expand the knowledge base and clinical skill of those who will work in the area of HNCa rehabilitation.

References

American Speech-Language-Hearing Association [ASHA]. (2016). *Scope of practice in speech-language pathology*. Rockville Pike, MD.

Benner, P. (1983). Uncovering the knowledge embedded in clinical practice. *Journal of Nursing Scholarship, 15*(2), 36–41.

Cantillon, P., & Jones, R. (1999). Does continuing medical education in general practice make a difference? *BMJ: British Medical Journal, 318*(7193), 1276.

Caty, M. È., Kinsella, E. A., & Doyle, P. C. (2009). Linking the art of practice in head and neck cancer rehabilitation with the scientists' art of research: A case study on reflective practice. *Canadian Journal of Speech-Language Pathology & Audiology, 33*(4), 183–188.

Caty, M. È., Kinsella, E. A., & Doyle, P. C. (2015). Reflective practice in speech-language pathology: A scoping review. *International Journal of Speech-Language Pathology, 17*(4), 411–420.

Caty, M. È., Kinsella, E. A., & Doyle, P. C. (2016a). Reflective practice in speech-language pathology: Relevance for practice and education. *Canadian Journal of Speech-Language Pathology & Audiology, 40*(1).

Caty, M. È., Kinsella, E. A., & Doyle, P. C. (2016b). Reflective processes of practitioners in head and neck cancer rehabilitation: A grounded theory study. *International Journal of Speech-Language Pathology, 18*(6), 580–591.

Centers for Disease Control and Prevention. (2019, January 14). Retrieved from https://www.cdc.gov/cancer/headneck/index.htm

Cooke, M., Irby, D. M., Sullivan, W., & Ludmerer, K. M. (2006). American medical education 100 years after the Flexner report. *New England Journal of Medicine, 355*(13), 1339–1344.

Davis, D. A. (1998). Global health, global learning. *BMJ, 316*, 385–389.

DiCarlo, L. M., Amster, W., & Herer, G. (1955). *Speech after laryngectomy.* Syracuse, NY: Syracuse University Press.

Diedrich, W. M., & Youngstrom, K. A. (1966). *Alaryngeal speech.* Springfield, IL: Charles C. Thomas.

Doyle, P. C. (1997). Foreword. In M. S. Graham (Ed.), *The clinician's guide to alaryngeal speech therapy.* Oxford, UK: Butterworth-Heinemann.

Frank, J. R., Snell, L. S., Cate, O. T., Holmboe, E. S., Carraccio, C., Swing, S. R., … Harden, R. M. (2010). Competency-based medical education: Theory to practice. *Medical Teacher, 32*(8), 638–645.

Gardner, W. H. (1971). *Laryngectomee speech and rehabilitation.* Springfield, IL: Charles C. Thomas.

Hawk, T. F., & Shah, A. J. (2007). Using learning style instruments to enhance student learning. *Decision Sciences Journal of Innovative Education, 5*(1), 1–19.

Holmboe, E. S., Sherbino, J., Long, D. M., Swing, S. R., Frank, J. R., & International CBME Collaborators. (2010). The role of assessment in competency-based medical education. *Medical Teacher, 32*(8), 676–682.

Leach, D. C. (2002). Competence is a habit. *JAMA, 287*(2), 243–244.

Leinhardt, G., Young, K. M., & Merriman, J. (1995). Integrating professional knowledge: The theory of practice and the practice of theory. *Learning and Instruction, 5*(4), 401–408.

Lenchus, J. D. (2010). End of the "see one, do one, teach one" era: The next generation of invasive bedside procedural instruction. *The Journal of the American Osteopathic Association, 110*(6), 340–346.

Logemann, J. A., & Bytell, D. E. (1979). Swallowing disorders in three types of head and neck surgical patients. *Cancer, 44*(3), 1095–1105.

Martin, I. G., Stark, P., & Jolly, B. (2000). Benefiting from clinical experience: The influence of learning style and clinical experience on performance in an undergraduate objective structured clinical examination. *Medical Education, 34*(7), 530–534.

Maudsley, G., & Strivens, J. (2000). Promoting professional knowledge, experiential learning and critical thinking for medical students. *Medical Education, 34*(7), 535–544.

McAllister, L. (2005). Issues and innovations in clinical education. *Advances in Speech Language Pathology, 7*(3), 138–148.

McAllister, S., Lincoln, M., Ferguson, A., & McAllister, L. (2010). Issues in developing valid assessments of speech pathology students' performance in the workplace. *International Journal of Language & Communication Disorders, 45*(1), 1–14.

McConnel, F., Mendelsohn, M. S., & Logemann, J. A. (1986). Examination of swallowing after total laryngectomy using manofluorography. *Head & Neck, 9*(1), 3–12.

McGaghie, W. C., Issenberg, S. B., Petrusa, E. R., & Scalese, R. J. (2006). Effect of practice on standardised learning outcomes in simulation-based medical education. *Medical Education, 40*(8), 792–797.

McWilliam, C. L. (2007). Continuing education at the cutting edge: Promoting transformative knowledge translation. *Journal of Continuing Education in the Health Professions, 27*(2), 72–79.

Morison, S., Boohan, M., Jenkins, J., & Moutray, M. (2003). Facilitating undergraduate interprofessional learning in healthcare: Comparing classroom and clinical learning for nursing and medical students. *Learning in Health and Social Care, 2*(2), 92–104.

Norman, G. R., & Schmidt, H. G. (2000). Effectiveness of problem-based learning curricula: Theory, practice and paper darts. *Medical Education, 34*(9), 721–728.

Rodger, S., Webb, G., Devitt, L., Gilbert, J., Wrightson, P., & McMeeken, J. (2008). Clinical education and practice placements in the allied health professions: An international perspective. *Journal of Allied Health, 37*(1), 53–62.

Rodriguez-Paz, J., Kennedy, M., Salas, E., Wu, A. W., Sexton, J. B., Hunt, E. A., & Pronovost, P. J. (2009). Beyond "see one, do one, teach one": Toward a different training paradigm. *BMJ Quality & Safety, 18*(1), 63–68.

Sandars, J. (2009). The use of reflection in medical education: AMEE Guide No. 44. *Medical Teacher, 31*(8), 685–695.

Schoen, D. A. (1983). *The reflective practitioner: How professionals think in action.* New York, NY: Basic Books.

Sheepway, L., Lincoln, M., & Togher, L. (2011). An international study of clinical education practices in speech-language pathology. *International Journal of Speech-Language Pathology, 13*(2), 174–185.

Singer, M. I., & Blom, E. D. (1980). An endoscopic technique for restoration of voice after laryngectomy. *Annals of Otology, Rhinology, and Laryngology, 89,* 529–533.

Skelly, M. (1973). *Glossectomee speech rehabilitation.* Springfield, IL: Charles C. Thomas.

Smith, C. S., & Irby, D. M. (1997). The roles of experience and reflection in ambulatory care education. *Academic Medicine, 72*(1), 32–35.

Snidecor, J. C. (Ed.). (1968). *Speech Rehabilitation of the laryngectomized.* Springfield, IL: Charles C. Thomas.

Spencer, J. (2003). ABC of learning and teaching in medicine: Learning and teaching in the clinical environment. *BMJ: British Medical Journal, 326*(7389), 591.

ten Cate, O. (2005). Entrustability of professional activities and competency-based training. *Medical Education, 39*(12), 1176–1177.

ten Cate, O. (2013). Competency-based education, entrustable professional activities, and the power of language. *Journal of Graduate Medical Education, 5*(1), 6–7.

Teunissen, P. W., Scheele, F., Scherpbier, A. J. J. A., Van Der Vleuten, C. P. M., Boor, K., Van Luijk, S. J., & Diemen-Steenvoorde, V. (2007). How residents learn: Qualitative evidence for the pivotal role of clinical activities. *Medical Education, 41*(8), 763–770.

Weller, J. M. (2004). Simulation in undergraduate medical education: Bridging the gap between theory and practice. *Medical Education, 38*(1), 32–38.

Ziv, A., Wolpe, P. R., Small, S. D., & Glick, S. (2006). Simulation-based medical education: An ethical imperative. *Simulation in Healthcare, 1*(4), 252–256.

Well-Being and Quality of Life in Head and Neck Cancer

27

Philip C. Doyle and Chelsea MacDonald

...Not every illness can be overcome. But, there is always a margin
within which life can be lived with meaning and even with a certain
measure of joy, despite illness. (Cousins, 1979, p. 149)

Introduction

Head and neck cancer (HNCa) may serve to challenge an individual's ability to live a life filled with full meaning and joy. Moreover, the experience of HNCa has the potential to challenge one's capacity to participate fully and find continued purpose as life proceeds forward (Lee, Ready, Davis, & Doyle, 2017). HNCa is a disease that, along with the myriad consequences of its treatment, carries a significant and long-term potential for reductions in an individual's quality of life (QoL) and

well-being (WB). It is, therefore, reasonable to identify QoL as being characterized by a sense that life is worth living and that living has meaning (Doyle, 1994). Reductions in QoL or WB often denote that a significant gap exists between an individual's ideal functional status and their current level of functioning (Semple, Sullivan, Dunwoody, & Kernohan, 2004). For individuals who have received a diagnosis of HNCa, this gap may be particularly expansive due to the profound biopsychosocial challenges that influence the most basic and vital elements of life.

As such, this chapter seeks to delineate the constructs of QoL and WB in the context of HNCa. For the purposes of the chapter to follow, QoL and WB will be used interchangeably. In the sections to follow, we have sought to define issues in a more generic fashion, rather than to provide intricate details by cancer subsite within the head and neck region or relative to the modality of treatment undertaken. In light of the highly individualized, multidimensional, and dynamic nature of QoL and WB, definitional caveats will also be considered and contextualized. Subsequently, a review of current QoL methodology and associated challenges will be presented. Finally, generic consideration of the impact of disease and treatment on an individual's QoL must always be recognized and addressed if the best possible outcomes are to be facilitated. Thus, clinical

P. C. Doyle (✉)
Voice Production and Perception Laboratory & Laboratory for Well-Being and Quality of Life, Department of Otolaryngology – Head and Neck Surgery and School of Communication Sciences and Disorders, Western University, Elborn College, London, ON, Canada
e-mail: pdoyle@uwo.ca

C. MacDonald
Laboratory for Well-Being and Quality of Life in Oncology, Health and Rehabilitation Sciences, Western University, London, ON, Canada

© Springer Nature Switzerland AG 2019
P. C. Doyle (ed.), *Clinical Care and Rehabilitation in Head and Neck Cancer*,
https://doi.org/10.1007/978-3-030-04702-3_27

applications of QoL will be outlined in the context of the disablement and rehabilitation concomitant with HNCa.

Initial Considerations in Head and Neck Cancer

Owing to the complexity of the anatomical location where HNCa occurs, treatment for the disease has the potential to result in substantial physical, psychological, and social consequences that are highly interrelated (Newell, Sanson-Fisher, Girgis, & Ackland, 1999). More specifically, the treatment for HNCa may result in physical morbidity that can include the experience of pain, xerostomia, and physical disfigurement, as well as deficits in the individual's ability to breathe, swallow, and eat (Hansson, Carlstrom, Olsson, Nyman, & Koinberg, 2017; Howren, Christensen, Karnell, & Funk, 2012; Kearney & Cavanagh, Chap. 20; Reeve et al., 2016; Richardson, Morton, & Broadbent, 2016; Smith, Chap. 22). The extensive array of physical sequelae of HNCa treatment is paralleled by substantial psychological dysfunction such as distress, depression, anxiety, negative body image, and reduced self-esteem (Bornbaum & Doyle, Chap. 5; Bornbaum et al., 2012; Cohen et al., 2015; Dropkin, 1981; Howren, Christensen, Karnell, & Funk, 2010; Nash, Scott, Fung, Yoo, & Doyle, 2014). Correspondingly, the physical and psychological impairments associated with HNCa, both during and following treatment, also exert an interdependent influence on the individual's social functioning. This will often be evidenced by the potential for disrupted social interaction and participation and the experience of stigma (Reeve et al., 2016; Vartanian, Rogers, & Kowalski, 2017). Thus, the real impact of HNCa is truly interdependent and multidimensional.

In the context of HNCa, an additional factor is of critical importance in the consideration of functioning and QoL posttreatment. Namely, the diagnosis of HNCa may often hold the very real potential for verbal communication (voice and speech) to be disrupted at least in some manner.

Given that verbal communication is likely the primary vehicle from which one can directly address concerns, worries, and fears, a substantial agent of optimizing QOL may be significantly challenged (Doyle, 2005; Evitts, Chap. 28; Ma & Yiu, 2001). It also holds the potential to limit effective communication between the person with the disease and those who are most important to them. Coping and psychological adjustment to cancer as an illness almost certainly find their foundation in having the capacity to communicate one's concerns and expectations for what lies ahead. In light of the potential for posttreatment biopsychosocial morbidity and the profound influence of cancer on functioning, it is, therefore, critical to consider QoL within the context of HNCa (Gritz et al., 1999).

It is also important to remember that the impact of HNCa and its treatment is not directly proportional to the sum of the biopsychosocial consequences. More accurately, the consequences exert a reciprocal influence between each of the domains of functioning producing somewhat of a multiplicative effect. In essence, physical or psychological consequences commonly render an individual unable to undertake activities within the social realm of functioning; however, the impact of such changes can exert reciprocal negative influences on both physical and psychological functioning. For example, the presence of physical symptoms or changes in body image may in turn foster isolation from others, with this type of social restriction creating additional anxiety and distress. Thus, the interdependent nature of the consequences of HNCa and its treatment becomes increasingly evident. It is, therefore, reasonable to suggest that the influence of HNCa and its treatment on an individual's QoL may be devastating (Doyle, 2005) and, perhaps most important, a challenge that will, to some extent, persist throughout an individual's life.

Regardless of anatomic site, all individuals who are diagnosed with a malignancy will face a unique set of challenges. However, it is widely recognized that when compared to individuals diagnosed with a malignant neoplasm outside the head and neck region, those who receive treatment for HNCa experience the most substantial posttreatment morbidity (Mochizuki, Matsushima, & Omura, 2008; Ninu et al., 2015). Concomitantly, individuals with HNCa also face more extensive detriments to all domains of functioning that influence QoL (Gritz et al., 1999). This is not to say that cancers originating outside the head and neck region are without significant concerns but, rather, that HNCa carries a unique set of challenges. The changes that occur secondary to HNCa may significantly disrupt the most rudimentary human functions that are vital to daily living and, thus, represent an unparalleled impact on one's QoL and WB. Accordingly, HNCa is commonly considered to be the most emotionally traumatic cancer diagnosis (Bornbaum et al., 2012; Doyle, 2005; Eadie, 2007; Myers, 2005).

Despite substantial advancements in oncologic detection and treatment efficacy (Giuliani et al., 2016; Stanton, Rowland, & Ganz, 2015; Wells, Semple, & Lane, 2015), as well as the emergence of a more favorable prognosis for HPV-positive oropharyngeal carcinomas (Maxwell et al., 2014; Michaelson, Gronhoj, Michaelson, Frigborg, & von Buchwald, 2017; Ringash, 2015; Theurer, Chap. 4), morbidity and dysfunction remain high among those diagnosed with and treated for HNCa (Cohen et al., 2015). This ultimately equates to an increasing number of survivors who must face the potentially disabling long-term biopsychosocial consequences of HNCa and the potential for diminished QoL. In light of the increasing survival rates and growing HNCa survivorship population, period of survival post-diagnosis can no longer be the primary outcome measure of oncological treatment efficacy (Doyle, 1994; Lawford & Eiser, 2001). The resultant shift in the perception of HNCa as a chronic illness instead of a life-threatening disease (Ferrell & Hassey Dow, 1997) necessitates that QoL is categorically distinct from the rate of biomedically defined survival. In essence, increasing the period of posttreatment survival may equate to increasing *quantity* of life but by no means does the extended period of survival equate to increasing *quality* of life (MacDonald, 2017). Thus, there is a need for increased under-standing and consideration of the concepts of QoL and WB in oncological research and care delivery to facilitate the potential to "not only add years to life but life to years" (Sayed et al., 2009, p. 397).

Defining Quality of Life and Well-Being

The terms QoL and WB are both omnibus terms that represent a large array of behaviors and functions with considerably complex boundaries specific to functioning (Aaronson, 1991). Definitions of QoL have historically been guided by the assumption that physical, psychological, and social domains of functioning must be considered as the core domains of the construct. However, considerations of symptoms and pain, as well as spirituality and sexuality, have also been explicitly added to the larger framework that represents the conceptualization of QoL (Gritz et al., 1999).

The World Health Organization (WHO) (1997) arguably provides the most widely cited definition of QoL. According to the WHO, QoL can be conceptualized as individuals':

> … perception of their position in life in the context of the culture and value systems in which they live and in relation to their goals, expectations, standards, and concerns. It is a broad ranging concept affected in a complex way by the person's physical health, psychological state, level of independence, social relationships, personal beliefs, and their relationship to salient features of their environment. (p. 1)

The definition provided by the WHO seeks to guide one's consideration of QoL as a concept, and, thus, it is not meant to be interpreted as inflexible and/or prescriptive. By definition, QoL represents a highly personalized and dynamic construct that cannot be uniformly defined for all. Rather, QoL associated with health, illness, disease entity, or condition is both personally and contextually bound. Morton and Izzard (2003) have provided a more flexible definition when they suggest that QoL "encompasses an extensive range of physical and psychological characteristics and limitations that describe ability to function and derive satisfaction in doing so" (p. 884). It is, therefore, suggested that QoL is "best defined as the perceived discrepancy between the reality of what a person has and the concept of what that person wants, needs, or expects" (Morton & Izzard, 2003, p. 884). Within the notably equivocal QoL literature, there appears to be some level of agreement around this conceptualization of the construct; the notion that QoL reflects a self-perceived comparison between current and ideal levels of functioning has been mirrored and adopted by other authors (e.g., Cella & Cherin, 1988; Semple et al., 2004).

In this sense, QoL is truly in the "eye of the beholder" as one's status can only be accurately contextualized by the individual. This also denotes that despite the individualized nature of QoL, it is not a static entity but one that will vary (sometimes considerably) over time. It follows that definitional boundaries and personal perception may also lead to mismatches or ambiguity in how QoL and WB may be defined. While the definitional challenges associated with QoL and WB are acknowledged, what is at times lacking is the concomitant acknowledgment that sources of definitional ambiguity also directly influence how QoL is measured, how data are interpreted, and, perhaps most critically, how such information is applied. Thus, definitional ambiguity carries with it downstream risks that must be considered.

Definitional ambiguity in the HNCa literature The origin of the modern-day study of QoL evolved from the pioneering work of Karnofsky and colleagues (Karnofsky, 1961; Karnofsky, Abelmann, Craver, & Burchenal, 1948; Karnofsky et al., 1951; Karnofsky & Burchenal, 1949). Briefly, this body of work emerged as an outgrowth of clinical observations of the toxic effects of chemotherapeutic agents on individuals who were receiving treatment for lung cancer. Karnofsky and Burchenal (1949) identified that changes in one's "performance status" secondary to treatment needed to be quantified. In essence, their clinical observations suggested that the cancer *treatment* had substantial negative consequences on both physical and psychological

functioning. From that starting point in the middle of the twentieth century, the idea of looking beyond the disease itself became of increasing importance to others.

Although much has changed in the intervening decades since the work of Karnofsky and colleagues, many questions and definitional challenges remain. Unfortunately, what is consistent in the QoL literature that followed is that the construct of QoL is inconsistently defined and conceptualized.[1] A clear definition is rarely articulated in the HNCa QoL literature, and, thus, the conceptualization of QoL is eclipsed with considerable confusion (Morton & Izzard, 2003; Murphy, 2009). Since QoL is an omnibus term, a significant source of the confusion that complicates the establishment of a concrete definition comes from the common occurrence of different terms being used interchangeably. The lexicon of QoL and WB is not always clear and uniform. For instance, QoL has been used implicitly to convey the broad concepts of functional or performance status, symptom burden, or health outcomes (Karnofsky et al., 1948; Murphy, 2009; Sayed et al., 2009; Singer, Langendijk, & Yarom, 2013).

Notably, the term *health-related quality of life* (HRQoL) is often used by HNCa researchers in place of the more generic term: QoL. In the context of oncology, HRQoL denotes a more specific realm within the larger construct of QoL (Singer et al., 2013). The term HRQoL provides a distinct subcategory under the larger classification of QoL in order to specifically identify the individual's perception of their health (Singer et al., 2013). It is commonly used to reflect the reality that demographic variables such as household income or social support are peripheral to the variables that can be controlled and modified

---

[1] As an interesting side note to this concern, we would suggest that some proportion of this problem is borne of a push to develop new QoL instruments, rather than attempts which seek to expand and/or refine existing tools. Additionally, QoL measurement continues to be challenged by the underlying mismatch between the desire of healthcare systems and their need to quantitate, in some form, what are essentially qualitative aspects of personal functioning.

during oncological treatment (Sayed et al., 2009). In addition to one's perception of disease- and treatment-related variables (Klein, Livergant, & Ringash, 2014; Singer et al., 2013), HRQoL also takes into consideration the limitation or disruption of an individual's daily behaviors, social participation, and psychological functioning secondary to physical dysfunction, pain, and related psychosocial distress (Bornbaum et al., 2012; Eadie, Chap. 29; Lawton, 2001). When considered collectively, factors noted by Sayed et al. (2009), Klein et al. (2014), Singer et al. (2013), and Lawton (2001) provide a template of issues which include those that have been historically identified as forming QoL (physical, psychological, and social functioning), in addition to the influence of treatment and, finally, the larger, more individualized array of demographic variables.

Evidently, there exists unavoidable overlap between the conceptualizations of HRQoL and QoL that only serves to further confound efforts at the establishment of a clear-cut definition for QoL research and clinical practice. This suggests that findings from the literature, whether related to HNCa or any other cancer site or disease category, must be scrutinized relative to how any given variable or factor has been defined. Without such efforts to understand potential definitional discrepancies or overlaps, interpretation of data will be limited at best. Consequently, these definitional challenges may unfortunately discourage clinicians from considering the use of formal (HR)QoL measures in clinical practice.

Universal Caveats for QoL Definitions

Despite the equivocal nature of QoL definitions in the literature, there exist several caveats for QoL that are widely agreed upon and may serve to center one's understanding of the construct. It is universally recognized that the constructs of QoL and WB are highly individualized and subjective, multidimensional, and dynamic. For this reason, each of these requisites will be addressed in subsequent sections.

QoL is individualized and subjective   Inherent in the definition of QoL is that it "implies value based on subjective functioning in comparison with personal expectations and is defined by subjective experiences, states, and perceptions. Quality of life, by its very nature, is idiosyncratic to the individual" (Revicki et al., 2000, p. 888). There is a considerable body of QoL research that supports the notion that the entities of both WB and QoL cannot be indexed without gathering a given individual's subjective impression of his or her situation (Aarstad, Aarstad, & Olofsson, 2008; Bjordal & Bottomley, 2016; Sayed et al., 2009; Vartanian et al., 2017). In all WB or QoL explorations, regardless of the disease or illness being studied, it is uniformly agreed that the *target* of the investigation is also the *source* of the information from which determinations are made. In essence, when all elements of QoL definitions are addressed collectively, the impression of the person who experiences the problem is primary. It is critical to remember that any effort to understand the impact of a disease and its treatment will be solely incomplete without the direct and explicit input of the person who has the problem.

Although it clearly can be expected that one's QoL is negatively influenced by HNCa, no simple or linear relationship exists between the experience of the disease and dimensions of QoL (Lawford & Eiser, 2001). For instance, two individuals with comparable objective experiences of HNCa (e.g., site and stage of disease, etc.) may vary substantially in their perceived QoL as a function of the subjective nature of the construct. It is critically important to acknowledge that the range of biopsychosocial consequences associated with HNCa and its treatment are highly individualized. Even in situations where stages of disease, site, treatment modality, etc. are the same, the ultimate outcome will be unique to every person with HNCa. In essence, it is unlikely that a given disease class or entity, particularly a malignant disease, will have a predictable pattern of performance relative to QoL outcomes, whether real or perceived. Further, there is no predictable trajectory of how or when QoL may be disrupted. As a result, individuals' subjective experiences of surviving HNCa and their appraisal of its overall impact on functioning will influence perceived QoL in an idiosyncratic manner (Lawford & Eiser, 2001).

If the inevitably subjective nature of the disease and concomitant disablement are considered from the perspective of the more traditional, albeit limited, biomedical framework, complications inevitably arise. For example, QoL and WB do not conform to categorical assumptions. Although a "functional" category may be identified, it will be incomplete because of the clearly recognized, individual nature of QoL. Similarly, there is no predictable or corresponding QoL or performance status expectation which coincides with survival data, such as those generated through use of the "product-limit estimation" method or what is more commonly known as a Kaplan-Meier curve (Kaplan & Meier, 1958).

In the realm of the types of assessment information that can be gathered in healthcare, the concern of objective versus subjective information often emerges. Although valuable data about a disease or treatment modality can be garnered from clinical tests, dichotomization of the objective aspects of the disease or treatment and the individual's subjective contextualized experience is often impossible (Sayed et al., 2009; Ueda & Okawa, 2003). While HNCa research often revolves around objective measures such as recurrence of disease, length of survival, or treatment toxicity (Klein et al., 2014), objective outcomes undoubtedly interact with the intrinsic attributes and subjective perceptions of the individual to idiosyncratically modify QoL. Similarly, common indices for the classification and categorization of HNCa, for example, tumor site, clinical and pathological staging, etc., are necessary, but they have little predictive value relative to the impact of the disease and treatment on QoL. The dynamic and interactive nature of the human elements that underlie perceived QoL and WB are highly variable and are influenced by multiple factors over the course of one's life.

Thus, since WB and QoL are subjective indices that are borne of those who directly experience the problem, a singular focus on objective outcomes may prevent the potential for maximiz-ing *quality* of life in addition to maximizing *quantity* of life. As such, avoiding dichotomous consideration of subjective and objective variables would seem to represent QoL most completely, though the continuum between these dichotomies will be judged individually. Objective indices of *quantity* of life cannot be assumed to represent perceived quality. Perhaps it is this recognition that has driven our increasing understanding of palliative and end-of-life care; in such circumstances, a key component to QoL is seen in reducing pain and suffering. Accordingly, a high QoL can exist when one is nearing the end of life (Singer, Martin, & Kelner, 1999). Separation of the objective from the subjective is further complicated by the notion that individuals' experiences with HNCa do not exist in a vacuum, as evidenced by the "medical, psychosocial, interpersonal, financial, and functional consequences of disease and its therapies [that] all contribute to [their] experience" (Miller & Shuman, 2016, p. 1). These multiple dimensions cannot be discounted nor excluded from investigation since they idiosyncratically interrelate to contribute to the individual's perceived QoL throughout the course of a disease and into the period of end of life.

QoL is multidimensional It is also universally accepted that QoL is by definition a multidimensional construct (Curran et al., 2007; Ninu et al., 2015; Sayed et al., 2009; Singer et al., 2013). The multidimensionality of the construct reflects the countless facets of functioning that are central to an individual's valuation of QoL. For instance, one's perception of QoL is influenced by functional dimensions that may include physical functioning, social activity and participation, psychological and emotional well-being, as well as the dimensions of cognitive, spiritual, and role functioning (Carlson & Bultz, 2004; Curran et al., 2007; Eadie, 2003; Myers, 2005; Tschiesner et al., 2009). Among the many domains that may affect one's QoL, health-related issues and the experience of disease are critical (Doyle, 1994; Murphy, Ridner, Wells, & Dietrich, 2007). A prime example lies with one's experience of HNCa which may result in severely disabling effects on the three traditional core domains of functioning that contribute to one's valuation of QoL. Consider the following concerns that are common in those treated for HNCa: dysphagia, xerostomia, and pain contribute to dysfunction in the physical domain; distress, depression, and visible disfigurement result in dysfunction in the psychological domain; and detriments to eating, communication, and speech functions lead to dysfunction in the social domain. Accordingly, since an individual's experience with HNCa has the potential to influence the biopsychosocial dimensions of functioning that are central to an individual's perceived QoL, the consideration and assessment of QoL in those with HNCa is of notable relevance (Gritz et al., 1999; Myers, 2005).

QoL is dynamic Not only does QoL vary drastically between individuals, but the same individual's QoL also has the potential to vary substantially over time (Mount & Cohen, 1995). As outlined previously, QoL is a construct that is fluid and changes relative to different contexts and over the course of one's life (Semple et al., 2004). In the context of health or illness, an individual's perceived QoL undergoes continuous changes. The diagnosis of HNCa commences with what may often be an overwhelming amount of new information. This exposure to unfamiliar information and the inundation of potentially adverse encounters and experiences is likely to evoke a fluctuating range of responses that may directly influence perceived QoL. Thus, the same individual's QoL is likely to vary as he or she faces different challenges (e.g., symptoms of the disease, treatment sequelae, etc.) over the course of the clinical pathway. For this reason, efforts that seek to quantify QoL must be guided by the fact that each individual will dictate his or her own status specific to one or more features of interest and, perhaps most importantly, that changes are not presumed to be static in all cases.

The very nature of these three caveats (i.e., QoL is individualized and subjective, multidimensional, and dynamic) also presents challenges that complicate quantifying this inherently qualitative construct. However, the evaluation and measurement of QoL is critical in individuals diagnosed with HNCa given the range and chronicity of disability that is likely to occur, as well as the extensive impact of the disease and its treatment on numerous domains of biopsychosocial functioning (Vartanian et al., 2017).

QoL Methodology

Review of the current literature reveals that the assessment of QoL and WB has evolved into a bountiful and organized scientific discipline that has captured individuals' nuanced experiences concomitant with myriad states of disease or illness (Sayed et al., 2009). A plethora of standardized, valid, and reliable measurement instruments are now available to researchers and clinicians; such tools are intended to provide insight into the multitude of factors that contribute to QoL and WB. Results obtained from QoL measures have become a critical element of the appraisal of health outcomes, particularly in the context of oncology (Rogers, Scott, Chakrabati, & Lowe, 2008; Sayed et al., 2009). While assessment methods for QoL may involve qualitative interviews or quantitative measurement instruments, the later are more commonly utilized at the clinical level, most frequently taking the form of self-administered questionnaires (Singer et al., 2013).

Despite the challenges of quantifying individuals' perceptions, the number of instruments available to psychometrically assess QoL has rapidly increased (Sayed et al., 2009). QoL questionnaires tend to consist of items that pose questions to elicit the individual's perception of various functional behaviors that are assumed to influence QoL or WB. Individuals typically indicate their responses to an instrument's questions using Likert-type scales or visual analogue scales (Vartanian et al., 2017). Generally, an individual's responses to singular items are subsequently categorized into multiple domains of functioning, which usually are collapsed in some manner as an aggregated score for "global" QoL (Vartanian et al., 2017). Yet, just as valuations of particular questions may not be fully sensitive to a given individual's functioning, the aggregate score may also carry similar limitations. That is, an identical total score of X on QoL instrument Y does not represent identical functioning; thus, interpretation or collation of data must be done with care.

Table 27.1 displays a selection of QoL questionnaires that are frequently used in HNCa research and clinical practice. Questionnaires that assess QoL can be categorized according to the level of specificity of factors measured. For instance, generic questionnaires are designed to evaluate QoL irrespective of a specific disease or illness (Singer et al., 2013; Vartanian et al., 2017). In contrast, disease-specific QoL tools seek to assess QoL by measuring concerns

common to individuals who have been diagnosed with a specific disease or illness (e.g., cancer). Disease-specific QoL questionnaires in oncology may be further categorized into site-specific questionnaires. These site-specific measures are designed to increase sensitivity to unique domains of functioning that are particularly affected by the site of the disease and its associated treatment. Since the site of the disease commonly affects a distinctive array of functional abilities, some QoL measurement instruments that are specific to particular areas of functioning (e.g., swallowing) also exist; instruments of this type are referred to as domain-specific QoL questionnaires.

Table 27.1 Widely used HNCa QoL measurement instruments

Category	QoL instrument	Content summary
Disease specific	European Organization for Research and Treatment of Cancer Quality of Life Questionnaire (EORTC QLQ-C30)	30-item core questionnaire Domains: 5 functioning scales (physical, role, cognitive, emotional, social), 6 single-item measures (dyspnea, insomnia, appetite loss, constipation, diarrhea, financial difficulties), 1 global health status/QoL scale Strong psychometric properties
	Functional Assessment of Cancer Therapy – General (FACT-G)	27-item core questionnaire Domains: physical, social/family, emotional, functional, relationship with physician Sound psychometric properties
Site specific	The European Organization for Research and Treatment of Cancer Head and Neck Cancer Module (EORTC QLQ-H&N35)	35 items (supplements QLQ-C30) Domains: 7 multi-item scales (pain, swallowing, senses, speech, social eating, social contact, sexuality) and 11 single items (teeth, mouth opening, dry mouth, sticky saliva, coughing, felt ill, pain killers, nutritional supplements, feeding tube, weight loss, weight gain) Strong psychometric properties
	Functional Assessment of Cancer Therapy – Head and Neck Module (FACT-H&N)	11-item subscale (supplements FACT-G) Domains: HNCa-specific concerns (not intended for use without FACT-G) Sound psychometric properties
	University of Washington Quality of Life Instrument (UW-QoL)	12 items Domains: 9 disease specific (pain, chewing, swallowing, speech, shoulder disability, appearance, activity, recreation, employment), 3 general items (global HRQoL, change in HRQoL since diagnosis, overall QoL) Strong psychometric properties
Domain specific	Voice-Related Quality of Life (V-RQoL)	10 items Domains: physical functioning, social emotional Sound psychometric properties

Adapted from Morton and Izzard (2003), Ojo et al. (2012), Pusic et al. (2007), Ringash and Bezjak (2000), Singer et al. (2013)

Since questionnaires that are specific to disease, site, or domain (i.e., physical, psychological, or social) only include items that reflect the measure's specific category (Sayed et al., 2009), they may be more precise and sensitive to both clinical changes and the individual's lived illness experience (Vartanian et al., 2017). Nevertheless, there is undeniable value in utilizing a combination of both specific and generic QoL measurement instruments to provide a more comprehensive depiction of the individual's perceived QoL (Howren, Christensen, Karnell, Van Liew, & Funk, 2013; Mount & Cohen, 1995; Vartanian et al., 2017). In such instances, measures obtained over time may serve as means of better characterizing the dynamic nature of QoL and, thus, reflect changes that may be contextually bound.

Many existing HNCa-specific QoL measurement instruments include and address an array of issues specific to the cancer site and the consequences of treatment.[2] However, a complete index of which factors are indeed of critical importance in individuals' assessments of their QoL is not always clear nor guided by universal agreement. Further, in light of the conceptually complex nature of QoL, paired with the myriad biopsychosocial domains that are commonly affected by HNCa, a "gold standard" questionnaire does not exist for the measurement of QoL in those with HNCa (Vartanian et al., 2017). Yet defining features that contribute to the conceptualization of QoL serve to guide the potentially challenging task of selecting a suitable instrument to accurately quantify QoL. For instance, QoL questionnaires should be constructed to include multiple domains or dimensions to better assess the multidimensional nature of QoL (Singer et al., 2013). Additionally, since QoL is by definition, a subjective construct, QoL questionnaires should assess QoL from the perspective of the target of the measurement instrument. In other words, it is recommended that QoL

questionnaires be self-administered to allow individuals to identify and prioritize their own idiosyncratic challenges and concerns in the context of their unique experience with HNCa. Not only will this provide a more illuminating depiction of the individual's holistic circumstances and functioning, it has also been suggested that the patient's self-rating of QoL is more sensitive and reliable than that of the clinician (Sayed et al., 2009). When considered broadly, and knowing that no perfect tool exists, efforts to assess QoL or measure the impact of a disease on one's functioning require careful consideration. In the context of clinical practice, this suggests that clinicians must strive to identify the measure that will provide the most useful information.[3]

In light of the absence of a gold standard QoL questionnaire, researchers and clinicians should be aware of several additional practical and methodological attributes when selecting an appropriate measurement instrument; the QoL questionnaire should be valid, reliable, sensitive, brief, and interpretable (Ringash, 2015; Sayed et al., 2009). Additionally, floor and ceiling effects should be absent from a dependable QoL questionnaire (Sayed et al., 2009). In essence, a QoL questionnaire must also be able to detect changes in the upper and lower extremes of QoL, or in other words, it must be able to measure the worsening of already low QoL, as well as improvement of high levels of QoL (Sayed et al., 2009; Ware et al., 1995). While a working knowledge of attributes of dependable QoL measurement instruments is important, understanding the psychometric properties of all measurement instruments, as well as vulnerable areas of QoL questionnaires that may threaten to introduce measurement error, is arguably just as critical.

---

[2]It is important to acknowledge that a variety of supplemental measures may also be employed. Although specifically developed to identify symptoms (physical or psychosocial), "symptom screening" tools can be used in combination with other more extensive QoL measures.

[3]At times, clinicians may utilize sections of larger QoL measures in an effort to document or monitor particular aspects of functioning. While the objective of this type of exploration may serve to facilitate specific types of intervention and follow-up, and is not discouraged, it must be recognized that doing so does threaten the validity of the measure(s) obtained.

Sources of Measurement Error

There are well-recognized concerns specific to threats to the validity of any assessment instrument, and such concerns remain of considerable importance relative to the measurement of WB and QoL. In the subsections to follow, threats to validity will be discussed briefly and contextualized through application to a frequently reported QoL trajectory in the HNCa literature.

Application of Sources of Measurement Error to QoL Trajectory

The HNCa literature repeatedly reports that QoL tends to decline after diagnosis of the cancer, reach a nadir following treatment completion, and gradually recover to near baseline levels approximately 1 year after diagnosis (Astrup, Rustoen, Hofso, Gran, & Bjordal, 2016; Curran et al., 2007; Goldstein, Karnell, Christensen, & Funk, 2007; Howren et al., 2010; Howren et al., 2013; Infante-Cossio et al., 2009; Klein et al., 2014; Michaelson et al., 2017; Richardson et al., 2016; Singer et al., 2014). Although this trajectory of QoL is widely reported, concerns regarding threats to validity may serve to confound the underlying reasons of this common finding.

Awareness of potential threats to validity, paired with critical appraisal of both past and current literature, serves to enhance both clinicians' and researchers' understanding of the intricacies of QoL measurement. Such efforts may ultimately enable them to be better prepared to maximize QoL in those they serve. Without psychometric measurement of QoL objective, quantified improvement of QoL is unlikely. Thus, pursuits to measure QoL are of the utmost importance, particularly in a population that is at risk for such substantial detriments to QoL and WB. In light of the following discussion of potential threats to validity, drawing attention to the potential sources of measurement error in QoL research is not intended to undermine the value or worth of pursuits to measure this vital construct. Conversely, discussion of sources of measurement error is intended to better prepare consumers of the data to maximize the QoL of those individuals who are vulnerable to the effects of disease or illness. There is no perfect measure; however, an awareness of the potential limitations of any given QoL measure will serve to provide the best possible information that is as free as possible from confound and erroneous assumptions in interpretation.

Response shift Measurement error may be introduced into the quantification of individuals' perceived QoL through the phenomenon termed *response shift*. The concept of the response shift may be defined as the tendency for quantified self-rated QoL to return to scores that resemble baseline reference QoL scores with no clinically relevant difference, despite clinically significant detriments to biopsychosocial domains of functioning and WB (Michaelson et al., 2017). In the context of a diagnosis of a critical illness, response shift may be observed when individuals subjectively adjust their values, recalibrate internal standards of measurement, reprioritize domains of WB, or reconceptualize QoL (Michaelson et al., 2017; Ringash, 2015). All of these concerns may limit the ability to accurately interpret the measure gathered.

For individuals who have been diagnosed with HNCa, their entire existence is commonly influenced and transformed by the disease and its treatment. This may in turn translate into a shift in one's frame of reference as adjustment to a new normal occurs (Singer et al., 2014). The changing of one's internal metric of assessment over time limits the comparative capacity of measures obtained. This is not a willful act but rather one that emerges as a function of adaptation, coping, adjustment, and resilience (Blood, Luther, & Stemple, 1992; MacDonald, 2017). As an individual adapts to changes in his or her health status, a response shift may confound a finding that suggests the absence of a reasonable reduction in quantified QoL scores despite severe biopsychosocial dysfunction (Sayed et al., 2009). As a result of the potential for response shifts, the paradoxical finding of a return to baseline QoL scores may be reported in populations of individuals who continue to experience persistent disablement (Singer et al., 2014).

Maturation An additional factor that jeopardizes the validity of QoL studies is a concept referred to as *maturation*. Campbell and Stanley (1963) described maturation as "processes within the respondents operating as a function of the passage of time per se (not specific to the particular events)" (p. 5). In the context of QoL research pertaining to individuals diagnosed with HNCa, participants' QoL "scores" may show an upward trajectory that could represent recovery or improvement; however, the concept of maturation may suggest that QoL has increased solely as a function of the passage of time. In essence, the gap between a survivor's ideal and actual level of perceived QoL that may have become expansive following the diagnosis of HNCa may have become smaller as a simple function of the passage of time, not because QoL outcomes have improved (Payakachat, Ounpraseuth, & Suen, 2012).

Selection bias of long-term survivors The trajectory of assumed eventual recovery of QoL scores in HNCa survivors may also be falsely elevated because of *selection bias.* Owing to the realities of the disablement faced by participants, longitudinal QoL studies among HNCa survivors are particularly susceptible to selection bias (Maxwell et al., 2014; Singer et al., 2014). More specifically, the commonly reported trajectory of QoL may be misleading because short-term survivors are likely to have a different experience of disablement and unique profiles of QoL scores when compared to long-term survivors (Goldstein et al., 2007). Unfortunately, the reality is that selection bias may select against these short-term HNCa survivors since they are more likely to drop out of studies as a result of substantial health problems, treatment-related side effects, or death (Klein et al., 2014; Sayed et al., 2009). Thus, the reported return of QoL to baseline may reflect only those individuals who are retained as participants at the time of follow-up, a fact which inevitably excludes the lowest-performing individuals who were included at baseline.

Stated differently, because of the absence of the contributions of deceased participants, an inflated, "apparent" improvement in longer-term follow-up QoL scores (e.g., data collected at 12 months) may be reported. The presence of selection bias would suggest that this change occurs because the low QoL scores from participants who die before study completion may lower the mean QoL scores at the short-term follow-up points (Goldstein et al., 2007). Conversely, the high QoL scores contributed by the long-term survivors may mask the low QoL scores of those individuals who drop out early in longitudinal studies if the data gathered from all participants are averaged (Goldstein et al., 2007). Thus, long-term, high-performing participants in HNCa QoL studies may represent only a minority of those accrued at study inception. If this occurs, data may not be generalizable to the majority of those individuals who face the challenges and disablement concomitant with HNCa (Goldstein et al., 2007). In other words, the external validity of such findings is directly threatened.

Thus, while this commonly reported QoL trajectory may serve as a source of optimism and encouragement for survivors who are faced with uncertainty surrounding their future, clinicians and researchers must be conscientious of the unique needs of those short-term survivors who may not conform with the trajectory. In this regard, the ultimate data obtained must be interpreted in a manner that similarly reflects the individualized and dynamic nature of QoL and one's perception of it. Therefore, the importance of awareness of threats to validity is underscored. If QoL measures are gathered carefully and with an understanding of relative strengths and limitations, there is no reason to invalidate or devalue information obtained to assess QoL or discount the use of such evaluative approaches. Ultimately, researchers have an ethical obligation to collect, analyze, publish, translate, and implement data to ensure that participants' efforts in serving as the target of the investigation give back to the population to which they belong (Ringash, 2016).

Clinical Application

The consideration and assessment of QoL holds considerable utility in the clinical setting. The potential for detriments to HNCa survivors' perceived QoL is profound. For this reason, the assessment of QoL is critical in terms of ensuring optimal provision of care. However, extending QoL assessments to address the potential longer-term consequences of the disease and its treatment is essential. The evaluation of QoL facilitates a more holistic understanding of the impact of HNCa and its treatment on the multiple facets of an individual's functioning and WB (Richardson et al., 2016). Given the aforementioned interdependent nature of the challenges associated with HNCa, in combination with its clearly multidimensional nature, the identification of factors that reduce perceived QoL is critical. Without this type of information, efforts that seek to improve HNCa survivors' recovery and rehabilitation will be insufficient. For example, physical disfigurement that is visually apparent, or auditorily apparent deficits in one's voice, speech, and one's efficiency in communication (Evitts, Chap. 28) may be associated with social isolation and depression. These types of changes may in turn negatively influence an individual's desire and adherence with self-care and rehabilitation regimes (Howren et al., 2013; Starmer, Chap. 24). Thus, the simple identification of a specific deficit on a QoL measure holds great potential of altering QoL in larger aspects of psychosocial functioning. Quantitative assessment of QoL may serve to identify more significant underlying issues (e.g., social isolation, depression) that may not be directly apparent if a HNCa survivor initially presents with a single concern (e.g., speech deficits). Attending to a survivor's holistic experience of disablement may allow for the identification of individuals who are not forthcoming with psychosocial issues and, yet, are struggling to cope (Carlson & Bultz, 2004).

Moreover, screening and identifying individuals that may be vulnerable to reduced QoL presents as a proactive approach that serves to minimize the influence of the challenges faced by individuals diagnosed with HNCa. If reductions in QoL are identified, pre-existing biopsychosocial morbidity may not become as firmly manifested. Moreover, the identification of vulnerability facilitates identified individuals to be directed toward interventions proactively, before dysfunction or morbidity can become deeply rooted. Thus, measurement of QoL has the reciprocal effect of having the potential to ultimately improve HNCa survivors' QoL by informing and guiding intervention and rehabilitative efforts that are led by the survivor's subjective perceptions, needs, and priorities.

In effect, an enhanced understanding of the holistic impact of HNCa on the individual enables the clinician to uncover and establish a clearer picture of the patient's subjective priorities for recovery. This information may then be used to guide treatment decisions and may ultimately serve to improve and optimize outcomes (Richardson et al., 2016). In light of recent developments and advancements in HNCa treatment, QoL assessment in those diagnosed with HNCa may be implemented in the clinical setting to guide the planning of treatment strategy (Vartanian et al., 2017). QoL data serve a central role in treatment decision-making, particularly when two treatment modalities have purported equivalent survival rates (Rogers et al., 2008; Vartanian et al., 2017). For instance, in the case of early-stage glottic tumors, definitive radiotherapy, conservation laryngectomy, or endoscopic laser resection are feasible curative options with similar rates of survival; however, each of these approaches may very well generate distinct morbidities and subsequent functional deficits (Vartanian et al., 2017). Thus, an explicit understanding of the patient's fears, goals, values, and beliefs (all vital components of one's valuation of QoL) allows treatment decisions to be more reflective of the outcomes that may be best tolerated by the individual patient. Ultimately, fostering direct and ongoing communication between the patient and members of the HNCa team is likely to foster cooperative efforts with the goal of facilitating the best possible QoL outcomes over time.

Not only does the use of QoL data place the patient in the center of clinical considerations, but it also may better equip them to actively participate in their own care (Klein et al., 2014; Vartanian et al., 2017). Increased participation in medical decisions may in part be related to the improved communication and enhanced relationship between the healthcare professional and their patient, which is reported to result from the utilization of QoL measurement instruments in the clinical setting (Murphy et al., 2007; Vartanian et al., 2017). Ultimately, QoL assessment moves the provision of oncological treatment toward a more person-centered model of care delivery, which facilitates the identification of the individual's ideal outcomes and goals of treatment (Sayed et al., 2009). The consequential amplification of the physician's understanding of the individual's expectations of care affects not only treatment adherence but also the individual's satisfaction with the care they receive (Sayed et al., 2009). Somewhat reciprocally, when patients are satisfied with the care they receive, there exists a correlation with improved QoL outcomes (Fröjd, Lampic, Larsson, & Essen, 2009; Ong, Visser, Lammes, & De Haes, 2000).

The Role of the Clinician in the Application of QoL Research to Clinical Practice

Despite the numerous advantages and benefits of considering QoL in the context of HNCa, QoL data are most frequently presented within research formats that may be challenging and time consuming for healthcare professionals to understand, interpret, and incorporate into their routine clinical practices (Rogers et al., 2008). In order to maximize the uptake of QoL findings by healthcare professionals, there is a critical need for the findings of HNCa QoL research to be presented in a clinically useful way that is both interpretable and practical (Ringash, 2015; Rogers et al., 2008). The most significant challenge associated with the use of QoL measures as integral components of the clinical outcome process is often related to the translation of *what* research findings mean and *how* they apply to one's caseload. In this regard, clinicians must be able to

appreciate that wide variability in perceived QoL is common and that findings from clinical studies should not seek to categorize patients. Rather, clinical information that is gleaned from QoL measures should be used as an acknowledgment of the range of deficits that may exist and their subsequent impact on the patient's functioning.

Future efforts must strive to not only obtain but present QoL data in a way that will bridge the gap between research and clinical practice (Sayed et al., 2009). The inability to bridge such a divide may only serve to maintain the judgment that research data have no direct relationship to clinical practice. Because QoL instruments typically sample an array of domain-driven (i.e., physical, psychological, social) functional abilities, the clinician must be able to integrate disparate pieces of QoL data. However, perhaps of greater importance is the ability of the clinician to make logical steps in understanding relationships, real or anticipated, between specific areas of assessment and their ultimate manifestation.

For example, treatment of HNCa may often result in physical disfigurement. While such changes may vary from relatively minor to those that are more significant in appearance (e.g., creation of permanent tracheostoma), the potential for such changes to influence QoL is substantial. It is the clinician's responsibility to also anticipate the impact of physical disfigurement in the larger context of potential concomitant changes in functioning. Accordingly, in those instances where disfigurement is judged by the patient to be an important QoL factor, the clinician may proactively seek information on how this influences one socially. If one has withdrawn to some extent from interactions with others because of the changes in one's body image, psychological sequelae (e.g., distress, depression) may also emerge.

Clinicians must, therefore, consider how one deficit may extend to other areas of functioning with the collective cascade of difficulties having a dramatic influence on QoL. Consequently, determining the QoL impact in those with HNCa is often incomplete or insufficient if only "hard" data are considered. In essence, the most valuable clinical application relies on the clinician's logical interpretation of the collected data and ability to proactively raise suspicion of potential downstream challenges that may emerge. Clinical intuition may lead to verification of a problem as part of an open clinician-patient dialogue. If areas of concomitant impact are identified, then the clinician can actively and collaboratively work with the patient to understand the problems they experience and, ideally, provide access to information or other professional resources to minimize the problem. Furthermore, while the potential relationship between some problems may be relatively obvious (e.g., the loss of one's ability to communicate effectively following HNCa treatment and the subsequent avoidance of interactions with others), other clusters of deficits may not be as readily apparent (e.g., a withdrawal from social gatherings because of the deficits in one's ability to eat and swallow efficiently). The most valuable clinical approaches to addressing challenges to QoL will be guided by the clinician's willingness to ask questions pertaining to a range of biopsychosocial functioning and then seek to contextualize reported difficulties and identify the idiosyncratic impact on the patient. The clinician's ability to gather individual information and interpret identified losses specific to each patient (Doyle, 1994) arguably holds the greatest potential for targeted efforts to improve QoL in those with HNCa.

vidual's QoL (MacDonald, 2017). In essence, increased *quantity* of life provided by advanced treatment for HNCa does not mean that an individual's struggle to cope with the profound functional losses will cease when the transition is made from cancer patient to cancer survivor (MacDonald, 2017). In some respects, the emotional burden of disease or illness may mirror the challenges associated with the death of a loved one; this includes responses such as denial, fear, and anger (Kubler-Ross, 1969, 1975). For this reason, chronic illness and the potential disability that occurs secondary to treatment also may be seen as creating a process of personal response that is not inconsistent with grieving. Thus, efforts that consider changes in one's health status should be careful to also consider associated emotional responses and the concomitant impact on QoL.

In conclusion, this chapter has addressed and defined factors specific to QoL and WB in those who are diagnosed and treated for HNCa. Current approaches to QoL methodology and associated sources of measurement error were discussed. Clinical applications of QoL and the role of the clinician in the application of QoL research in clinical practice were outlined. Finally, this chapter has sought to promote facilitation of the best possible outcomes through consideration of the profound impact of HNCa and its treatment on survivors' QoL.

Conclusions

It is well recognized that the diagnosis of any serious disease or illness will be met with difficult and potentially persistent challenges of disablement, particularly in situations where chronic problems occur (Shook, 1983; Smith, 1981). In the case of a diagnosis of HNCa, individuals are often at risk for substantial biopsychosocial dysfunction that may create significant detriments to QoL. The extensive array of the biopsychosocial treatment sequelae associated with advanced treatment modalities illustrates that achieving curative intent in the context of HNCa is often done at the expense of the indi-

References

Aaronson, N. K. (1991). Methodologic issues in assessing the quality of life of cancer patients. *Cancer, 63*(3 Suppl), 844–850. https://doi.org/10.1002/1097-0142(19910201)67:3+<844::AID-CNCR2820671416>3.0.CO;2-B

Aarstad, A. K., Aarstad, H. J., & Olofsson, J. (2008). Personality and choice of coping predict quality of life in head and neck cancer patients during follow-up. *Acta Oncologica, 47*(5), 879–890. https://doi.org/10.1080/02841860701798858

Astrup, G. L., Rustoen, T., Hofso, K., Gran, J. M., & Bjordal, K. (2016). Symptom burden and patient characteristics: Association with quality of life in patients with head and neck cancer undergoing radiotherapy. *Head & Neck, 39*(10), 2114–2126. https://doi.org/10.1002/hed.24875

Bjordal, K., & Bottomley, A. (2016). Making advances in quality of life studies in head and neck cancer. *International Journal of Radiation Oncology, 97*(4), 659–661. https://doi.org/10.1016/j.ijrobp.2016.11.051

Blood, G. W., Luther, A. R., & Stemple, J. C. (1992). Coping and adjustment in alaryngeal speakers. *American Journal of Speech-Language Pathology, 1*(2), 63–69.

Bornbaum, C. C., Fung, K., Franklin, J. H., Nichols, A., Yoo, J., & Doyle, P. C. (2012). A descriptive analysis of the relationship between quality of life and distress in individuals with head and neck cancer. *Supportive Care in Cancer, 20*, 2157–2165.

Campbell, D. T., & Stanley, J. C. (1963). *Experimental and quasi-experimental designs for research*. Boston, MA: Houghton Mifflin Company.

Carlson, L., & Bultz, B. (2004). Efficacy and medical cost offset of psychosocial interventions in cancer care: Making the case for economic analyses. *Psycho-Oncology, 13*(12), 837–849. https://doi.org/10.1002/pon.832

Cella, D. F., & Cherin, E. A. (1988). Quality of life during and after cancer treatment. *Comprehensive Therapy, 14*(5), 69–75.

Cohen, E. E. W., LaMonte, S. J., Erb, N. L., Beckman, K. L., Sadeghi, N., Hutcheson, K. A., … Pratt-Chapman, M. L. (2015). American cancer society head and neck cancer survivorship care guidelines. *CA: a Cancer Journal for Clinicians, 66*(3), 204–239. https://doi.org/10.3322/caac.21286

Cousins, N. (1979). *Anatomy of an illness as perceived by the patient*. New York, NY: Norton.

Curran, D., Giralt, J., Harari, P. M., Ang, K. K., Cohen, R. B., Kies, M. S., … Bonner, J. A. (2007). Quality of life in head and neck cancer patients after treatment with high-dose radiotherapy alone or in combination with cetuximab. *Journal of Clinical Oncology, 25*(16), 2191–2197. https://doi.org/10.1200/JCO.2006.08.8005

Doyle, P. C. (1994). *Foundations of voice and speech rehabilitation following laryngeal cancer*. San Diego, CA: Singular Publishing Group.

Doyle, P. C. (2005). Rehabilitation in head and neck cancer: Overview. In P. C. Doyle (Ed.), *Contemporary considerations in the treatment and rehabilitation of head and neck cancer* (pp. 3–15). Austin, TX: PRO-ED.

Dropkin, M. J. (1981). Changes in body image associated with head and neck cancer. In L. B. Marino (Ed.), *Cancer nursing* (pp. 560–581). St Louis, MO: Mosby.

Eadie, T. L. (2003). The ICF: A proposed framework for comprehensive rehabilitation of individuals who use alaryngeal speech. *American Journal of Speech-Language Pathology, 12*(2), 189–197.

Eadie, T. L. (2007). Application of the ICF in communication after total laryngectomy. *Seminars in Speech and Language, 28*(4), 291–300. https://doi.org/10.1055/s-2007-986526. ISSN 0734-0478.

Ferrell, B., & Hassey Dow, K. (1997). Quality of life among long-term cancer survivors. *Oncology, 11*(4), 565–571.

Fröjd, C., Lampic, C., Larsson, G., & Essen, L. V. (2009). Is satisfaction with doctors' care related to health-related quality of life, anxiety and depression among patients with carcinoid tumours? A longitudinal report. *Scandinavian Journal of Caring Sciences, 23*(11), 107–116.

Giuliani, M., Mcquestion, M., Jones, J., Papadakos, J., Le, L. W., Alkazaz, N., … Ringash, J. (2016). Prevalence and nature of survivorship needs in patients with head and neck cancer. *Head & Neck, 38*(7), 1097–1103. https://doi.org/10.1002/HED

Goldstein, D. P., Karnell, L. H., Christensen, A. J., & Funk, G. F. (2007). Health-related quality of life profiles based on survivorship status for head and neck cancer patients. *Head & Neck, 29*(3), 221–229. https://doi.org/10.1002/hed

Gritz, E. R., Carmack, C. L., de Moor, C., Coscarelli, A., Schacherer, C. W., Meyers, E. G., & Abemayor, E. (1999). First year after head and neck cancer: Quality of life. *Journal of Clinical Oncology, 17*(1), 352–360.

Hansson, E., Carlstrom, E., Olsson, L., Nyman, J., & Koinberg, I. (2017). Can a person-centred-care intervention improve health-related quality of life in patients with head and neck cancer? A randomized, controlled study. *BMC Nursing, 16*(9), 1–12. https://doi.org/10.1186/s12912-017-0206-6

Howren, M. B., Christensen, A. J., Karnell, L. H., & Funk, G. F. (2010). Health-related quality of life in head and neck cancer survivors: Impact of pretreatment depressive symptoms. *Health Psychology, 29*(1), 65–71. https://doi.org/10.1037/a0017788

Howren, M. B., Christensen, A. J., Karnell, L. H., & Funk, G. F. (2012). Psychological factors associated with head and neck cancer treatment and survivorship: Evidence and opportunities for behavioral medicine. *Journal of Consulting and Clinical Psychology*. https://doi.org/10.1037/a0029940

Howren, M. B., Christensen, A. J., Karnell, L. H., Van Liew, J. R., & Funk, G. F. (2013). Influence of pretreatment social support on health-related quality of life in head and neck cancer survivors: Results from a prospective study. *Head & Neck, 35*(6), 779–787. https://doi.org/10.1002/hed.23029

Infante-Cossio, P., Torres-Carranze, E., Cayuela, A., Hens-Aumente, E., Pastor-Gaitan, P., & Gutierrez-Perez, J. L. (2009). Impact of treatment on quality of life for oral and oropharyngeal carcinoma. *International Journal of Oral and Maxillofacial Surgery, 38*(10), 1052–1058. https://doi.org/10.1016/j.ijom.2009.06.008

Kaplan, E. L., & Meier, P. (1958). Nonparametric estimation from incomplete observations. *Journal of the American Statistical Association, 53*, 457–481.

Karnofsky, D. A. (1961). Meaningful clinical classifications of therapeutic responses to anticancer drugs. *Clinical Pharmacology & Therapeutics, 2*(6), 709–712.

Karnofsky, D. A., Abelmann, W. H., Craver, L. F., & Burchenal, J. H. (1948). The use of the nitrogen mustards in the palliative treatment of carcinoma. With particular reference to bronchogenic carcinoma. *Cancer, 1*(4), 634–656.

Karnofsky, D. A., & Burchenal, J. H. (1949). The clinical evaluation of chemotherapeutic agents in cancer. In C. M. MacLeod (Ed.), *Evaluation of chemotherapeutic agents* (pp. 191–205). New York, NY: Columbia University Press.

Karnofsky, D. A., Burchenal, J. H., Armstead, G. C., Southam, C. M., Bernstein, J. L., Craver, L. F., & Rhoads, C. P. (1951). Triethylene melamine in the treatment of neoplastic disease: A compound with nitrogen-mustard-like activity suitable for oral and intravenous use. *AMA Archives of Internal Medicine, 87*(4), 477–516.

Klein, J., Livergant, J., & Ringash, J. (2014). Health related quality of life in head and neck cancer treated with radiation therapy with or without chemotherapy: A systematic review. *Oral Oncology, 50*(4), 254–262. https://doi.org/10.1016/j.oraloncology.2014.01.015

Kubler-Ross, E. (1969). *On death and dying*. New York, NY: Macmillan.

Kubler-Ross, E. (1975). *Death, the final stage of growth*. Englewood Cliffs, NJ: Prentice-Hall.

Lawford, J., & Eiser, C. (2001). Exploring links between the concepts of quality of life and resilience. *Pediatric Rehabilitation, 4*(1), 209–216.

Lawton, M. P. (2001). Quality of life and end of life. In J. E. Birren & K. W. Schaie (Eds.), *Handbook of the psychology of aging* (5th ed., pp. 593–616). San Diego, CA: Academic Press.

Lee, J. Y., Ready, E. A., Davis, E. N., & Doyle, P. C. (2017). Purposefulness as a critical factor in functioning, disability and health. *Clinical Rehabilitation, 31*(8), 1005–1018. https://doi.org/10.1177/0269215516672274

Ma, E. P. M., & Yiu, E. M. L. (2001). Voice activity and participation profile: Assessing the impact of voice disorders on daily activities. *Journal of Speech, Language, and Hearing Research, 44*, 511–524.

MacDonald, C. (2017). *Minimizing the impact of disease while maximizing quality of life: An exploration of resilience in head and neck cancer survivors*. Retrieved from Electronic Thesis and Dissertation Repository. (4790). https://ir.lib.uwo.ca/etd/4790

Maxwell, J. H., Mehta, V., Wang, H., Cunningham, D., Duvvuri, U., Seungwon, K., ... Ferris, R. L. (2014). Quality of life in head and neck cancer patients: Impact of HPV and primary treatment modality. *The Laryngoscope, 124*(7), 1592–1597. https://doi.org/10.1002/lary.24508

Michaelson, S. H., Gronhoj, C., Michaelson, J. H., Frigborg, J., & von Buchwald, C. (2017). Quality of life in survivors of oropharyngeal cancer: A systematic review and meta-analysis of 1366 patients. *European Journal of Cancer, 78*, 91–102. https://doi.org/10.1016/j.ejca.2017.03.006

Miller, M. C., & Shuman, A. G. (2016). Survivorship in head and neck cancer – A primer. *JAMA Otolaryngology – Head & Neck Surgery, Special Communication*, 1–7. https://doi.org/10.1001/jamaoto.2016.1615

Mochizuki, Y., Matsushima, E., & Omura, K. (2008). Perioperative assessment of psychological state and quality of life of head and neck cancer patients undergoing surgery. *International Journal of Oral and Maxillofacial Surgery, 38*(2), 151–159. https://doi.org/10.1016/j.ijom.2008.11.007

Morton, R. P., & Izzard, M. E. (2003). Quality-of-life outcomes in head and neck cancer patients. *World Journal of Surgery, 27*(7), 884–889. https://doi.org/10.1007/s00268-003-7117-2

Mount, B. M., & Cohen, S. R. (1995). Quality of life in the face of life-threatening illness: What should we be measuring? *Current Oncology, 2*(3), 121–125.

Murphy, B. A. (2009). Advances in quality of life and symptom management for head and neck cancer patients. *Current Opinion in Oncology, 21*(3), 242–247. https://doi.org/10.1097/CCO.0b013e32832a230c

Murphy, B. A., Ridner, S., Wells, N., & Dietrich, M. (2007). Quality of life research in head and neck cancer: A review of the current state of the science. *Critical Reviews in Oncology/Hematology, 62*(3), 251–267. https://doi.org/10.1016/j.critrevonc.2006.07.005

Myers, C. (2005). Quality of life and head and neck cancer. In P. C. Doyle & R. L. Keith (Eds.), *Contemporary considerations in the treatment and rehabilitation of head and neck cancer* (pp. 697–736). Austin, TX: Pro-ed.

Nash, M. M., Scott, G. M., Fung, K., Yoo J., & Doyle, P. C. (2014, July). An exploration of perceived body image in adults treated for head and neck cancer. 5th World Congress of International Federation of Head and Neck Oncologic Society (IFNOS) Annual Meeting (AHNS), New York. NY.

Newell, S., Sanson-Fisher, R. W., Girgis, A., & Ackland, S. (1999). The physical and psycho-social experiences of patients attending an outpatient medical oncology department: A cross-sectional study. *European Journal of Cancer Care, 8*(2), 73–82.

Ninu, M. B., Miccinesi, G., Bulli, F., De Massimi, A., Muraca, M. G., Franchi, G., & Saraceno, M. S. (2015). Psychological distress and health-related quality of life among head and neck cancer patients during the first year after treatment. *Tumori Journal, 102*(1), 96–102. https://doi.org/10.5301/tj.5000448

Ong, L. M., Visser, M. R., Lammes, F. B., & De Haes, J. C. (2000). Doctor-patient communication and cancer patients' quality of life and satisfaction. *Patient Education and Counseling, 41*(2), 145–156.

Ojo, B., Genden, E. M., Teng, M. S., Milbury, K., Misiukiewicz, K. J., & Badr, H. (2012). A systematic review of head and neck cancer quality of life assessment instruments. *Oral Oncology, 48*(10), 923–937. https://doi.org/10.1016/j.oraloncology.2012.03.025

Payakachat, N., Ounpraseuth, S., & Suen, J. Y. (2012). Late complications and long-term quality of life for survivors (>5 years) with history of head and neck cancer. *Head & Neck, 35*(6), 819–825. https://doi.org/10.1002/hed.23035

Pusic, A., Liu, J. C., Chen, C. M., Cano, S., Davidge, K., Klassen, A., … Cordeiro, P. G. (2007). A systematic review of patient-reported outcome measures in head and neck cancer surgery. *Otolaryngology – Head and Neck Surgery, 136*(4), 525–535. https://doi.org/10.1016/j.otohns.2006.12.006.

Reeve, B. B., Cai, J., Hongtao, Z., Weissler, M. C., Wisienwski, K., Gross, H., & Olshan, A. F. (2016). Factors that impact health-related quality of life over time for individuals with head and neck cancer. *The Laryngoscope, 126*, 2718–2725. https://doi.org/10.1002/lary.26073

Revicki, D. A., Osoba, D., Fairclough, D., Barofsky, I., Berzon, R., Leidy, N. K., & Rothman, M. (2000). Recommendations on health-related quality of life research to support labeling and promotional claims in the United States. *Quality of Life Research, 9*(8), 887–900.

Richardson, A. E., Morton, R. P., & Broadbent, E. A. (2016). Changes over time in head and neck cancer patients' and caregivers' illness perceptions and relationships with quality of life. *Psychology & Health, 31*(10), 1203–1219. https://doi.org/10.1080/08870446.2016.1203686

Ringash, J. (2015). Survivorship and quality of life in head and neck cancer. *Journal of Clinical Oncology, 33*(29), 3322–3328. https://doi.org/10.1200/JCO.2015.61.4115

Ringash, J. (2016). Quality of life in head and neck cancer: Where we are, and where we are going. *International Journal of Radiation Oncology, 97*(4), 662–666. https://doi.org/10.1016/j.ijrobp.2016.12.033

Ringash, J., & Bezjak, A. (2000). A structured review of quality of life instruments for head and neck cancer patients. *Head & Neck, 23*(3), 201–213.

Rogers, S. N., Scott, J., Chakrabati, A., & Lowe, D. (2008). The patients' account of outcome following primary surgery for oral and oropharyngeal cancer using a 'quality of life' questionnaire. *European Journal of Cancer Care, 17*(2), 182–188. https://doi.org/10.1111/j.1365-2354.2007.00832.x

Sayed, S. I., Elmiyeh, B., Rhys-Evan, P., Syrigos, K. N., Nutting, C. M., Harrington, K. J., & Kazi, R. (2009). Quality of life and outcomes research in head and neck cancer: A review of the state of the discipline and likely future directions. *Cancer Treatment Reviews, 35*(5), 397–402. https://doi.org/10.1016/j.ctrv.2009.03.001

Semple, C. J., Sullivan, K., Dunwoody, L., & Kernohan, W. G. (2004). Psychosocial interventions for patients with head and neck cancer: Past, present and future. *Cancer Nursing, 27*(6), 434–441.

Shook, R. (1983). *Survivors: Living with cancer.* New York, NY: Harper & Row.

Singer, P. A., Martin, D. K., & Kelner, M. (1999). Quality end-of-life care: Patients' perspectives. *Journal of the American Medical Association, 28*(2), 163–168. https://doi.org/10.1001/jama.281.2.163

Singer, S., Danker, H., Guntinas-Lichius, O., Oeken, J., Pabst, F., Schock, J., … Dietz, A. (2014). Quality of life before and after total laryngectomy: Results of a multicenter prospective cohort study. *Head & Neck, 36*(3), 359–368. https://doi.org/10.1002/hed.23305

Singer, S., Langendijk, J., & Yarom, N. (2013). Assessing and improving quality of life in patients with head and neck cancer. *American Society of Clinical Oncology Educational Book*, 230–235. https://doi.org/10.1200/EdBook_AM.2013.33.e230

Smith, D. (1981). *Survival of illness.* New York, NY: Springer.

Stanton, A. L., Rowland, J. H., & Ganz, P. A. (2015). Life after diagnosis and treatment of cancer in adulthood. *The American Psychologist, 70*(2), 159–174. https://doi.org/10.1037/a0037875

Tschiesner, U., Linseisen, E., Coenen, M., Rogers, S., Harreus, U., Berghaus, A., & Cieza, A. (2009). Evaluating sequelae after head and neck cancer from the patient perspective with the help of the international classification of functioning, disability and health. *European Archives of Oto-Rhino-Laryngology, 266*(3), 425–436.

Ueda, S., & Okawa, Y. (2003). The subjective dimension of functioning and disability: What is it and what is it for? *Disability and Rehabilitation, 25*(11–12), 596–601.

Vartanian, J. G., Rogers, S. N., & Kowalski, L. P. (2017). How to evaluate and assess quality of life issues in head and neck cancer patients. *Current Opinion in Oncology, 29*, 159–165. https://doi.org/10.1097/CCO.0000000000000369

Ware, J. E., Jr., Kosinski, M., Bayliss, M. S., McHorney, C. A., Rogers, W. H., & Raczek, A. (1995). Comparison of methods for the scoring and statistical analysis of SF-36 health profile and summary measures: Summary of results from the medical outcomes study. *Medical Care, 33*, AS264–AS279.

Wells, M., Semple, C. J., & Lane, C. (2015). A national survey of healthcare professionals' views on models of follow-up, holistic needs assessment and survivorship care for patients with head and neck cancer. *European Journal of Cancer Care, 24*(6), 873–883.

World Health Organization. (1997). *WHOQOL: Measuring quality of life.* Retrieved from http://www.who.int/mental_health/media/68.pdf

The Impact of Postlaryngectomy Audiovisual Changes on Verbal Communication

28

Paul M. Evitts

Introduction

There is a long and rich history of research on the effects of surgical treatment for laryngeal cancer dating back nearly 70 years. While much of this literature has focused on the changes associated with the speaker and the resultant acoustic signal, there is a subset of research which has been devoted to the impact of the newly acquired post-laryngectomy voice on the listener. Considering that communication involves both a speaker and a listener, the inclusion of this component is clearly warranted. The purpose of this chapter seeks to provide a structured overview of the impact of alaryngeal speech on the listener with particular attention directed toward the influence of audiovisual information.

Following a laryngectomy, there are marked changes in both auditory and visual information. Voicing is no longer accomplished through vibration of the vocal folds, and the new vibratory source, either mechanically or surgically created, results in a disordered acoustic signal. The acoustic change associated with alaryngeal voice and speech is easily recognized by the listener. Visual

changes include alterations to the face and neck due to surgery, as well as the presence of different hand movements required for speech production. Considering that a significant amount of communication takes place in person, it is imperative for all those involved to have an awareness and genuine understanding of the impact that the surgical treatment of laryngeal cancer will have on communication. This increased understanding should be shared by the person with the laryngectomy, his/her spouse or caregiver, as well as related health-care professionals.

Acoustic Changes Associated with Alaryngeal Speech

As discussed in additional detail elsewhere in this text, there are primarily three communication options available to replace the loss of normal voice following total laryngectomy. Briefly, electrolaryngeal (EL) speech involves a mechanical, vibrating device which is can either be held to the neck/face or have the mechanical vibration sent inside the oral cavity via an intraoral device. This vibration can then be "shaped" into sounds using the articulators (Nagle, Chap. 9; Salmon, 1999). Esophageal (ES) speech production requires the speaker to move air from the oral cavity into the esophagus and then return that air back into the oral cavity, thus, setting the newly created pharyngoesophageal segment (PES) into vibration (Doyle & Finchem, Chap. 10; Duguay,

P. M. Evitts (✉)
Department of Audiology, Speech-Language Pathology, & Deaf Studies, Towson University, Towson, MD, USA

Department of Otolaryngology – Head and Neck Surgery, Johns Hopkins School of Medicine, Baltimore, MD, USA
e-mail: pevitts@towson.edu

© Springer Nature Switzerland AG 2019
P. C. Doyle (ed.), *Clinical Care and Rehabilitation in Head and Neck Cancer*,
https://doi.org/10.1007/978-3-030-04702-3_28

1989). The PES consists of blended muscle fibers from the inferior pharyngeal constrictor, the upper esophageal sphincter, and the cricopharyngeus (Diedrich, 1991). Lastly, tracheoesophageal (TE) speech is a surgical-prosthetic method of alaryngeal speech that involves the speaker redirecting pulmonary airflow through a one-way TE puncture voice prosthesis, thus setting the newly created PES into vibration (Graville, Palmer & Bolognone, Chap. 11; Knott, Chap. 12; Singer & Blom, 1980; Wetmore, Krueger, & Wesson, 1981). In addition to the use of a different vibratory source (external mechanical with EL speech and the internal biological PES with ES and TE), there are also significant alterations to the vocal tract following total laryngectomy (e.g., Liao, 2016; Searl & Evitts, 2004). These changes to both the voicing source and the filter (i.e., the vocal tract) result in marked acoustic changes across modes of alaryngeal speech resulting in a disordered acoustic signal (e.g., Globlek, Stajner-Katusic, Musura, Horga, & Liker, 2004; Liao, 2016; Robbins, Fisher, Blom, & Singer, 1984). Aside from the impact on the acoustic signal, these fundamental changes to the vibratory source and vocal tract following a total laryngectomy are also associated with visual changes during communication.

Visual Changes Associated with Alaryngeal Speech

Postlaryngectomy visual changes may be related to either the surgery itself or with the particular method of alaryngeal speech production that a given speaker uses. As a result of surgery, inherent changes across modes of alaryngeal speech will include reduction of vocal tract volume (Liao, 2016; Searl & Evitts, 2004), potential scarring of neck or orofacial region, and the presence of a permanent tracheostoma. While not as overt, changes in respiratory patterns associated with speech production following total laryngectomy may also be present (e.g., Bohnenkamp, Chap. 7; Bohnenkamp, Stowell, Hesse, & Wright, 2010; Lewis, Chap. 8; Stepp, Heaton, & Hillman, 2008), and potentially these

changes will be visible to the listener.[1] Changes to the "rhythmically organized" respiratory patterns (Warner, 1979) may, in part, contribute to a disruption in the flow of communication for persons with a laryngectomy.

The presence of a permanent tracheostoma following total laryngectomy warrants special attention due to its impact on quality of life. Numerous studies have shown individuals with a laryngectomy identify the "stoma" or factors related to the tracheostoma (e.g., daily sputum production, coughing, need for forced expectoration) as having a significant impact on their quality of life (e.g., De Santo, Olsen, Perry, Rohe, & Keith, 1995; Hilgers, Ackerstaff, Aaronson, Schouwenburg, & Van Zandwijk, 1990). More specific to voicing and communication, Weinstein, El-Sawy, Ruiz, et al. (2001) attributed increased "voice-related quality of life" scores for persons who underwent conservation surgery[2] to their lack of a tracheostoma. Similarly, Evitts, Kasapoglu, Demerici, and Miller (2011) used a quality of life (QOL) assessment specifically designed for persons with a laryngectomy (Self-Evaluation of Communication Experiences after Laryngeal Cancer [SECEL], Blood, 1993) and found improved communication adjustment (i.e., how well the person "feels they have adjusted to their new voice") for those persons who underwent conservation surgery relative to those who received a total laryngectomy. This improved adjustment was attributed to the lack of a permanent tracheostoma and preserved laryngeal tissue. Thus, aside from the overt visual impact on the listener, the presence of a tracheostoma clearly has a substantial overall impact on the

---

[1]Research on the respiratory patterns of healthy individuals shows that communication partners are in synchrony with their communication partner (e.g., McFarland, 2001). That is, inspiratory and expiratory patterns follow a predictable pattern based on linguistic and pragmatic factors. It is plausible that these respiratory patterns are visible to the listener, either implicitly or explicitly.

[2]Conservation surgery (e.g., supracricoid laryngectomy, supraglottic laryngectomy, vertical partial laryngectomy) includes only the partial removal of laryngeal structures with the primary purpose to preserve swallowing and vocal functions without the need for a permanent tracheostoma (Kempster, 2005).

person with the laryngectomy by interfering with such basic physical functions as respiration, voicing, eating, and deglutition. Furthermore, the presence of the stoma may act as a visual distractor to the listener (Evitts & Gallop, 2011), thus, negatively impacting communication.

Additional visual changes for individuals who use an EL include the presence of a highly visible, vibrating, mechanical device which is typically held on the neck or face, the potential presence of a tube from an intraoral EL device placed in the person's oral cavity, and hand movements associated with placement of the device. In contrast, the most salient changes for individuals who use ES include orofacial movements associated with the movement of air into the esophagus (see Doyle, 1994). Rather than pulmonary airflow driving vocal fold vibration during typical, laryngeal speech, ES requires air to be moved into the esophagus from the oral cavity which then sets the PES into vibration. To accomplish this movement of air, there are three main methods: inhalation, tongue injection, and glossopharyngeal press (Doyle & Finchem, Chap. 10; Travis, 1957; Snidecor, 1962). While the inhalation method does not typically require muscular contractions of the facial region, both the tongue injection and the glossopharyngeal press require such contractions of the neck, face, and mouth.

Visual changes for TE speech include hand movements and, in some instances, digital occlusion of the tracheostoma to redirect airflow from the airway into the TE prosthesis during speech production.[3] Regardless of the mode of alaryngeal speech, other visual changes associated with total laryngectomy may also include peripheral equipment such as heat and moisture exchangers (HMEs) and adhesive housings, among others (Lewis, Chap. 8). While not directly related to speech production, these optional pieces of airway equipment have been shown to result in improved QOL (e.g., Hilgers et al., 1990; Quail et al., 2016). Thus, for many people with a laryn-

gectomy, the use of these devices is an important and required in addition to their daily routine. As noted earlier, visual changes for a person with a laryngectomy are frequently a result of the surgical procedure which will substantially alter regions of the neck and potentially one's facial appearance. However, many of the changes in visual information are also attributable to speech production itself.

Speech-Related Visual Changes

In addition to those visual changes noted previously, there are also other inherent visual changes associated with a total laryngectomy. These changes to the visual information a listener receives are unrelated to the surgery itself or associated treatment but rather may be associated with the speech production process. For example, common nonverbal behaviors may include facial grimacing, squinting, erratic head movements, and loss of eye contact. Graham (1997) astutely notes that when the laryngectomee appears relaxed and free from these behaviors, the listener is more likely "to attend to *what* the laryngectomee is saying rather than to *how* he or she is saying it" (p. 122).

In general, all methods of alaryngeal speech are marked by reduced and variable levels of speech intelligibility. For this reason, individuals with a laryngectomy are commonly instructed to use compensatory strategies to improve the quality of the acoustic speech signal for the listener, thereby, improving communication. One of these common strategies to address the reduction in speech intelligibility is the use of "clear speech" (Krause & Braida, 2002; Picheny, Durlach, & Braida, 1985, 1986; Smiljanić & Bradlow, 2009; Uchanski, 2005).

Clear speech is commonly employed by a speaker in order to increase listener understanding, and this approach represents a popular therapeutic method to increase speech intelligibility in both typical, healthy and disordered speakers and with people with hearing impairments (e.g., Dromey, 2000; Ferguson, 2012; Hustad & Weismer, 2007). Aside from the acoustic changes

---

[3]Please note that while hands-free tracheoesophageal valves are available, the most common form of tracheoesophageal voicing is with digital occlusion (Evitts et al., 2010).

associated with clear speech relative to conversational communication (Ferguson & Kewley-Port, 2007; Smiljanić & Bradlow, 2009; Uchanski, 2005), there are also potential changes to the visual information presented to the listener.

For instance, clear speech typically involves volitional efforts to increase articulatory precision on the part of the speaker, which is in turn associated with increased oral air pressures and articulatory contact pressures. Specific to alaryngeal speakers, Searl (2002) adds that those speakers who produce perceptually accurate phonemes generate significantly higher oral air pressures than laryngeal speakers. Increased pressures during clear speech have been shown in both typical, laryngeal (Searl & Evitts, 2012) and TE (Searl, 2002) speakers; these changes have also been suggested by Doyle, Danhauer, and Reed (1988) to result in differential intelligibility profiles between esophageal and TE speech modes. Even without the directed goal of clear speech, accurate production of various sound classes (i.e., obstruents) requires strong articulatory contacts (Graham, 1997). To the listener, the corresponding visual effect of this would be the observation of longer and more pronounced lip and tongue movements, thus, adding to the potential visual benefit of clear speech. Alternatively, since these prolonged articulatory movements are not routinely used during typical conversation, they may act as a visual distractor to the listener and be counter to the original intended purpose of improving intelligibility. Thus, attempts to clarify speech may result in overall reductions to communication due to the visual changes that may emerge.

Alaryngeal Speech and the Listener

The information presented up to this point has primarily focused on visual and acoustic changes from the speakers' perspective. However, since communication requires a speaker *and* a listener, it is also important to consider the impact of all of the changes following treatment for laryngeal cancer on the listener specifically. In a model depicting factors related to speech intelligibility

for speakers with dysarthria, Yorkston, Strand, and Kennedy (1996) identified various factors which influence the acoustic signal, thus, altering the information available to the listener (see Fig. 28.1). This model also can be applied to all methods of alaryngeal speech as there are not only negative influences on the acoustic signal, but alaryngeal speakers also use compensatory strategies in an effort to enhance the acoustic signal. In fact, much of therapy to enhance speech intelligibility for alaryngeal speakers often focuses on employing those compensatory strategies of reduced rate and increased articulatory precision (i.e., clear speech).

As noted, central to Fig. 28.1 is the concept that communication involves both a speaker and a listener and both have been investigated in the alaryngeal speech literature using various outcome measures. The following section provides a brief review of frequently used outcome measures, including reaction times, speech intelligibility, listener comprehension, speech acceptability, voice quality, and listener attitudes. These specific measures are also discussed in relation to Fig. 28.1, along with proposed changes to the model in order to provide additional insight into the nature of alaryngeal speech processing.

Reaction Time

In their original model of factors which may influence speech intelligibility, Yorkston and colleagues (1996) showed that there is an area labeled "listener processing" (see Fig. 28.1). While not explored in the context of the original article, this area on the figure implies that the listener is utilizing cognitive-perceptual processes to decode the disordered acoustic signal (Liss, Spitzer, Caviness, & Adler, 2002). That is, these cognitive-perceptual strategies are the processes used by the listener to decode and analyze the incoming speech signal, as well as including the amount of cognitive effort required by the listener to process spoken information (Liss et al., 2002). Thus, the demand placed on a listener in the context of less-than-intelligible speech cannot be disregarded. If a speech signal is degraded,

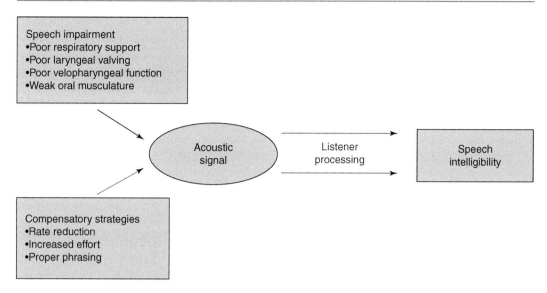

Fig. 28.1 A model of factors that contribute to comprehensibility of speakers with dysarthria. Adapted with permission from Yorkston et al. (1996). Copyright by the American Speech-Language-Hearing Association

a listener will need to attend in a more focused and demanding manner which can detract from the efficiency of communication.

Furthermore, these processes then provide the foundation for the listener to extract both phonetic units (i.e., elements of intelligibility) and ultimately derive the overall meaning (i.e., comprehension) of the spoken signal. Results obtained from a series of studies from the dysarthria literature (Liss, Spitzer, Caviness, Adler, & Edwards, 1998, 2000; Liss et al., 2002) suggest that manipulating features of the listener rather than that of the speaker or the signal can influence how the signal is processed (Evitts & Searl, 2006). Ironically, while the laryngeal and alaryngeal voice and speech disorder literature is replete with studies on speech intelligibility, there is a dearth of information on *how* listeners process the resultant disordered signal. This is especially pertinent from a therapeutic perspective as it provides an evidence-based foundation for either training or educating the listener on strategies to improve the perception of a disordered signal. The construct of "listener processing," therefore, provides a rich area of research that has yet to be fully cultivated in the alaryngeal literature.

Evitts and Searl (2006) explored reaction times to investigate the cognitive effort or workload required by typical, healthy listeners when presented with different modes of alaryngeal speech. Cognitive workload here was defined as the amount of mental demand placed on the listener during an activity (Pass, Tuovinen, Tabbers, & Gerven, 2003). Results showed that listeners required significantly more cognitive workload when presented with ES, EL, and synthetic speech, and no difference in cognitive workload demand for comparisons between typical laryngeal and TE speech (Evitts & Searl, 2006). Overall, results mirror numerous studies which have found TE speech to be more similar to laryngeal speech in intelligibility and acceptability (e.g., Clark & Stemple, 1982; Most, Tobin, & Mimran, 2000; Robbins et al., 1984; Yiu, van Hasselt, Williams, & Woo, 1994). These results in part may have been observed because TE speech places the least amount of demand (cognitive workload) from the listener, while both ES and EL speech require relatively more demand or effort from the listener (Evitts & Searl, 2006). In comparison to laryngeal speakers, recent results suggest that the amount of cognitive workload required to process ES speech is similar to the amount required to process dysphonic voices (Evitts et al., 2016).

Similar to cognitive workload, the amount of "effort" required on the part of the listener to process alaryngeal speech has also been investigated. Listener effort has been defined as the amount of attention required to process speech (Downs, 1982; Feuerstein, 1992; Hicks & Tharpe, 2002). In this context, listener effort may be considered the subjective correlate to the objective measure of cognitive workload as listeners rate the amount of effort required to process various speech stimuli (Nagle & Eadie, 2012). To provide insight into this concept, Nagle and Eadie (2012) presented speech stimuli from 14 highly intelligible TE speakers and asked 20 listeners to rate the amount of effort required to process the signal, as well as to rate the acceptability of the stimuli. Results showed a strong correlation between listener ratings of speech acceptability and listener effort (Nagle & Eadie, 2012). Since the TE speakers used in the study were all highly intelligible and there was a large variation in ratings for both effort and acceptability, the overall results endorse the notion that intelligibility is a separate and distinct construct from that of listener effort and speech acceptability (Nagle & Eadie, 2012; Shipp, 1967).

Interestingly, Nagle and Eadie (2012) also highlighted the fact that neither their study nor the earlier findings of the Evitts and Searl (2006) study included the effect of visual information on either cognitive workload or listener effort. While the author is not aware of any published research within the alaryngeal literature, there is research from the speech perception literature which may shed further light on the relationship between visual information and cognitive workload. For example, Fraser, Gagné, Alepins, and Dubois (2010) investigated the impact of audiovisual information as compared to audio-only information on listener effort and reaction times in healthy, young adults. To adjust the amount of listener effort, Fraser et al. used different signal-to-noise ratios (SNR). Results showed that while speech recognition scores were more accurate when listeners were presented with audiovisual information, reaction times were significantly slower in the audiovisual condition regardless of the SNR (Fraser et al., 2010).

Similarly, Alsius, Navarra, Campbell, and Soto-Faraco (2005) investigated audiovisual integration of facial gestures and vocal sounds under different attentional loads by using a dual-task paradigm which requires the listener to attend to two different tasks, thus serving to increase attentional load. Results showed that visual information had a reduced influence on auditory information when the attentional load was increased, a finding that led the authors to conclude that integration of audio and visual information is subject to attentional demands placed on the listener.

Taken together, the findings from Alsius et al. (2005) and Fraser et al. (2010) suggest that as a result of the degraded acoustic signal and the altered visual information, listeners are required to use greater cognitive workload and effort. Since listeners tend to recruit more visual information from the speaker when presented with a degraded auditory stimulus (Keintz, Bunton, & Hoit, 2007), it then creates an additional burden for processing the alaryngeal voice and speech signal. Furthermore, an added confounding variable is that the median age of persons diagnosed with laryngeal cancer is 65 years (SEER, 2017). Considering that nearly 40% of persons aged 60–69 years have some level of hearing impairment (Hoffmann, Dobie, Losonczy, Themann, & Flamme, 2017) and that older persons have been shown to experience greater listener effort (e.g., Gosselin & Gagné, 2011; Desjardins & Doherty, 2013), alaryngeal speakers may be at an additional communication disadvantage due to the age of their peer group.

Overall, the negative effects that occur with interaction between audio and visual information along with increased cognitive demands placed on the listener may result in listeners choosing to either not engage in or at the least minimize communication with a person with a laryngectomy due to the increased burden they confront (Nagle & Eadie, 2012). In a related study, 31% of partners of persons with a laryngectomy reported reduced social interactions, and 51% of those partners expressed frustration that others would speak to the non-laryngectomized partner instead (Offermann, Pruyn, de Boer, Busschbach, &

Baatenburg de Jong, 2015). Evidence of reduced communication capacity from the speakers' perspective has been provided by Evitts et al. (2011) who reported that 64% of persons with a laryngectomy spoke less after their surgery compared to only 2% who reportedly spoke more. In sum, there is a plethora of research as well as anecdotal evidence suggesting that a laryngectomy has a negative impact in the realm of social interaction for both the person with the laryngectomy as well as their communicative partner(s). While multifaceted, reduced speech intelligibility also may be a contributing factor for this reduced social interaction. Thus, the complexity of challenges related to the alaryngeal speaker and his/her communicative partner(s) are substantial.

Speech Intelligibility

Speech intelligibility is perhaps the most frequently used outcome measure in the disordered speech literature, including a relatively large body of research on the intelligibility of alaryngeal speech. While numerous definitions exist, speech intelligibility is generally defined as the ability of a listener to recover a speaker's intended message based on the acoustic signal (Hustad, 2008; Kent, Weismer, Kent, & Rosenbek, 1989; Yorkston & Beukelman, 1980; Yorkston et al., 1996; and others). Indices of speech intelligibility are useful as they serve as an "index of the severity of the overall functional limitation" (Yorkston, Beukelman, Strand, Bell, & Hustad, 1999, p. 237). That is, the inability to accurately decipher a speaker's message will have a direct influence on communication interactions.

Although there is much debate surrounding the most appropriate measurement method (e.g., Kent, Miolo, & Bloedel, 1994), speech intelligibility is generally assessed by presenting words or sentences to a listener or group of listeners and calculating the number of orthographic transcription errors. The resultant score then speaks to the adequacy of the acoustic speech signal (Hustad & Beukelman, 2002). With regard to alaryngeal speech, the acoustic signal has been shown to be significantly different than laryngeal speech in

multiple acoustic parameters, including jitter, shimmer, intensity, formant values, and range of fundamental frequency (e.g., Ng & Chu, 2009; Robbins, 1984; Robbins et al., 1984). Therefore, it is not surprising that these marked acoustic differences contribute to a degraded signal which may subsequently impact overall speech intelligibility.

In fact, existing research has consistently shown that alaryngeal speakers who use an alternate form of postlaryngectomy voice (i.e., TE, ES, or EL) always demonstrate some level of reduced intelligibility (e.g., Cullinan, Brown, & Blalock, 1986; Doyle et al., 1988; McCroskey & Mulligan, 1963; Merwin, Goldstein, & Rothman, 1985; Most et al., 2000; Yiu et al., 1994). While a more complete discussion of alaryngeal speech intelligibility is explored elsewhere (see Doyle & Sleeth, Chap. 14), a summary is provided here with particular attention directed to the impact of audiovisual information. The inclusion of audiovisual information when assessing speech intelligibility is important as it is likely to more closely reflect typical day-to-day conversation and the interaction between a speaker and a listener. Thus, the inclusion of audiovisual information in research leads to increased ecological validity and may provide a more accurate measure of the speakers' ability to convey their intended message.

There is a large body of research demonstrating the positive effects of audiovisual information on speech perception in both typical, laryngeal speakers (e.g., Sumby & Pollack, 1954; Davis & Kim, 2004; Helfer, 1997; Rudner, Mishra, Stenfelt, Lunner, & Rönnberg, 2016) and for disordered speakers (e.g., Borrie, 2015; Garcia & Cannito, 1996; Garcia & Daegenais, 1998; Hustad, 2006; Hustad & Beukelman, 2001; Munhall, Jones, Callan, Kuratate, & Vatikiotis-Bateson, 2004). The most frequent explanation for this observed improvement is the fact that as an acoustic signal becomes more degraded, listeners will rely more on visual information during speech perception tasks (Sumby & Pollack, 1954; Sanders & Goodrich, 1971). This active perceptual process also has been supported by neuroimaging data showing increased cortical activation when an individual is presented with increasingly degraded acoustic stimuli (Kawase et al., 2005).

Since alaryngeal speech has been shown to be markedly different from typical, laryngeal speech in multiple areas including acoustics (e.g., Robbins, 1984; Robbins et al., 1984), aerodynamics (e.g., Searl & Evitts, 2004), and contact pressures (e.g., Searl, 2007), it should be no surprise that alaryngeal speech intelligibility also has been shown to benefit from visual information. Knox and Anneberg (1973) showed improved speech intelligibility of EL speech following video training for both naïve and experienced listeners. Similarly, Berry and Knight (1975) showed improved subjective ratings of listeners' impressions of speech intelligibility in the audiovisual mode for ES speakers. Finally, Hubbard and Kushner (1980) compared good-to-superior ES speech with typical, laryngeal speech in three different conditions (visual-only, auditory-only, and combined audiovisual) and showed improved intelligibility scores for the ES speakers during audiovisual mode of presentation. These results are consistent with those of other studies using healthy, laryngeal speakers (e.g., Davis & Kim, 2004; Helfer, 1997; Sumby & Pollack, 1954), as well as disordered speakers (e.g., Garcia & Cannito, 1996; Garcia & Daegenais, 1998; Hustad & Beukelman, 2001). These combined findings serve to highlight the beneficial impact of audiovisual information on speech intelligibility.

Such observed improvements in speech intelligibility noted previously provide support for an adapted version of the Yorkston et al. (1996) original model of factors with disordered speakers (see Fig. 28.2). That is, when provided with an adequate acoustic signal, listeners do not need to rely on additional cues (e.g., visual, linguistic, contextual) in order to accurately process the signal. However, when presented with a degraded auditory signal, listeners need to actively recruit additional cognitive-perceptual processes (Liss et al., 1998, 2000) which may result in increased cognitive workload (Munro & Derwing, 1995; Evitts & Searl, 2006) and/or increased listener effort (Fraser et al., 2010; Nagle & Eadie, 2012).

The adapted model, however, also suggests that the visual information being used by the listener may either be of positive or negative value (Fig. 28.2). Clearly, previous studies showing improved speech intelligibility would suggest that the additional visual information positively augmented the acoustic signal (Davis & Kim, 2004; Garcia & Cannito, 1996; Garcia & Daegenais, 1998; Helfer, 1997; Hustad & Beukelman, 2001; Sumby & Pollack, 1954). Conversely, there is research to suggest that visual information may distort the acoustic signal or potentially distract the listener. The classic example of this negative interaction between auditory and visual information is demonstrated by what is termed the McGurk effect (McGurk & MacDonald, 1976). For this, a listener is presented with an auditory stimulus (e.g., /ga/) paired with an incongruent visual stimulus (e.g., /ba/). This results in a distortion of the auditory signal where listeners either hear a combination token (/bga/) or a fusion token (/da/) (McGurk & MacDonald, 1976). This effect has been proven to be robust across numerous populations and in multiple experimental designs (e.g., Massaro, 1998; Munhall, Gribble, Sacco, & Ward, 1996; Norrix, Plante, Vance, & Boliek, 2007). Overall, these results provide evidence that visual information clearly has the capacity to influence a listeners' perception of an incoming acoustic signal.

In addition to the previously noted influences on listener perception, there is research from the dysarthric and hearing-impaired literature demonstrating either a negative or neutral impact of audiovisual information on speech intelligibility (e.g., Brentari & Wolk, 1986; Garcia & Cannito, 1996; Nelson & Hodge, 2000; Hustad & Cahill, 2003; Keintz et al., 2007; Yi, Phelps, Smiljanic, & Chandrasekaran, 2013). In an attempt to explain this apparent negative impact of audiovisual information on speech intelligibility, it has been suggested that speakers with high baseline intelligibility only receive minimal benefit from the inclusion of audiovisual information (Hustad & Cahill, 2003; Keintz et al., 2007). In fact, Keintz et al. (2007) proposed a possible "ceiling effect" where highly intelligible speakers (>88%)

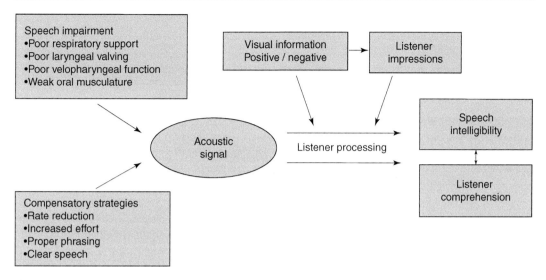

Fig. 28.2 A proposed model of factors that impact intelligibility and listener comprehension of alaryngeal speech. Adapted with permission from Yorkston et al. (1996). Copyright by the American Speech-Language-Hearing Association

may not benefit from the inclusion of audiovisual cues. Thus, while alaryngeal speakers with reduced speech intelligibility may directly benefit from audiovisual information, this beneficial effect may elude highly proficient alaryngeal speakers. Thus, the relative advantages of audiovisual cues for alaryngeal speech remain in question.

There is also limited evidence from the alaryngeal speech literature which suggests that the inclusion of audiovisual information may have a deleterious effect on speech intelligibility. For example, while overall results from Hubbard and Kushner's (1980) study showed a positive benefit from access to audiovisual information, three ES speakers in that study actually experienced small decreases in speech intelligibility in the audiovisual mode. Hubbard and Kushner (1980) posited the extraneous facial movements associated with the injection of air required for ES speech, may have served in some manner to distract the listeners. Furthermore, Evitts, Cohen, and Wysokinski (2007) investigated viseme recognition by presenting video-only recordings of highly intelligible alaryngeal and laryngeal speakers to a group of 33 young, healthy listeners. Results showed that when presented with syllables from these alaryngeal speakers, listeners had higher accuracy

scores with more visible phonemes (i.e., bilabial, labiodental) but decreased accuracy with less visible phonemes (i.e., alveolar, linguapalatal) compared to the laryngeal speakers (Evitts, Cohen, & Wysokinski, 2007).

Finally, Evitts and colleagues (2009) investigated the speech intelligibility of all three modes of alaryngeal speech in both audio-only and audiovisual modes of presentation and showed a small but significant 3% increase in intelligibility across modes for the audiovisual condition. However, the only significant increase within mode of speech was observed for the EL speaker who experienced a 10% increase in intelligibility from a baseline level of 71%. In fact, the ES speaker included in this study actually experienced a small decrease in intelligibility in the audiovisual mode. Since the ES speaker had a high baseline intelligibility, this may have been related to the ceiling effect mentioned earlier (Keintz et al., 2007). Alternatively, the observed decrease may have been related to the extraneous facial movements associated with superior ES speech production (Evitts, Portugal, Van Dine, & Holler, 2010) which was visible to the listeners in the audiovisual condition.

In summary, there is an abundance of literature from a variety of disciplines demonstrating the benefit of audiovisual information on speech intelligibility. While the limited results available from alaryngeal speakers appear to be similar, it is important to note that this positive impact on speech intelligibility as a result of the added visual information may not apply to all alaryngeal speakers. Specifically, the facial movements required to inject air into the esophagus for ES production may actually distract the listener and negatively impact a speakers' intelligibility. The auditory analog of this air injection was labeled "klunking" by Shanks (1977). When this "klunking" is paired with the extraneous facial movements, the result may be both a visual and auditory distractor to the listener (Hyman, 1979). Furthermore, it is plausible that any compensatory articulatory movements (e.g., use of clear speech) or other auditory or visual differences that the listener may find salient may actually override perception of the acoustic stimulus even when that acoustic signal is not degraded (Kent, 1996). Clearly, more research is needed to better elucidate the impact of visual information on alaryngeal speech intelligibility across different modes of alaryngeal speech, as well as across different levels of speaking proficiency.

Listener Comprehension

The third objective outcome measure used in the speech disorder literature pertains to listener comprehension. While speech intelligibility refers to the ability of a listener to retrieve a speakers' intended message from an acoustic signal (e.g., Hustad, 2008), listener comprehension measures a listeners' ability to acquire the overall meaning of a speakers' intended message. However, this retrieval of the message may not be dependent on accurate perception of phonetic or lexical elements (Hustad & Beukelman, 2002). One could argue that listener comprehension involves a much more dynamic process whereby listeners utilize any and all available cues, including visual, contextual, and/or shared knowledge with the speaker, to arrive at the gist of the speakers' intended message (Hustad, 2008; Miller & Selfridge, 1950). Consequently, speech intelligi-

bility may require greater cognitive workload or effort on the part of the listener. This increase may be required in order to accurately retrieve individual phonetic units, rather than using all available cues (e.g., contextual, shared knowledge) in order to "comprehend" the signal (Evitts et al., 2016).

In the adapted version of Yorkston and colleagues' model of speech perception (Fig. 28.2), listener comprehension is not solely an extension of speech intelligibility, but rather it is complementary in nature and may not necessarily require adequate speech intelligibility (Hustad, 2008). In fact, both Hustad and Beukelman (2002) and Evitts et al. (2016) reported a weak and nonsignificant relationship between the two providing further support for the proposal that intelligibility and listener comprehension "tap into different phenomenon" (Hustad, 2008).

The distinction between speech intelligibility and listener comprehension is important as it is well established that persons who undergo laryngectomy and use alaryngeal speech experience reduced intelligibility (e.g., Cullinan et al., 1986; McCroskey & Mulligan, 1963; Merwin et al., 1985; Most et al., 2000; Yiu et al., 1994). However, a review of the literature suggests that there is not any explicit research on listener comprehension and alaryngeal speech. However, information from related studies shows that listeners have demonstrated reduced comprehension when presented with speech stimuli from speakers who have dysarthria (e.g., Hustad & Beukelman, 2008; Hustad, 2008), dysphonia (Morton & Watson, 2001; Lyberg-Åhlander, Haake, Brännström, Schötz, & Sahlén, 2015), or those speakers with a foreign accent (Wilson & Spaulding, 2010).

For example, Wilson and Spaulding (2010) compared listener comprehension scores for native and Korean-accented speech that was presented with increased levels of background noise. Their results showed a 3% decrease in listener comprehension scores for native speech but a 34% decrease in comprehension scores with foreign-accented speech. This suggests that listeners' cognitive workload may be operating at a maximum when presented with a different or disordered acoustic signal and when further taxed (e.g., with increased background noise), the system falters.

Although there is no direct research on alaryngeal speech and listener comprehension, evidence from the speech intelligibility and reaction time literature may provide some insights relative to the potential impact. For example, when presented with moderately intelligible foreign-accented speech, listeners have been shown to exhibit significantly longer reaction times than when presented with both highly intelligible foreign-accented speech and native speech (Wilson & Spaulding, 2010). As described previously, alaryngeal speech also has been repeatedly shown to result in reduced speech intelligibility relative to typical, laryngeal speech (e.g., Merwin et al., 1985; Most et al., 2000; Yiu et al., 1994). Furthermore, listeners have been shown to have significantly longer reaction times with both ES and EL speech relative to typical, laryngeal speech (Evitts & Searl, 2006); this finding would indicate that a greater cognitive workload or that additional time must be devoted by the listener to processing these unique speech signals. Based on these findings, it is reasonable to conclude that listeners will have increasing difficulty extracting the overall message (comprehension) from an alaryngeal speaker and, in particular, from those speakers who are less proficient in their speech production.

Alternatively, Evitts and colleagues (2016) presented healthy listeners with dysphonic voices and reported increased cognitive workload (i.e., longer reaction times) and decreased speech intelligibility for those speakers with dysphonia. However, there were no significant differences in the listeners' ability to comprehend the overall message. This finding led Evitts et al. to suggest that while listeners may have difficulty processing the individual phonetic segments required in an intelligibility task (i.e., transcription), listener comprehension may not be affected due to the additional processing time and subsequent increased cognitive workload dedicated to the incoming message. This suggests a trade-off between intelligibility and comprehension; that is, rather than dedicating cognitive resources to identifying individual phonetic components, additional listener effort is recruited to arrive at the overall meaning of the signal as evidenced by longer reaction times. While this suggestion is based on exposure to dysphonic voices, similar results may be observed with alaryngeal speakers.

Given the degraded acoustic nature of alaryngeal speech, it is conceivable that listeners may have more difficulty with intelligibility as compared to comprehension. Increases in cognitive workload are then dedicated to comprehension at the expense of intelligibility. Ideally, future research on alaryngeal speech and listener comprehension would demonstrate that regardless of the reduced speech intelligibility, alaryngeal speakers are still able to successfully convey their overall message to their audience.

Listeners' Impressions of Paralinguistic Information

To this point, the content of this chapter has primarily focused on the impact of alaryngeal speech on the listener by using objective measures (i.e., reaction times, speech intelligibility, listener comprehension). However, the use of subjective measures to determine how the altered speech signal and visual information is perceived by the listener is also vitally important. In fact, in addition to processing linguistic information, listeners also make numerous perceptual judgments regarding the acceptability of the voice, the identity, and emotional state of the speaker, among other characteristics (Belin, Zatorre, & Ahad, 2002; Nusbaum, Schwab, & Pisoni, 1984). These judgments are sometimes referred to as "paralinguistic" and are processed by the listener in a parallel fashion along with the linguistic information. Evidence for this dual processing is provided by neuroimaging data showing that following initial processing by the primary auditory cortex, numerous other parts of the brain, bilaterally, are activated (Mummery, Ashburner, Scott, & Wise, 1999; Thivard, Belin, Zilbovicius, Poline, & Samson, 2000; Belin et al., 2002).

Depending on the nature of the signal, the additional processing of this paralinguistic information may lead to increased cognitive workload for the listener. Figure 28.2 depicts the potential influence of the inclusion of this paralinguistic information (listener impressions), its proposed influence on cognitive workload (listener processing), and its subsequent influence on both speech intelligibility and listener comprehension. For example, the auditory and visual signal sent to a listener from a person with a laryngectomy is marked by a degraded acoustic stimulus, altered paralinguistic information, and different visual characteristics. It is, therefore, reasonable to deduce that those features influence the listeners' ability to process the signal. As a result, the ability of the listener to extract the specific phonemes (intelligibility) or the overall, intended message of the speaker (comprehension) may be impacted. While more subjective in nature, paralinguistic information is an essential component of efficient verbal communication.

As depicted in Fig. 28.2, paralinguistic information may have a substantial influence on the processing of an alaryngeal speech signal. The importance of this paralinguistic information and its impact on the listener is evidenced by the substantial body of research into alaryngeal speech. Two of the more popular subjective outcome measures of paralinguistic information include listeners' impressions of speech acceptability and voice quality. To address these issues, researchers typically present running speech stimuli to the listener and ask them to record their subjective opinion on a variety of factors. Survey instruments differ from one another, and debate exists as to which tool may be the most appropriate (e.g., Eadie & Doyle, 2002, 2005), but most methods commonly include direct magnitude estimation or equal-appearing interval rating scales. The following section contains information on three different subjective methods of investigating paralinguistic information: speech acceptability, voice quality, and listener attitudes.

Speech Acceptability Since the focus of this chapter includes the impact of audiovisual information associated with alaryngeal speech, it should be duly noted that researchers investigat-

ing listeners' attitudes and impressions of alaryngeal speakers have long recognized the importance of including visual information. This was first exemplified by Hyman (1955) who stated that additional "research is needed in testing the *visual* aspects of these two types [EL and ES] of speech, to determine whether or not listeners object to seeing the artificial-larynx and how detrimental it is to the effectiveness of the speaker" (p. 299). Hyman (1955) then provides a foundation from which future researchers can investigate its potential impact.

There are multiple studies which have addressed the potential impact of audiovisual information and alaryngeal speech. For example, Hartman and Scott (1974) observed gas station attendants during face-to-face conversation with an EL speaker. Their results showed that the attendants stared more at the EL speaker and either spoke louder or slower during the interaction. Gilmore (1974) compared the social and vocational acceptability of esophageal speakers to laryngeal speakers in three different modes of presentation, audio-only, audiovisual, and visual-only. Results consistently showed that listeners perceived the esophageal speakers as less favorable than the laryngeal speakers across modes. Results also showed that listeners had more negative perceptions of the esophageal speakers in the audiovisual mode. Gilmore noted that there is a "negative visible concomitant of esophageal speech" (p. 605), most likely those features related to facial muscular contractions, and that the reduction of such visible stigmas should be targeted in therapy. Green and Hults (1982) compared listener preferences for three types of alaryngeal speech (pneumatic aid speech, EL speech, and poor esophageal speech) and showed that the use of an EL was rated as most preferred with regard to visual appearance and that poor ES was judged by listeners to be the least preferred overall when compared to EL speech. When considered together, these studies highlight the importance of audiovisual information and provide additional support for the inclusion of visual information when investigating the impact of alaryngeal speech on listeners.

The alaryngeal speech literature also contains other studies related to the acceptability of alaryngeal speech using audio-only stimuli (e.g., Bennett & Weinberg, 1973; Trudeau, 1987; Pindzola & Cain, 1988; Finizia, Lindström, & Dotevall, 1998; Evitts, Gabel, & Searl, 2007). While not all of these studies using either the audiovisual or audio-only mode directly investigated "acceptability" per se, they do speak to some of the paralinguistic features present in the alaryngeal speech signal. As such, the data obtained provide insight into the complex, multidimensional relationship among perceptual measures observed in alaryngeal speech (Doyle & Eadie, 2005). Clearly, the differences observed via perceptual measures of alaryngeal speech relative to laryngeal speech have a significant impact on the processing of the signal by listeners and are predicated on both audio and visual information.

Furthermore, the majority of studies using either audiovisual or audio-only modes of presentation are in concert with other auditory-perceptual comparisons of the different modes of alaryngeal speech (e.g., Clark & Stemple, 1982; Doyle et al., 1988; Evitts et al., 2010; Merwin, 1985; Most et al., 2000; Cullinan et al., 1986; Shames, Font, & Matthews, 1963; Yiu et al., 1994). That is, TE speech is generally judged to be more acceptable than ES, and ES speech is generally more acceptable than EL speech. Finally, however, all modes of alaryngeal speech are frequently rated as less acceptable than typical, laryngeal speech (e.g., Pindzola & Cain, 1988). Thus, the unique features that characterize all modes of alaryngeal speech do appear to have salient perceptual consequences to the listener as evidenced by the relative consistency of these results.

Voice Quality Previous reports have consistently indicated that regardless of alaryngeal mode, listeners can still distinguish between an alaryngeal and a laryngeal speaker (Doyle & Eadie, 2005). Sadly, this difference remains even after years of advances in surgery, as well as following improvements in alaryngeal communication that have been achieved over the years, (e.g., Doyle & Eadie, 2005; Eadie, Day, Sawin, Lamvik, & Doyle, 2013). This ability to distinguish between

the two is primarily based on a speakers' voice quality. Although numerous studies exist on the voice quality of alaryngeal speech, Snidecor (1962) and Hartman (1979) stated that there is no agreed upon definition and that there are a multitude of different terms used to describe this concept. Kreiman and Gerratt (1998) have even suggested that listeners may have an unstable internal representation of perceptual voice attributes, thus, rendering their impressions of voice quality in general as being unreliable.

Regardless, the ear still provides the gold standard for voice quality assessment and "one cannot underestimate the importance of perceptually derived information" (Hartman, (1979), p. 88). As such, a brief review of the literature on alaryngeal speech voice quality generally shows that listeners perceive quality of TE speech as more favorable than ES speech and ES speech as more favorable than EL (e.g., Williams & Watson, 1987). However, there are exceptions to this general hierarchy. For instance, Ng, Kwok, and Chow (1997) found that listeners rated EL speech as more favorable than either TE or ES. In addition, Green and Hults (1982) also found that listeners preferred the voice quality of EL over ES speech. The explanation for these inconsistencies may be related to individual speaker characteristics, rather than mode of speech alone (Kalb & Carpenter, 1981).

Listener Attitudes In addition to listener impressions of acceptability and voice quality, it is also important to understand how all postlaryngectomy changes, including those that result in auditory and visual attributes, affect listeners' attitudes toward the person with the laryngectomy. In fact, there is a great deal of research from a variety of fields within communication disorders, including stuttering (e.g., Susca & Healey, 2001), voice disorders (e.g., Blood, Mahan, & Hyman, 1979), speech disorders (e.g., Lass, Ruscello, & Lakawicz, 1988; von Tiling, 2011), and in people with hearing impairment (e.g., Blood, Blood, & Danhauer, 1978). The consensus of this literature unequivocally supports the notion that listeners have less favorable impressions of a speaker who presents with a speech, hearing, or voice impairment relative to healthy speakers.

Although there is less research on the listeners' attitudes of people who have had a laryngectomy and now use an alternate form of voice, the limited research available appears to be encouraging. For example, Evitts, Gabel, and Searl (2007) used audio-only stimuli to study listeners' perceptions of the personality of male, alaryngeal speakers and reported no difference among the three modes and that overall mean judgments of personality for all modes were considered favorable. In a similar study using audiovisual information, Evitts, Van Dine, and Holler (2009) showed that listeners judged the personality of alaryngeal speakers more favorably in the audiovisual mode when compared to the audio-only mode. Those same listeners also rated the personality of the TE and EL speakers as more favorable than the ES speaker in the audiovisual mode (Evitts et al., 2009). This last finding is pertinent as it may be related to the extraneous facial movements that occur in relation to air insufflation during the production of ES as noted by Hubbard and Kushner (1980).

Regardless, the findings from Evitts et al. (2009) as well as Evitts Gabel and Searl (2007) should not detract from the large body of literature indicating that persons with a laryngectomy report significant decreases in overall quality of life, social acceptance, and social activity (e.g., Deshmane, Parikh, Pinni, Parikh, & Rao, 1995; Doyle & MacDonald, Chap. 27; Pereira da Silva et al., 2015; Relic, Mazemda, Arens, Koller, & Glanz, 2001). Additional research is, however, warranted in order to provide more insight into listeners' broad judgments of alaryngeal speakers. Similar to listener comprehension, this area represents an importance to both those with a laryngectomy and health-care professionals who seek to better understand the impact of laryngectomy on social communication.

Eye Gaze and Alaryngeal Speech Thus far, this chapter has presented extensive evidence of the impact of audiovisual information on alaryngeal speech perception. While the majority of the evidence has shown a positive benefit of the inclusion of visual information (e.g., Keintz et al., 2007; Sumby & Pollack, 1954), there have been studies to the contrary which demonstrate that the inclusion of visual information may either distort the incoming auditory signal (e.g., McGurk Effect) or may distract the listener from the incoming signal (Hustad & Cahill, 2003; Hyman, 1955; McGurk & MacDonald, 1976). However, these studies have failed to identify what specific visual features listeners found salient during speech perception. To shed light on which visual features listeners attend to during speech perception tasks, researchers have investigated the eye gaze of the listener. That is, efforts have been undertaken to determine where a listener directs their visual gaze during their monitoring of a speaker's communication. Previous investigations into the gaze of the listener used subjective data acquisition to determine a listeners' gaze (e.g., Argyle & Cook, 1976; Argyle & Dean, 1965; Mirenda, Donnellan, & Yoder, 1983). However, recent advances in eye-gaze technology have allowed researchers to precisely and objectively identify those visual features that listeners find salient during a speech perception task.

In the alaryngeal literature, there is one study to date which used eye-gaze tracking to determine which visual features listeners find salient during face-to-face interaction with an alaryngeal speaker. Evitts and Gallop (2011) had 60 participants engage in a 10-min conversation with one of four highly proficient speakers representing the three modes of alaryngeal speech and a typical, laryngeal speaker. Results showed significantly different eye-gaze patterns during conversation with an ES speaker (i.e., more gaze directed at lower face) and similar eye-gaze patterns during conversation with the TE and typical, healthy speakers (Evitts & Gallop, 2011). Such changes in gaze patterns associated with ES speech may be related to the muscular contractions and facial contortions (e.g., lip pursing, head movements, etc.) required for successful ES speech production (e.g., Doyle, 1994; Graham, 1997).

These results, coupled with previous reports of decreased speech intelligibility for ES in the audiovisual condition (e.g., Evitts et al., 2010; Ng et al., 1997) and less favorable impressions of an ES speaker in the audiovisual mode of presentation (Evitts et al., 2009), provide support for the notion that the extraneous facial movements associated with ES speech production may distract the listener (Hubbard & Kushner, 1980). In addition, results also endorse the notion that of the three alaryngeal modes of speech, listeners perceive TE speech as most similar to typical, laryngeal speech.

Summary

The overarching goal of this chapter has attempted to provide the reader with detailed information on the impact of audiovisual information associated with alaryngeal speech on the listener. Following a total laryngectomy, numerous changes to the visual scene may be present. These changes may include the presence of a tracheostoma, altered articulatory patterns, and the presence of nonverbal behaviors, among many others. Although the inclusion of visual information is generally associated with improved speech perception, alaryngeal speakers may pose a unique challenge to this refrain. That is, audiovisual information inherent with alaryngeal speech may actually *distract* the listener or distort the already challenged acoustic signal. Thus, it is imperative for those involved with alaryngeal speech rehabilitation to have a better understanding of the impact of these audiovisual changes in hopes of minimizing the potential negative impact on the listener.

References

Alsius, A., Navarra, J., Campbell, R., & Soto-Faraco, S. (2005). Audiovisual integration of speech falters under high attention demands. *Current Biology, 15,* 839–843.

Argyle, M., & Cook, M. (1976). *Gaze and mutual gaze.* New York, NY: Cambridge University Press.

Argyle, M., & Dean, J. (1965). Eye-contact, distance, and affiliation. *Sociometry, 28,* 289–304.

Belin, P., Zatorre, R. J., & Ahad, P. (2002). Human temporal-lobe response to vocal sounds. *Cognitive Brain Research, 13,* 17–26.

Bennett, S., & Weinberg, B. (1973). Acceptability ratings of normal, esophageal, and artificial larynx speech. *Journal of Speech and Hearing Research, 16,* 608–615.

Berry, R. A., & Knight, R. E. (1975). Auditory versus auditory-visual intelligibility measurements of alaryngeal speech: A preliminary report. *Perceptual and Motor Skills, 40,* 915–918.

Blood, G. W. (1993). Development and assessment of a scale addressing communication needs of patients with laryngectomies. *American Journal of Speech-Language Pathology, 2,* 82–90.

Blood, G. W., Blood, I. M., & Danhauer, J. L. (1978). Listeners' impressions of normal-hearing and hearing-impaired children. *Journal of Communication Disorders, 11,* 513–518.

Blood, G. W., Mahan, B. W., & Hyman, M. (1979). Judging personality and appearance from voice disorders. *Journal of Communication Disorders, 12,* 63–68.

Bohnenkamp, T. A., Stowell, T., Hesse, J., & Wright, S. (2010). Speech breathing in speakers who use an electrolarynx. *Journal of Communication Disorders, 43,* 199–211.

Borrie, S. A. (2015). Visual speech information: A help or hindrance in perceptual processing of dysarthric speech. *The Journal of the American Acoustical Society of America, 137,* 1473–1480.

Brentari, D., & Wolk, S. (1986). The relative effects of three expressive methods upon the speech intelligibility of profoundly deaf speakers. *Journal of Communication Disorders, 19,* 209–218.

Clark, J. G., & Stemple, J. C. (1982). Assessment of three modes of alaryngeal speech with a synthetic sentence identification task in varying message to competition ratios. *Journal of Speech and Hearing Research, 25,* 322–333.

Cullinan, W. L., Brown, C. S., & Blalock, P. D. (1986). Ratings of intelligibility of esophageal and tracheoesophageal speech. *Journal of Communication Disorders, 19,* 185–195.

Davis, C., & Kim, J. (2004). Audio-visual interactions with intact clearly audible speech. *The Quarterly Journal of Experimental Psychology, 57A,* 1103–1121.

De Santo, L., Olsen, K., Perry, W., Rohe, D., & Keith, R. (1995). Quality of life after surgical treatment of cancer of the larynx. *The Annals of Otology, Rhinology, and Laryngology, 104,* 763–769.

Deshmane, V., Parikh, H., Pinni, S., Parikh, D., & Rao, R. (1995). Laryngectomy: A quality of life assessment. *Indian Journal of Cancer, 32,* 121–130.

Desjardins, J., & Doherty, K. (2013). Age-related changes in listening effort for various types of masker noises. *Ear and Hearing, 34,* 261–272.

Diedrich, W. M. (1991). Anatomy and physiology of esophageal speech. In S. J. Salmon & K. H. Mount (Eds.), *Alaryngeal speech rehabilitation: For clinicians by clinicians* (pp. 1–26). Austin, TX: Pro-Ed.

Downs, D. W. (1982). Effects of hearing aid use on speech discrimination and listening effort. *The Journal of Speech and Hearing Disorders, 47*, 189–193.

Doyle, P., & Eadie, T. (2005). The perceptual nature of alaryngeal voice and speech. In P. C. Doyle & R. L. Keith (Eds.), *Contemporary considerations in the treatment and rehabilitation of head and neck cancer: Voice, speech, and swallowing* (pp. 113–142). Austin, TX: Pro-Ed.

Doyle, P. C. (1994). *Foundations of voice and speech rehabilitation following laryngeal cancer*. San Diego, CA: Singular.

Doyle, P. C., Danhauer, J., & Reed, C. (1988). Listeners perceptions of consonants produced by esophageal and tracheosophageal talkers. *The Journal of Speech and Hearing Disorders, 53*, 400–407.

Dromey, C. (2000). Articulatory kinematics in patients with Parkinson disease using different speech treatment approaches. *The Journal of Medical Speech-Language Pathology, 8*, 155–161.

Duguay, M. J. (1989). Esophageal speech: An historical review. *Journal of Voice, 3*, 264–268.

Eadie, T. L., & Doyle, P. C. (2002). Direct magnitude estimation and interval scaling of naturalness and severity in tracheoesophageal (TE) speakers. *Journal of Speech, Language, and Hearing Research, 45*, 1088–1096.

Eadie, T. L., & Doyle, P. C. (2005). Scaling of voice pleasantness and acceptability in tracheoesophageal speakers. *Journal of Voice, 19*, 373–383.

Eadie, T. L., Day, A. M., Sawin, D. E., Lamvik, K., & Doyle, P. C. (2013). Auditory-perceptual speech outcomes and quality of life after total laryngectomy. *Otolaryngology Head Neck Surgery, 148*(1), 82–88.

Evitts, P., Cohen, H., & Wysokinski, J. (2007). *The McGurk effect and disordered speech: Effects of altered visual information on disordered speech intelligibility*. Poster presentation at the annual convention of the Pennsylvania Speech and Hearing Association (PSHA), State College, PA.

Evitts, P., Gabel, R., & Searl, J. (2007). Listeners' perceptions of the personality of male, alaryngeal speakers. *Logopedics, Phoniatrics, Vocology, 32*, 53–59.

Evitts, P., & Searl, J. (2006). Reaction times of normal listeners to alaryngeal speech. *Journal of Speech, Language, and Hearing Research, 49*(6), 1380–1390.

Evitts, P., Starmer, H., Teets, K., Montgomery, C., Calhoun, L., Schulze, A., … Adams, L. (2016). The impact of dysphonic voices on healthy listeners: Listener reaction times, speech intelligibility, and listener comprehension. *American Journal of Speech-Language Pathology, 25*(4), 561–575.

Evitts, P. M., & Gallop, R. (2011). Objective eye-gaze behavior during face-to-face communication with proficient alaryngeal speakers: A preliminary study. *International Journal of Language and Communication Disorders, 46*, 535–549.

Evitts, P. M., Kasapoglu, F., Demerici, U., & Miller, J. (2011). Communication adjustment of patients with a laryngectomy in Turkey: Analysis by type of surgery and mode of speech. *Psychology, Health & Medicine, 16*, 650–660.

Evitts, P. M., Portugal, L., Van Dine, A., & Holler, A. (2010). Effects of audiovisual information on alaryngeal speech intelligibility. *Journal of Communication Disorders, 43*, 92–104.

Evitts, P. M., Van Dine, A., & Holler, A. (2009). Effects of audio-visual information and mode of speech on listener perceptions of alaryngeal speakers. *International Journal of Speech-Language Pathology, 11*(6), 1–11.

Ferguson, S. H. (2012). Talker differences in clear and conversational speech: Vowel intelligibility for older adults with hearing loss. *Journal of Speech, Language, and Hearing Research, 55*, 779–190.

Ferguson, S. H., & Kewley-Port, D. (2007). Talker differences in clear and conversational speech: Acoustic characteristics of vowels. *Journal of Speech Language and Hearing Research, 50*, 1241–1255.

Feuerstein, J. F. (1992). Monaural versus binaural hearing: Ease of listening, word recognition, and attentional effort. *Ear and Hearing, 13*(2), 80–86.

Finizia, C., Lindström, J., & Dotevall, H. (1998). Intelligibility and perceptual ratings after treatment for laryngeal cancer: Laryngectomy vs. radiotherapy. *Laryngoscope, 108*, 138–143.

Fraser, S., Gagné, J. P., Alepins, M., & Dubois, P. (2010). Evaluating the effort expended to understand speech in noise using a dual-task paradigm: The effects of providing visual cues. *Journal of Speech, Language, and Hearing Research, 53*, 18–33.

Garcia, J. M., & Cannito, M. P. (1996). Influence of verbal and nonverbal contexts on the sentence intelligibility of a speaker with dysarthria. *Journal of Speech and Hearing Research, 39*, 750–760.

Garcia, J. M., & Daegenais, P. A. (1998). Dysarthric sentence intelligibility: Contribution of iconic gestures and message predictiveness. *Journal of Speech, Language, and Hearing Research, 41*, 1282–1293.

Gilmore, S. I. (1974). Social and vocational acceptability of esophageal speakers compared to normal speakers. *Journal of Speech and Hearing Research, 17*, 599–607.

Globlek, D., Stajner-Katusic, S., Musura, M., Horga, D., & Liker, M. (2004). Comparison of alaryngeal voice and speech. *Logopedics, Phoniatrics, Vocology, 29*, 87–91.

Gosselin, P., & Gagné, J. (2011). Older adults expend more listening effort than young adults recognizing audiovisual speech in noise. *International Journal of Audiology, 50*, 786–792.

Graham, M. S. (1997). *The clinicians guide to alaryngeal speech therapy*. Boston, MA: Butterworth – Heinemann.

Green, G., & Hults, M. (1982). Preferences for three types of alaryngeal speech. *The Journal of Speech and Hearing Disorders, 47*, 141–145.

Hartman, D. E., & Scott, D. A. (1974). Overt responses of listeners to alaryngeal speech. *The Laryngoscope, 84*, 410–416.

Hartman, D. E. (1979). Perceptual and acoustic characteristics of esophageal speech. In R. L. Keith & F. L. Darley (Eds.), *Laryngectomee rehabilitation* (pp. 87–106). Houston, TX: College Hill Press.

Helfer, K. S. (1997). Auditory and auditory-visual perception of clear and conversational speech. *Journal of Speech, Language, and Hearing Research, 40*, 432–443.

Hicks, C., & Tharpe, A. (2002). Listening effort and fatigue in school-age children with and without hearing loss. *Journal of Speech, Language, and Hearing Research, 45*, 573–584.

Hilgers, F., Ackerstaff, A., Aaronson, N., Schouwenburg, P., & van Zandwijk, N. (1990). Physical and psychosocial consequence of total laryngectomy. *Clinical Otolaryngology, 15*, 421–425.

Hoffmann, H., Dobie, R., Losonczy, K., Themann, C., & Flamme, G. (2017). Declining prevalence of hearing loss in US adults aged 20 to 69 years. *JAMA Otolaryngology. Head & Neck Surgery, 143*, 274–285.

Hubbard, D., & Kushner, D. (1980). A comparison of speech intelligibility between esophageal and normal speakers via three modes of presentation. *Journal of Speech and Hearing Research, 23*, 909–916.

Hustad, K. (2006). A closer look at transcription intelligibility for speakers with dysarthria: Evaluation of scoring paradigms and linguistic errors made by listeners. *American Journal of Speech-Language Pathology, 15*, 268–277.

Hustad, K., & Beukelman, D. (2001). Effects of linguistic cues and stimulus cohesion on intelligibility of severely dysarthric speech. *Journal of Speech, Language, and Hearing Research, 44*, 497–510.

Hustad, K., & Beukelman, D. (2002). Listener comprehension of severely dysarthric speech: Effects of linguistic cues and stimulus cohesion. *Journal of Speech, Language, and Hearing Research, 45*, 545–558.

Hustad, K. C., & Cahill, D. R. (2003). Effects of presentation mode and repeated familiarization on intelligibility of dysarthric speech. *American Journal of Speech-Language Pathology, 12*, 198–208.

Hustad, K. C., & Weismer, G. (2007). Interventions to improve intelligibility and communicative success for speakers with dysarthria. In G. Weismer (Ed.), *Motor speech disorders* (pp. 217–228). San Diego, CA: Plural Publishing.

Hustad, K. (2008). The relationship between listener comprehension and intelligibility scores for speakers with dysarthria. *Journal of Speech, Language, and Hearing Research, 51*, 562–573.

Hyman, M. (1955). An experimental study of artificial-larynx and esophageal speech. *The Journal of Speech and Hearing Disorders, 20*, 291–299.

Hyman, M. (1979). Factors influencing intelligibility of alaryngeal speech. In R. L. Keith & F. L. Darley (Eds.), Laryngectomee rehabilitation (pp. 165–179). Houston, TX: College Hill Press.

Kalb, M. B., & Carpenter, M. A. (1981). Individual speaker influence on relative intelligibility of esophageal speech and artificial larynx speech. *The Journal of Speech and Hearing Disorders, 46*, 77–80.

Kawase, T., Yamaguchi, K., Ogawa, T., Suzuki, K., Suzuki, M., Itoh, M., … Fujii, T. (2005). Recruitment of fusiform face area associated with listening to degraded auditory-visual speech perception: A PET study. *Neuroscience Letters, 382*, 254–258.

Keintz, C., Bunton, K., & Hoit, J. (2007). Influence of visual information on the intelligibility of dysarthric speech. *American Journal of Speech-Language Pathology, 16*, 222–234.

Kempster, G. B. (2005). Recent advances in conservation laryngectomy procedures. In P. Doyle & R. Keith (Eds.), *Contemporary considerations in the treatment and rehabilitation of head and neck cancer* (pp. 223–236). Austin, TX: Pro-Ed.

Kent, R. (1996). Hearing and believing: Some limits to the auditory-perceptual assessment of speech and voice disorders. *American Journal of Speech-Language Pathology, 5*, 7–23.

Kent, R., Miolo, G., & Bloedel, S. (1994). The intelligibility of children's speech: A review of evaluation procedures. *American Journal of Speech-Language Pathology, 3*, 81–95.

Kent, R. D., Weismer, G., Kent, J. F., & Rosenbek, J. C. (1989). Toward phonetic intelligibility testing in dysarthria. *The Journal of Speech and Hearing Disorders, 54*, 482–499.

Knox, A. W., & Anneberg, M. (1973). The effects of training in comprehension of electrolaryngeal speech. *Journal of Communication Disorders, 6*, 110–120.

Krause, J. C., & Braida, L. D. (2002). Investigating alternative forms of clear speech: The effects of speaking rate and speaking mode on intelligibility. *The Journal of the Acoustical Society of America, 112*(5), 2165–2172.

Kreiman, J., & Gerratt, B. R. (1998). Validity of rating scale measures of voice quality. *Journal of the American Acoustical Society of America, 104*(3 Pt 1), 1598–1608.

Lass, N. J., Ruscello, D. M., & Lakawicz, J. A. (1988). Listeners' perceptions of nonspeech characteristics of normal and dysarthric children. *Journal of Communication Disorders, 21*, 385–391.

Liao, J. (2016). An acoustic study of vowels produced by alaryngeal speakers in Taiwan. *American Journal of Speech-Language Pathology, 25*(4), 481–492. https://doi.org/10.1044/2016_AJSLP-15-0068. Downloaded 30 September 2016.

Liss, J. M., Spitzer, S. M., Caviness, J. N., & Adler, C. (2002). The effects of familiarization on intelligibility and lexical segmentation in hypokinetic and ataxic dysarthria. *Journal of the Acoustical Society of America, 112*, 3022–3030.

Liss, J. M., Spitzer, S. M., Caviness, J. N., Adler, C., & Edwards, B. (1998). Syllabic strength and lexical boundary decisions in the perception of hypokinetic dysarthric speech. *Journal of the Acoustical Society of America, 104*, 2457–2466.

Liss, J. M., Spitzer, S. M., Caviness, J. N., Adler, C., & Edwards, B. (2000). Lexical boundary error analysis in hypokinetic and ataxic dysarthria. *Journal of the Acoustical Society of America, 107*, 3415–3424.

Lyberg-Åhlander, V., Haake, M., Brännström, J., Schötz, S., & Sahlén, B. (2015). Does the speaker's voice quality influence children's performance on a language comprehension test? *International Journal of Speech-Language Pathology, 17*, 63–73.

Massaro, D. W. (1998). *Perceiving talking faces: From speech perception to a behavioral principle.* Cambridge, MA: MIT Press.

McCroskey, R., & Mulligan, M. (1963). The relative intelligibility of esophageal speech and artificial-larynx speech. *The Journal of Speech and Hearing Disorders, 28*, 37–41.

McFarland, D. (2001). Respiratory markers of conversational interaction. *Journal of Speech, Language, and Hearing Research, 44*, 128–143.

McGurk, H., & MacDonald, J. (1976). Hearing lips and seeing voices. *Nature, 264*, 746–748.

Merwin, G. E., Goldstein, L. P., & Rothman, H. B. (1985). A comparison of speech using artificial larynx and tracheosophageal puncture with valve in the same speaker. *Laryngoscope, 95*, 730–734.

Miller, G. A., & Selfridge, J. A. (1950). Verbal context and the recall of meaningful material. *American Journal of Psychology, 63*, 176–185.

Mirenda, P., Donnellan, A., & Yoder, D. (1983). Gaze behavior: A new look at an old problem. *Journal of Autism and Developmental Disorders, 13*, 397–409.

Morton, V., & Watson, D. (2001). The impact of impaired vocal quality on children's' ability to process spoken language. *Logopedics, Phoniatrics, Vocology, 26*, 17–25.

Most, T., Tobin, Y., & Mimran, R. C. (2000). Acoustic and perceptual characteristics of esophageal and tracheoesophageal speech production. *Journal of Communication Disorders, 33*, 165–180.

Mummery, C. J., Ashburner, J., Scott, S. K., & Wise, R. J. (1999). Functional neuroimaging of speech perception in six normal and two aphasic subjects. *Journal of the Acoustical Society of America, 106*, 449–457.

Munhall, K., Gribble, P., Sacco, L., & Ward, M. (1996). Temporal constraints on the McGurk effect. *Perception & Psychophysics, 58*, 351–352.

Munhall, K., Jones, J., Callan, D., Kuratate, T., & Vatikiotis-Bateson, E. (2004). Visual prosody and speech intelligibility. *American Psychological Society, 15*, 133–137.

Munro, M., & Derwing, T. (1995). Processing time, accent, and comprehensibility in the perception of native and foreign-accented speech. *Language and Speech, 38*, 289–306.

Nagle, K., & Eadie, T. (2012). Listener effort for highly intelligible tracheoesophageal speech. *Journal of Communication Disorders, 45*, 235–245.

Nelson, M. A., & Hodge, M. M. (2000). Effects of facial paralysis and audiovisual information on stop place identification. *Journal of Speech, Language, and Hearing Research, 43*, 158–171.

Ng, M., Kwok, C., & Chow, S. (1997). Speech performance of adult Cantonese-speaking laryngectomees using different types of alaryngeal phonation. *Journal of Voice, 11*, 338–344.

Ng, M. L., & Chu, R. (2009). An acoustical and perceptual study of vowels produced by alaryngeal speakers of Cantonese. *Folia Phoniatrica et Logopedics, 61*, 9–104.

Norrix, L., Plante, E., Vance, R., & Boliek, C. (2007). Auditory-visual integration for speech by children with and without specific language impairment. *Journal of Speech, Language, and Hearing Research, 50*, 1639–1651.

Nusbaum, H. C., Schwab, E. C., & Pisoni, D. B. (1984). *Subjective evaluation of synthetic speech: Measuring preference, naturalness, and acceptability* (Research on Speech Perception, Progress Report No. 10). Bloomington, IN: Indiana University.

Offermann, M., Pruyn, J., de Boer, M., Busschbach, J., & Baatenburg de Jong, R. (2015). Psychosocial consequences for partners of patients after total laryngectomy and for the relationship between patients and partners. *Oral Oncology, 51*, 389–398.

Pereira da Silva, A., Feliciano, T., Vaz Freitas, S., Esteves, S., Almeida, E., & Sousa, C. (2015). Quality of life in patients submitted to total laryngectomy. *Journal of Voice, 29*, 382–388.

Picheny, M. A., Durlach, N. I., & Braida, L. D. (1985). Speaking clearly for the hard of hearing. I. Intelligibility differences between clear and conversational speech. *Journal of Speech, Language, and Hearing Research, 28*, 96–103.

Picheny, M. A., Durlach, N. I., & Braida, L. D. (1986). Speaking clearly for the hard of hearing. II. Acoustic characteristics of clear and conversational speech. *Journal of Speech, Language, and Hearing Research, 29*, 434–446.

Pindzola, R. H., & Cain, B. C. (1988). Acceptability ratings of tracheoesophageal speech. *Laryngoscope, 98*, 394–397.

Quail, G., Fagan, J., Raynham, O., Krynauw, H., John, L., & Carrara, H. (2016). Effect of cloth stoma covers on tracheal climate of laryngectomy patients. *Head & Neck, 38*, E480–E487.

Relic, A., Mazemda, P., Arens, C., Koller, M., & Glanz, H. (2001). Investigating quality of life and coping resources after laryngectomy. *European Archives of Oto-Rhino-Laryngology, 258*, 514–517.

Robbins, J. (1984). Acoustic differentiation of laryngeal, esophageal, and tracheoesophageal speech. *Journal of Speech and Hearing Research, 27*, 577–585.

Robbins, J., Fisher, H. B., Blom, E. C., & Singer, M. I. (1984). A comparative study of normal, esophageal, and tracheoesophageal speech production. *The Journal of Speech and Hearing Disorders, 49*, 202–210.

Rudner, M., Mishra, S., Stenfelt, S., Lunner, T., & Rönnberg, J. (2016). Seeing the talker's face improves free recall of speech for young adults with normal hearing but not older adults with hearing loss. *Journal of Speech, Language, and Hearing Research, 59*, 590–599.

Salmon, S. J. (1999). Artificial larynx devices and their use. In S. J. Salmon (Ed.), *Alaryngeal speech rehabilitation* (pp. 79–104). Austin, TX: Pro-Ed.

Sanders, D. A., & Goodrich, S. J. (1971). The relative contribution of visual and auditory components of speech to speech intelligibility as a function of three conditions of frequency distortion. *Journal of Speech, Language, and Hearing Research, 14*, 154–159.

Searl, J. (2007). Bilabial contact pressure and oral air pressure during tracheoesophageal speech. *The Annals of Otology, Rhinology, and Laryngology, 116*, 304–311.

Searl, J., & Evitts, P. (2004). Velopharyngeal aerodynamics of /m/ and /p/ in tracheoesophageal speech. *Journal of Voice, 18*, 557–566.

Searl, J., & Evitts, P. M. (2012). Tongue-palate contact pressure, oral air pressure and acoustics of clear speech. *Journal of Speech, Language, and Hearing Research, 56*, 826–839.

Searl, J. P. (2002). Magnitude and variability of oral pressure in tracheoesophageal speech. *Folia Phoniatrica et Logopedia, 54*, 312–328.

Shanks, J. C. (1977). Variations on a vocal theme through interpersonal therapy with alaryngeal patients. In M. Cooper & M. H. Cooper (Eds.), *Approaches to vocal rehabilitation*. Springfield, IL: Charles C. Thomas.

Shames, G. H., Font, J., & Matthews, J. (1963). Factors related to speech proficiency of the laryngectomized. *Journal of Speech and Hearing Disorders, 28*, 273–287.

Shipp, T. (1967). Frequency, duration, and perceptual measures in relation to judgments of alaryngeal speech acceptability. *Journal of Speech and Hearing Research, 10*, 417–427.

Singer, M. I., & Blom, E. D. (1980). An endoscopic technique for restoration of voice after laryngectomy. *Annals of Otology, Rhinology, and Laryngology, 89*, 529–533

Smiljanić, R., & Bradlow, A. (2009). Speaking and hearing clearly: Talker and listener factors in speaking style changes. *Lang & Ling Compass, 3*, 236–264.

Snidecor, J. C. (1962). *Speech rehabilitation of the laryngectomized*. Springfield, IL: Charles C. Thomas.

Stepp, C. E., Heaton, J., & Hillman, R. (2008). Postlaryngectomy speech respiration patterns. *The Annals of Otology, Rhinology, & Laryngology, 117*, 557–563.

Sumby, W., & Pollack, I. J. (1954). Visual contribution to speech intelligibility. *Journal of the Acoustical Society of America, 26*, 212–215.

Surveillance, Epidemiology, and End Results (SEER) Program. *SEER*Stat Database: Cancer of the larynx (1973–2014)*. www.seer.cancer.gov. Accessed 25 Oct 2017.

Susca, M., & Healey, E. C. (2001). Perceptions of simulated stuttering and fluency. *Journal of Speech, Language, and Hearing Research, 44*, 61–72.

Thivard, L., Belin, P., Zilbovicius, M., Poline, J. B., & Samson, Y. (2000). A cortical region sensitive to auditory spectral motion. *Neuroreport, 11*, 2969–2972.

Travis, L. E. (1957). *Handbook of speech pathology*. New York, NY: Appleton-Century-Crofts.

Trudeau, M. D. (1987). A comparison of speech acceptability of good and excellent esophageal and tracheoesophageal speakers. *Journal of Communication Disorders, 20*, 41–49.

Uchanski, R. M. (2005). Clear speech. In D. B. Pisoni & R. E. Remez (Eds.), *The handbook of speech perception* (pp. 207–235). Malden, MA: Blackwell Publishing.

Von Tiling, J. (2011). Listener perceptions of stuttering, prolonged speech, and verbal avoidance behaviors. *Journal of Communication Disorders, 44*, 161–172.

Warner, R. M. (1979). Periodic rhythms in conversational speech. *Language and Speech, 22*, 381–396.

Weinstein, G., El-Sawy, M. M., Ruiz, C., et al. (2001). Laryngeal preservation with supracricoid partial laryngectomy results in improved quality of life when compared to total laryngectomy. *The Laryngoscope, 111*, 191–199.

Wetmore, S. J., Krueger, K., & Wesson, K. (1981). The Singer-Blom speech rehabilitation procedure. *Laryngoscope, 91*, 1109–1117.

Williams, S., & Watson, J. (1987). Speaking proficiency variations according to method of alaryngeal voicing. *Laryngoscope, 97*, 737–739.

Wilson, E. O., & Spaulding, T. J. (2010). Effects of noise and speech intelligibility on listener comprehension and processing time of Korean-accented English. *Journal of Speech and Hearing Research, 53*, 1543–1554.

Yi, H. G., Phelps, J., Smiljanic, R., & Chandrasekaran, B. (2013). Reduced efficiency of audiovisual integration for nonnative speech. *Journal of the Acoustical Society of America, 134*, EL387–EL393.

Yiu, E. M., van Hasselt, C. A., Williams, S. R., & Woo, J. J. (1994). Speech intelligibility in tone language (Chinese) laryngectomy speakers. *European Journal of Disorders of Communication, 29*, 339–347.

Yorkston, K. M., & Beukelman, D. R. (1980). A clinician-judged technique for quantifying dysarthric speech based on single-word intelligibility. *Journal of Communication Disorders, 13*, 15–31.

Yorkston, K. M., Beukelman, D. R., Strand, E. A., Bell, K. R., & Hustad, K. C. (1999). Optimizing communication effectiveness: Bringing it together. In *Management of motor speech disorders in children and adults* (2nd ed., pp. 483–541). Austin, TX: Pro-Ed Publishing.

Yorkston, K. M., Strand, E. A., & Kennedy, M. R. (1996). Comprehensibility of dysarthric speech. *American Journal of Speech-Language Pathology, 5*, 55–66.

Communicative Participation After Head and Neck Cancer

Tanya L. Eadie

Introduction

One of the most significant difficulties experienced by survivors of head and neck cancer (HNC), as well as those who are undergoing HNC treatment, relates to deficits in verbal communication. Difficulties with speech and voice may lead to withdrawal and social isolation that can affect relationships and the ability to return to work and daily activities and, ultimately, impact the person's quality of life (Dwivedi et al., 2009; Karnell, Funk, & Hoffman, 2000). For these reasons, communication outcomes are important for measuring both the impact and success of HNC treatment, as well as providing directions for follow-up care.

Traditional methods of assessing communication after HNC include both objective and subjective measures. For example, objective measures of speech and voice include measures that capture aspects related to the acoustic signal, air pressure, or airflow through the larynx and vocal tract. Subjective measures include perceptual judgments made by unfamiliar listeners as well as experienced listeners. These measures typically include auditory-perceptual ratings of speech understandability or roughness of the

voice or visual-perceptual ratings of vocal fold function using various types of laryngeal imaging. However, to understand the functional consequences of a speech or voice difficulty that may arise from HNC, it also is necessary to include the patient's perspective, which often entails the use of a patient-reported outcome (PRO) measure. As per the US Department of Health and Human Services Food and Drug Administration (2009), a PRO is any report of the status of a patient's health condition that comes directly from the patient, without interpretation of the patient's response by a clinician or others, such as family members or other proxies. PRO measures are increasingly used to document treatment- and disease-related effects after the diagnosis and treatment of HNC (Ringash et al., 2015). These measures may be disease-specific (i.e., investigating the influence of specific HNC symptoms on quality of life) or discipline- or area-specific such as measuring characteristics within a discipline or area, for example, vocal function or swallowing on quality of life (QOL) or other areas of functioning (see Doyle & MacDonald, Chap. 27).

Until recently, no tool was solely dedicated toward measuring communication in everyday life situations, or what is called communicative participation (Eadie et al., 2006). Communicative participation "is defined as taking part in life situations where knowledge, information, ideas or feelings are exchanged… [and occur across

T. L. Eadie (✉)
Department of Speech and Hearing Sciences, Department of Otolaryngology – Head and Neck Surgery, University of Washington, Seattle, WA, USA
e-mail: teadie@uw.edu

© Springer Nature Switzerland AG 2019
P. C. Doyle (ed.), *Clinical Care and Rehabilitation in Head and Neck Cancer*,
https://doi.org/10.1007/978-3-030-04702-3_29

multiple life situations related to]... personal care, household management, leisure, learning, employment, and community life" (Eadie et al., 2006, p. 309). For example, communicative participation includes talking to strangers, ordering a meal in a restaurant, talking to a friend on the telephone, or discussing end-of-life care wishes with family members. These areas are long-standing areas of concern for those who are undergoing or who have undergone treatment for HNC. The purpose of this chapter is to provide a summary of potential challenges to communicative participation in the HNC population. Methods of measuring communicative participation will be outlined for both clinical and research use, as well as how this type of PRO measure differs from other measures of speech and voice. Finally, implications for HNC rehabilitation will be discussed.

Defining Communicative Participation

For many healthcare fields, the World Health Organization's (WHO's) *International Classification of Functioning, Disability and Health* (ICF; WHO, 2001) has provided a framework and terminology for understanding the different ways that individuals experience health conditions, as well as the range of factors that contribute to those experiences (American Speech-Language-Hearing Association, 2004, 2016). The ICF has compelled us to broaden our views of health from traditional biomedical models, in which disability is regarded as being driven primarily by the nature and the severity of impairments, to biopsychosocial models, in which disability is construed as a complex construct influenced by a combination of impairments, activity limitations, participation restrictions, as well as personal and environmental factors (see Borrell-Carrió, Suchman, & Epstein, 2004; Eadie, 2007).

The usefulness of the ICF is highlighted in the following example, as a means for understanding the impact of a health-related condition such as HNC on a person's functioning, disability, and

health. Consider an individual who is deemed "disease-free," 10 years after HNC treatment. In a quiet environment with a familiar listener, that person may be able to produce relatively understandable speech (e.g., exhibiting a mild speech impairment). However, that same individual may continue to experience difficulty in everyday activities such as communicating with store clerks or co-workers because of the unfamiliarity of communication partners, attitudes of partners (e.g., related to facial disfigurement or changes in speech or voice quality), or because of the presence of background noise (Doyle & Keith, 2005). Thus, how communication difficulties affect one's participation in life situations depends not only on the degree of the impairment but also on the interaction between participation and factors related to the person and the environment. In this example, personal factors may include characteristics such as a person's sex, age, or even coping style. All of these factors may affect the communication outcome. Similarly, environmental factors also affect the success of a communicative interaction; these factors may include physical characteristics of the environment such as background noise or attitudinal features such as the familiarity of a person's communication partner (Eadie, 2003, 2007).

The paradigm shift from the biomedical model to the biopsychosocial model underlying the ICF has led researchers and clinicians to reexamine how well current assessment and intervention practices address each component of the ICF. By making direct comparisons between current practice and the ICF theoretical model, we can better identify gaps in service and how we might better address the multifactorial components of health and disability. In fact, the American Speech-Language-Hearing Association (ASHA) has adopted the ICF as the framework for the preferred practice patterns in assessing and treating those with communication disorders, including individuals with HNC (ASHA, 2004). In making comparisons between clinical practice and the ICF model, researchers and clinicians have noted that standard instruments assessing individuals with speech and voice difficulties secondary to HNC are primarily focused at the impairment level (Eadie, 2003; Eadie, 2007). Yet, patients often state that communicating in everyday settings remains a priority after HNC treatment (Baylor, Burns, Eadie, Britton, & Yorkston, 2011; Tschiesner et al., 2013). As a result, there appears to be a gap in assessment methods that capture communication outcomes that are meaningful to both clinicians and patients alike.

While there are numerous PRO measures available for assessing outcomes after HNC (Ringash et al., 2015), results from a literature review revealed that no instrument was available that independently measured communicative participation (Eadie et al., 2006). Whereas the concept of communicative participation is reflected in several QOL instruments used in the HNC population, it is intertwined with other dimensions such as emotional, physical, and social functioning. Eadie et al. (2006) also identified a lack of PRO instruments that measured functional *speech* difficulties, as opposed to *voice-related* function. While voice-related QOL measures may sensitively capture difficulties for those with laryngeal cancer, those with oral and oropharyngeal-based tumors may have more difficulty in *speech*-related tasks due to surgical or radiation effects on structures in the oral and pharyngeal cavities (Funk, Karnell, & Christensen, 2012). This leaves a large gap in our ability to evaluate functional communication outcomes in this growing number of patients. While a few instruments subsequently have been developed to capture difficulties related to speech, such as the *Speech Handicap Index* (Rinkel et al., 2008), an additional challenge remains. With the adoption of multiple instruments, comparisons of outcomes are difficult within and across HNC populations, who may experience deficits across speech, voice, or both areas. The use of multiple instruments in clinical practice also introduces additional burden on patients who ultimately are impacted in communicative participation, regardless of its contributing factors (i.e., speech, voice, or others). All of these factors bear consideration when developing an instrument that may measure a construct such as communicative participation.

Measuring Communicative Participation

The gap between patient priorities and clinical and research practice led our interdisciplinary team to begin the development of a novel and valid PRO measure called the *Communicative Participation Item Bank* (CPIB; Baylor, Yorkston, Eadie, Miller, & Amtmann, 2009; Baylor et al., 2013). The CPIB is intended to measure communicative participation in community-dwelling adults with a range of communication disorders. It was developed using best practices in application of modern psychometric theory (item response theory, IRT). The statistical approach used in this case is one that allows the measurement of a construct and so-called latent trait using probabilistic equations.

A latent trait, such as a person's interference in communicative participation, is one that is not directly measured but must be inferred from a person's discrete responses to items measuring that construct. The goal in developing an item bank such as the CPIB is to (a) ensure that the items represent a unidimensional construct (e.g., communicative participation) across a broad range of trait or difficulty levels and (b) establish local independence of the items, such that a participant's response to any given item in the item bank is independent from that person's response to any other item. One of the key advantages of this approach is that once an item bank has been developed to measure the latent trait such as communicative participation, any combination or subset of items (e.g., 6–7 items) can be used for individual assessment needs, reducing the burden on participants (Hays, Morales, & Reise, 2000). A shortened test is usually accomplished using computerized adaptive testing – a test in which the next item or set of items selected to be administered depends on the accuracy or ability of the test taker's responses to the most recently administered items. In addition, short forms of the instrument may be created; in doing so, it is possible to measure the construct across a range of trait levels using a selected subset of calibrated items. Readers who are interested in IRT-based scales are referred to Baylor et al. (2010) for a tutorial that outlines the steps and advantages of using such an approach.

Items in the CPIB were developed on the basis of a literature review (Eadie et al., 2006) and multiple qualitative studies of people with communication disorders, including those with HNC (Baylor et al., 2011; Yorkston et al., 2007; Yorkston et al., 2008). The CPIB was initially validated in 208 individuals with a neurogenic voice disorder (spasmodic dysphonia; Baylor et al., 2009). Results revealed strong psychometric properties in that a large number of items met the criteria of unidimensionality (i.e., all items measured the same construct), good item fit to the model, a lack of local dependence, a wide and even measurement range (suggesting that the instrument measured the construct across a wide range of communicative participation "levels"), and good function of the response categories. In other words, the items that were created appeared to measure different levels of communicative participation, they were not redundant, and there were an adequate number of response options that were able to differentiate those with different levels of communicative participation. This was a vital first step in establishing the reliability and validity of the instrument. Yet, at this point, it was still not known whether individuals who exhibit different types of communication disorders might respond differently to the same items and whether a different instrument was needed to be developed for different patient populations.

As a result, construct validity of the CPIB was then investigated using a large cross-sectional sample ($N = 701$) of individuals with a variety of communication disorders, including 197 patients who had undergone treatment for HNC (Baylor et al., 2013). A core item bank was developed that met IRT criteria, demonstrating unidimensionality, local independence, good item fit, and good measurement precision across the range of the scale. Interestingly, Baylor et al. (2013) also showed that the items in the CPIB did not function differently across diagnostic groups. That is, when responses from people with multiple sclerosis, Parkinson's disease, and HNC were compared, the analysis revealed no meaningful differences in *how* the items in the CPIB functioned. These results were consistent with previous qualitative studies that revealed that despite differences in their underlying impairments, people with different communication disorders experience similar difficulties in life participation (Baylor et al., 2011). For example, regardless of the communication disorder, individuals revealed that they all had difficulty in fast-paced environments or in situations involving background noise. As a result, a disorder-generic instrument was proposed and validated, and it included participants with both voice and speech difficulties.

A follow-up study by our team established the concurrent validity of the CPIB by examining relationships between communicative participation and global QOL, HNC-specific QOL, and discipline-specific QOL (i.e., voice-related QOL) in 195 individuals treated for HNC (Eadie et al., 2014). As hypothesized, correlations between the CPIB and global and disease-specific QOL scores were relatively weak ($r = 0.37 - 0.38$), suggesting that the CPIB was measuring a unique construct not represented on PRO measures typically used in HNC. However, not surprisingly, a stronger relationship ($r = -0.79$) was found between the CPIB and a QOL measure related to voice function called the *Voice Handicap Index-10* (Jacobson et al., 1997; Rosen, Lee, Osborne, Zullo, & Murry, 2004). These findings suggest that communicative participation is measuring a construct more similar to voice handicap than global QOL; yet, while the relationship is moderately strong, the advantage of the CPIB over a voice-specific PRO measure is that the CPIB may capture difficulties that may be voice- or speech-specific (or both), as one might expect in a broader HNC population.

The CPIB currently consists of a 46-item bank of questions with computer-based administration (CAT) parameters ready for implementation and a 10-item short form currently available for clinical and research use (Baylor et al., 2013). The items ask individuals to rate how much their condition (e.g., HNC) interferes with participation in a wide range of daily speech communication activities (e.g., making a telephone call to get information). Ratings range from "not at all" to "very much" on a 4-point Likert-type scale (see Table 29.1 for items in the CPIB short form; Baylor et al., 2013).

Table 29.1   The Communicative Participation Item Bank short form

Item stem	Response options			
Does your condition interfere with:	Not at all	A little	Quite a bit	Very much
1. Talking with people you know?	O	O	O	O
2. Communicating when you need to say something quickly?	O	O	O	O
3. Talking with people you do NOT know?	O	O	O	O
4. Communicating when you are out in your community (e.g., errands; appointments)?	O	O	O	O
5. Asking questions in a conversation?	O	O	O	O
6. Communicating in a small group of people?	O	O	O	O
7. Having a long conversation with someone you know about a book, movie, show, or sports event?	O	O	O	O
8. Giving someone DETAILED information?	O	O	O	O
9. Getting your turn in a fast-moving conversation?	O	O	O	O
10. Trying to persuade a friend or family member to see a different point of view?	O	O	O	O

Adapted from Baylor et al. (2013)
From The Communicative Participation on Item Bank (CPIB): Item Bank Calibration and Development of a Disorder-Generic Short Form, JSLHR, 56, 1190-1208,

Appendix B, with permission of ASHA; https://doi.org/10.1044/1092-4388(2012/12-0140

For each question, the participant is asked to mark how much his/her condition interferes with his/her participation in that situation. If speech varies, the participant is asked to think about an AVERAGE day for his/her speech (i.e., not best or worst days

To score the short form, the user adds the scores for the 10 items (Not at all = 3; A little = 2; Quite a bit = 1; Very much = 0) to create a summary score (range = 0 – 30). Summary scores from the CPIB are converted either to logits (a unit of measurement usually found in IRT), with scores typically ranging from −3.0 to 3.0 logits ($M = 0$), or to standardized T-scores ($M = 50$ and SD = 10; see Baylor et al., 2013). In both scoring systems, the mean score is the average of the calibration sample used when developing the CPIB, which included HNC patients. Higher scores represent better communicative participation (Baylor et al., 2013). For example, if T-scores are used, clinicians may interpret a person's score of 60 as a level of communicative participation that is one standard deviation above the mean of the original calibration sample, which included a group of long-term HNC survivors.

The development of the CPIB now permits the use of a meaningful PRO measure related to communication outcomes for HNC patients. As a result, the CPIB is not confined solely to voice-related QOL but also includes interference in communicative participation related to speech difficulties. Interestingly, preliminary outcomes have shown that the CPIB scores appear to vary with site of diagnosis, with more interference in communicative participation reported for individuals with tumors across multiple sites (e.g., spanning from the base of the tongue to hypopharynx to larynx) or for those with laryngeal cancer and better scores for those with oral and oropharyngeal cancers (Eadie et al., 2014). However, more research is needed to determine how these PRO measures relate to impairment-based measures of voice and speech, as well as for determining what is the smallest difference in scores that patients perceive as beneficial. While the instrument will offer additional insight into communicative participation after HNC in the future, we must consider the source of those challenges when interpreting the results and providing directions for clinical care.

Challenges in Communicative Participation After HNC

Individuals who have undergone treatment for HNC often report difficulties in communication, regardless of the site of the tumor or the treatment type. For example, Danker et al. (2010) found that up to 40% of patients postlaryngectomy reported that they spoke as little as possible, left things unsaid, and spoke only if there was no other way to communicate. Baylor, Yorkston, Bamer, Britton, and Amtmann (2010) also reported changes in the way communication goals are achieved in participants who had undergone total laryngectomy. While changes in communication postlaryngectomy are perhaps obvious, one group who has received less attention in the area of speech and voice includes those individuals with oral and oropharyngeal cancers (see Constantinescu & Rieger, Chap. 16). One important review by Dwivedi and colleagues (2009) identified this as an area of significant concern. They concluded that because most general and HNC-specific questionnaires only included a few questions related to speech, that evaluation of speech in this group was insufficient and that "we need to assess a patient's speech and its impact on [a] patient's daily life by using speech-specific questionnaires" (Dwivedi et al., 2009; p. 420).

Other researchers have identified speech and voice outcomes as being overlooked in patients who have undergone concurrent radiotherapy or advanced HNC with the aim of organ preservation (Jacobi, Molen, Huiskens, Rossum, & Hilgers, 2010). In their systematic review, Jacobi and colleagues (2010) established that speech and voice in this HNC group also deteriorate during treatment but improve progressively after treatment. Importantly, however, typical values for voice and speech are not reached, not even in the long term (Jacobi et al., 2010; Van der Molen et al., 2012). As highlighted in a qualitative study, changes in communication for all types

of HNC patients manifest at home, work, and social and community settings (Fletcher, Cohen, Schumacher, & Lydiatt, 2012). As a result, these outcomes are important to assess for all individuals affected by HNC and should not solely be limited to those with laryngeal-based tumors or those who have undergone laryngectomy.

Many factors affect self-reported communication success in everyday contexts for people with communication disorders, including those with HNC (Baylor et al., 2011; Eadie, 2007; Fletcher et al., 2012). The variables may range from physical symptoms and reduced capacity for performing tasks (e.g., reduced speech intelligibility, fatigue, etc.) to individual coping responses (Baylor et al., 2011; Eadie & Bowker, 2012) to changes in body image (Chen et al., 2015; Nash, 2014) to environmental facilitators and barriers. Factors in the environment may include reactions of communication partners and social support, as well as physical barriers such as background noise (Eadie, 2007). Thus, self-reported communication success is influenced by multiple variables, and it may change over time. Knowing which variables are related to communicative participation is essential for building empirical models upon which future interventions may be founded. A hypothetical model for predictors of communicative participation after HNC is presented in Fig. 29.1.

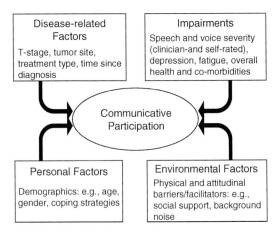

Fig. 29.1 A hypothetical model for predictors of communicative participation after HNC

Communicative participation also may be influenced by one's overall health, as well as other health conditions such as loss of mobility or vision (Yorkston et al., 2007; Yorkston et al., 2001). Most of the research examining factors that are predictive of communicative participation has been qualitative (Baylor et al., 2011; Fletcher et al., 2012). However, using an early version of the CPIB, Baylor, Yorkston, et al. (2010) followed a cohort of community-dwelling adults with multiple sclerosis over a period of 2 years. Results revealed no significant change in communicative participation in the group as a whole over the duration of the study. However, further statistical analysis revealed three distinct subgroups of participants: (a) those reporting good communicative participation demonstrated low incidence of communication disorder symptoms, as well as low levels of fatigue and depression; (b) the significant predictor of membership in a subgroup reporting midrange participation scores was low social support; and (c) the subgroup reporting the most problems with participation was predicted by a combination of higher incidence of self-reported cognitive symptoms and low social support. How all of these factors might predict communicative participation after HNC also needs to be determined. One way to better understand the nature of these relationships in the HNC population is to differentiate relationships between speech and voice factors and communicative participation on the one hand and contrast those with relationships between nonspeech and voice factors and communicative participation on the other hand. Studies summarizing those relationships are presented next.

Influence of speech and voice severity on communicative participation Some studies in the HNC literature have examined the relationship between indices of speech and voice severity, usually measured by clinician- or listener-rated speech intelligibility or voice quality, and PRO measures, such as QOL or voice-related QOL (see Doyle & Sleeth, Chap. 14; Eadie & Doyle, 2004; Meyer et al., 2004). In general, these studies have found weak to moderate relationships between clinician- or listener-rated measures and

PRO measures (e.g., Law, Ma, & Yiu, 2009; Meyer et al., 2004). Results reveal that there is often a disassociation between how speech or voice is rated by listeners and how a patient self-assesses his or her own speech or voice. For example, some patients may be 100% intelligible, or their speech may sound highly acceptable to an unfamiliar communication partner, yet some of these same patients may report significant difficulties in their own QOL. Likewise, some individuals who exhibit significantly impaired speech intelligibility or have significant dysphonia may report few problems in their overall QOL or voice-related QOL, suggesting that these individuals may have developed good compensatory strategies or coping mechanisms for dealing with these situations. These results again highlight the underlying differences in clinician-rated speech or voice impairments as compared to PRO measures.

Our team previously investigated associations among alaryngeal speech intelligibility in 25 individuals who had undergone total laryngectomy and who used different alaryngeal speech modes with both disease- and voice-specific QOL measures (Eadie, Day, Sawin, Lamvik, & Doyle, 2013). Results of this study revealed weak correlations among the measures: the relationship between speech intelligibility (percentage of words understood from the *Sentence Intelligibility Test*; Yorkston, Beukelman, & Tice, 1996) and the VHI-10 (Rosen et al., 2004) was extremely weak to nonexistent ($r = 0.04$). The correlation between speech intelligibility and one item measuring self-rated speech understandability on a disease-specific scale was also weak ($r = 0.22$). Again, these results highlight differences between measures derived from clinicians, other listeners, and patients with HNC.

In a follow-up study, we investigated similar relationships between communicative participation and postlaryngectomy speech outcomes, including listener-rated speech intelligibility and acceptability and patient-rated speech acceptability and perceived voice handicap (Eadie, Otero, Cox, et al., 2016). Thirty-six laryngectomized individuals completed the CPIB short form and the VHI-10.

These patients also provided recordings from the *Sentence Intelligibility Test* (SIT; Yorkston et al., 1996) and a reading passage and then rated their own speech acceptability. Forty-eight inexperienced listeners then transcribed the SIT sentences in order to derive speaker intelligibility scores. Eighteen additional listeners judged the speech acceptability using rating scales. Consistent with previous literature, weak, nonsignificant relationships were found between communicative participation and listener-rated outcomes. We may therefore consider PRO measures and listener-rated measures as complementary and not redundant. By using all of these measures together, we may capture a broad perspective of a person's communication function across different levels of the ICF (WHO, 2001).

While relatively weak relationships have been found between listener-rated measures such as speech intelligibility and PRO measures, it is necessary to consider how they are both obtained. For example, clinical assessment of speech intelligibility for people with speech disorders is typically performed in a quiet environment. Yet in daily life, events often occur in suboptimal listening conditions which may negatively affect a communication partner's ability to process the speech signal during a communication exchange. Further, it is well known that the presence of noise adversely affects speech intelligibility, even for healthy control speakers (Sperry, Wiley, & Chial, 1997). Results from several studies also appear to show that background noise may differentially penalize speakers with communication disorders. McColl, Fucci, Petrosino, Martin, and McCaffrey (1998) examined the different impacts of noise levels on one healthy control speaker and one tracheoesophageal speaker. Unsurprisingly, results of the study revealed that the tracheoesophageal speaker was significantly less intelligible than the control speaker across all conditions; however, both speakers had significantly lower intelligibility in noise. Interestingly, there was a significant interaction between the variables: the tracheoesophageal speaker's intelligibility was more affected by noise than was that of the healthy control speaker. These results may suggest that relationships between speech

intelligibility and PRO measures of communication may be weak because the method used to assess speech intelligibility does not reflect everyday situations that often include background noise. In terms of the ICF (WHO, 2001), this means that the relationship between a speech impairment and communicative participation may be mediated somewhat by factors related to the environment, such as background noise.

As a result of the previously noted findings, we sought to examine how sentence intelligibility relates to self-reported communication in tracheoesophageal speakers when speech intelligibility was measured in quiet and noise (Eadie, Otero, Bolt, et al., 2016). Twenty-four tracheoesophageal speakers who were at least 1 year postlaryngectomy provided audio recordings of five sentences from the SIT (Yorkston et al., 1996). Speakers also completed self-reported measures of communication including the VHI-10 (Rosen et al., 2004) and the CPIB short form (Baylor et al., 2013). Speech recordings were presented to two groups of inexperienced listeners who heard sentences in quiet or noise, and listeners transcribed the sentences to yield speech intelligibility scores. Consistent with past studies, results revealed very weak relationships between listeners' ratings of speech intelligibility in quiet and patient-reported measures of voice handicap and communicative participation (Eadie, Otero, Bolt, et al., 2016). Slightly stronger but still weak and nonsignificant relationships were observed between measures of intelligibility in noise and both self-reported measures. However, 12 speakers who were more than 65% intelligible in noise showed strong and statistically significant relationships with both self-reported measures ($r^2 = 0.76 - 0.79$). These results suggest that listeners' ratings of speech intelligibility in noise may be a better metric of self-reported communicative function for a subset of speakers who demonstrate higher speech intelligibility in noise.

While listener-rated measures may not strongly predict PROs such as communicative participation, most studies examining speech and voice outcomes have found that if both measures are patient-rated, then the outcomes are more strongly correlated. For example, Eadie, Otero, Cox, et al. (2016) compared self-judgments of speech acceptability from 36 individuals who had undergone total laryngectomy with judgments of 18 inexperienced listeners. This comparison revealed that speakers judged their own speech acceptability to be significantly better than did the inexperienced listeners, a finding that is similar to those reported by Finizia and colleagues (Finizia, Hammerlid, Westin, & Lindstrom, 1998; Finizia, Lindstrom, & Dotevall, 1998). This result suggests that speakers and listeners may be using different standards with which to judge speech acceptability. These different standards also affect PROs such as communicative participation; as a result, patient-reported speech acceptability would appear to be more strongly related to voice-related QOL or communicative participation than that of listener-rated speech acceptability (Eadie et al., 2013; Eadie et al., 2016).

One recent study investigated factors that could predict communicative participation in a group of individuals (n = 197) who were at least 6 months post-diagnosis of HNC (Bolt, Eadie, Yorkston, Baylor, & Amtmann, 2016). Demographic information and PRO measures were gathered for participants. Among 17 predictor variables, regression analysis revealed that the strongest predictor of communicative participation was self-rated speech severity, accounting for 22.7% of the variance in scores: patients with worse self-rated speech reported worse communicative participation. To a lesser extent, though still statistically significant, better communicative participation was also associated with not having undergone total laryngectomy surgery and longer time since diagnosis. These data are consistent with findings from others who have reported lower levels of voice-related QOL for those who have undergone total laryngectomy compared to those with laryngeal preservation procedures (Fung et al., 2005; Stewart, Chen, & Stach, 1998). In addition, prior research supports the idea that quality of life improves over time as people adapt to a "new normal." Increased time since diagnosis also has been positively associated with other outcomes in HNC (Terrell et al., 2004).

Perhaps the most surprising finding from the Bolt et al. (2016) study was that the second strongest predictor of communicative participation, accounting for 19.3% of the variance, was self-reported cognitive function. This variable was not hypothesized to be an a priori predictor because cognitive symptoms have not traditionally been considered to be a problem in those who have undergone treatment for non-nasopharyngeal HNC. However, results from neuropsychological testing and brain imaging are beginning to suggest that there are changes in memory, concentration, and word-finding that are not solely attributable to chemotherapy (Gan et al., 2011; Wilbers et al., 2015). Therefore, results from Bolt et al. (2016) suggest that there are other factors, such as cognitive function, that may impact communicative participation in those diagnosed with HNC.

The results from the Bolt et al. (2016) study are interesting not only for what they found was significantly related to communicative participation but also for what was *not* found to significantly contribute to the model. For example, variables such as cancer location, age, sex, and self-reported pain, among others, did not emerge as significant predictors. Thus, in HNC survivors, many of the contributing factors remain unknown, with 54% of the variance remaining unaccounted for in the model. Among the variables that were not explored in that study were many nonspeech and voice-related factors, including measures of depression, coping strategies, or measures related to social support. These nonspeech and voice-related impairments, as well as psychosocial factors, are examined subsequently.

Influence of nonspeech and voice-related factors Communicative participation may be influenced by a variety of factors related to the person (e.g., coping, sex, age), factors related to the environment (e.g., background noise, social support from others), as well as other nonspeech and voice-related impairments (e.g., fatigue, depression; Eadie, 2003; see Fig. 29.1). Results from other clinical populations (e.g., multiple sclerosis, Parkinson's disease, aphasia, etc.) suggest that factors beyond voice and speech, such as fatigue, depression, social support, and cognitive symptoms, also are related to communicative participation (Baylor, Yorkston, et al., 2010; Hilari, Needle, & Harrison, 2012; McAuliffe, Baylor, & Yorkston, 2017). While such factors have not been extensively examined in relation to communicative participation after HNC, they have been identified as strong predictors of other patient-reported outcomes, such as QOL. While health-related QOL outcomes are not synonymous with communicative participation, the constructs are related (Eadie et al., 2014). Thus, we might hypothesize that these non-voice and speech-related factors also may affect communicative participation in the HNC patient population. A few of these examples are provided in the subsequent section.

First, one physical impairment that has been shown to affect communicative participation in other health populations is that of fatigue (Baylor, Yorkston, et al., 2010; McAuliffe et al., 2017). Fatigue may occur secondary to radiation therapy in HNC but also from sequelae related to changes in respiratory function, obstructive sleep disturbances, and coincidentally with untreated depression (see Bohnenkamp, Chap. 7). With increased fatigue, patients report a decreased ability or desire to participate in social activities and relationships with others (Yorkston et al., 2001), with implications for reduced communicative participation. How strongly this affects communicative participation in HNC deserves further study.

A second impairment of great consequence to HNC is that of depression (Howren, Christensen, Karnell, & Funk, 2013).

Given the importance that is placed on the appearance of the head and neck, coupled with the visibility of the disease and treatment sequelae, HNC is arguably one of the most psychologically traumatic cancers to experience (Bjorklund, Sarvimaki, & Berg, 2010; Doyle & Keith, 2005). Depression is a significant factor to consider not only at the time of cancer diagnosis but also during treatment and recovery. In fact, a recent cross-sectional study identified 19.5% of HNC patients with depression, either in the 2 years prior to their cancer diagnosis or in the year following diagnosis (Rieke et al., 2016).

Given the high prevalence of depression in this population, it is perhaps unsurprising that it is a significant predictor of poor QOL and distress in HNC patients (Bornbaum et al., 2012; Llewellyn, McGurk, & Weinman, 2005). It also has been shown to affect speech, eating, and social functioning (Funk, Karnell, Christensen, Moran, & Ricks, 2003). How depression affects communicative participation also warrants future study.

Beyond other impairments, personal factors within the WHO (2001) ICF must be considered in how they relate to communicative participation outcomes (see Fig. 29.1). For example, in one large population-based study of HNC patients, Rieke et al. (2016) found that significant differences in depression were based on gender. Specifically, gender was significantly associated with a diagnosis of depression before and after cancer diagnosis, with females having higher likelihood of depression. This factor is especially salient to consider, since females are increasingly (at least proportionately) being diagnosed with HNC and because aspects related to voice, speech, and facial disfigurement may differentially affect females (Eadie & Doyle, 2004).

Another personal factor within the ICF includes individual coping strategies, which also may affect HNC outcomes. How individuals make sense of HNC and its treatment is variable; much information may be gleaned from qualitative studies in this regard. For example, Isaksson, Salander, Lilliehorn, and Laurell (2016) interviewed 56 patients with HNC at 6, 12, and 24 months posttreatment about how they lived their lives. Four different trajectories and transitions emerged from the data. The first group (n = 15) of participants evaluated their illness experience as a past event in their life, suggesting that they had psychologically left the illness behind. The second group (n = 9) of participants was to some extent still affected by side effects, although they regarded these factors as "no big deal." The cancer itself made a significant difference in the third group (n = 12), in both positive and negative ways, and reflected a balance between such effects. Finally, in the fourth group (n = 20), physical and/ or psychological problems predominated their lives, with these participants perceiving a change for the worse. These types of studies are important for understanding which patients may be more or less vulnerable to certain outcomes, including difficulties in communication in everyday settings. These topics deserve further study and have implications for identifying targets for intervention, including the use of active coping strategies.

Finally, how environmental factors within the ICF (WHO, 2001) affect communicative participation should be considered and needs further study. For example, Rieke et al. (2016) showed that individuals who were divorced/separated or widowed at the time of cancer diagnosis were at greater risk for depression prior to HNC compared to those who were married. This may be related to a lack of social support, an environmental factor which has been found to be an important predictor of communicative participation in other health populations (Baylor, Yorkston, et al., 2010), as well as in relation to broader HNC outcomes. Karnell, Christensen, Rosenthal, Magnuson, and Funk (2007) found that greater perceived social support measured at 1 year post-diagnosis was related to more favorable global QOL and HNC-specific QOL. When measured prior to the initiation of oncological treatment, Howren, Christensen, Karnell, Van Liew, and Funk (2013) also reported that perceived social support was associated with increased global and HNC-specific QOL outcomes 1 year later after controlling for other clinical and demographic variables. Finally, in their qualitative study of individuals with HNC, Fletcher et al. (2012) reported that not only did changes in communication affect relationships among their participants and their families but that family, friends, and healthcare providers also acted as facilitators for adaptations in communication. In other words, it appeared that social support also affected communication outcomes such as communicative participation in this HNC population. This topic deserves future study, and could have implications for developing future interventions that include aspects related to social support.

Implications for Rehabilitation and Future Research

In speech-language pathology, there has been increasing attention on participation-focused interventions to optimize participation in valued life roles (Torrence, Baylor, Yorkston, & Spencer, 2016). This is of obvious importance because communicative participation is significantly affected in populations with communication disorders, including those with HNC. Yet one recent survey of 66 speech-language pathologists (SLPs) revealed that while a large proportion of their rationale for therapy was significantly related to improving participation, only 8% of the SLP's goals for therapy specifically referenced "participation" (Torrence et al., 2016). Thus, while important, it remains difficult for SLPs to incorporate elements specifically related to participation into current therapy approaches. In the survey by Torrence et al. (2016), SLPs also identified many barriers to implementation including time and productivity constraints, limits of clinical settings, and documentation challenges. Further, providing an evidence-based outcome measure related to participation was identified as a challenge. With the adoption of the CPIB (Baylor et al., 2013) in both clinical and research practice, it is hoped that this type of challenge for SLPs may be reduced.

Results from all studies summarized in this chapter suggest a need for interventions to enhance all aspects of communication in HNC survivors. Although the HNC literature boasts abundant examples of speech and QOL interventions, there are very few intervention studies in HNC that focus on communicative participation. However, the first implication is that interventions that directly target communicative participation must be implemented and their efficacy and effectiveness determined. There is an obvious role for education and counseling in this type of approach. For example, many patients compare their current speech and voice outcomes with their pre-HNC function. SLPs can help manage these expectations by working with patients to identify communication strengths and facilitate methods for compensating and coping with difficulties. Interestingly, there may be differences between those who have undergone total laryngectomy and other HNC treatments in this regard. For example, Moukarbel et al. (2011) suggest that although a higher level of disability may be anticipated for those using postlaryngectomy voice and speech, regardless of alaryngeal method used, the simple reacquisition of voice may change a person's perspective. Moukarbel et al. (2011) state that because these individuals have fully lost their normal method of verbal communication and then have regained it in some form, it may indicate they assess their ability relative to an acquisition, as opposed to a deficit, model. However, the manner in which this potentially relates to coping and expectations for communicating after all types of HNC warrants future study.

Communicative participation may not only be impacted by directly targeting participation outcomes with the HNC patient but also through other factors known to affect communicative participation. Maddelena and Pfrang (1993) used a psychological training program in a rehabilitation setting with 51 male laryngectomy patients and reported increased communication skills. Training over 6 months improved both the patients' speech and their perception of their partner's ability to understand them. In another study, Sharp, Laurell, Tiblom, Andersson, and Birksjo (2004) used care diaries to improve communication between patients, family/friends, and healthcare providers and to improve patient involvement in care. The authors reported that 85% of the respondents to a survey regarding the use of care diaries stated that the intervention, which primarily related to social support, had a positive effect on information in general and for communication. Thus, approaches that include families and caregivers, as well as others with HNC (e.g., support groups), continue to be powerful options. Finally, targeted approaches to diagnose or prevent depression as well as possible cognitive changes are urgently needed in patients undergoing therapy for HNC. All of these approaches need to be individualized to each patient to ensure the best possible outcomes.

Conclusions

This chapter has identified challenges to communicative participation in the HNC population. A novel PRO instrument, the CPIB and its short form (Baylor et al., 2013), appears to offer a promising new tool for measuring the impact of HNC on communicative participation for both research and clinical purposes. The CPIB clearly measures an aspect of function that is meaningful to HNC patients, including those with both speech and voice difficulties. Its value is that it addresses a gap in our current assessment practice and may complement other types of measures, including both traditional clinician-rated or other patient-reported measures (e.g., QOL questionnaires; Eadie et al., 2014; Eadie, Otero, Cox, et al., 2016). Directions for future research and clinical practice include using participation-based approaches, as well as targeting other factors (e.g., social support, coping strategies, etc.) known to affect participation. However, it is equally clear that all of these approaches need further study to promote the best possible practices in the care of those with HNC.

Acknowledgments I would like to thank hundreds of study participants for generously sharing their time and their experiences over the years. I also would like to acknowledge assistance from past and present members of the UW Vocal Function Laboratory, and intellectual contributions and support from co-investigators over the years including Kathryn Yorkston, Carolyn Baylor, Dagmar Amtmann, Robert Miller, Eduardo Mendez, Neal Futran, Philip Doyle, Devon Otero, Kristin Lamvik, Mara Kapsner-Smith, Susan Bolt, and Cara Sauder. Funding for this work is from the National Institutes of Health, National Cancer Institute (R01CA177635; PI: Eadie).

References

American Speech-Language-Hearing Association. (2004). *Preferred Practice Patterns for the Profession of Speech-Language Pathology* [Preferred Practice Patterns]. Available from www.asha.org/policy

American Speech-Language-Hearing Association. (2016). Scope of Practice in Speech Language Pathology [Scope of Practice]. Available from www.asha.org/policy.

Baylor, C., Burns, M., Eadie, T., Britton, D., & Yorkston, K. (2011). A qualitative study of interference with communicative participation across communication disorders in adults. *American Journal of Speech-Language Pathology, 20,* 269–287.

Baylor, C., Hula, W., Donovan, N. J., Doyle, P. J., Kendall, D., & Yorkston, K. (2010). An introduction to item response theory and Rasch models for speech-language pathologists. *American Journal of Speech-*

Language Pathology, 20(3), 243–259. https://doi.org/10.1044/1058-0360(2011/10-0079)

Baylor, C., Yorkston, K., Bamer, A., Britton, D., & Amtmann, D. (2010). Variables associated with communicative participation in people with multiple sclerosis: A regression analysis. *American Journal of Speech-Language Pathology, 19*(2), 143–153.

Baylor, C., Yorkston, K., Eadie, T., Kim, J., Chung, H., & Amtmann, D. (2013). The communicative participation item Bank (CPIB): Item bank calibration and development of a disorder-generic short form. *Journal of Speech, Language, and Hearing Research, 56*(4), 1190–1208. https://doi.org/10.1044/1092-4388(2012/12-0140

Baylor, C. R., Yorkston, K. M., Eadie, T. L., Miller, R. M., & Amtmann, D. (2009). Developing the communicative participation item Bank: Rasch analysis results from a spasmodic dysphonia sample. *Journal of Speech, Language, and Hearing Research, 52,* 1302–1320.

Bjorklund, M., Sarvimaki, A., & Berg, A. (2010). Living with head and neck cancer: A profile of captivity. *Journal of Nursing & Healthcare of Chronic Illness, 2,* 22–31.

Bolt, S., Eadie, T., Yorkston, K., Baylor, C., & Amtmann, D. (2016). Variables associated with communicative participation after head and neck Cancer. *JAMA-Otolaryngology Head & Neck Surgery.* https://doi.org/10.1001/jamaoto.2016.1198

Borrell-Carrió, F., Suchman, A. L., & Epstein, R. M. (2004). The biopsychosocial model 25 years later: Principles, practice, and scientific inquiry. *The Annals of Family Medicine, 2*(6), 576–582.

Bornbaum, C. C., Fung, K., Franklin, J. H., Nichols, A., Yoo, J., & Doyle, P. C. (2012). A descriptive analysis of the relationship between quality of life and distress in individuals with head and neck cancer. *Supportive Care in Cancer, 20,* 2157–2165.

Chen, S.-C., Yu, P.-J., Hong, M.-Y., Chen, M.-H., Chu, P.-Y., Chen, Y.-J., ... Lai, Y.-H. (2015). Communication dysfunction, body image, and symptom severity in postoperative head and neck cancer patients: Factors associated with the amount of speaking after treatment. *Supportive Care in Cancer, 23,* 2375–2382. https://doi.org/10.1007/s00520-014-2587-3

Danker, H., Wollbruck, D., Singer, S., Fuchs, M., Brahler, E., & Meyer, A. (2010). Social withdrawal after laryngectomy. *European Archives of Otorhinolaryngology, 267,* 593–600.

De Maddelena, H., & Pfrang, H. (1993). Improvement of communication behavior of laryngectomized and voice-rehabilitated patients by a psychological training program. *Head and Neck Oncology, 41*(6), 289–295.

Dwivedi, R. C., Kazi, R. A., Agrawal, N., Nutting, C. M., Clarke, P. M., Kerawala, C. J., ... Harrington, K. J. (2009). Evaluation of speech outcomes following treatmetn of oral and oropharygeal cancers. *Cancer Treatment Reviews, 35,* 417–424. https://doi.org/10.1016/j.ctrv.2009.04.013

Doyle, P. C., & Keith, R. L. (Eds.). (2005). *Contemporary consideration in the Treament and Rehabiliation of head and neck Cancer: Voice, speech and swallowing.* Austin, TX: Pro-Ed.

Eadie, T. L. (2003). The ICF: A proposed framework for comprehensive rehabilitation of individuals who use alaryngeal speech. *American Journal of Speech-Language Pathology, 12*(2), 189–197.

Eadie, T. L. (2007). Application of the ICF after total laryngectomy. *Seminars in Speech and Language, 28*(4), 291–300.

Eadie, T. L., & Bowker, B. C. (2012). Coping and quality of life after total laryngectomy. *Otolaryngology-Head & Neck Surgery, 146,* 959–965.

Eadie, T. L., Day, A. M. B., Sawin, D. E., Lamvik, K., & Doyle, P. C. (2013). Auditory-perceptual speech outcomes and quality of life after total laryngectomy. *Otolaryngology-Head & Neck Surgery, 148,* 82–88.

Eadie, T. L., & Doyle, P. C. (2004). Auditory-perceptual scaling and quality of life in tracheoesophageal speakers. *The Laryngoscope, 114,* 753–759.

Eadie, T. L., Lamvik, K., Baylor, C. R., Yorkston, K. M., Kim, J., & Amtmann, D. (2014). Communicative participation and quality of life in head and neck cancer. *Annals of Otology, Rhinology, & Laryngology, 123*(4), 257–264. https://doi.org/10.1177/0003489414525020

Eadie, T., Otero, D. S., Bolt, S., Kapsner-Smith, M., & Sullivan, J. R. (2016). The effect of noise on relationships between speech intelligiblity and self-reported communication measures in tracheoesophageal speakers. *American Journal of Speech-Language Pathology, 25*(3), 393–407. https://doi.org/10.1044/2016_AJSLP-15-0081

Eadie, T. L., Otero, D., Cox, S., Johnson, J., Baylor, C. R., Yorkston, K. M., & Doyle, P. C. (2016). The relationship between communicative participation and postlaryngectomy speech outcomes. *Head & Neck, 38*((1), Suppl 1), E1955–E1961. https://doi.org/10.1002/hed.24353

Eadie, T. L., Yorkston, K. M., Klasner, E. R., Dudgeon, B. J., Deitz, J. C., Baylor, C. R., ... Amtmann, D. (2006). Measuring communicative participation: A review of self-report instruments in speech-language pathology. *American Journal of Speech-Language Pathology, 15*(4), 307–320. https://doi.org/10.1044/1058-0360(2006/030

Finizia, C., Hammerlid, E., Westin, T., & Lindstrom, J. (1998). Quality of life and voice in patients with laryngeal carcinoma: A posttreatment comparison of laryngectomy (salvage surgery) versus radiotherapy. *Laryngoscope, 108*(10), 1566–1573.

Finizia, C., Lindstrom, J., & Dotevall, H. (1998). Intelligibility and perceptual ratings after treatment for laryngeal cancer: Laryngectomy versus radiotherapy. *Laryngoscope, 108*(1 Pt 1), 138–143.

Fletcher, B. S., Cohen, M. Z., Schumacher, K., & Lydiatt, W. (2012). A blessing and a curse: Head and neck cancer survivors' experiences. *Cancer Nursing, 35*(2), 126–132.

Funk, G. F., Karnell, L. H., & Christensen, A. J. (2012). Long-term health-realted quality of life in survivors of head and neck cancer. *Archives of Otolaryngology Head & Neck Surgery, 138*(2), 123–133.

Funk, G. F., Karnell, L. H., Christensen, A. J., Moran, P. J., & Ricks, J. (2003). Comprehensive head and neck oncology health status assessment. *Head & Neck, 25*(7), 561–575.

Fung, K., Lyden, T. H., Lee, J., Urba, S. G., Worden, F., Eisbruch, A., … Wolf, G. T. (2005). Voice and swallowing outcomes of an organ-preservation trial for advanced laryngeal cancer. *International Journal of Radiation Oncology Biology Physics, 63*, 1395–1399. https://doi.org/10.1016/j.ijrobp.2005.05.004

Gan, H. K., Bernstein, L. J., Brown, J., Ringash, J., Vakilha, M., Wang, L., … Siu, L. L. (2011). Cognitive functioning after radiotherapy or chemoradiotherapy for head-and-neck cancer. *Interntational Journal of Radiation, Oncology, Biology, & Physiology, 81*(1), 126–134. https://doi.org/10.1016/j.ijrobp.2010.05.004

Hays, R. D., Morales, L. S., & Reise, S. P. (2000). Item response theory and health outcomes measurement in the 21st century. *Medical Care., 38*(9), SII28–SII42.

Hilari, K., Needle, J. J., & Harrison, K. L. (2012). What are the important factors in health-related quality of life for people with aphasia? A systematic review. *Archives of Physical Medicine and Rehabilitation, 93*(1 Suppl), S86–S95. https://doi.org/10.1016/j.apmr.2011.05.028

Howren, M. B., Christensen, A. J., Karnell, L. H., & Funk, G. F. (2013). Psychological factors associated with head and neck cancer treatment and survivorship: Evidence and opportunities for behavioral medicine. *Journal of Consulting and Clinical Psychology, 81*(2), 299–317.

Howren, M. B., Christensen, A. J., Karnell, L. H., Van Liew, J. R., & Funk. (2013). Influence of pretreatment social support on health-related quality of life in head and neck cancer survivors: Results from a prospective study. *Head & Neck, 35*(6), 779–787. https://doi.org/10.1002/hed.23029

Isaksson, J., Salander, P., Lilliehorn, S., & Laurell, G. (2016). Living an everyday life with head and neck cancer 2-2.5 years post-diagnosis-a qualitative prospective study of 56 patients. *Social Science & Medicine, 154*, 54–61.

Jacobi, I., Molen, L., Huiskens, H., Rossum, M., & Hilgers, F. (2010). Voice and speech outcomes of chemoradiation for advanced head and neck cancer: A systematic review. *European Archives of Oto-Rhino-Laryngology, 267*(10), 1495–1505.

Jacobson, B. H., Johnson, A., Grywalsky, C., Silbergleit, A., Jacobson, G., Benninger, M. S., & Newman, C. W. (1997). The voice handicap index (VHI): Development and validation. *American Journal of Speech-Language Pathology, 6*, 66–70.

Karnell, L. H., Funk, G. F., & Hoffman, H. T. (2000). Assessing head and neck cancer patient outcome domains. *Head & Neck, 22*(1), 6–11.

Karnell, L. H., Christensen, A. J., Rosenthal, E. L., Magnuson, J. S., & Funk, G. F. (2007). Influence of social support on health-related quality of life outcomes in head and neck cancer. *Head & Neck, 29*(2), 143–146.

Law, I. K. Y., Ma, E. P. M., & Yiu, E. M. L. (2009). Speech intelligibility, acceptability, and communication-related quality of life in Chinese alaryngeal speakers. *Archives of Otolaryngology–Head & Neck Surgery, 135*(7), 704–711.

Llewellyn, C. D., McGurk, M., & Weinman, J. (2005). Are psycho-social and behavioural factors related to health related-quality of life in patients with head and neck cancer? A systematic review. *Oral Oncology, 41*, 440–454.

McAuliffe, M. J., Baylor, C. R., & Yorkston, K. M. (2017). Variables associated with communicative participation in Parkinson's disease and its relationship to measures of health-related quality-of-life. *International Journal of Speech-Language Pathology, 19*(4), 407–417.

McColl, D., Fucci, D., Petrosino, L., Martin, D. E., & McCaffrey, P. (1998). Listener ratings of the intelligibility of tracheoesophageal speech in noise. *Journal of Communication Disorders, 31*(4), 279–288; quiz 288–289.

Meyer, T. K., Kuhn, J. C., Campbell, B. H., Marbella, A. M., Myers, K. B., & Layde, P. M. (2004). Speech intelligibility and quality of life in head and neck cancer survivors. *The Laryngoscope, 114*, 1977–1981.

Moukarbel, R. V., Doyle, P. C., Yoo, J. H., Franklin, J. H., Day, A. M., & Fung, K. (2011). Voice-related quality of life (V-RQOL) outcomes in laryngectomees. *Head & Neck, 33*, 31–36.

Nash, M. M., Body Image and Quality of Life: An Exploration Among Individuals with Head and Neck Cancer (2014). Electronic Thesis and Dissertation Repository. 2295. http://ir.lib.uwo.ca/etd/2295

Rieke, K., Boilesen, E., Lydiatt, W., Schmid, K. K., Houfek, J., & Watanabe-Galloway, S. (2016). Population-based retrospective study to investigate preexisting and new depression diagnosis among head and neck cancer patients. *Cancer Epidemiology, 43*, 42–48.

Rinkel, R. N., Verdonck-de Leeuw, I. M., van Reij, E. J., Aaronson, N. K., & Leemans, C. R. (2008). Speech handicap index in patients with oral and pharyngeal cancer: Better understanding of patients' complaints. *Head & Neck, 30*, 868–874. https://doi.org/10.1002/hed.20795

Ringash, J., Bernstein, L., Cella, D., Logemann, J., Movsas, B., Murphy, B., … Ridge, J. (2015). Outcomes toolbox for head and neck cancer research. *Head & Neck, 37*(3), 425–439. https://doi.org/10.1002/hed.23561

Rosen, C. A., Lee, A. S., Osborne, J., Zullo, T., & Murry, T. (2004). Development and validation of the voice handicap index-10. *Laryngoscope, 114*(9), 1549–1556.

Sharp, L., Laurell, G., Tiblom, Y., Andersson, A., & Birksjo, R. M. (2004). Care diaries: A way of increasing head and neck cancer patient's involvement in their own care and the communication between clinicians. *Cancer Nursing, 27*(2), 119–126.

Sperry, J. L., Wiley, T. L., & Chial, M. R. (1997). Word recognition performance in various background competitors. *Journal of the American Academy of Audiology, 8*, 71–80.

Stewart, M. G., Chen, A. Y., & Stach, C. B. (1998). Outcomes analysis of voice and quality of life in patients with laryngeal cancer. *Archives of Otolaryngology-Head & Neck Surgery, 124*(2), 143–148.

Terrell, J. E., Ronis, D. L., Fowler, K. E., Bradford, C. R., Chepeha, D. B., Prince, M. E., ... Duffy, S. A. (2004). Clinical predictors of quality of life in patients with head and neck cancer. *Archives of Otolaryngology-Head & Neck Surgery, 130*(4), 401–408.

Torrence, J. M., Baylor, C. R., Yorkston, K. M., & Spencer, K. A. (2016). Addressing communicative participation in treatment planning for adults: A survey of U.S. speech-language pathologists. *American Journal of Speech-Language Pathology, 25*(3), 355–370. https://doi.org/10.1044/2015_AJSLP-15-0049

Tschiesner, U., Sabariego, C., Linseisen, E., Becker, S., Stier-Jarmer, M., Cieza, A., & Harreus, U. (2013). Priorities of head and neck cancer patients: A patient survey based on the brief ICF core set for HNC. *European Archives of Otorhinolaryngology, 270*(12), 3133–3142. https://doi.org/10.1007/s00405-013-2446-8

Van der Molen, L., Rossum, M. A., Jacobi, I., van Son, R. J. J. H., Smeele, L. E., Rasch, C. R. N., & Hilgers, F. J. M. (2012). Pre- and posttreatment voice and speech outcomes in patients with advanced head and neck cancer treated with chemoradiotherapy: Expert listeners' and patients' perception. *Journal of Voice, 26*, 664.e25-664.e33. https://doi.org/10.1016/j.jvoice.2011.08.016

U.S Department of Health and Human Services Food and Drug Administration Guidance for Industry: Patient-Reported Outcome Measures: Use in Medical Product Development to Support Labeling Claims. [Last Accessed on 2011 Apr 20];U.S. FDA, Clinical/Medical. 2009. available from: http://www.fda.gov/downloads/Drugs/GuidanceComplianceRegulatoryInformation/Guidances/UCM193282.pdf]

Wilbers, J., Kappelle, A. C., Versteeg, L., Tuladhar, A. M., Steens, S. C. A., Meijer, F. J. A., ... van Dijk, E. J. (2015). Cognitive function, depression, fatigue and quality of life among long-term survivors of head and neck cancer. *Neuro-Oncology Practice, 2*(3), 144–150. https://doi.org/10.1093/nop/npv012

World Health Organization. (2001). *International classification of functioning, disability and health: ICF*. Geneva, Switzerland: World Health Organization.

Yorkston, K. M., Baylor, C. R., Deitz, J., Dudgeon, B. J., Eadie, T., Miller, R. M., & Amtmann, D. (2008). Developing a scale of communicative participation: A cognitive interviewing study. *Disability and Rehabilitation, 30*, 425–433.

Yorkston, K. M., Baylor, C. R., Klasner, E. R., Deitz, J., Dudgeon, B. J., Eadie, T., ... Amtmann, D. (2007). Satisfaction with communicative participation as defined by adults with multiple sclerosis: A qualitative study. *Journal of Communication Disorders, 40*, 433–451.

Yorkston, K. M., Klasner, E. R., & Swanson, K. M. (2001). Communication in context: A qualitative study of the experiences of individuals with multiple sclerosis. *American Journal of Speech-Language Pathology, 10*, 126–137.

Yorkston, K., Beukelman, D., & Tice, R. (1996). *Sentence intelligibility test (version 1.0) [speech analysis]*. Lincoln, NE: Tice Technology Services.

Index

© Springer Nature Switzerland AG 2019
P. C. Doyle (ed.), *Clinical Care and Rehabilitation in Head and Neck Cancer*,
https://doi.org/10.1007/978-3-030-04702-3

Printed by Printforce, the Netherlands